Nutrition 101: Choose Life!

A Family Nutrition and Health Program

Enjoy great health! Debra Raybern

Debra Raybern, N.D.
Sera Johnson
Laura Hopkins
Karen Hopkins

ISBN: 978-0-9816954-2-6
Printed in the United States of America
First printing.

Growing Healthy Homes LLC
837 Crown Drive
Bartlesville, OK 74006

To obtain additional copies of this book, please visit
www.GrowingHealthyHomes.com.

Required disclaimer: The information given in this book is for educational purposes only and is not intended as diagnosis, treatment or prescription for any disease. This is a compilation of the author's beliefs based on independent reseach and professional and personal experiences. The reader is advised to seek the advice of his or her chosen health professional before adhering to any health regimen. The authors and publisher bear no responsibility for the use or misuse of any of this information. The decision to use or not to use any of this information is the sole responsibility of the reader.

If you have a health-related question or a health challenge, please seek the guidance of the health professional of your choice. Growing Healthy Homes LLC is not able to answer health questions.

Dedicated to all the families who read and implement the healthy living suggestions outlined in **Nutrition 101: Choose Life!**, so they may have the physical and emotional health to fulfill God's calling on their lives.

Nutrition 101: Choose Life!

" I call heaven and earth to record this day against you, that I have set before you life and death, blessing and cursing: therefore choose life, that both thou and thy seed may live:"
Deuteronomy 30:19

Introduction

The study of nutrition is more than just a look into food and its nutrients. It is an in-depth look at how we eat, what we eat, how the body works and how these foods affect the body. This program is not a rehash of biology or science, but a discovery of how the body systems are affected by the foods – good or bad – we eat. Research, recipes and projects will make **Nutrition 101: Choose Life!** fun for the whole family and establish lifelong habits and desires to eat wholesome foods that support great health. This corroborates III John 2: "Beloved, I wish above all things that thou mayest prosper and be in health, even as thy soul prospereth."

The 12 main body systems will be covered in six units.

Unit 1 – The Brain and Nervous System

Unit 2 – The Digestive System

Unit 3 - The Respiratory, Olfactory, Auditory and Visual Systems

Unit 4 - The Muscular and Skeletal Systems

Unit 5 - The Cardiovascular and Immune Systems

Unit 6 - The Endocrine System & Emotions

If the principles in **Nutrition 101: Choose Life!** are already a part of your family's lifestyle, use it to enhance your food preparation and meal time experiences. This teaches the whys of eating the way you do. Rather than, "Mom said I can't have that," they can say "I choose not to eat that because I know what it does to my body."

This program was written for you.

"Train up a child in the way he should go: and when he is old, he will not depart from it." Proverbs 22:6

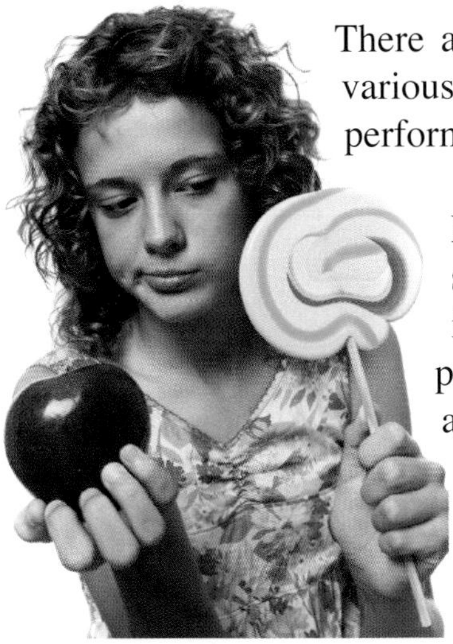

There are many textbooks written on the subjects of science and biology, explaining the various body systems and organs, how they work, where they are located and the jobs they perform. Still more books cover health issues and various theories about longevity.

Every student, whether public, private or home educated, is required to read and study these subjects. If this is so, then why is disease increasing at an alarming rate in this country? Why are children stricken with cancers today more than in years past? Why has diabetes risen to near epidemic levels? Why is heart disease, even with advancements in modern medicine, still the number one killer in America and now prevalent in our teenagers? Why, with a myriad of pharmaceutical drugs and state-of-the art diagnostic tools, are we sicker now than ever before? (See Health Statistics in the United States in Appendix A.)

The American Diabetes Association, the American Heart Association and the National Institutes of Cancer all state the most important thing we can do to prevent and even "cure" these diseases is ... CHANGE THE WAY WE EAT!

If we are listening to these experts, why are we not making progress?

This is precisely why **Nutrition 101: Choose Life!** was created. We, the authors, have a mandate to assist families, especially those with children, to understand the real relationship food has on our "fearfully and wonderfully made" bodies, as referenced in Psalm 139:14.

The Bible gives us clear direction about taking instruction and gaining wisdom. "My people are destroyed for a lack of knowledge," states Hosea 4:6. So we encourage families to heed the advice of Proverbs 4:13, "Take firm hold of instruction, do not let go; Keep her, for she is your life."

Would you like to feed your family more nutritiously, but have no idea where to start? Have you tried telling your family the importance of eating right, only to slip back into the fast food maze? Do you think the cost of eating nutritiously is out of your budget? Would you like some biblically sound help from real families and expert counsel about real food and real world eating?

That is the purpose of **Nutrition 101: Choose Life!** Written by a team of four mothers, this program is designed for positive, effective, long-term, healthy lifestyle changes.

Is This Even Possible?

Absolutely! Romans 8:28-39 is well known for encouraging believers that they are more than conquerors, but the preceding statement in verses 26 and 27 are less quoted and equally contextual for this program. "In the same way, the Spirit helps us in our weakness. We do not know what we ought to pray for, but the Spirit himself intercedes for us with groans that words cannot express. And He who searches our hearts knows the mind of the Spirit, because the Spirit intercedes for the saints in accordance with God's will."

Perhaps you have prayed for the answers you will find in this study without even knowing it. When we pray for wisdom and discernment and healing, God loves us and wants to grant our request. When He grants it, he does so knowing that we are fully equipped to receive it.

As you equip your family by implementing the information in this program, you most likely will encounter adversity and be tempted in moments of weakness. The following sections are intended to encourage you in those times and prepare you with ideas for your own proactive action plan.

About the Authors

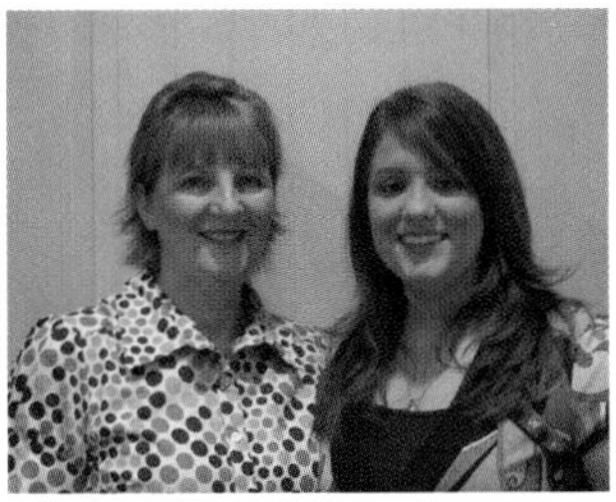

Debra Raybern, N.D., M.H., C.N.C., I.C.A. (Naturopathic Doctor, Master Herbalist, Certified Nutritional Counselor, Internationally Certified Aromatherapist) is a veteran home school mom and shares from nearly two decades of personal and professional experience in helping families just like yours to regain and maintain optimum health. Assisting thousands of people overcome minor and life threatening illness, Debra knows the importance of proper, body system specific nutrition and supplementation.

"I know that **Nutrition 101: Choose Life!** will change your life, as the information shared has already been proven to change the way people look at food and has given them the health to enjoy life and serve their community, church and God. Since I cannot personally counsel everyone, this program is a way for me to enter your home and help you be successful in keeping your family feeling their best and "be-ing in health."

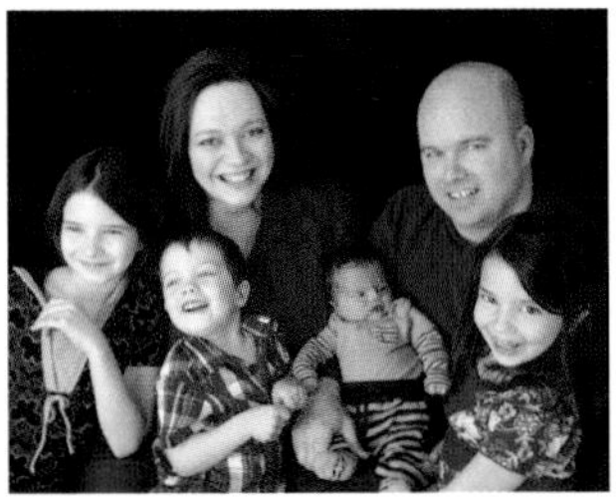

Sera Johnson, B.Mu. is a home school mother of four, private music teacher and the president of operations for Growing Healthy Homes LLC. As the former self-labeled "Fast Food Queen," she and her husband realized their family's health was in great jeopardy and sought the Lord for wisdom about what to do. After being introduced to Debra Raybern and learning about better health through eating God's food, Sera's family is now healthier than ever and looking forward to living out full, healthy, abundant lives for the Glory of God. Her heart is to share with mothers what she has learned and that it is never too late to teach your family how to eat *and* love God's food.

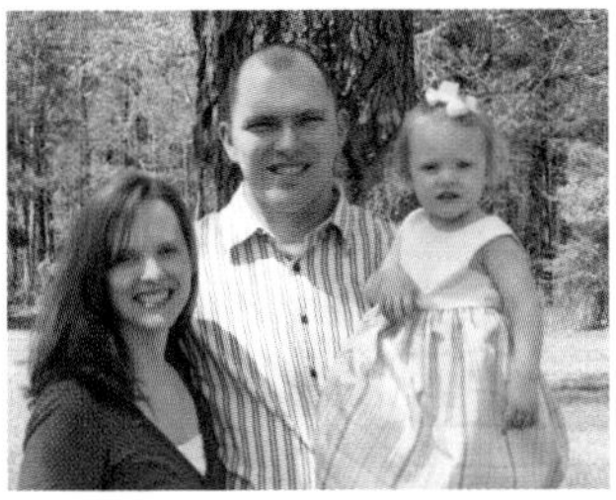

Laura Hopkins, B.S. is a professional communicator with a decade of experience in the public and private sectors, including a Fortune 8 global energy company. As president of communications for Growing Healthy Homes LLC, she is responsible for content and Internet management, preparing material so families may easily consume the concept of true wholeness as God prescribes. She strives to model for her own family that, as children of God, it is crucial to maintain a hunger for His provision and make daily choices that impact abundant living.

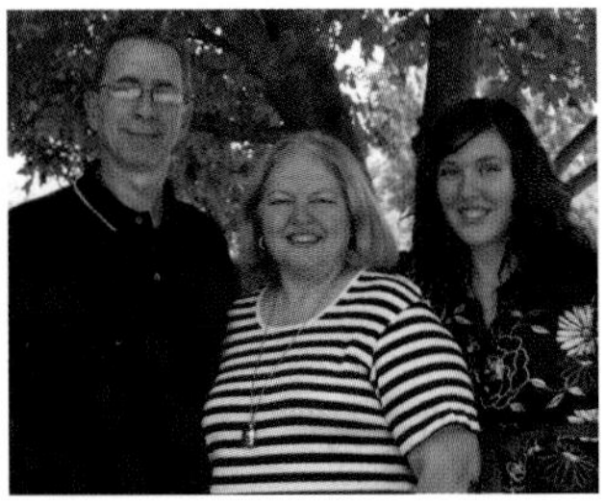

Karen Hopkins, B.S. is a former Home Economics teacher and published author who developed diabetes at the age of 45 due to S.A.D (Standard American Diet). Traditional nutrition courses did not prepare her for the onslaught of processed, fast food eating habits and the busy lifestyle of a growing family. Forced to face the reality of a short lifespan due to excessively high blood sugar levels, Karen reversed the prognosis in six short months without medication through the use of specific natural supplements, diet and exercise. She founded Growing Healthy Homes LLC in 2007 to educate and train families about God's desire for His children to prosper in health even as their souls prosper (III John 2).

Table of Contents

Getting Started

Nutrition 101: Choose Life! is a unit study in that it encompasses all ages from toddlers to adults, covers a wide variety of subjects like science, anatomy, biology, nutrition and health and can be implemented in a daily or weekly schedule. Use grocery shopping, meal preparation and meal time as opportunities to incorporate the program to allow children to learn as they live. This should be an organic process that makes healthy choices second-nature.

This program can be utilized daily by all families whether as a curriculum or during meal planning and food preparation. Other ways to use the program include in homeschool co-ops, private schools, church groups, family home groups and extracurricular clubs, like the Girls Scouts and Boy Scouts. Multiple licenses and permission to print more than one copy of the program can be obtained from the publisher by e-mailing editor@growinghealthyhomes.com.

Some of the material throughout the study may be too in depth for some children. In such cases, parents should read through the material in each chapter, highlight the important parts with the children and enforce these simple facts through the activities.

Chapters are structured to be completed in a week. However, feel free to extend it an extra week for the longer, more in-depth chapters. It is fine to focus on a particular chapter if your family enjoys that topic or wants to do extra activities. All six units were designed to be completed in a year. Because there are so many activities, the entire program can repeated and modified each year to reinforce or refresh what already has been learned.

Each unit contains:

Chapters - Each one includes information about body systems or how food affects them.

Discussion Questions - Try to answer these questions with the whole family. See how answers vary from children to adults.

Activities - Pick and choose... or do them all. Extend the time spent in the chapter to finish activities or save them for next year as reinforcement. The activities are structured to allow children to progress as they mature.

Additional Resources - These are optional and can be a great way to dive deeper into learning, especially if a family member takes a particular interest in something.

"Power" Recipes and Additional Recipes - Use the "Power" Recipe to enhance the topics covered in the chapter and incorporate the additional recipes throughout the course of the unit.

Activity Guide - Located before the Appendix, this is an answer key for all activities.

Appendix - This contains charts, tables and articles that elaborate on the text and give direction for some of the discussion and activities.

Here is an example of how to implement a chapter in a week:

Monday - Read over the chapter and discussion questions and choose activities.

Tuesday - Review chapter highlights and shop for or collect ingredients for the "Power" Recipe.

Wednesday - Prepare the "Power" Recipe for snack or meal time.

Thursday - Choose activities from the "Power" Recipe.

Friday - Share highlights from the week during family meal time.

As your family progresses through **Nutrition 101: Choose Life!**, we want each person to be encouraged to take responsibility for his or her health. With a plethora of recipes, activities and resources for independent study, every member of the family can get involved and understand how food affects the human body. Now is the best time to start making necessary changes to the family diet that will have long-term, positive and habit-forming benefits.

What About Picky Eaters?

Co-author Sera Johnson is the self proclaimed former "Fast Food Queen." She dealt with the struggles of introducing completely new foods and a new healthy lifestyle to her family. Over the past several years, it was not easy, but her family is eating healthier than ever and has made huge strides toward better health. People ask her all the time, "How did you do it? My child is so picky! They will NEVER eat healthy food!" Here are Sera's suggestions in her own words.

"I had the princess of picky eaters! My oldest daughter, Julia, only ate three kinds of food at home – boxed mac and cheese, frozen personal size pizzas and ramen noodles – all of which I introduced to her and allowed her to become addicted to. Yes, addicted. The only other food she would eat were chicken nuggets from only two particular fast food restaurants and none others. If I ever attempted to offer her a vegetable at dinner and ask her to take one bite, we were in for several hours of agony for the whole family. The Lord opened my eyes and showed me that several of my children were already headed down a path to destruction in their health. I learned that my responsibility to my family included their health and helping them establish long-term healthy eating habits. I knew I had to make drastic changes! Here are some of the initial things I did to help us get on the right track:

1. **Get rid of the junk!** - I immediately got rid of all the processed food and junk food in my house. I knew that it would be better if those choices were completely taken out of the picture.

2. **Make a list.** - Then, I sat down with each of my children, and we wrote down all the vegetables, fruits, grains and healthy proteins that they liked. At first the list was very short, especially for Julia, but it was a start. We focused on what she did like – broccoli, apples, grapes and oranges.

3. **Eat the healthy foods you do like.** - For the next several days and even weeks, we ate lots of broccoli, apples, grapes and oranges. Julia did get very upset that her normal choices were no longer available, but I knew that she would at least eat the things she did like and would probably eat just about anything if she got hungry enough. I knew she wouldn't starve.

4. **Make positive confessions.** – At mealtime, I had Julia pray aloud with me, "Lord, thank you for this good food You made and thank you for helping me to love Your food." At first, she didn't believe her own words, but the more we prayed and the more she spoke those positive words out of her own mouth, the more it helped her in trying new foods and opening up her heart to what God had provided for her to eat for her health.

5. **Try at least one new thing at each meal.** – Statistics say that if a child doesn't like a new food at first, trying it again at least ten more times in a row will help him develop a taste for it. The more new foods Julia tried, the more she realized she did, in fact, like. She didn't like everything and still doesn't, but she started developing a confidence in at least trying new foods. After a while, she took pride in her ever-growing list of good food. Children will pick up on your language and facial expressions, so parents should be leaders in trying foods on their not-so-favorite list. This curriculum will guide you in healthy ways to make some foods more palatable.

6. **Find healthy alternatives to those old favorites.** – Although Julia didn't like them as much at first, I found and created healthier, homemade versions of those old foods she once loved. The chicken nugget recipe featured in Unit 4 helped take the place of the fast food version and is now a beloved family favorite, even for Julia. We now make homemade pizza with freshly made crust and sauce, which the children help make and tout as being the best ever made.

"The next steps were to work on me. Although I do like just about everything, except for turnips and liver, my challenge was changing my mindset that I was just too busy to cook. When I did find the time, I didn't know what to cook. That is where I asked the Lord to help me change my thinking, help me to prioritize my life to find time to plan some meals and to basically teach me about what my family needed to eat for their health. I felt like I was at ground zero and had so much to learn and so much to unlearn, but the Lord led me to some great resources that included my mother, Karen Hopkins, and Debra Raybern. I truly wish I had **Nutrition 101: Choose Life!** back then! It would have made things easier and a lot more fun! However, we have come a long way and are still a work in progress. My family is healthier than ever, and I give God all the glory for it. I hope you can learn from my experiences and be encouraged that change can happen!"

Let's Get Started ...

By the time your family completes this program and implements new food choices and strategies, you may be surprised by the improvements you may begin to experience. Some families may choose to keep a journal or photo essay of their journey. We pray God's blessings on your family as you learn to love His food and respect your bodies as He has created them to function. May this Scripture encourage you, "Who satisfies thy mouth with good things, so that thy youth is renewed like the eagle's." Psalm 103:5

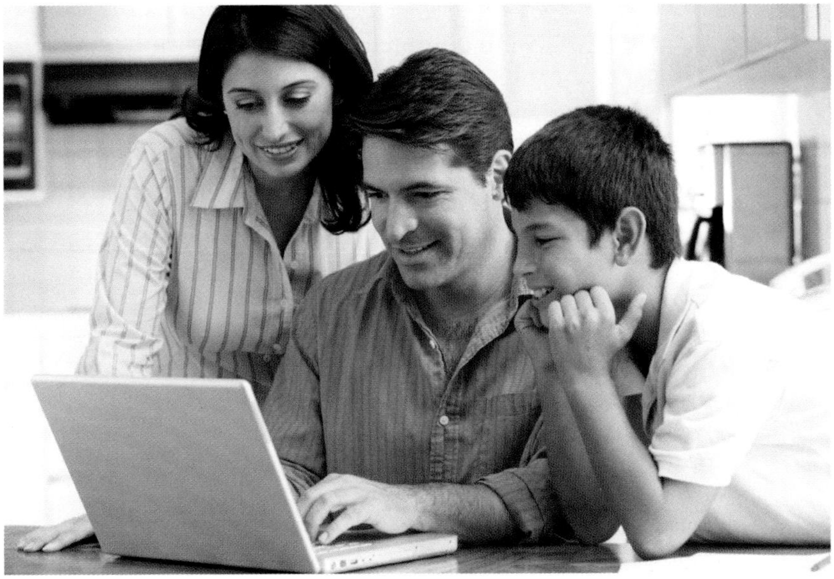

Unit 1

The Brain and Nervous System

Without our brains and nervous systems, we would not be alive. The brain and nervous system are the control centers for everything – thinking, learning, walking, talking, breathing and more. They tell the heart to beat and the muscles to contract when we want to run. They tell us to quickly move our hands away if we have touched something hot. Psalm 139:14 declares "I praise you because I am fearfully and wonderfully made; your works are wonderful, I know that full well." God made our brains and nervous systems to do some amazing things! But they cannot do those things alone.

We all need good air to breathe, good water to drink and good food to eat. Along with exercise and proper sleep, the food we put into our body affects how well it functions. This is especially true for the brain and nervous system. Not all food is the same; some foods help us and other foods hurt us. As good stewards of the bodies God has given us, we need to learn how our bodies work and how food affects them. This knowledge will allow us to make wise choices about what to eat and in turn we can have long, healthy, abundant lives.

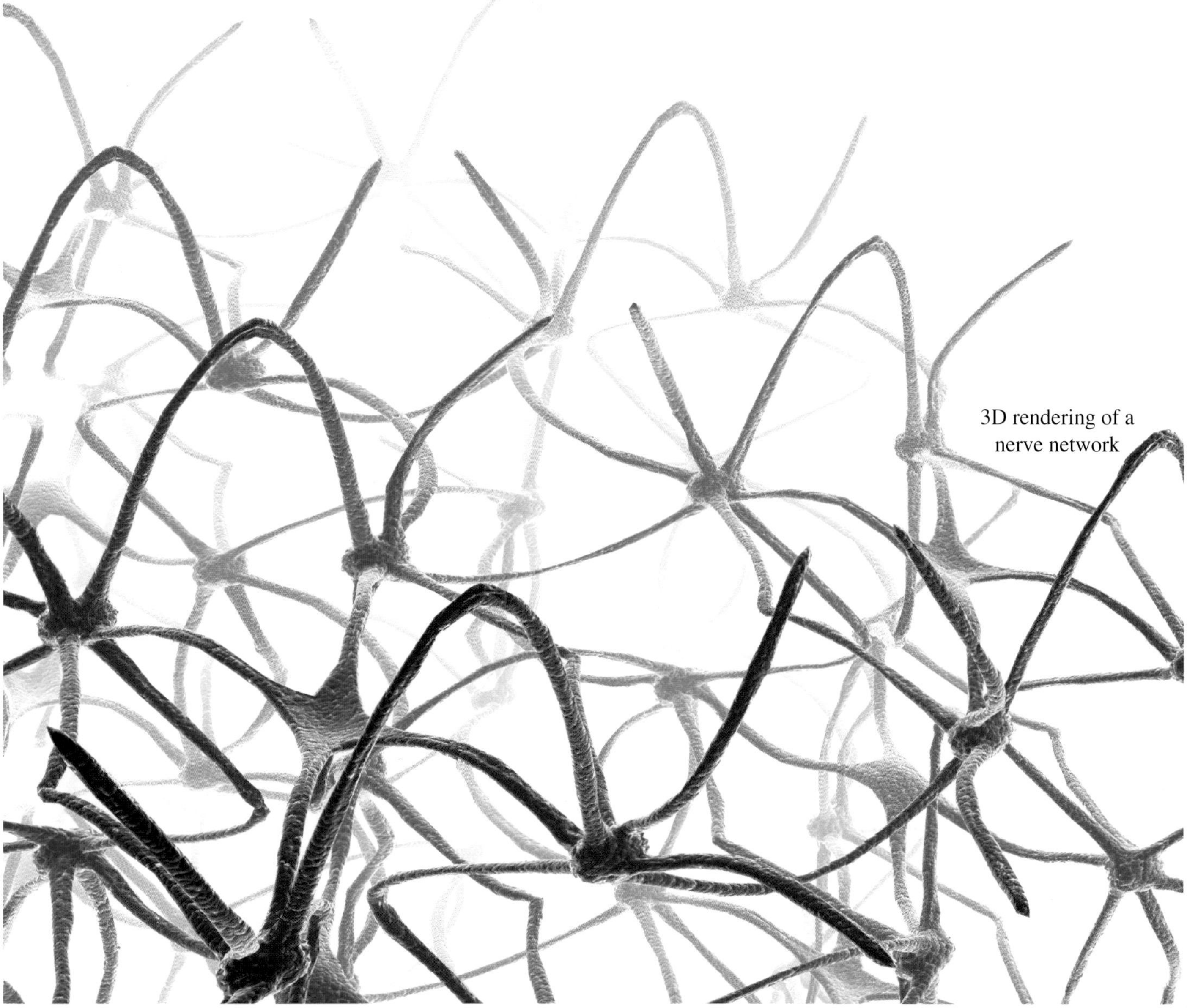

3D rendering of a nerve network

Chapter 1

The Brain

"Let this mind be in you which was also in Christ Jesus." Philippians 2:5

Our brain is so amazing and complex that experts don't even fully understand how it works. However, they agree that good nutrition is key to healthy brain development. This process begins as a baby develops in his mother's womb and is dependent upon her diet. Fats (Omega-3, Omega-6, and Omega-9), protein, complex carbohydrates, vitamins, minerals and water are crucial for proper brain development. If nutrients are scarce for the developing baby, then his brain will receive them at the expense of the other organs. Some part of the baby's brain development will be curtailed, some structures will go unbuilt, and some functions will not be performed if proper nutrition is not available.

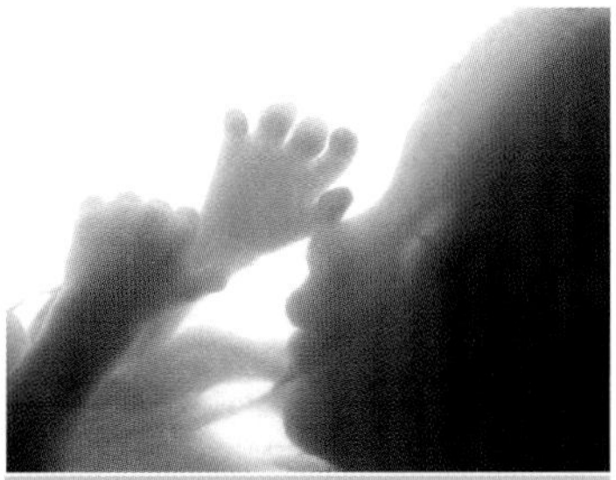

Fun Fact

At only 31 days post conception, the brain of a developing baby is already forming. The very first of over 100 billion neurons is being formed.

Fun Fact

In 1998, a team of American and Swedish scientists demonstrated for the first time that new brain cells are generated in the hippocampus (memory and learning area) of adult humans ages 55 to 70. (November 1998, Nature Medicine).

The nutrient requirements of the brain are constant and continue all the way through adulthood, meaning nutrition is vital for a healthy brain no matter a person's age. To fully understand the needs of this fascinating organ and how nutrition affects it, we must first know more about the structure and function of the brain.

What is the Brain?

Weighing about three pounds in the average adult, the brain is part of the nervous system. It has been likened to a computer with its many functions. However, no computer – not even a super computer – has ever come close to matching the human brain's capabilities. The brain is the site of thinking and the control center for the rest of the body. The brain coordinates our ability to move, walk, jump, run, touch, smell, hear, speak and see. It allows us to understand and to perform functions such as adding and subtracting, thinking ahead, reasoning and even daydreaming. The brain receives input -- what we hear, see, touch, smell and taste – analyzes the input and then responds. The brain also adjusts to emotions and mood.

Word Power

Cognitive
Pronunciation: \käg-nə-tiv\
Function: adjective
Date: 1586
1 : of, relating to, being, or involving conscious intellectual activity (as thinking, reasoning, or remembering) <cognitive impairment> 2 : based on or capable of being reduced to empirical factual knowledge
— **cog·ni·tive·ly** adverb

The brain is estimated to have about 10 trillion cells! One hundred billion of these cells are called neurons. The neurons act as on and off switches, similar in function to light switches and produce chemicals that trigger other neurons. Different neurons require and use different types of chemicals. These chemicals are called neurotransmitters or messengers and are given names like epinephrine, norepinephrine or dopamine.

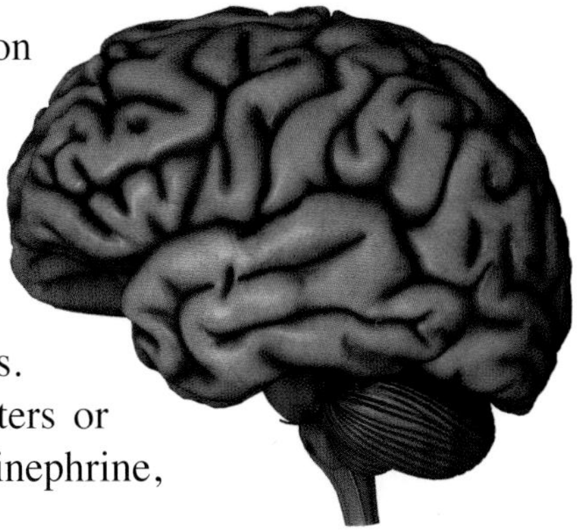

The brain needs a constant stream of nourishment and oxygen. About 20 percent of our oxygen-rich blood continuously flows from the heart to the brain. A loss of blood flow to the brain for more than 10 seconds can lead to a loss of consciousness. Abnormally low blood levels or high levels of a toxic substance can cause the brain to malfunction within seconds, but thankfully

God has created within the brain a built-in mechanism called the blood-brain barrier (BBB) to keep most toxins from causing severe damage. It is important to note that the BBB was made to protect us from unknown harmful toxins, not as a filter for the known toxins to which we may choose to expose or overload our bodies.

What are the parts of the brain and what do they do?

The brain has three main components: the cerebellum, cerebrum and brain stem.

The **cerebellum** (Fig. 1) is the bottom part of the brain. It controls balance and coordination and helps the body make smooth, precise movements when reaching, throwing, walking, turning and bending.

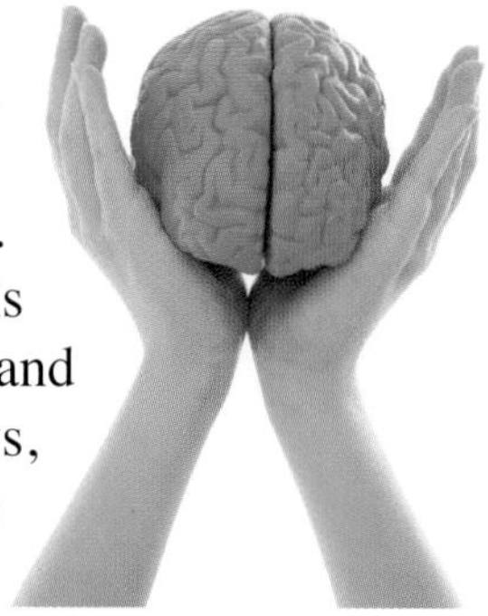

The **cerebrum** or cerebral cortex is the top and largest portion of the brain. It is divided into two halves – the right hemisphere or right brain and the left hemisphere or left brain. The right hemisphere of the brain deals with visual activities and plays a role in identification. It takes visual information, puts it together, and says "That is a dog." The left hemisphere is the analytical portion. It manages details, analyzes information collected by the right brain and applies critical thinking to it. The right hemisphere sees a dog, but the left hemisphere says, "I know whose dog that is." The cerebral hemispheres account for 85 percent of the brain's weight and are further divided into **four lobes**.

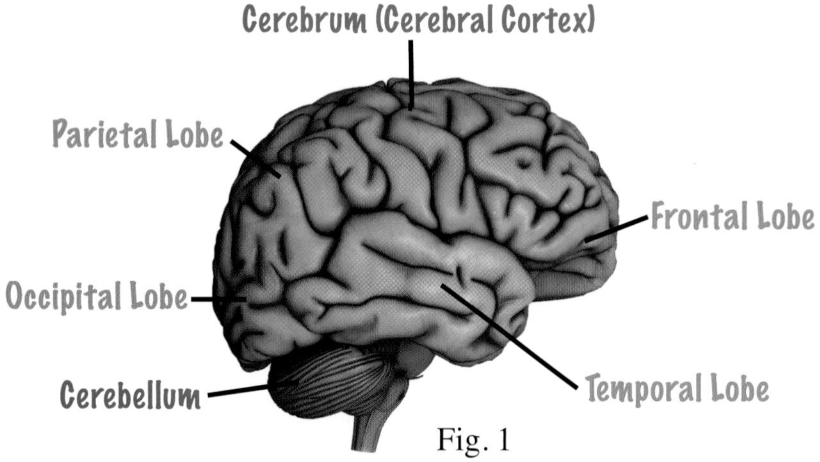

Fig. 1

The **frontal lobes** are involved in motor function, speech, thoughts, planning and mood. In most people, the left frontal lobe controls language-related movement, while the right frontal lobe controls non-verbal skills. The frontal lobes also are where we process organizational skills and the completion of simple tasks. If this area of the brain is damaged or undernourished a person may become less motivated, lethargic and struggle just to get out of bed. The frontal lobes also have a role in behavior and prevent people from saying things that may be threatening, inappropriate or bizarre. Damage to the frontal lobes may result in people doing things that are completely out of character, like swearing, undressing or urinating in public and other inappropriate behavior.

The **parietal lobe** interprets sensory data input from the rest of the body. It has an important role in dealing with our senses. In most people, the left side of the parietal lobe is considered dominant because of the way it helps us to do everyday tasks such as reading, writing, making calculations and speaking. Areas within the parietal lobe on the non-dominant side of the brain -- the right side – control spatial orientation. From these areas we derive our ability to know where we are in space, and we know how to find our way from one place to another. Damage to the non-dominant parietal hemisphere may result in the inability to read maps and the loss of the ability to stay oriented even in familiar places. A peculiar condition called spatial neglect causes victims of parietal damage to ignore one half of the environment. They may neglect to shave one half the face, eat portions on one half of the dinner plate only, or ignore people conversing standing or sitting on one side of the body, but not the other.

The **occipital lobe** processes our vision. While it is the eyes that see objects, it is the occipital lobe that makes sense of what we are seeing. Damage to this lobe may lead to loss of vision or the inability to fully comprehend what is being seen.

The **temporal lobe** generates emotions and memory. It allows us to recognize objects and people, process short- and long-term memory and initiate communication. Because of the temporal lobe, we can remember where we left a book or recall details from last year's picnic.

At the base of the cerebrum lie a collection of nerve cells called the basal ganglia, thalamus and hypothalamus. See Figure 2 below.

The **basal ganglia** help to smooth out movement.

The **thalamus** organizes sensory data messages to and from the highest level of the brain - the cerebrum.

The **hypothalamus** lies under the thalamus and coordinates the more automatic functions of the body like sleep, temperature and water balance. It issues instructions to correct any imbalances, including hormone irregularity.

The **limbic system** links the brain stem with the higher reasoning elements of the cerebral cortex. It controls emotions and instinctive behavior. This also is where the sense of smell is located.

The **hippocampus** is important for learning and short-term memory. This part of the brain is considered to be the site where short-term memories are converted into long-term memories for storage in other brain areas.

The **brain stem** lies at the base of the brain near the top of the neck. Even though it is the smallest segment of the brain, it is critical to our survival. It connects the brain and spinal cord. All information to and from the body passes through the brain stem. It controls our heart rate, blood pressure, breathing and sense of balance. Sleeping and daydreaming also are functions controlled by the brain stem.

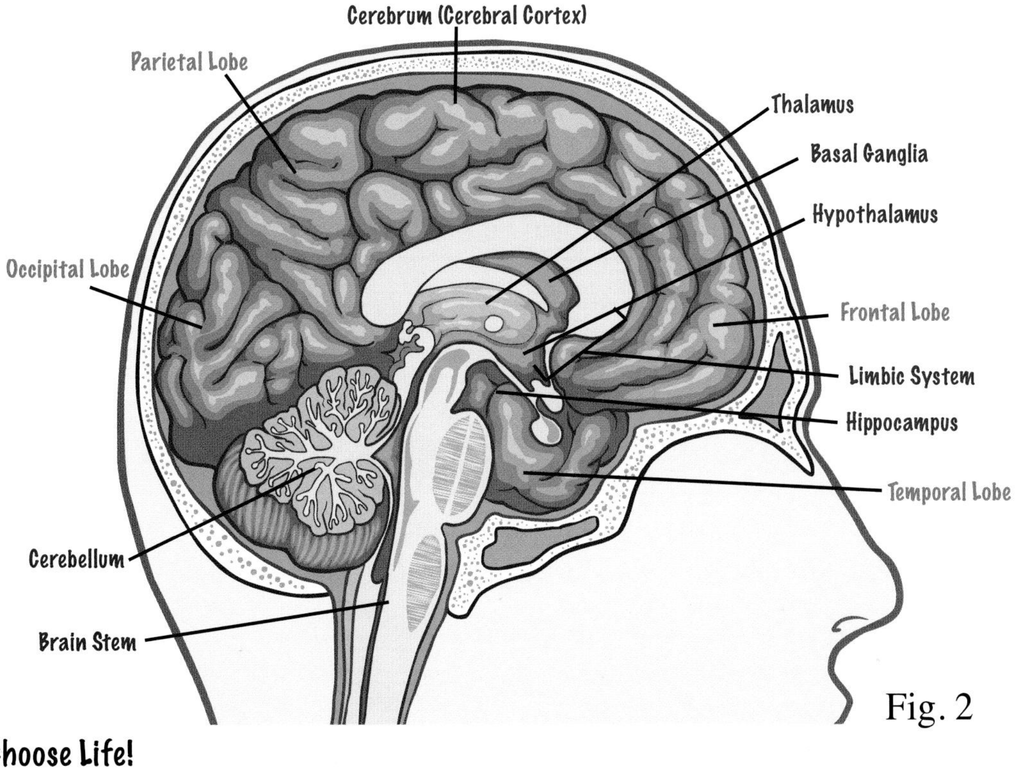

Fig. 2

Unit 1 Chapter 1
Discussion Questions

1. What does it mean to be “fearfully and wonderfully made?”
2. What other scripture references support what we’ve learned about the brain?
3. How does a healthy brain make a healthy body? How healthy is your brain?
4. Why is it so important to wear your helmet while bicycling or roller blading?
5. How is your brain like a computer? How is your brain better than a computer?
6. Do you think playing video games exercises your brain? Why or why not?

Activities - plus the Guacamole “Power” Recipe and activities.

Elementary

1. In the morning, brush your teeth with your non-dominant hand. At night, brush your teeth with your dominant hand. Was this hard or easy? Why? Try to use your non-dominant hand at other tasks, such as eating and writing.
2. Using the game 20 Questions as a framework, families can use their own memories to stimulate the brain and have fun. Have one family member recall a family memory and let others ask questions and guess. In addition to recollecting good memories, younger family members get to hear stories they may not remember first hand.
3. One family member should collect five household items that are used or known by every family member. Try to find objects that stimulate all of the senses, except sight. Using a blindfold, the other family members should take turn identifying the objects.
4. Find and memorize three scriptures associated with the mind.
5. Play the game Memory.

Secondary

Choose any from above plus

1. Read the article at the following link: http://www2.scholastic.com/browse/article.jsp?id=3629. Take the Cognitive Style Quiz at the bottom of the page to help you understand your style and how those around you learn.
2. Research the word lobe. From which language was it derived?
3. What are the careers specifically focused on the brain or the study of the brain?
4. Watch an interesting move about the brain: www.youtube.com/watch?v=FZ3401XVYww

Additional Resources

Web sites:

1. Neuroscience for kids by Eric Chudler, Ph.D., University of Washington – http://faculty.washington.edu/chudler/neurok.html
2. Brain teasers for older children: http://www.brainbashers.com/index.asp
3. Try the free trial for http://www.brainpop.com/

Books:

1. “Keep Your Brain Alive” Katz Lawrence C., Ph.D. and Rubin Manning, Workman Publishing Inc. 1999, www.keepyourbrainalive.com
2. “Unlock the Einstein Inside: Applying New Brain Science to Wake Up the Smart in Your Child” Gibson, Ken, Hanson, Kim and Mitchell Tanya, LearningRx, 2007.

"Power" Recipes and Activities

Proverbs 9:10 says "The fear of the Lord is the beginning of wisdom: and the knowledge of the holy is understanding." It is very important to learn how our bodies work and how food affects them; it is even more important to apply that knowledge. The best way to do that is to get in the kitchen!

This may be the most popular portion of **Nutrition 101: Choose Life!**

The following **"Power" Recipe** and the subsequent **"Power" Recipes** following each chapter are accompanied by engaging and exciting activities that will enhance the learning experience beyond the recipes. Start by reading about the basic food groups as defined in the **Nutrition 101: Choose Life! Food Pyramid** in Appendix B. Then, prepare the "Power" recipe from the week's corresponding chapter. Feel free to make any of the other recipes in the Additional Recipes section. Another option is to pick out some of your favorite family recipes and see how you can incorporate any of the good brain or nervous system foods from the lists in the previous chapters or how you can make healthier substitutions for some of the ingredients.

This will help you equip your children with incredibly valuable tools such as planning a meal, selecting fresh produce (see Appendix D), following a recipe and preparing a meal. Then, the entire family can enjoy the fruits and vegetables of your collective labor.

1. Study the **Nutrition 101: Choose Life! Food Pyramid** (Appendix B).
2. Pick out one of the "Power" Recipes with activities.
3. Use "How to Select Fresh Produce" (Appendix D) and the "**Nutrition 101: Choose Life!** Shopping List" (Appendix C) when shopping for your ingredients. Buy **organic** and local when possible. See Appendix D to find out more about organic and local food.
4. Read through "Kitchen Safety" (Appendix E).
5. Get in the kitchen!
6. "Kitchen talk" while preparing the meal. Emphasize and reinforce the things learned in that week's chapter. Meal preparation and/or meal times are great opportunities for the discussion questions from the chapter. Talk about how each ingredient is beneficial. Point out skills used to complete a recipe once the ingredients are gathered. This includes knowing kitchen materials/tools, reading, comprehending, counting, measuring, telling time and appropriate portions for all family members.
7. Pick and choose from the listed activities that go along with the recipes.
8. Enjoying your time cooking? Choose more recipes to make from the Additional Recipes section.
9. Pick favorite family recipes, incorporate good body system supporting foods and make healthy substitutions where necessary.
10. Make up your own recipes from the good foods lists.
11. Have fun!

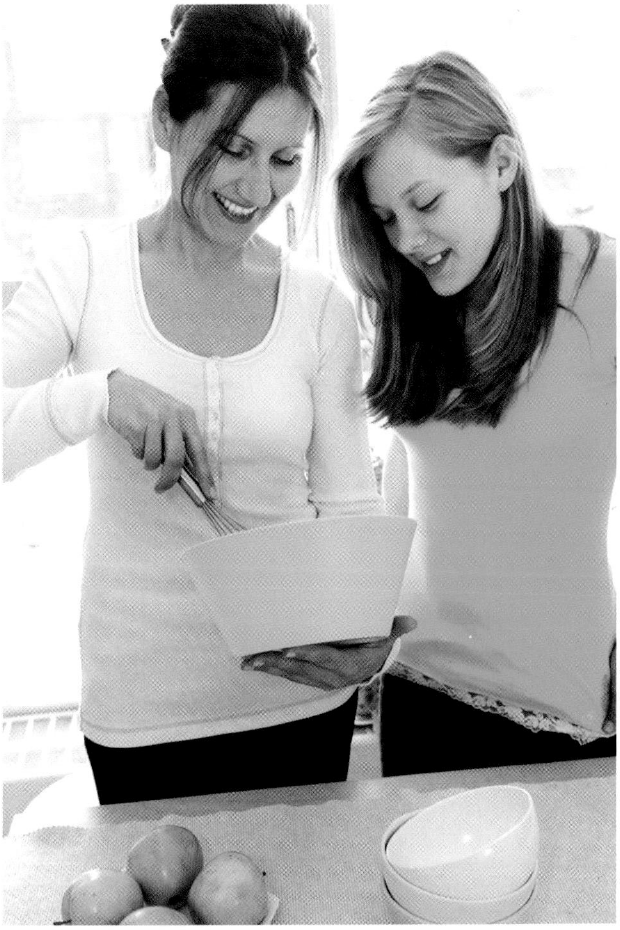

Brain Power

AVOCADOS

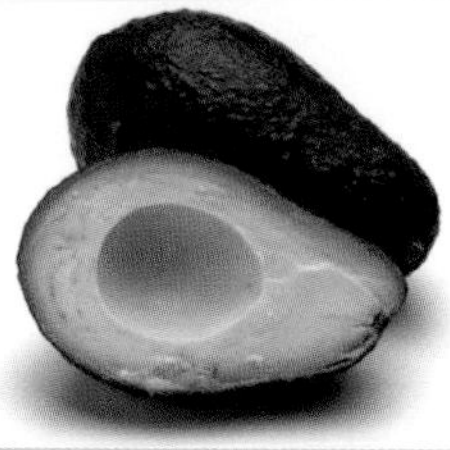

Did you know that avocados are fruit and NOT vegetables?
Avocados are a source of good, Brain Power fat!

Guacamole

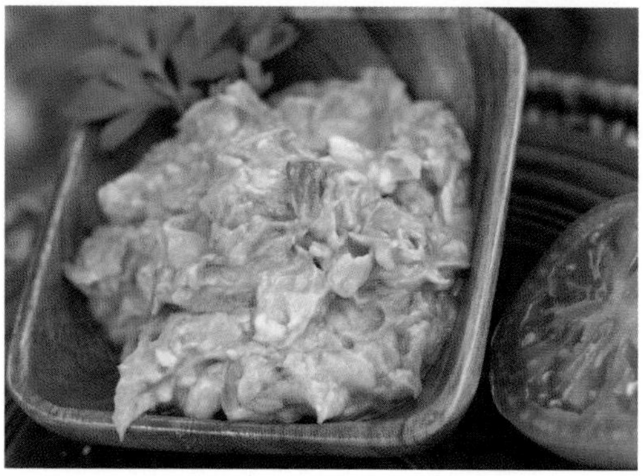

4 - 5 ripe avocados
2 Tbs. fresh cilantro finely chopped
2 Tbs. onion finely chopped
½ cup tomato finely chopped
Juice of one small lemon
1 clove garlic or ½ tsp. minced garlic
Salt and pepper to taste

Peel and scoop out the flesh of the avocado into a bowl and mash with a fork. Add remaining ingredients and stir. Serve with fresh veggies and/or baked whole grain pita chips. Makes eight servings.

Activities

Elementary

1. At the grocery store, learn how to pick out fresh, ripe and ready-to-eat produce for the recipe (refer to Appendix D).
2. Help make the guacamole by measuring and adding the ingredients while learning or reviewing fractions.
3. Experiment to find out how to make avocados ripen faster with some unripened avocados, an apple and a small paper bag. Compare the process with a regular avocado sitting by itself next to the bag. Is there a difference? Give your findings in an oral or written report.
4. Grow an avocado plant.

Secondary

Choose any from above plus

1. Why and how does activity #3 above work? Give your findings in an oral or written report.
2. Use a banana rather than an avocado in the experiment and see if it changes your results and why. Give your findings in an oral or written report.
3. Calculate how many grams of fat are in one serving of the guacamole above.
4. Find out what kind of fat is an avocado.

Chapter 2

Brain Health and Nutrition

"He that walketh with wise men shall be wise: but a companion of fools shall be destroyed." Proverbs 13:20

Nutrition plays a large role in the development and performance of our brains. For example, short-term memory depends on adequate intake of vitamin B12, vitamin C and vitamin E. Problem solving tasks rely on adequate intake of riboflavin, folate, B12 and vitamin C. Overall mental health relies on thiamin, niacin, zinc and folate. Cognitive functions work best with folate, vitamin B6, vitamin B12, iron and vitamin E. Without proper nutrition, the brain cannot function optimally and is left vulnerable to various health issues.

Brain Health Issues

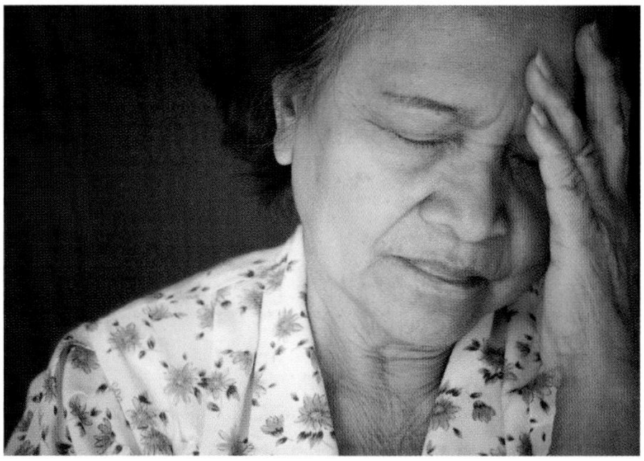

Dementia is a decline in mental ability which generally progresses slowly. Memory, thinking, judgment, even the ability to learn and pay attention also may deteriorate. For some individuals even their personality changes. While there are many causes (age, injury, toxins that destroy brain cells, disease), dementia is not considered to be a normal part of aging.

Alzheimer's is the most common form of dementia in which certain parts of the brain degenerate, destroying brain cells. Remaining brain cells are no longer responsive to chemicals that transmit signals to the brain. Alzheimer's can be caused by successive strokes, the formation of plaque in the brain, abnormal proteins in the brain and neurofibrillary tangles which have been seen in the autopsies of Alzheimer's patients. While diagnosis is about 85 percent correct, only an autopsy after death can confirm Alzheimer's.

Autism is a disorder in young children usually appearing within the first year of life and always before the age of three in which the child does not develop normal social skills and relationships. They generally behave in compulsive and ritualistic ways and many fail to develop normal intelligence, though some are classified as high functioning and exhibit above normal intelligence in certain areas. Causes still are largely unknown. Many have suspected a link between autism and mercury in childhood vaccinations; while for other children genetics or chromosomal damage is the cause.

Attention Deficit Disorder (ADD) generally is not regarded as an illness, but rather the tendency to exhibit poor concentration and focus, generally observed during the early school years. At times, inappropriate and impulsive behavior also is exhibited with or without hyperactivity. ADD is diagnosed 10 times more often in boys than girls and in an estimated five to 10 percent of school-aged children.

Epilepsy is a disorder characterized by the tendency to have seizures that reoccur randomly. The cause in adults is related to abnormal electrical activity in the brain due to scarring. In many young people no reason can be found for the seizures. These seizures can be triggered by certain sounds, flashing lights and even video games. Low blood sugars also have been implicated in some epileptic seizures. Some seizers can be very mild and affect only certain parts of the body such as hands or feet. The most severe form, status epilepticus, requires immediate medical attention to avoid permanent organ damage or even death.

Nutrition and the Brain

Because our brains are more than 60 percent fat, fats are the most important nutrient for optimal brain power. Fats are often considered bad for us – causing weight gain or high cholesterol – as the wrong kinds of fats can do. However, the right kinds of fats are highly important to maintaining healthy brains and bodies.

What are fats?

Fats are compounds made up of oxygen, hydrogen and carbon and belong to a group of substances called lipids. **Lipids** have three basic forms, which are all found in some combination in most foods.

1. Triglycerides - includes fats and account for about 95 percent of the weight of fats in foods. Fatty acids are components of triglycerides and are the simplest forms of fat.
2. Phospholipids, which act as emulsifiers that break up fats.
3. Sterols, the most well known of which is cholesterol.

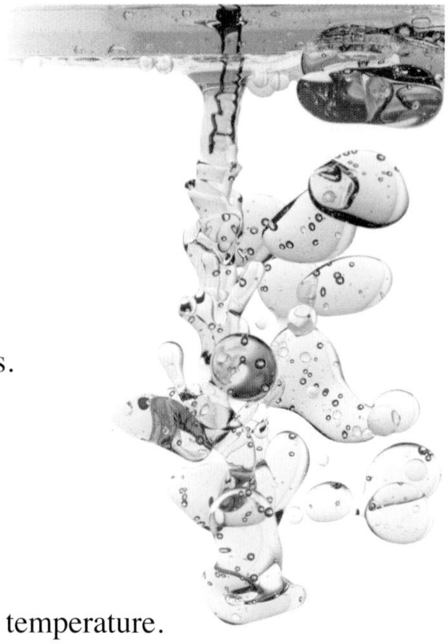

Fats are a common name for triglycerides and can be split into two groups:

1. **Saturated fats**
2. **Unsaturated fats** - includes monounsaturated and polyunsaturated fats, which can be further split into fatty acids.
   a. **Omega-3 fatty acids**
   b. **Omega-6 fatty acids**

Is fat different from oil?

Generally, **fats** are solid at room temperature, while **oils** are liquid at room temperature. However, some oils like coconut oil have a very low melting point at 76° F, so in a cool room, it appears as a solid.

What does unsaturated and saturated mean?

The terms unsaturated and saturated have to do with the chemistry of fats. Basically, it comes down to hydrogen atoms.

Unsaturated fats are not saturated with hydrogen atoms. They have one or more double bonds in the fatty acid chain. Where there are double bonds, hydrogen atoms are eliminated. Monounsaturated fats have one bond, and polyunsaturated fats have two or more bonds. As polyunsaturated fats include Omega-3 and Omega-6 fatty acids, they are essential to the diet. Sources of monounsaturated fats are olive, canola and peanut oils and avocados. Sources of polyunsaturated fats are safflower, sesame, soy, corn and sunflower seed oils, and nuts and seeds.

Word Power

Metabolism

Pronunciation: \mə-ta-bə-li-zəm\ Function: noun, Date: 1878

1 a: the sum of the processes in the buildup and destruction of protoplasm; specifically : the chemical changes in living cells by which energy is provided for vital processes and activities and new material is assimilated b: the sum of the processes by which a particular substance is handled in the living body c: the sum of the metabolic activities taking place in a particular environment <the metabolism of a lake>

Saturated fats have no double bonds, thus they are saturated with hydrogen atoms. Hydrogen-carbon bonds are broken down through cellular metabolism to create energy. So saturated fats, which have more hydrogen atoms, create more energy and have more calories. Saturated fats are found in foods from animals, such as dairy products and meat, and in plant sources, such as coconut, palm fruit and palm kernel. While much modern dietary advice says to avoid saturated fats altogether, significant research supports the contrary.[1] Saturated fats from coconut oil and from animals raised organically in their natural surroundings do have health benefits.

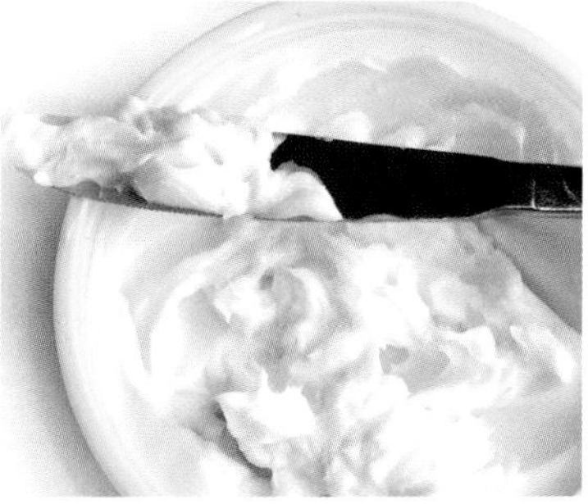

Be a Label Reader!
Avoid trans fatty foods with the words "partially hydrogenated" and "hydrogenated"on their labels.

What are hydrogenated and trans fats?

Hydrogenation occurs in a laboratory when hydrogen is added to unsaturated vegetable oils to create fully or partially hydrogenated fat, or **trans fat**. Margarine and shortening contain trans fats as do most processed, commercially baked and fried foods.

Trans fat has a longer shelf life, which is why so many commercial food manufacturers use it in their processed food products in place of unsaturated fats. The molecules of unsaturated fats can break down and go rancid through a process known as **oxidation**. This is when oxygen molecules mix with atoms in the fat. Trans fat molecules are more stable and can make processed food last so much longer.

No amounts of trans fats from hydrogenated oils are healthy because they are unnatural to the human body.

The body does not even recognize trans fats as food and cannot use them for any type of nutrition. They cannot be metabolized, so they are stored as toxins in the body's fat cells. Trans fats raise bad LDL cholesterol and lower good HDL cholesterol in the blood.[2] European studies have shown that women with breast cancer have higher levels of trans fats in their tissues than those without the disease.[3]

Fun Fact - Free radicals are produced during oxidation and cause cell damage and promote disease. Antioxidants protect cells by removing free radicals. Eating foods rich in antioxidants, like berries, will help minimize the damage oxidation causes.

Fun Fact - When most vegetable oils, including olive oil, are heated to 400° F or more for frying, their molecular structures change making them unhealthy fats. One exception is coconut oil, which can withstand high temperatures without becoming an unhealthy fat. See more information on fats and oils in Appendix J.

What do our bodies do with fat?

- Fats supply a continuing source of fuel. They are converted into energy for the ability to function throughout the day – move, walk, and exercise. Energy from excess foods eaten and not used is stored as fat. Fat surrounds vital organs, such as kidneys, acting as a shock absorber and providing structural support.
- Fats, or lipids, are the components of cell membranes.
- Fats help insulate us, holding in heat, and are present in all cells.

---

1 "The Importance of Saturated Fats for Biological Functions" Mary G. Enig, PhD http://www.westonaprice.org/knowyourfats/import_sat_fat.html
2 "Trans fat is double trouble for your heart health" MayoClinic.com, June 16, 2009.
3 "Dietary Fat and Cancer Trends-A Critique" M G Enig, et al, Federation Proceedings, July 1978, 37:(9):2215-2220.

- Fats help us absorb fat soluble vitamins A, E, D and K.
- Body fat can hold unabsorbed drugs, even those taken years ago.
- Fats hold toxins that our bodies were unable to eliminate.

How much fat and what kind do we need?

On average, Americans consume 142 grams of fat per day, whereas the Japanese consume only 42 grams. Since there are no actual guidelines for fat intake, a reasonable amount for most Americans would be 50 grams or less per day. No more than one-third of our total intake of fat should be saturated or hard fats, and at least one-third should be polyunsaturated Omega-6 and the Omega-3 fatty acids. See Appendix J for more detailed information about the different types of fats and oils.

What are Omega Fatty Acids?

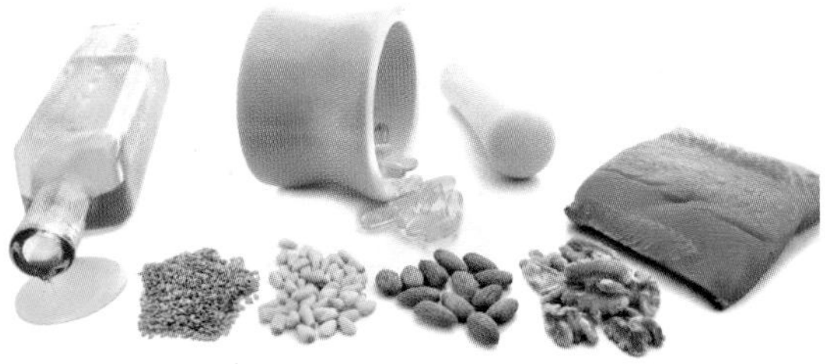

Omega-3 and Omega-6 – also known as essential fatty acids – were given their name when researchers found they were essential to normal growth in young children and animals.

Omega-3 Fatty Acids

There are three types of Omega-3 fatty acids: eicosapentaenoic acids **EPA**, docosahexaenoic acids **DHA** and alpha-linolenic acids **ALA**. They are termed essential because the body cannot make Omega-3 fatty acids and they are needed for our growth, development and general health.

EPA and DHA can be found primarily in fish, beef and wild game and are synthesized by the body from ALA. ALA is found in the oil of nuts and seeds from plants. However, ALA is poorly converted to DHA and EPA with only a small percent being converted.

DHA is essential for brain development, brain function and vision. It can positively affect learning abilities, coordination and mood. A diet rich in DHA is necessary for a pregnant woman because it is vital to the development of her baby's growing brain. Lower DHA content in mother's milk and lower consumption of seafood have been linked with higher rates of postpartum depression[4].

EPA is needed for hormone production. EPA and DHA reduce blood stickiness, control cholesterol and fat levels, improve immune function and metabolism, reduce inflammation and provide water balance.

The best source for Omega-3 is fish. Adequate plant sources are chia, flax and pumpkin, all of which contain ALA and must under go conversion to EPA and DHA. Again, only a small percent of the ALA actually is converted to EPA and DHA.

Omega-6 Fatty Acids

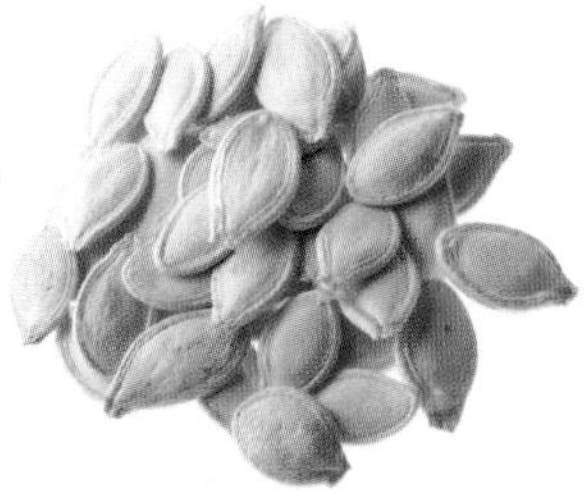

Key Omega-6 fatty acids are arachidonic acid **AA** and linoleic acid **LA**, which is a precursor to AA. LA is also converted in the body to gamma-linolenic acid **GLA**. However, not everyone has the enzymes necessary for the conversion to GLA. Evening primrose and borage oil are the richest source of GLA. Daily intake of GLA should be about 150 mg.

4 "Seafood consumption, the DHA content of mothers' milk and prevalence rates of postpartum depression: a cross-national, ecological analysis" Hibeln, Jr. http://www.ncbi.nlm.nih.gov/pubmed/12103448

Omega-6 oils help keep the blood thin, balance elevated blood pressure, improve nerve and immune system function, relax blood vessels and aid in blood sugar balance.

The Omega-6 fatty acids come from vegetable oils such as pumpkin, safflower, sesame, corn, walnut, soybean and wheat germ.

How much Omega-3 and Omega-6 should we have in our diets?

Our ancestors ate much better than we do today by growing many of their vegetables and fruits and raising livestock. A diet with a 1:1 ratio of Omega-3 to Omega-6 was the norm.

Currently, with fast food addictions, eat-out-of-a-box mentalities and the commercially raised beef we consume, it is estimated that we now have a ratio closer to 1:15 Omega-3 to Omega-6. This imbalance increases the risk of coronary heart disease and also heightens the body's natural inflammatory process.

The optimum ratio suggested by today's health professionals is 1:3 to 1:5 Omega-3 to Omega-6.

So why do we need to eat more Omega-3 fatty acids?

First of all, Omega-3's are heart protective, nourish the brain, skin, nails and hair, and support the immune system.

Secondly, it is too easy to get too much Omega-6 in our diet. Chips, fries, fried foods, commercially baked goods, cookies, cakes, crackers and commercially raised beef all have excess Omega-6. Another reason why we get too much Omega-6 is due to the slow conversion process of the plant based ALA Omega-3 into EPA and DHA.

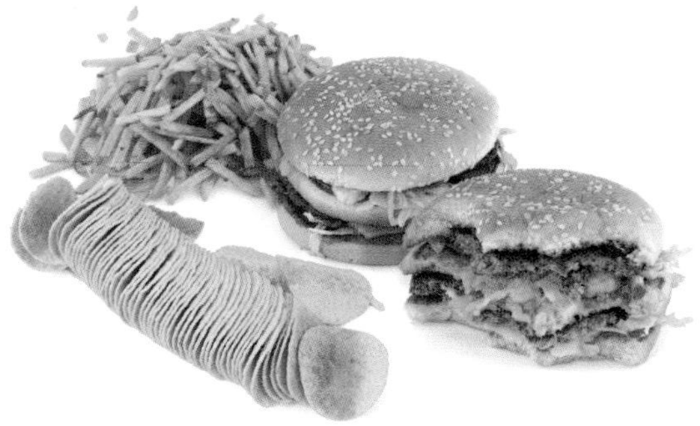

Omega-6's **when not in proper balance to Omega-3's** can stir up toxins in our bodies and can cause inflammation. Arachidonic acid (AA), which is a form of Omega-6, was discovered in 1965 to be converted by the body into prostaglandins – a pro-inflammatory agent.[5] AA is found in high levels in beef products.

Disorders of the brain that have a link to Omega-3 deficiency include Attention Deficit Disorder (ADD), Attention Deficit Hyperactive Disorder (ADHD), Alzheimer's Disease and Parkinson's Disease.

The American Heart Association says Omega-3's reduce the risk of cardiovascular disease.[6] With heart disease the number one killer of American adults,[7] and childhood heart disease on the rise, we can safely assume that we should all be consuming more Omega-3's.

Even if we take drastic measures to reduce the amount of Omega-6's we eat, and increase Omega-3's, most likely we will need to supplement our diets with a quality Omega-3. This is especially true for those who do not like the taste of fish.

---

5 "Biosynthesis of Prostaglandins from Arachidonic Acid in Guinea Pig Lung, Prostaglandins And Related Factors", Erik Rd And Bengt Samuelsson, From the Department of Chemistry, Karolinska Insifutet, Stockholm 60, Sweden, The Journal of Biological Chemistry, Vol. 240, No. 9, September 1965.

6 http://www.americanheart.org/presenter.jhtml?identifier=4632

7 http://www.americanheart.org/presenter.jhtml?identifier=3054076

How to Choose the Right Supplements for Your Brain

Omega-3 Supplements

Fun Fact

While the U.S. has not established a Recommended Daily Allowance (RDA) Omega-3 fatty acids, nutritionists recommend one to three grams per day for the general population.
100 grams (3.5 oz.) of fish gives you 1 gram combined EPA and DHA.

Fish Sources

Most supplements, even if using pharmaceutical grade fish oil, must remove toxins and heavy metals from the fish oil. Then a flavoring is added to lessen the fishy taste during digestion or indigestion (burping).

A better choice is a supplement that:

1. Uses fish oil from fish with higher concentrations of EPA-DHA, where the fish live in clean water free of heavy metals and toxins.
2. Is enteric coated so digestion doesn't begin until it reaches the small intestine.
3. Is enhanced with a blend of plant compounds known to fight inflammation, a chief culprit of excess Omega-6 consumption.

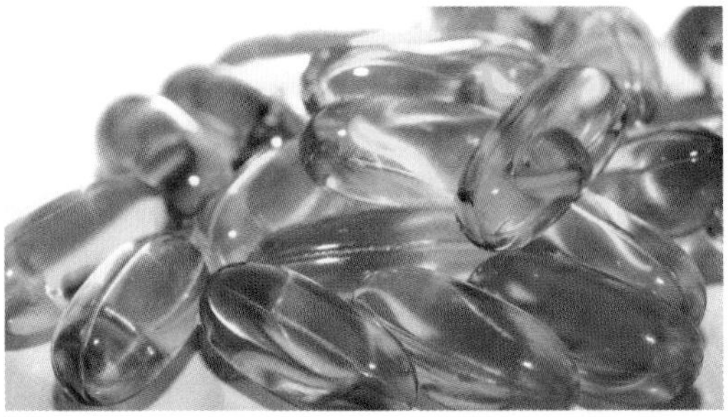

Vegetarian Sources

While it is true that fish are the best food source of EPA- and DHA-rich Omega-3's, several plants have rich sources of ALA, which a properly functioning body can convert a small percentage into usable EPA and DHA through several processes. Be aware, though, that these sources alone might not end up providing enough of the daily required EPA and DHA.

Flaxseed

In 1955, German biochemist Dr. Johanna Budwig became the first author to publish information on the role of flax oil in healing cancer and degenerative disease. She also warned about the detrimental effects of trans fats.[8]

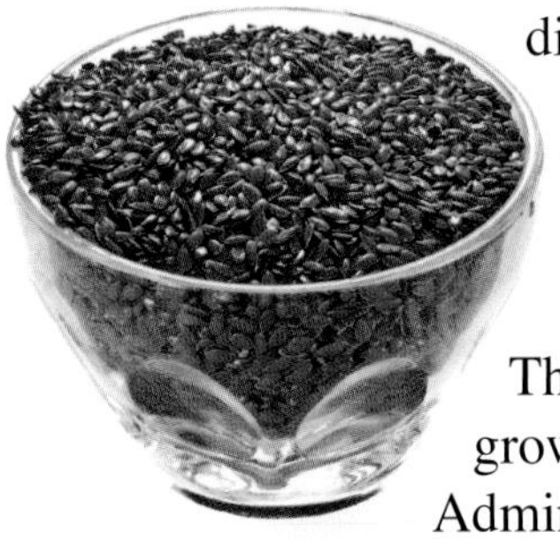

Flaxseed has long been researched for its potential to fight diseases such as cancer and digestive disorders. Constipation and intestinal issues often are abated by adding either ground flax or flax oil to the diet because of its high fiber content. See the Fiber Chart in Appendix K. It is an affordable addition to daily meals, due to its relatively low cost and availability in the market.

The University of Toronto's Dr. Stephen Cunnane showed that flax prevented the growth of new cancer cells and lowered blood cholesterol levels.[9] The U.S. Food and Drug Administration has endorsed flaxseed as a possible food for prevention of disease.

Flaxseed soaked in warm water will turn into a mucilaginous, or slimy, gruel. As strange as it may look, when eaten this gruel brings gentle relief from all sorts of intestinal discomfort.

Flaxseed is approximately 48 to 64 percent ALA Omega-3 and 26 to 34 percent Omega-6.

---

8 "Flax Oil as a True Aid Against Arthritis, Heart Infarction, Cancer, and Other Diseases" Budwig, Dr. Johanna, 1992, pages 5-59.

9 "Flaxseed in Human Nutrition" Dr. Cunnane, Stephen and Dr. U Thompson, Lillian. Champaign, Illinois: AOCS Press. ISBN: 0-935315-60-8.

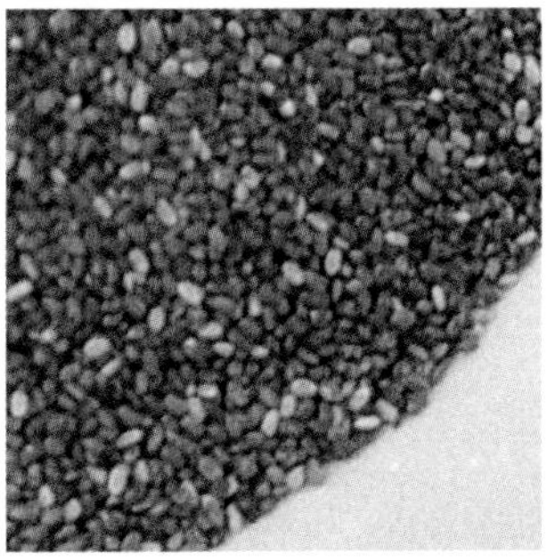

Chia Seed

Chia seed is emerging as an even better plant choice than flax. As Chia (Salvia hispanica L.) seed is very high in soluble fiber, it is the richest plant source of Omega-3 fatty acids known and contains natural antioxidants. Originating in southern Mexico and Guatemala, the plant is a member of the mint family. There are two seed colors: white and black. Both seeds contain essentially the same amount of Omega-3, protein, fiber, etc.

As part of an effort lead by the University of Arizona in the 1990's to establish new crops in northwestern Argentina[10], the chia plant was brought back after being lost for five centuries. This project led to successful commercialization of chia as a crop, making it more widely available today.

Unlike flax, chia seeds do not need to be ground. They can be eaten as is, or they can be added to juices, yogurt, broths, salads, omelets and cereals. They can also be mixed, either ground or whole, with flour and used for making baked goods like bread, pizza dough and muffins. Chia seeds may be found in most health food stores. For more information on chia seeds, see the Additional Resources at the end of this chapter.

As the daily recommended amount of Omega-3 is one to three grams per day for the general population, two tablespoons of chia seed provide **four grams of ALA Omega-3**. Although the body may not convert all of the ALA into EPA and DHA, chia also are a great source of fiber, protein, calcium and other nutrients.

Fun Fact - Combine two tablespoons of each flaxseed, chia seed, sesame seed, sunflower seed and pumpkin seed. Grind them together and store in a jar in the refrigerator. Consume one tablespoon daily by taking it alone or adding it to a smoothie.

Omega-3 Deficiency Symptoms

Hampered growth
Change in behavior
Leaky gut
Water retention
Dry or inflamed skin
Low energy and general weakness
High triglycerides
Tingling in the arms and legs
Poor motor coordination
Insulin resistance
Depression
Learning problems
High blood pressure
Allergies
Low metabolism
Low thyroid function
Low adrenal function
Hyperactivity
Psoriasis
Eczema
Acne

Good Brain Foods

Avocados, bananas, lean beef, brewer's yeast, broccoli, brown rice, Brussels sprouts, cantaloupe, chia seeds, chicken, collard greens, eggs, flaxseed oil, legumes, oatmeal, oranges, almonds, cashew or walnut butter, peas, potatoes, romaine lettuce, salmon, spinach, tuna, turkey and wheat germ

Bad Brain Foods

Alcohol, artificial colors and flavors†, artificial sweeteners†, caffeine, cakes, candy, corn syrup†, dairy, fried foods, hydrogenated fats and oils†, high fructose corn syrup†, margarine, partially hydrogentated oils†, shortenings, sodas, sugar, sweet baked goods and trans fats†.

†These are chemcials and because they cannot be digested, they turn to toxins in the body.

10 "Chia: Rediscoverying a forgotten crop of the Aztecs" Ayerza, R. and W. Coates, The University of Arizona Press, Tucson, 2005. Arizona., http://www.bajaaz.org/chia.php

Attention deficit
Platelets sticking, which causes clots to form and leads to heart attack or stroke
Poor vision
Slow wound healing

Omega-6 Supplements

Omega-6 fatty acids come from some vegetable sources like corn, sunflower, safflower, soybean, cottonseed, nuts and seeds. Omega-6 also is common from lean meat, eggs and poultry. Animals fed diets rich in flaxseed meal will have better Omega-3 to Omega-6 ratios, but it is known that grass-fed, free-ranging animals have better ratios naturally.

Omega-6 Deficiency Symptoms

Eczema
Sterility in males
Dry skin and hair
Dry eyes
Elevated cholesterol
Susceptible to infection
Kidney malfunction
Drying up of the glands
Fatty liver
Miscarriage in females
Hair loss
Excessive sweating

Fun Fact
Olive oil contains no appreciable amounts of Omega-3 or Omega-6, but it is an excellent heart protective oil, none the less.

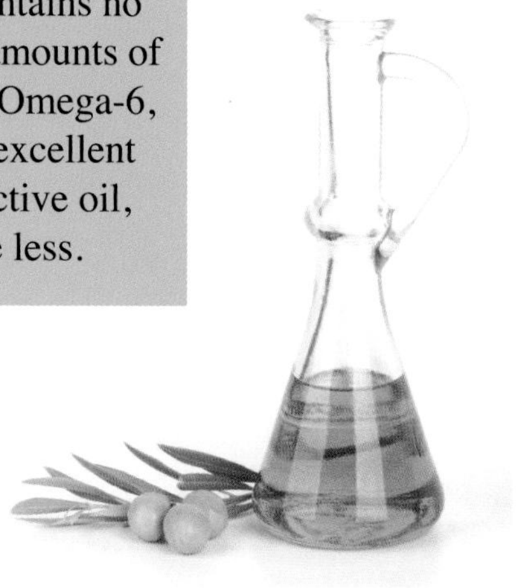

Having the right balance of both Omega-3 and Omega-6 fatty acids is crucial for our health. A deficiency of the Omega-6 is more difficult to identify because Omega-3 can cover for an Omega-6 deficiency, but Omega-6 cannot cover for Omega-3. Proper intake of Omega-3 rich foods, which contain both Omega-3 and Omega-6, is essential.

For a healthier body, better brain function and to prevent disease, there may be no better health choice than to eat foods rich in both Omega-3 and Omega-6 with a predominance of Omega-3's and supplement with either a quality fish oil supplement and/or chia or flaxseed.

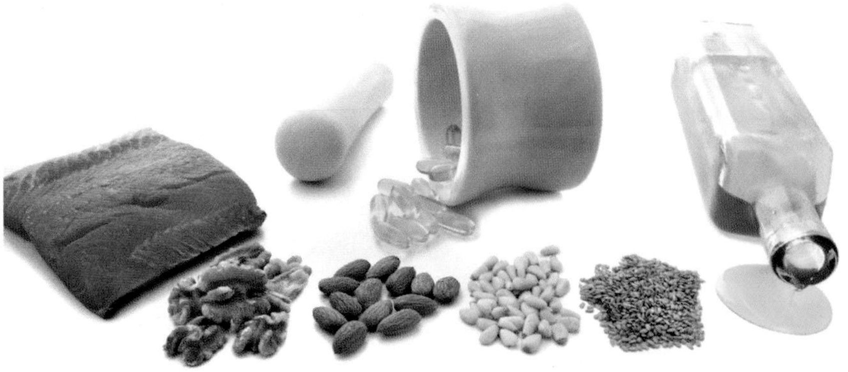

Unit 1 Chapter 2
Discussion Questions

1. Do you think that what you eat as a child affects your brain when you are an adult? Why or why not?
2. Can you think of health problems in the elderly that may suggest brain conditions?
3. Why are hydrogenated and trans fats bad for us and detrimental to future health? What happens when an oil is heated above 400° F?
4. Of the good brain foods listed in Chapter 3, which ones are your favorites?

Activities - plus the Greek Salad "Power" Recipe and activities.

Elementary

1. To download coloring pages, go to www.dole5aday.com. Select "Games & More" from the top tool bar. Scroll down that page and the SuperKids Coloring Pages are located under Games, then Comics & Puzzles.
2. Eat one of the foods from the "Good Brain Foods" list each day for a week. You must eat a different food each day. Describe their taste, texture, smell, etc. Make a chart to keep track.
3. Write or give an oral presentation on the best three foods for the brain.
4. If you can find an item with trans fat or hydrogenated fat in your cupboard, experiment to see how long it takes until it begins to go bad. If you do not have any selections in the house, you can purchase a small bag of French fries from most fast food chains. Put the item in a plastic bag and use a permanent marker to write the date the item was purchased.
5. Write a poem about your favorite brain food. It can be funny or serious.
6. Visit your local produce stand and identify all of the good brain foods. If you have the opportunity, ask an employee how the fruits and vegetables are grown.

Secondary

Choose any from above plus

1. Create a breakfast using three of the foods from the Good Brain Foods list.
2. Refer to the Omega Chart in Appendix J. List the highest Omega-3 plant and fish source.
3. Look up the meaning of the word "omega." Based on the meaning, why do you believe scientists named them Omega fatty acids? Research the naming and see if you are correct. Share this information with your family during a meal or snack that includes good Omega-3s.
4. Interview someone (preferably over 70) who grew up on a farm. Ask him or her what kind of foods they grew, what animals they raised and what it was like to live on a farm. Write a report about how it is similar to or different from how your family gets food.
5. Create a daily menu including the highest Omega-3 foods. Use the **Nutrition 101: Choose Life! Food Pyramid** to include a variety of foods from all of the food groups and make sure it contains the daily recommendation of one to three grams of Omega-3. It should also be tasty. Refer to the charts in Appendices B and E.
6. Research the process used to remove oil from a seed. How does this impact the price of various types of products, such as vegetable oil, sunflower seed oil, olive oil and flaxseed oil?
7. Research chia seeds to learn what is required to grow them. Provide your findings in a written report.
8. Print out Appendix J and the Bad Brain Food List. Go to the grocery store and find three packaged foods that are labeled as containing added Omega-3. Compare the label to Appendix J to find the Omega-3 ingredient. Then, compare it to the Bad Brain Foods List to see if it contains any of those ingredients. Do you feel this food would promote better brain power?

Additional Resources

Web sites: http://www.healthdiaries.com/eatthis/15-facts-about-chia-seeds.html

Books: "The Crazy Makers: How the food industry is destroying our brains and harming our children" Carol Simontacchi. Jeremy P. Tarcher/Putnam. New York. 2000.

Brain Power

Olive Oil

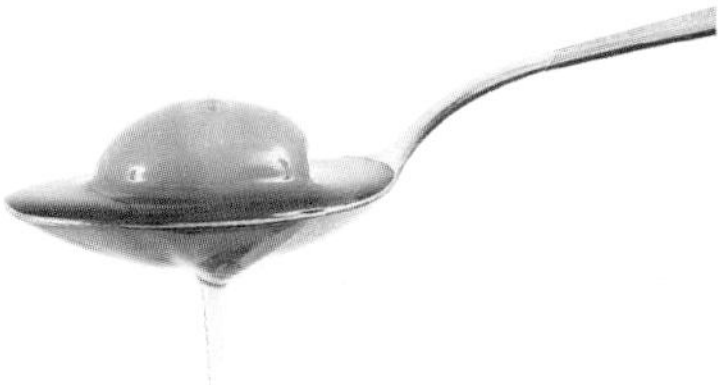

While olive oil has minimal amounts of Omega-3 and Omega-6 fatty acids, it is still a great Brain Power fat and helps protect the heart.

Greek Salad

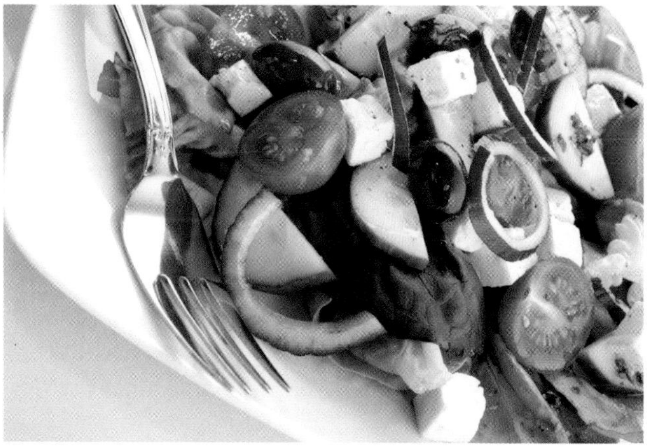

One head of green or red leaf lettuce, washed and crisped, torn into small pieces.
3 tomatoes, diced or 10-12 cherry tomatoes halved
1 cucumber, diced
10-20 green or black olives
1 Tbs. fresh oregano, finely diced
1 red onion, sliced thin and cut into half rings
1 cup feta cheese
1 tsp. balsamic vinegar
5 Tbs. olive oil
Salt, pepper and garlic powder to taste

Combine all ingredients in a salad bowl and toss.

Activities

Elementary

1. Experiment with the oil and vinegar in a smaller bowl. Do they combine or separate?
2. Find the expiration date on the bottle of olive oil. Why does this product have an expiration date? What other ingredients can go rancid?
3. Use two lettuce leaves to try an extended experiment. Take one leaf and tear it in half. Then use a pen or marker to label both pieces with "T" for tear. Cut the other leaf in half with a knife and mark both pieces with "C" for cut. Refrigerate the pieces on a plate. For the next three days, check the leaves and note any differences. The object is to see whether tearing or cutting the lettuce will allow it to last longer.

Secondary

Choose any from above plus

1. Experiment with the oil and vinegar in a smaller bowl. Then, observe what the ingredients do when mixed with the other ingredients in the recipe. Explain what happens in a written or oral report.
2. What are the different varieties of green leafy vegetables available at your local market? Research the nutritional value of each one.
3. Create your own healthy salad using at least 10 of your favorite ingredients (good brain foods and no bad brain foods). If you are pleased with the results, send it to editor@growinghealthyhomes.com for possible future publication.

Chapter 3

The Nervous System

"Why art thou cast down, O my soul? and why art thou disquieted within me? hope thou in God: for I shall yet praise him, who is the health of my countenance, and my God." Psalm 42:11

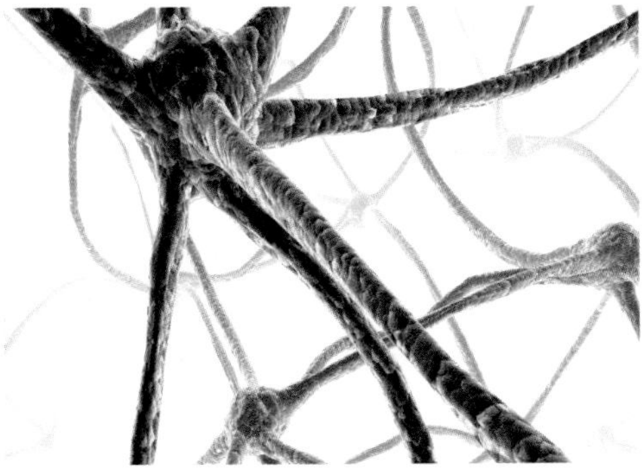

Like other systems in the body, the nervous system is composed of organs, principally the brain, spinal cord and a huge network of threadlike nerves. Together with the endocrine system, which we will learn more about in Unit 6, the nervous system is responsible for regulating and maintaining homeostasis – a normal state of the body. Just like our brains, our nervous system needs proper nutrition and certain key nutrients to function optimally. In order to understand how nutrition affects it, we need to first understand what our nervous system is and does how it works.

What are Nerves?

Nerves are communication pathways connecting the brain and spinal cord to various parts of your body. These threadlike nerve cells are called **neurons.** Your nervous system has billions of neurons and your brain alone has 100 billion! These neurons run all throughout your body and transmit information in the form of electrical signals, kind of like telephone lines. As a matter of fact, your nervous system has as many connections as in the world's telephone system, one of the most complex networks on the planet.

Neurons have many different, specialized jobs or functions. These various functions can be divided into three groups: sensory, integrative and motor.

Sensory

Through its specialized neurons called **sensory receptors**, the nervous system keeps us in touch with our environment, both external through our sense organs or receptor organs (eyes, ears, nose, tongue and skin) and internal organs. They monitor things outside the body such as temperature, sound and light, as well as those inside the body like pH (see Unit 2 Chapter 2), pressure, carbon dioxide concentration and levels of various electrolytes. This sensory input is converted into electrical signals called nerve impulses that travel across **synapses** (see Fig. 1 below) from one sensory neuron to the next and then to the brain. Here the signals are brought together to create sensations, to produce thoughts or to add to memory. This is the **sensory function**.

Integrative

Decisions, or integrations, are made by a system of cells, tissues and organs that regulate the body's response to sensory information. This system, or integration center, consists of the brain, spinal cord, nerves, ganglia and parts of the receptor and effector organs. They decide what messages or signals will be sent to the rest of the body. This is the **integrative function**.

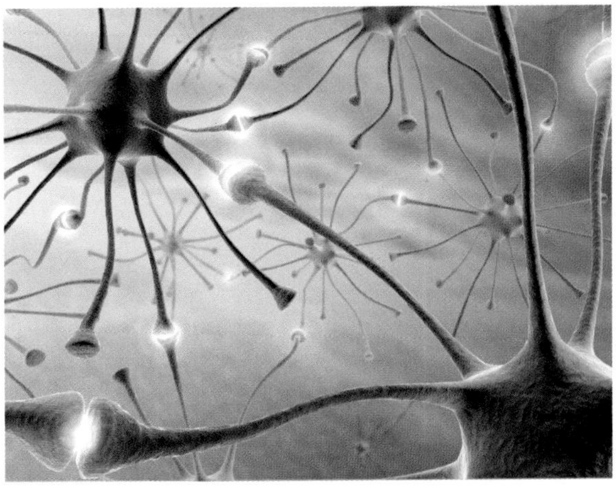

Fig. 1

Motor

The nervous system then sends signals away from the brain to muscles and glands through **motor neurons**. The motor neurons cause muscles to contract or glands to produce secretions based on the sensory integration (decisions) from the brain. Muscles and glands are called effector organs because they cause an effect in response to directions from the nervous system. This is the motor output or **motor function**.

When learning about neurons, **glial cells**, or simply glia, cannot be ignored. While they do not carry messages in the brain, they are the heroes of neurons. The glia's job is to support neurons by transporting nutrients to them, holding the neurons in place, cleaning up debris in the brain and even digesting parts of other dead neurons.

Fun Fact
In the Greek language, glia means glue or putty.

Fun Fact
Did you know that there are 10 to 50 times MORE glia in the brain than there are neurons?

What are the parts of the Nervous System and what do they do?

The nervous system is comprised of two separate systems: the **central nervous system** and the **peripheral nervous system.**

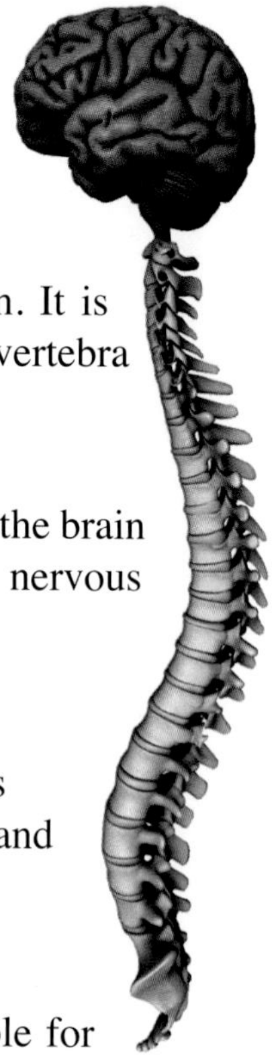

The **central nervous system (CNS)** includes the **brain** and **spinal cord**.

The **brain:** see Chapter 1 of this unit.

The **spinal cord** acts as the pathway for sending messages to and from the brain. It is protected by the spinal or vertebral column, which is a collection of bones known as vertebra that run down the center of the back.

The **peripheral nervous system (PNS)** is the network of nerves that lead to and from the brain and the spinal cord (see Fig. 2 on next page). It is divided into two major parts: the somatic nervous system and the autonomic nervous system.

The **somatic nervous system**, or voluntary nervous system, controls conscious movements of the skeletal muscles. When a person picks up an apple to take a bite, his somatic nervous system is at work telling the muscles in his arm and hand to contract and actually pick up the apple to put it in his mouth.

The **autonomic nervous system**, or involuntary nervous system, is responsible for controlling unconscious body processes. This includes the actions we almost never need to think about, like breathing, digestion, sweating and shivering. After the central nervous system has received information from the outside environment, the autonomic system responds by regulating the internal environment. For instance, if a person goes outside on a hot summer day, her central nervous system would gather that information and say, "Hey, it's hot outside!" Her autonomic nervous system would sense the body temperature rising and then tell her sweat glands to produce sweat to cool off the body.

The autonomic nervous system has three parts: the sympathetic, the parasympathetic and the enteric nervous systems.

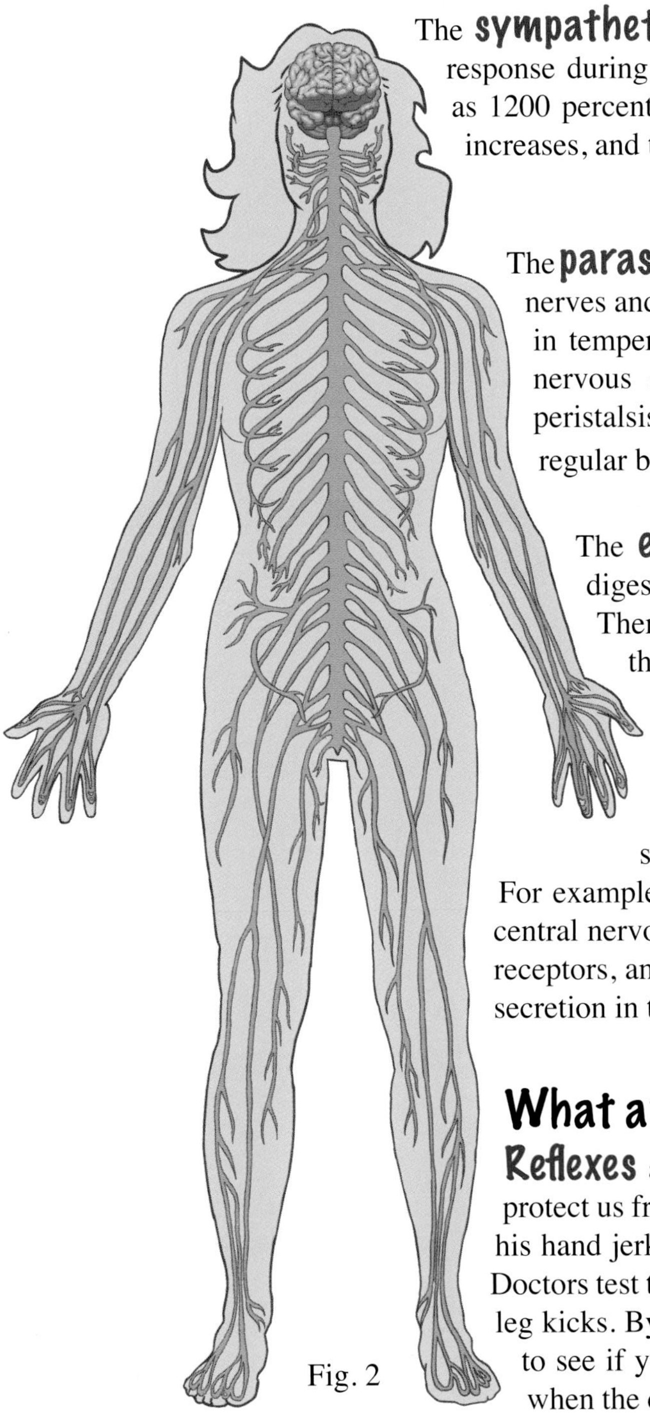

Fig. 2

The **sympathetic nervous system** is what gives us our fight-or-flight response during stressful conditions. Blood flow is increased up to as much as 1200 percent, the lungs open for greater oxygen exchange, the heart rate increases, and the pupils dilate.

The **parasympathetic nervous system** promotes a calming of the nerves and causes them to return to their normal state. It also is involved in temperature control, heart rate and digestion. The parasympathetic nervous system stimulates salivary gland secretion and accelerates peristalsis – the wave like motion of the intestines helping you to have regular bowel movements.

The **enteric nervous system** is not well known. It is the digestive system's very own nervous system and is very complex. There are as many neurons in the enteric nervous system as there are in the spinal cord. The enteric nervous system works autonomously, or by itself, but it is also linked to the central nervous system via the sympathetic and parasympathetic nervous systems. While it can function by itself to carry out regular digestive processes, sometimes the central nervous system carries a message directly to the digestive system. For example, the sight of good food can make your stomach growl. The central nervous system received external information via the sight sensory receptors, and then the central nervous system sent a message to stimulate secretion in the stomach.

What are reflexes?

Reflexes are involuntary, or automatic, actions that our bodies take to protect us from harm. For example, when a person touches something hot, his hand jerks away before his brain even gets the message, "That's hot!" Doctors test the reflexes by hitting a rubber hammer on the knee to see if the leg kicks. By testing that reflex, called the **knee-jerk reflex**, he is able to see if your central nervous system is functioning properly. Likewise, when the doctor shines a bright light into the eye, he is checking to make sure that the pupil constricts to protect the eye from being damaged by the bright light. If it does not constrict, then he knows that there is a problem with the nervous system. The body has many reflexes. Some other reflexes are coughing and sneezing; these are the body's way of clearing excess mucus from the system.

Fun Fact

Because nerves connect the spine to all body parts and end at the hands and feet, massage and reflexology are very effective in alternative healthcare.

Unit 1 Chapter 3

Discussion Questions

1. What is homeostasis? What do you think that means for our bodies?
2. If there are 100 billion neurons in the brain, then about how many glial cells are there? About how many neurons and glia are there together?
3. Name some receptor organs.
4. Name some effector organs.
5. Why do we have reflexes? What are some of the other reflexes of our body not mentioned in this chapter?
6. When does your sympathetic nervous system respond? Give an example of the fight or flight response.

Activities - plus the Potato Salad "Power" Recipe and activities.

Elementary

1. Using your fingernail, gently poke on your forearm, big toe, outer thigh and shoulder to see which place is the most sensitive.
2. Using a feather, stroke the faces of your family members with their eyes closed. Use the lightest touch possible. Ask them how it feels. Most people will report that the tickling sensation lingers several minutes.
3. Roll out a large piece of butcher paper on the floor, have a partner trace your body. Then, draw your brain and nervous system.
4. Have an adult check your reflexes by using his or her hand in a karate chop motion on the knee. Completely relax and see how much the leg jerks. Record the findings on all family members.
5. Take a piece of ice and place it in the palm of your hand. Using a stop watch or second hand on the watch, see how long before the area goes numb. Repeat on your calf.

Secondary

Choose any from the above plus

1. Give a specific example illustrating the three functions of neurons.
2. Learn more about neurons by going to http://faculty.washington.edu/chudler/cells.html, read the fascinating information about neurons and then take the quiz, the review test or even build a neuron!
3. Learn more about glia at http://faculty.washington.edu/chudler/glia.html
4. Test your reflexes at http://faculty.washington.edu/chudler/chreflex.html.

Additional Resources

Web sites:

1. Neuroscience For Kids Web site: http://faculty.washington.edu/chudler/neurok.html
2. http://pennhealth.com/health_info/body_guide/reftext/html/nerv_sys_fin.html
3. http://www.kidshealth.org/teen/your_body/body_basics/brain_nervous_system.html
4. http://www.juliantrubin.com/fairprojects/medicine/nervoussystem.html

Nervous System Power

Flaxseed Oil

Potato Salad with Flaxseed Oil - Hold the Mayo

8 medium sized golden Yukon potatoes, or 20 Red Russet potatoes, cooked, peeled and diced
3 hard boiled eggs, peeled and diced
4 Tbs. flaxseed oil
2 Tbs. nut oil (walnut, sesame, pumpkin)
1 tsp. apple cider vinegar
1 medium onion, diced
1 stalk celery, chopped fine
1 tsp. vegetable or beef broth powder
Salt, pepper and garlic powder to taste
Tomato slices and parsley to garnish

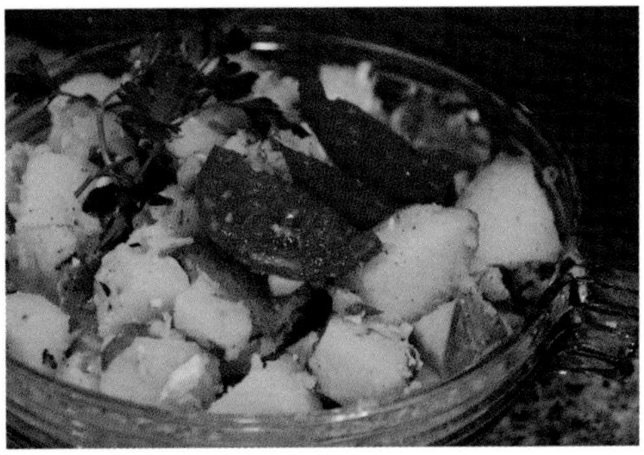

Combine all items in a large bowl. Garnish with 2 Tbs. fresh chopped parsley chopped and tomato wedges.

Activities

Elementary

1. Identify which specific ingredients in the recipe are good for the brain.
2. A nut is a seed, but a seed is not necessarily a nut. True or false? How is a seed different from a nut?
3. What is flax? Where does it grow? How is it harvested and processed?
4. Find the amount of ounces contained in the bottle of flaxseed oil. Find out how many tablespoons equal an ounce. Now find out how many tablespoons are in the container.

Secondary

Choose any from above plus

1. Research how oil is taken from seeds, nuts and vegetables. Are the processes similar or different?
2. In what kind of containers are your flaxseed oil and nut oil? Research the difference between glass and plastic containers. Is one superior?
3. What is the difference between a fluid ounce and a dry ounce?

Chapter 4

Nervous System Health and Nutrition

"For I delight in the law of God after the inward man: But I see another law in my members, warring against the law of my mind, and bringing me into captivity to the law of sin which is in my members." Romans 7:22-23

While there are some specific nutrients to consider, all known nutrients in our diets can influence the function of our nervous system. Some of the most important are proteins, amino acids, the B-complex vitamins and minerals – iron, iodine, calcium and magnesium. Without these important nutrients, the nervous system may not be able to function optimally.

Nervous System Health Issues

Multiple Sclerosis (MS) is a disorder where the nerves in the eye, brain and spinal cord lose patches of myelin. It is so named because of the multiple areas of scarring (sclerosis) representing these patches. Brain and spinal scans often show lesions, which are indicators that the symptoms match the diagnosis. Symptoms usually appear between the ages of 20 and 40 years of age and include tingling, numbness and weakness in the arms and legs. Sudden double vision, loss of vision and pain in one eye also are first indicators. While the exact cause is unknown, it is widely accepted that some virus or unknown antigen triggers an autoimmune process. Interestingly, MS occurs in one out of 2,000 people who spend the first decade of life in a temperate climate, but only one out of 10,000 of those born in a tropical climate and almost never occurs in people who grow up near the equator.

Word Power

Neurology
Pronunciation: nu˙r-ə-lä-jē
Function: noun
Etymology: New Latin neurologia, from neur- + -logia -logy
Date: circa 1681
: the scientific study of the nervous system especially in respect to its structure, functions, and abnormalities

Parkinson's is a slow progressing disease of the nervous system. It is characterized by shaking when at rest, sluggish movements and muscle rigidity. It affects one in 250 people over 40 and one in 100 people over 65 years old. The area of the brain affected is the basal ganglia where movement and coordination initiate.

Nutrition and the Nervous System

Proteins and **amino acids** play an important role in normal brain and nervous system function, particularly before birth when the concentrations in the blood of the developing baby can be three times greater than in the mother. Most of the essential chemical substances in the brain and central nervous system are neurotransmitters, such as dopamine and serotonin. These are produced in the body from amino acids.

It is essential for newborn infants and young children to have an adequate supply of amino acids, which are derived from proteins. Foods that are complete proteins with these essential amino acids include meat, fish, eggs, milk and dairy products*. Plants also have protein, but may not contain as much or may not exist in a complete state providing the amino acids. Vegans (those who do not eat animals or animal products) or strict vegetarians should supplement with specific foods or food combinations to achieve the complete proteins the body needs, like eating legumes and grains together, such as beans and rice.

*Fun Fact

While organic, raw, non-homogenized or unpasteurized cow's or goat's milk is better than their counterparts, dairy is mucus forming. For those who have a chronic runny nose, upper respiratory issues, allergies and other similar symptoms, you should consider eliminating them from your diet as they may contribute to these issues.

Conditions that affect adequate protein intake (very low energy diets, vegan or macrobiotic diets, alcoholism, anorexia) or conditions that increase the requirement for protein when intakes may be inadequate (pregnancy, lactation, periods of growth, illnesses that exhaust protein supplies), can lead to an imbalance in the supply of amino acids to the brain and central nervous system. This can result in neurological symptoms and damage.

What are Amino Acids?

Amino acids are the building blocks of the body; constructing cells, forming nerves and repairing tissue, they also form antibodies to combat invading bacteria and viruses. They also build nucleoproteins (RNA & DNA), carry oxygen throughout the body and participate in muscle activity.

When protein is broken down properly by digestion, the result is 21 known amino acids of proteins. Amino acids are found in all meats (beef, pork, chicken, fish, turkey, eggs, etc.), dairy products (milk, yogurt, cottage cheese, etc.) and in smaller amounts in fruits and vegetables. Vegetarians need to be sure and supplement with natural amino acids, as many times their protein intake is to low to supply all the necessary amino acids.

The body, through assimilation of amino acids, produces over 50,000 proteins and over 15,000 enzymes. Amino acids not only are responsible for the production of all the body's enzymes, including digestive enzymes, but they also play a key role in the nervous system in normalizing moods, concentration, aggression, attention and sleep.

Digestive enzymes break down the proteins we consume into amino acids. Then, individual amino acids are used to create necessary body proteins and enzymes. Scientists, experts and medical professionals agree that getting enough amino acids in our diets is an important factor in maintaining good nutrition.

Nervous system disorder symptoms

Anxiety, convulsions, depression, numbness, muscles twitching, muscle weakness, pain, paralysis, feeling of pins and needles, ticks and tremors

Textbooks differ as to the exact number -- either eight or nine -- of essential amino acids, ones that cannot be manufactured by the body. Non-essential amino acids can be manufactured by the body with proper nutrition.

Some plant food sources of amino acids

apple, papaya, apricot, pineapple, pears, grapes, pomegranates, wolfberry, brazil nuts, almonds, hazelnuts, olive, flax, legumes, hemp, carrots, radish, parsley, celery, okra, tomato, green vegetables, Brussels sprouts, spinach and avocado

What are the 21 amino acids and what do they do?

1. Tryptophan (Essential Amino Acid)

A natural relaxant, tryptophan helps alleviate insomnia by inducing normal sleep and reduces anxiety and depression. It helps treat migraine headaches, boost the immune system, reduce the risk of artery and heart spasms and also works with lysine in reducing cholesterol levels.

2. Lysine (Essential Amino Acid)

This amino acid ensures the adequate absorption of calcium and helps form collagen, which makes up bone cartilage and connective tissues, and also aids in the production of antibodies, hormones and enzymes. Recent studies have shown that lysine may be effective against herpes by improving the balance of nutrients that reduce viral growth. A deficiency may result in tiredness, the inability to concentrate, irritability, bloodshot eyes, retarded growth, hair loss, anemia and reproductive problems.

3. **Methionine** (Essential Amino Acid)

A principle supplier of sulfur, which prevents disorders of the hair, skin and nails, methionine helps lower cholesterol levels by increasing the liver's production of lecithin, reduces liver fat and protects the kidneys. Serving as a natural chelating agent for heavy metals, it regulates the formation of ammonia and creates ammonia-free urine, which reduces bladder irritation, and also influences hair follicles and promotes hair growth.

4. **Phenylalaine** (Essential Amino Acid)

Used by the brain to produce norepinephrine, a chemical that transmits signals between nerve cells and the brain, phenylalaine keeps us awake and alert, reduces hunger pains, functions as an antidepressant and helps improve memory.

5. **Threonine** (Essential Amino Acid)

This is an important constituent of collagen, elastin, and enamel protein. Threonine also aids the prevention of fat build-up in the liver, helps the digestive and intestinal tracts function more smoothly and assists metabolism and assimilation.

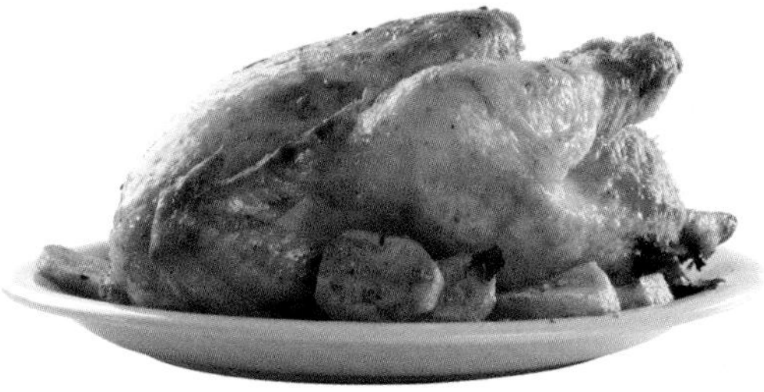

6. **Valine** (Essential Amino Acid)

It promotes mental vigor, muscle coordination and calm emotions.

7. **Histidine** (Essential Amino Acid)

Found abundantly in hemoglobin, histidine has been used in the treatment of rheumatoid arthritis, allergic diseases, ulcers and anemia. A deficiency can cause poor hearing.

8. **Leucine** and 9. **Isoleucine** (Essential Amino Acids)

These provide ingredients to manufacture other essential biochemical components in the body, some of which are utilized for the production of energy, as stimulants to the upper brain and to help us to be more alert.

10. **Arginine** (Non-Essential Amino Acid)

Studies have shown that it has improved immune responses to bacteria, viruses and tumor cells. Arginine promotes wound healing and regeneration of the liver, causes the release of growth hormones and is considered crucial for optimal muscle growth and tissue repair. It also has been shown to have significant cardiovascular benefits for restoring and retaining elasticity in blood vessels.

11. **Tyrosine** (Non-Essential Amino Acid)

This transmits nerve impulses to the brain, helps overcome depression, improves memory, increases mental alertness and promotes the healthy functioning of the thyroid, adrenal and pituitary glands.

12. **Glycine** (Non-Essential Amino Acid)

Glycine helps trigger the release of oxygen to the energy-requiring, cell-making process. It is important in the manufacturing of hormones responsible for a strong immune system.

13. **Serine** (Non-Essential Amino Acid)

A storage source of glucose by the liver and muscles, serine helps strengthen the immune system by providing antibodies and synthesizing fatty acid sheath around nerve fibers.

14. **Glutamic acid** (Non-Essential Amino Acid)

This amino acid is considered to be nature's brain food because it improves mental capacities. It also aids In the speed the healing of ulcers, gives a lift from fatigue and helps control alcoholism, schizophrenia and the craving for sugar.

15. **Glutamine** (Non-Essential Amino Acid)

The most abundant of all free amino acids, it aids in muscle building, recovery from surgery (especially abdominal) and it replenishes amino acid stores. This is the main reason glutamine is recommended during fasting or for people who suffer from physical trauma, immune deficiencies or cancer.

16. **Aspartic acid** and 17. **Asparagine** (Non-Essential Amino Acids)

These aid in the expulsion of harmful ammonia from the body. When ammonia enters the circulatory system it acts as a highly toxic substance, which can be harmful to the central nervous system. Recent studies have shown that aspartic acid may increase resistance to fatigue and increase endurance.

18. **Taurine** (Non-Essential Amino Acid)

It helps stabilize the excitability of membranes, which is very important in the control of epileptic seizures, and aids in the clearing of free radical wastes. Taurine and sulfur are considered to be factors necessary for the control of many biochemical changes that take place in the aging process.

19. **Cystine** (Non-Essential Amino Acid)

Cystine functions as an antioxidant and is a powerful aid to the body in protecting against radiation and pollution. It can help slow down the aging process, deactivate free radicals, neutralize toxins, aid in protein synthesis and present cellular change. It is necessary for the formation of the skin, which aids in the recovery from burns and surgical operations. Hair and skin are 10 to 14 percent cystine.

20. **Proline** (Non-Essential Amino Acid)

It is extremely important for the proper functioning of joints and tendons and helps maintain and strengthen heart muscles. Another non-proteinogenic amino acid is hydroxyproline, which plays a great role in collagen assembly, and is a derivative of proline.

21. **Alanine** (Non-Essential Amino Acid)

An important source of energy for muscle tissue, the brain and central nervous system, alanine strengthens the immune system by producing antibodies and aids in the metabolism of sugars and organic acids.

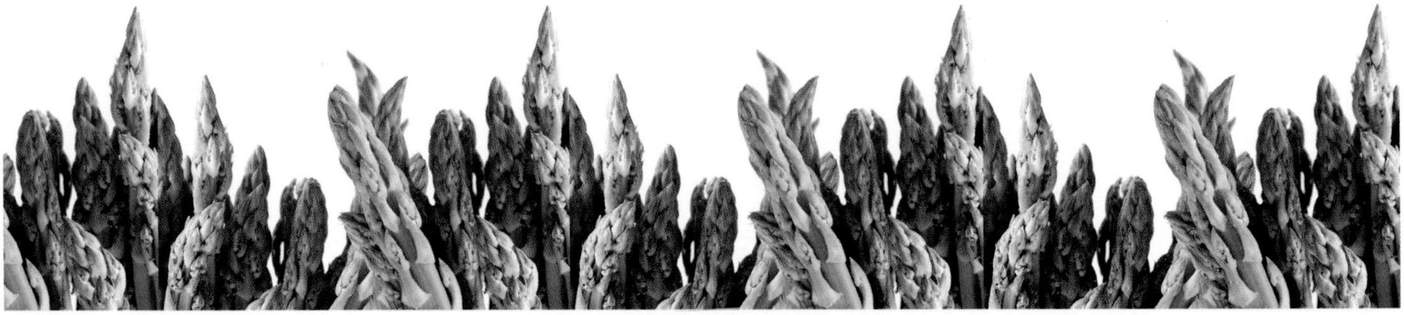

B-Complex Vitamins

The B-complex vitamins are a large group of water-soluble vitamins that play a role in healthy nerve function. There are three main B vitamins, namely thiamin, riboflavin and niacin that are the most important.

Thiamin - Vitamin B1

A deficiency in thiamin (vitamin B1) can interfere with the production of certain neurotransmitter amino acids, as well as glucose metabolism.

Mild **thiamin** deficiency can manifest as numbness in the legs, the feeling of pins and needles, calf muscle tenderness and loss of appetite. Extreme vitamin B1 deficiency causes beriberi, which is characterized by edema, shortness of breath and sensory disturbances with paralysis. Muscle weakness, irritability, loss of memory, convulsions and permanent brain damage also may develop. While beriberi is not very common, lack of adequate B1 does cause imbalances within the delicate nervous system.

Foods rich in thiamin: unrefined or minimally processed cereals and grains such as brown rice, whole wheat bread, nuts, legumes (dry beans, peas and lentils), romaine lettuce, asparagus, spinach, sunflower seeds, tuna, green peas, tomatoes, Brussels sprouts, cabbage, winter squash and black beans.

Niacin - Vitamin B3

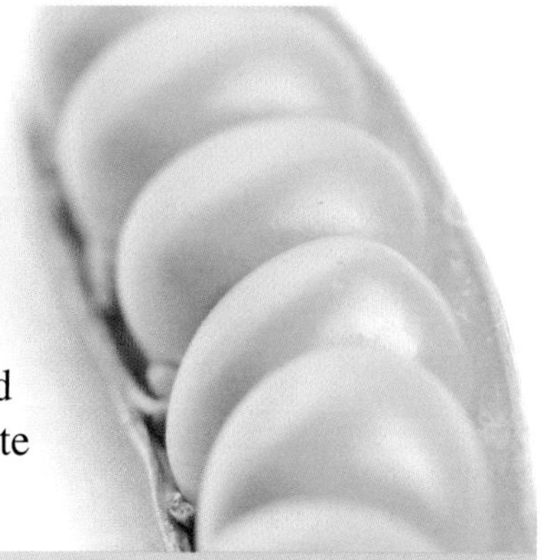

Niacin, or vitamin B3, is another one of the B-complex vitamins that is important to neurological function. Mild niacin deficiency is associated with weakness, tremor, anxiety, depression and irritability. In severe niacin deficiency a person may develop pellagra, characterized by the three D's - delirium, dementia and death. The human body is capable of manufacturing niacin from the amino acid **tryptophan**. Thus patients with a niacin deficiency will benefit from adequate intakes of high-quality protein foods.

Foods rich in niacin: tuna, chicken, turkey, salmon, green peas, peanuts, broccoli, whole grains, oats, brown rice or crushed wheat and tortillas made from maize treated with limewater. When maize is soaked in limewater it releases the tryptophan and makes it available for niacin production in the human body.

Riboflavin - Vitamin B2

A lack of riboflavin, or vitamin B2, can retard the growth of children and infants with typical symptoms such as anemia, rashes around the nose, cracks on the outer edges of the mouth and a red inflamed tongue. While a riboflavin deficiency is not as directly linked to neurological fallout and damage as thiamin and niacin, the anemia associated with a lack of B2 can have neurological consequences.

Foods rich in riboflavin: dairy products - milk, yogurt, cheese[11], lean meat and poultry, fish, eggs, broccoli, spinach, asparagus and whole grains.

---

11 Those who have a chronic runny nose, upper respiratory issues, allergies and other similar symptoms, should consider eliminating dairy from the diet as they may contribute to these issues.

Pyridoxine - Vitamin B6

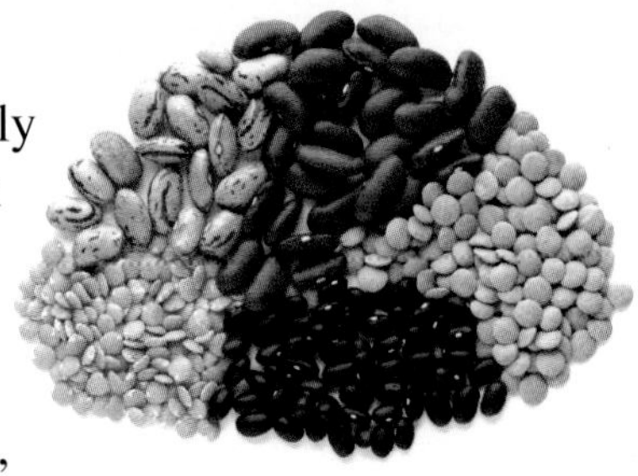

Pyridoxine, or vitamin B6, is essential for the synthesis or metabolism of practically all the neurotransmitters, which are chemicals which help to transmit messages in the central nervous system. Pyridoxine is especially important to women in that it helps to balance female hormones. Deficiency of pyridoxine causes symptoms such as tiredness, nervousness, irritability, depression, insomnia, and difficulty with walking. In addition, vitamin B6 deficiency is linked to dizziness, neuritis, neuralgia and carpal tunnel syndrome - the loss of feeling or pins and needles in the hands caused by swelling of connective tissue in the wrist which presses on nerves. Several drugs are known to lower pyridoxine levels in the blood and cause irritability, peripheral neuropathy and convulsions.

Food rich in pyridoxine: lean meat, tuna, potatoes, bananas and legumes, such as dry beans, peas and lentils.

How to Choose the Right Supplements for Your Nervous System

Protein

While many plant foods are high in protein, people who choose to supplement protein will find one of three types available: un-denatured whey (dairy), rice bran, or albumin (egg whites). Un-denatured whey protein is allergen free and easily digested even by people who are lactose free. Look for companies that use hormone-free whey. Rice bran protein powders use the protein found in rice bran for a vegetarian friendly version. Albumin or egg white protein powders typically are the best choice, except the price generally keeps people from supplementing with this form. It is important to read the many other ingredients listed in a protein powder to assure quality.

Fun Fact

Mix a protein powder with water, ice and frozen fruit for a delicious smoothie - a great way to start your day.

Amino acids

Amino acids come from protein rich sources such as meat, fish, dairy products and vegetables such as peas, legumes and grains. There are many types of amino acid supplements on the market. Many come primarily from a milk-protein source.

Those who could benefit from amino acid supplementation are vegetarians and those with allergies, stress-related fatigue or hypoglycemia. Trouble digesting food could be a signal of a diminishment in the production of digestive enzymes. This could lead to poor nutrition because the body cannot digest food at full capacity. In essence, our bodies need amino acids in order to obtain and utilize amino acids from food.

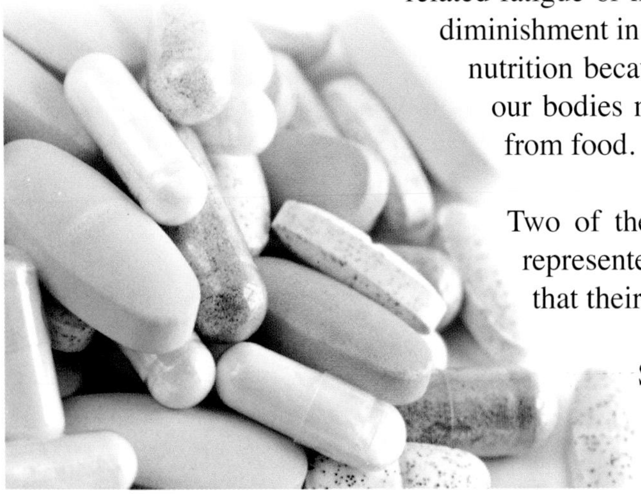

Two of the essential amino acids, lysine and tryptophan, are poorly represented in most plant proteins. Thus strict vegetarians should ensure that their diet contains sufficient amounts of these two amino acids.

Supplement amino acids by eating all the amino acid-rich food possible, but those who want an actual specific supplement should seek the advice of a trusted health care professional.

B-Complex Vitamin Supplements

When choosing a B vitamin to supplement, it is best to choose a whole food sourced B-complex rather than a synthetic. This is a tablet or capsule with all of the B vitamins in proper ratio to each other.

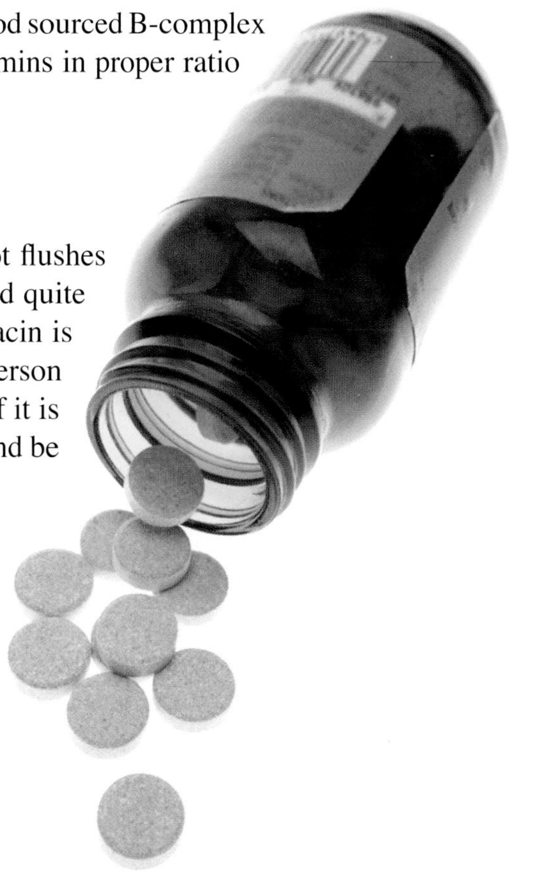

Avoid the hot pricklies!

Some people have taken B vitamins with niacin only to experience hot flushes and redness of the skin. No harm done, but it can be uncomfortable and quite a sight. This sensation is termed a niacin flush. It happens when the niacin is synthetic or out of proportion to the other B vitamins. If this occurs, a person should research the source of the niacin to determine if it is synthetic. If it is a quality product, cut back on future doses by cutting the tablet in half and be sure to take with adequate food.

Niacin is a blood vessel dilator and is often used to aid in cholesterol control. This means a niacin flush also can actually signal that the body's circulation is probably pretty good.

Good Nervous System Foods	Bad Nervous System Foods
asparagus	alcohol
cabbage	artificial colors and flavors
citrus fruit	artificial sweeteners
chia seeds	caffeine
eggs	cakes
fish	candy
flaxseed	dairy
kidney beans	excessive red meat
lecithin granules	fried foods
pine nuts	hydrogenated fats and oils
rice bran	margarine
sprouts	shortenings
sunflower seeds	sodas
turnips	sugar
vitamin C rich foods	sweet baked goods
vitamin B rich foods	trans fats
whole grains	
wheat germ	

Unit 1 Chapter 4
Discussion Questions

1. What is raw milk?
2. What is a vegetarian? What is a vegan?
3. Have you known anyone who has changed the way he or she feels by eating healthy food? If not, do you believe it is possible?
4. What does RDA stand for?

Activities - plus the Stuffed Eggs "Power" Recipe and activities.

Elementary

1. Eat one of the foods from the Good Nervous System Foods list each day for a week. You must eat a different food each day. Describe their taste, texture, smell, etc. Make a chart to keep track.
2. Comparing the list of good foods for the nervous system, try to find at least three things these have in common. Do the same thing for the bad foods list.
3. Write or give an oral presentation on three good foods for the nervous system and explain why they are good.
4. Do you have any plant sources of amino acids in your refrigerator? If so, draw a picture of them.
5. If there are any foods on the lists that you do not recognize, ask your parent/teacher to help you learn about them.
6. Write a song about how important food is for your nervous system and sing it for your family.
7. Create a lunch using three of the foods from the Good Nervous System Foods list.
8. Prepare a snack food using only three riboflavin-rich foods.
9. List three foods high in pyridoxine.

Secondary

Choose any from above plus

1. Refer to Appendix I. Create a complete dinner menu with four times the RDA of thiamin. Use a variety of foods, include all food groups and make it tasty. (refer to the chart below). You cannot use more than 2 servings of a single food. You may refer to other nutritional books and web sites for more foods rich in thiamin. Then, prepare the dinner for the family to eat.

Food	Serving	Thiamin Amount (mg)	Calories
Asparagus	1 cup	0.22 mg	43
Black beans	1 cup	0.4 mg	227
Brown rice	1 cup	0.19 mg	216
Brussels sprouts	1 cup	0.2 mg	61
Green peas	1 cup	0.4 mg	134
Spinach	1 cup	0.2 mg	41
Sunflower seeds	¼ cup	0.8 mg	205
Tuna	4 ounces	0.6 mg	158

2. For your next co-op or church event, prepare a side dish or snack that contains foods from the Good Nervous System Foods list.
3. Find out how the U.S. RDA standards are set and how often they are amended.
4. Help organize a family outdoor fun time that features games that utilize the nervous system. Check the following site for ideas: http://faculty.washington.edu/chudler/outside.html.
5. Look up the word locavore. Are you a locavore? What kind of effort does it take? Compile your findings in an oral or written report and share it with your family. After sharing, take a poll to see if they consider themselves locavores or want to do a locavore family trial for a set period of time.

Nervous System Power

Flaxseed Oil

Stuffed Eggs - Hold the Mayo

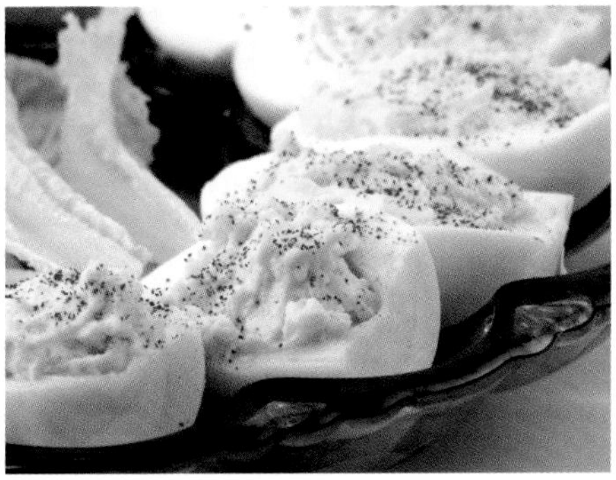

6-8 Hard boiled eggs, peeled, halved and the yolks set aside in a small bowl.
2 Tbs. sweet pickle relish
2 Tbs. diced white onion
1 Tbs. mustard
Salt and pepper to taste
Flaxseed or olive oil
Paprika (optional)

Combine the yolks, pickles, mustard and onions in a food processor or bowl. Slowly drizzle in the flaxseed or olive oil, just until mixture is smooth. Spoon into egg halves. Garnish with paprika or pepper.

Activities

Elementary

1. Using a blindfold, try to identify the ingredients with your other four senses.
2. Commonly mayonnaise is used for stuffed egg recipes. Look up the ingredients for a mayonnaise brand available at your local market. Does it contain good fats or bad fats?
3. Choose an ingredient from the recipe and make it an acronym with each letter representing a characteristic of the ingredient or with the letters combining to form a supporting sentence. For example: E.G.G.S. = Elliptical, gentle handling, good fatty acids, scrumptious! or Eating gets gooey … splat!
4. Identify other recipes that call for mayonnaise and substitute flaxseed oil or olive oil. Help prepare the dish and serve it at the next family meal.

Secondary

Choose any from above plus

1. Make a nutritional comparison between a mayonnaise brand available at your local market and both flaxeed oil and olive oil.
2. Determine the cost per ounce of the mayonnaise versus the flaxseed oil and olive oil. Which costs more per ounce? Considering the short- and long-term nutritional impact of the products, which has more value?
3. Research what happens when flaxseed oil and olive oil are heated.

Unit 1 Additional Recipes

Use organic ingredients when possible.

Chia Pancakes

1 cup of freshly milled whole wheat flour (soft wheat is best)
2 Tbs. Chia seeds
2 tsp. baking powder
Scant ¼ tsp. sea salt
1 Tbs. honey
1 Tbs. light olive oil
1 egg
1 cup water

Combine ingredients in a blender and mix at medium speed. May mix manually with a whisk – mix well, until batter is smooth. Ladle on hot griddle or waffle iron and cook until golden brown. Top with organic maple syrup, honey or Blue Agave Nectar, which has a glycemic index of 11.

Brain Power Smoothie

1 cup ice
1 cup frozen fruit (peaches, strawberries, grapes, blueberries, etc.)
2 Tbs. Chia Seeds
1 cup water
2 heaping Tbs. quality protein powder (Authors' preference is an un-denatured whey product such as Young Living Pure Protein, Dream Protein or an all vegetarian rice bran protein called Young Living Power Meal)

Blend well in blender.

Trail Mix

This is the most delicious, easiest to prepare granola/trail mix you can have for breakfast or snacks. Kids love to help prepare this one.

¼ cup flax seeds
¼ cup sunflower seeds
½ cup wheat germ
½ cup whole or sliced almonds
½ Tbs. cinnamon
2 ¼ cups fresh rolled oats
¼ cup honey or 2 Tbs. Blue Agave Nectar
¼ cup oil

Combine in large bowl and mix well. Spread on an un-greased cookie sheet and place in a pre-headed 300°F oven for 30 minutes. Halfway through the cooking, stir the granola. Remove and let cool. Store in airtight container. Keeps for about one month.

Unit 2

The Digestive System

Many common ailments associated with digestion can be resolved by making better food choices. Choosing good food is a must, but understanding how the body breaks down the foods we eat – known as digestion - may be even more important. In fact digestion and its corresponding elimination are key factors influencing your total wellbeing. Many health related books and researchers list digestive related disorders to include: acne, anemia, asthma, arthritis, constipation, eczema, fatigue, gall stones, infections, obesity, Type 2 diabetes and even some cancers.

People who have health challenges or who want to avoid sickness and prevent digestive-related issues should start at the beginning of the digestive process. Where does digestion begin? Some might say the stomach. Maybe others believe it is the mouth. Actually digestion begins the moment we see, smell or even think about food.

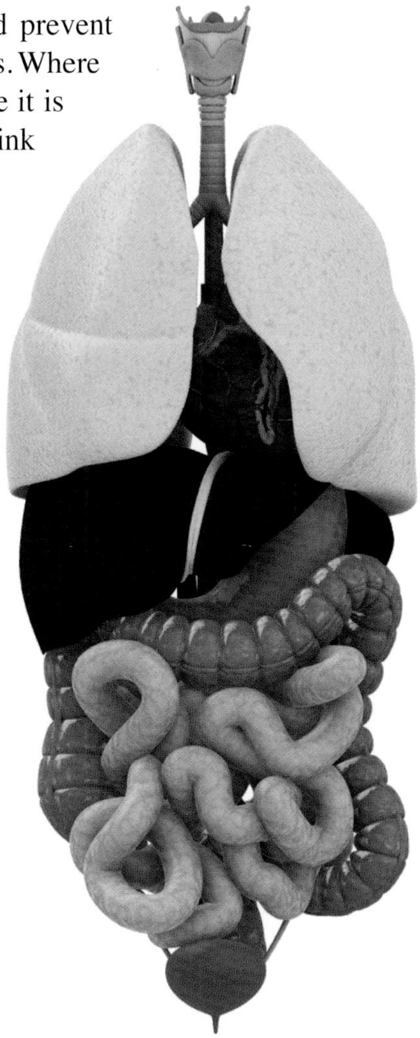

Fun Facts

What do Americans eat?

(according to the U.S. Department of Agriculture)

- One in four American's visit a fast food restaurant daily.
- French fries are the most eaten vegetable in America.
- The average American consumes 150 tablespoons of sugar and 566 cans of soda per year, which amounts to a whopping 52 teaspoons of sugar per day.
- One in five Americans suffer from constipation.
- Americans spend over $600 million on laxatives.

Chapter 1

The Digestive System

"If you fully obey the Lord your God and carefully follow all his commands I give you today, the Lord your God will set you high above all the nations on earth." Deuteronomy 28:1

Have you ever drooled at the sight of something tasty? Has your stomach ever growled at the thought of your upcoming lunch break? Your digestive system begins working even before you take your first bite of food and will work on that food for several hours.

What is digestion?

Digestion is the process of breaking down food for the absorption of nutrients.

What is the digestive system?

The **digestive system** is comprised of a long, twisting, turning tube, approximately 30 feet long, known as the **alimentary canal**. The canal is formed by several hollow organs known as the mouth, esophagus, stomach, small intestine, large intestine (colon), rectum and anus. The organs that make up this canal are lined with mucus and glands that produce enzymes.

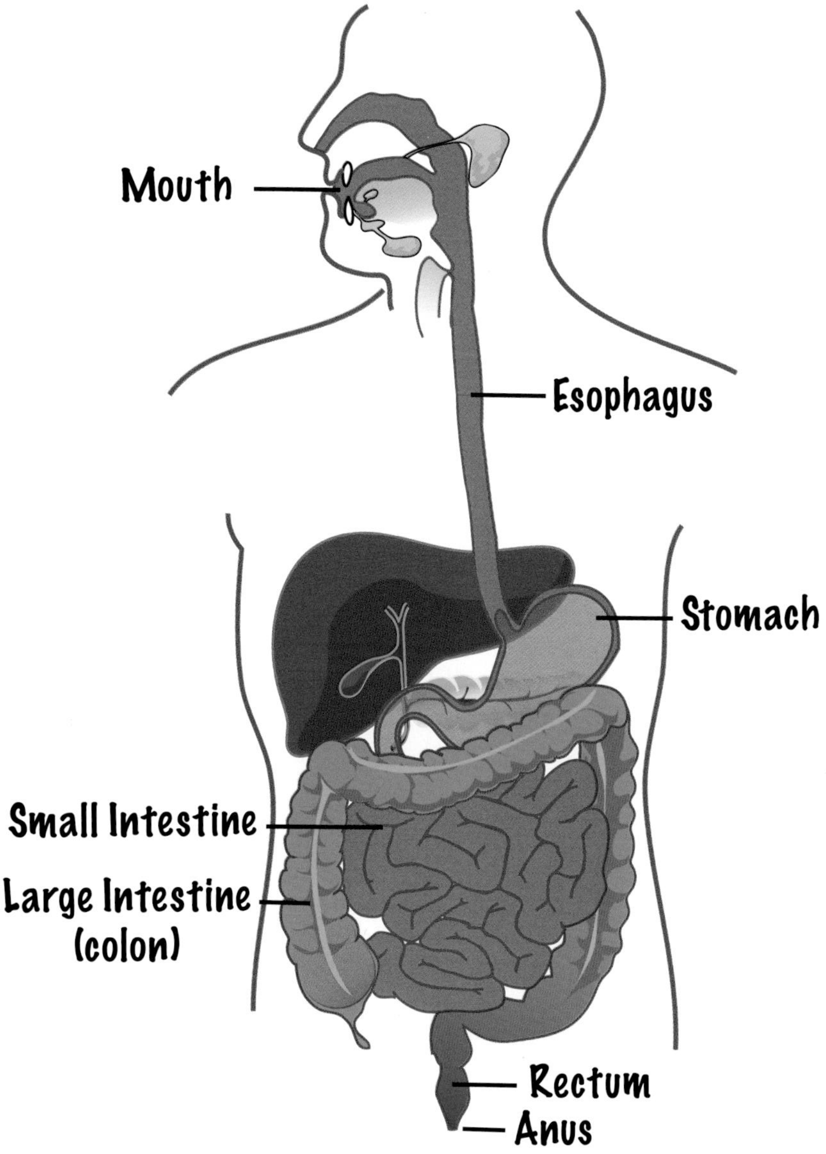

When does digestion start?

As mentioned earlier, digestion starts at the first sight, smell or even thought of food. The visual and thought stimulus goes to the cerebral cortex in the brain, and the smell stimulus goes to the hypothalamus in the brain. Then, the brain tells the salivary glands in the mouth to start producing **saliva** – or spit – and the digestive juices in the stomach to start churning.

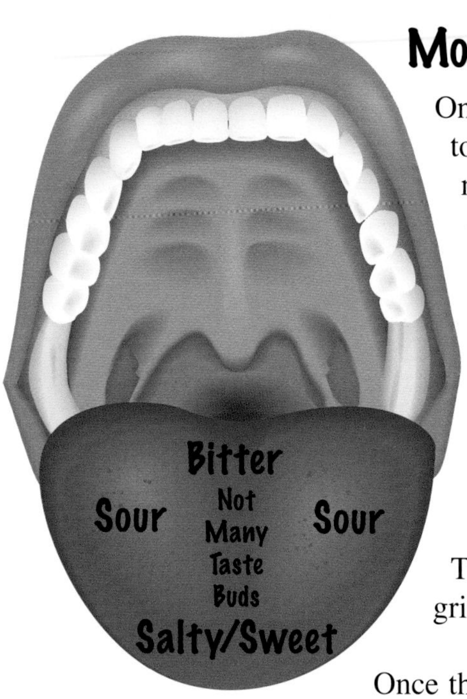

Mouth

Once you have taken your first bite of food, the salvia in the **mouth** starts to work. Saliva is made in the **salivary glands** and is made up of water, mucus, antibacterial compounds and various enzymes. As the first part of digestion, the enzymes break down some of the fat and starch in the food and make the food mushy, so it is easier to swallow. The saliva also protects the teeth, tongue and sensitive tissues in the mouth.

The **tongue** is a muscle that helps to grip food and move it around to the teeth while you chew. It is covered with a layer of tiny bumps called papillae that contain your taste buds. Taste buds can detect sweet, sour, bitter and salty flavors.

The **teeth** help break down the food into smaller particles by tearing and grinding, so the saliva and enzymes can do their job.

Once the food is broken down into a mushy ball called a **bolus**, you are ready to swallow and send it down to the esophagus.

Fun Fact

How many times should you chew your food before swallowing? The answer is in the next chapter.

Esophagus

The **esophagus** is a long, stretchy, muscular tube about nine to 10 inches long that takes the food from the back of the throat to the stomach. No enzymes are produced in the esophagus, but it does move food slowly into the stomach rather than food just dropping from the mouth and throat into the stomach. This process of the smooth muscles contracting and pushing the food down rather than allowing the food to go back up to the mouth is called **peristalsis**.

Sometimes when we eat too fast and get a twinge in the center of the chest, it is simply food backing up. Food takes two to three seconds to go down the esophagus; so slow down and give those organs enough time to do their jobs.

The esophagus is at the back of the throat right next to the windpipe, also called the trachea, which sends air to the lungs. When a ball of mushy food goes down the back of the throat, a small flap called the **epiglottis** closes so the food will go down the esophagus and not get caught in the windpipe. Have you ever tried to talk and eat at the same time only to suddenly start choking and coughing? The epiglottis didn't have enough time to close, and that food got sent down the wrong way. So swallow before you speak. Besides, no one wants to see your bolus!

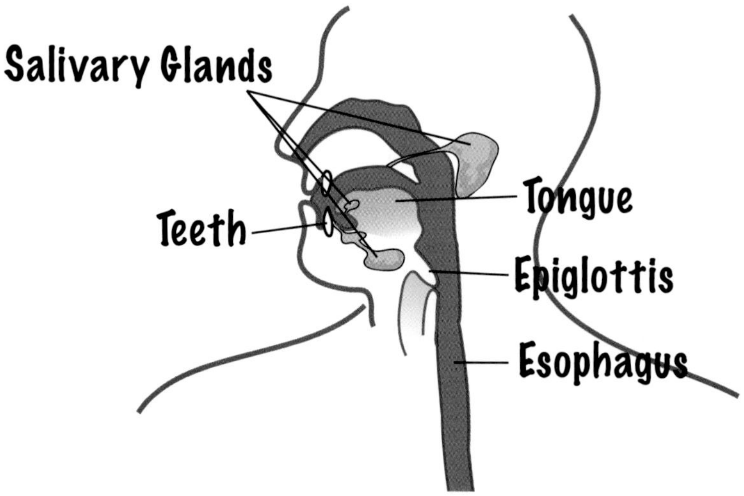

Stomach

Before the food enters into the **stomach**, it has to pass through a muscular one-way valve called the **esophageal sphincter** (pronounced sfeenk-ter). This muscle opens to let food pass to the stomach, but then closes so the acidic stomach juices don't get in the esophagus and cause a burning sensation often known as **heartburn**. It also keeps the bolus from going back up into the esophagus.

Fun Fact
The stomach can expand to hold between two to four liters of food.

The stomach is a muscular sac with a mucosal lining. It secretes HCI – hydrochloric acid - which sterilizes the food and is required for the breakdown and absorption of proteins, fats and minerals. Even though HCI is strong enough to dissolve concrete, it does not harm the stomach wall, which is protected by the mucous lining.

The stomach also secretes the enzyme pepsin for digestion, especially of proteins. Enzymes will be more thoroughly discussed in Chapter 3 of this Unit.

The mixture of the bolus and stomach juices – the HCI and enzymes – is known as **chyme**.

Fun Fact - The stomach produces 2.2 to 3 liters of gastric acid per day.

Small Intestine

The stomach squeezes and pushes the chyme into the **small intestine** through the **pyloric valve**, which triggers the release of hormones. These hormones stimulate the liver and gallbladder to release bile and the pancreas to release a mixture of enzymes called pancreatin.

The chyme then enters the first of three parts of the small intestine, which is called the **duodenum**. The other two parts are the **jejunum** and **ileum**. In the duodenum, the highly acidic chyme is now combined with bicarbonate from the pancreas changing the pH of the chyme from acidic to alkaline. There will be more information about pH in the next chapter.

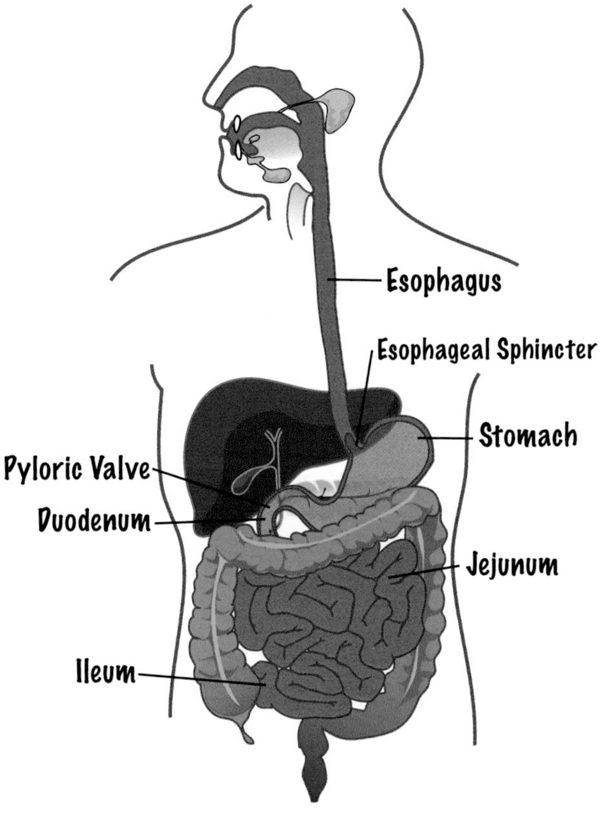

The small intestine is not just a 20 to 25 foot tube carrying food from one end to the other. It is the place where most of digestion happens. There are many nutrients like vitamins, minerals, amino acids and antioxidants that have been broken down from the food that need to get to cells. Once in the cells, they will provide energy, vitality and the building blocks for bone and tissue growth.

In order for these nutrients to gain access to the cells, they must be absorbed through millions of tiny fingerlike projections that line the small intestine which are called **villi**. Nutrients are absorbed through channels which run through the middle of the villi and are passed through the portal vein to the liver and then onward into your entire circulatory system to feed every cell in the body.

Fun Fact
The tiny villi increase the surface area of absorption in the small intestine to the size of a tennis court.

Think about this for a moment. Every morsel of food is destined for use by a cell in the body. So what are you feeding your cells - sugar, synthetic flavorings, colorants, dyes, chemical toxins? Or are you feeding your body quality, nutritious food that allows your body to thrive, grow and be healthy?

Throughout the Bible there is clear instruction on spiritual and physical nourishment, often as metaphors, but also to emphasize the importance of equal growth of the spirit and body. Isaiah 55:2 says "Wherefore do ye spend money for that which is not bread? And your labour for that which satisfieth not? Hearken diligently unto me, and eat ye that which is good, and let your soul delight itself in fatness."

Liver and Gallbladder

As the largest internal organ and gland, the **liver** is very important to your body. It is performs many different functions including the processing, or metabolizing, of the nutrient-rich blood coming from the small intestine. Some of the functions include:

- Filtering out old red blood cells.
- Detoxifying most of the harmful toxins and waste brought into the body from food, drugs, alcohol and the environment.
- Storing and metabolizing fats, including fatty acids, which are used for energy.
- Metabolizing and storing carbohydrates, which are the source for sugar – also called glucose – in the blood that red blood cells and the brain use.
- Creating bile to aid in the intestinal absorption of fats and the fat-soluble vitamins A, D, E and K.

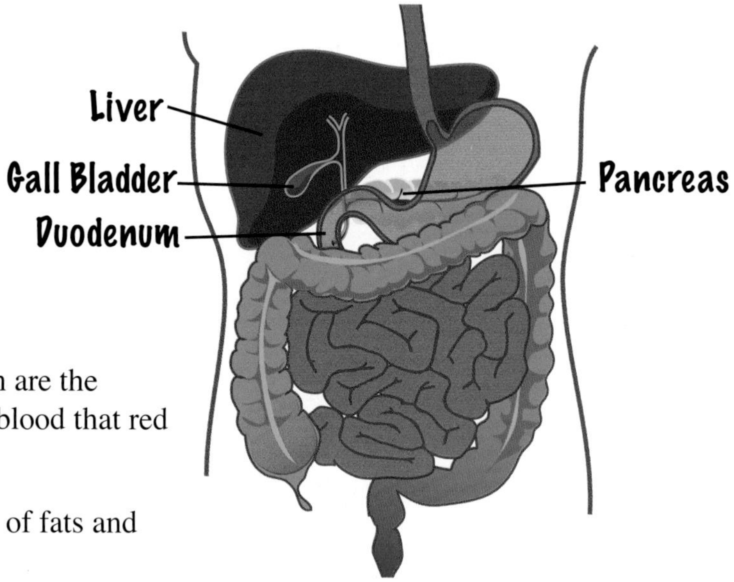

Bile is produced in the **liver** and is stored and secreted by the **gallbladder**. It acts as a detergent on fats by reducing them to smaller sizes so enzymes can more easily break them down. A healthy liver will produce about three cups of bile each day.

Pancreas

Many people think the **pancreas** is the gland responsible only for the production of hormones, specifically insulin, for blood sugar regulation. While this is true, it has a second job. The pancreas is actually a gland organ. As an organ, it secretes enzymes used to breakdown carbohydrates, fats and proteins in chyme while in the duodenum. The pancreas will be covered in more detail with the endocrine system in Unit 6.

Appendix

The **appendix** is a two- to four-inch pocket between the small and large intestines that can sometimes become clogged and infected through improper digestion and elimination, causing appendicitis. On Oct. 8, 2007, doctors at the Duke University Medical Center stated that the appendix is a safe house for good gut bacteria.[1] While there is still much debate as to the actual function of the appendix, God did not give us spare parts -- so taking care of the entire body, including the appendix, is our responsibility.

1 "Appendix Isn't Useless At All: It's A Safe House For Good Bacteria" Duke University Medical Center, ScienceDaily, October 8, 2007. Retrieved August 31, 2008, from http://www.sciencedaily.com /releases/2007/10/071008102334.htm

Large Intestine - Colon

The last stage of digestion happens in the large intestine, which is the last five feet of the intestinal tract and consists of the **cecum** and **colon**. Because of the way the colon goes up, bends and goes down in the body, it is comprised of several parts, known as the **ascending**, **transverse**, **descending** and **sigmoid colons**. The colon is where most water absorption takes place as two-thirds of the chyme's weight of water is squeezed out and absorbed. Any remaining vitamins or minerals also are absorbed at this stage. If there is adequate fiber in the diet, the colon is essentially scrubbed clean with the fiber.

A healthy colon is populated with some 100 trillion bacteria, which continually multiply. These organisms perform such activities as synthesizing vitamins, killing off harmful bacteria, stimulating the immune system and producing short-chain fatty acids, which are the energy source for cells lining the colon.

The **rectum** lies at the end of the colon and fills with unused food waste – or feces -- before being eliminated through the **anus**. Regular elimination – or bowel movement -- is critical for good health. Chapter 4 in this unit will have more important information about elimination.

From beginning to end the process of digestion takes between six to 18 hours.

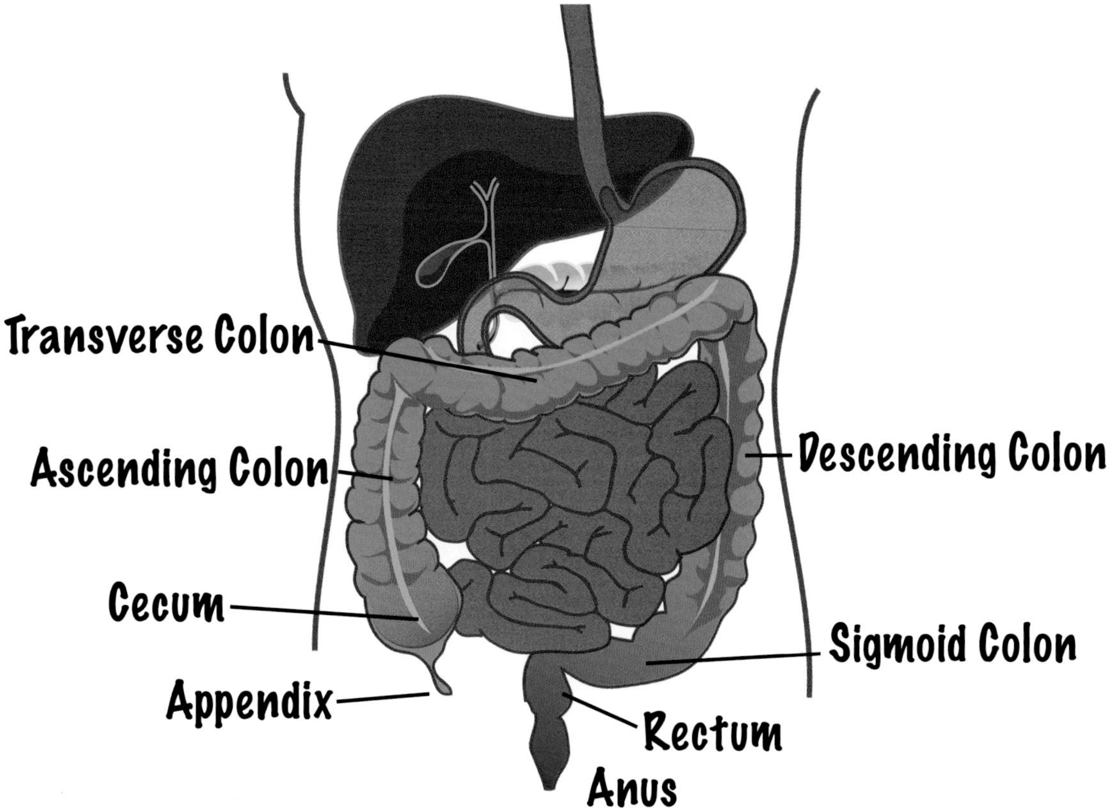

Unit 2 Chapter 1
Discussion Questions

1. What Scriptures support the information we have learned about digestion?
2. What part of this chapter did you already know? What facts surprised you?
3. How many times do you chew each bite? How can you help your family to remember to chew slowly?

Activities - plus the Fruit Salad "Power" Recipe and activities.

Elementary

1. Trace your body on a large sheet of butcher paper, draw in and label the parts of the digestive system.
2. Prepare four foods, one for each of the following: sweet, bitter, sour, bland. Examples: Sweet – watermelon, honey, agave, or maple syrup; Sour - lemons, limes, or some grapes; Bitter – vinegar; Bland: cracker, plain toast, plain white rice, noodle or potato. One at a time, look at the food. Think about eating it for one minute, place it in your mouth and suck on it, then chew and swallow. For each food log your answers:
   - When I was looking and thinking about the food, did my mouth begin to water? A little? A lot?
   - While the food was in my mouth, was more saliva being produced?
   - What was the sensation when the food was swallowed?
3. Download and do the Taste Tracker activity from the "How the Body Works: Tongue" page of the Web site www.kidshealth.org/kid/htbw.
4. Get a liquid measuring container that measures in liters to see how much one liter is. How many liters of food can your stomach hold? Is that more or less than a gallon?

Secondary

Choose any from above plus

1. Using yarn and a tape measure or other measuring device, snip the yarn once it reaches 30 feet. This is the length of the alimentary canal. Place the yarn on the butcher paper body as outlined in the first activity in the Elementary section.
2. After completing the second activity in the Elementary section, find three more foods that fit in each category. Test these foods according to the exercise and list in order of greatest saliva production.
3. To help you remember the digestive process, create a song about the organs involved in digestion and elimination, to the tune of "Dem Bones." ("the foot bone's connected to the ankle bone…")
4. Based on what you have learned about villi, measure the square footage of a regulation-size tennis court. If you do not have access to a tennis court, find a source that provides this information. You may have to calculate the square footage. How many rooms in your house does this equal?
5. Find a food mentioned this week in the news having a positive or negative effect on the digestive system. This can be newspaper, Internet, recently published book, television news, etc. Write a 500 word paper on this food with the reasons it is either beneficial or harmful to the digestive tract and why.
6. If the food from activity #5 is good for digestion, plan a meal using this food this week and record your family's reaction to eating it. If the food is bad for digestion, and your family has been eating it, talk about the reasons it is bad. If it meets with parental approval, eliminate this food from your diet.
7. Create flash cards for each of the hollow organs in the alimentary canal: mouth, esophagus, stomach, small intestine, liver, gallbladder, pancreas, appendix and large intestine (colon). On the opposite side of the card, write a brief description of the organ's function. After studying the cards, have a family member quiz you on your knowledge of the alimentary canal.

Additional Resources

Web sites:

1. www.kidshealth.org/kid/htbw
2. www.enchantedlearning.com/subjects/anatomy/digestive
3. http://faculty.washington.edu/chudler/coltaste.html

Digestive System Power

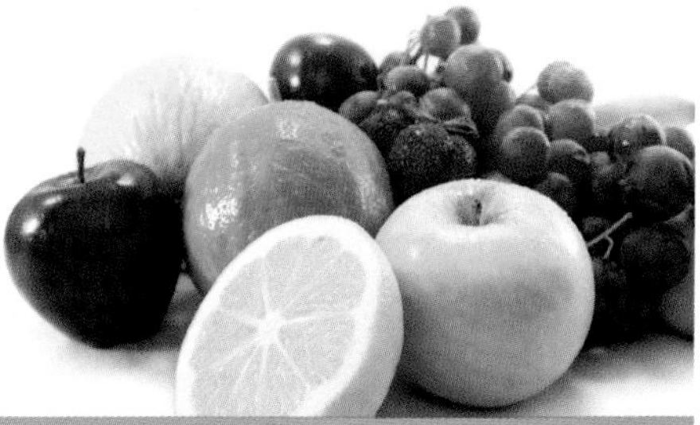

RAW FRUIT

Fruit contains vitamins, minerals, amino acids, enzymes and fiber for great digestive health.

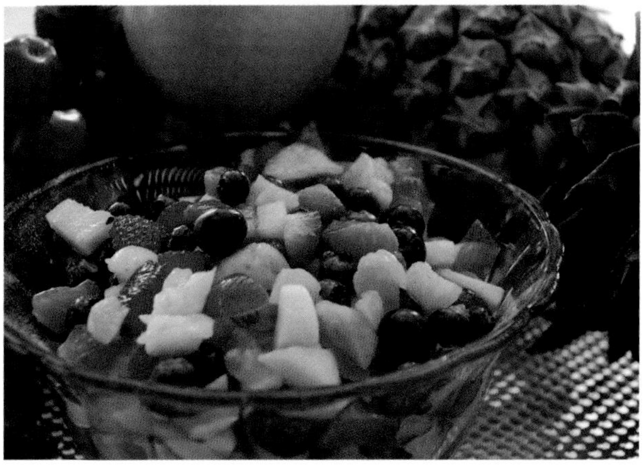

Fruit Salad

Use organic ingredients for best results.

Fresh peaches
Fresh apricots
Fresh blueberries
Fresh strawberries
Fresh pineapple
Fresh apples
Fresh grapes

Cut 1 cup each of the fruit into small pieces. Then, combine in a glass bowl. Enjoy as breakfast with some Trail Mix recipe from Unit 1 or alone as a delicious dessert. Cover and store in the refrigerator. It also can be stored in smaller containers for kids to grab as an afternoon snack.

Activities

Elementary

1. Pick three fruits from the bowl and find out how they grow – on a tree, vine or bush.
2. Look up the word antioxidant. What does it mean and why is it important?
3. The recipe says to use organic fruit. What does organic mean?
4. Choose one fruit in the recipe and prepare an oral or written a report about it.

Secondary

Choose any from above plus

1. Several of the fruits in the recipe are high in antioxidants. However, some of the antioxidants cannot be absorbed by the body. Look up bioavailability to learn why.
2. Find out which are the most chemically treated fruits and vegetables. Which are the least chemically treated?
3. With the information gathered about chemically treated fruit, prepare an oral or written report about the dangers of such foods and share this with your family.

Chapter 2

Digestive Health and Nutrition

"I will cure them, and will reveal unto them the abundance of peace and truth." Jeremiah 33:6

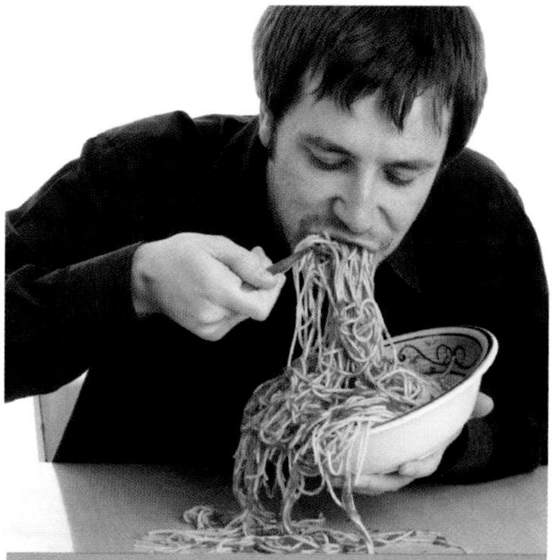

Many problems can occur in the digestive tract due to the wrong kind of foods entering the body; eating the right kinds of food can make a world of difference. Even the manner in which we eat can make a positive impact in our digestive health.

Fun Fact

While 20 times is a good average, there really is no set number to how many times you need to chew your food. The idea is to turn the food chuncks into mush no matter how many chews it takes. When the food is pureed, it may be swallowed for optimal digestion, absorption of nutrients and even better bowel movements.

Speed of Light

Do you eat at the **speed of light**? Do you chomp, swallow and finish your meal before anyone else has even filled a plate? Eating too fast can lead to overeating, weight gain and digestive disorders such as acid reflux, upset stomach, belching and bloating.

Slower than Molasses

Are you eating at a speed **slower than molasses**? Are you the last one to leave the table while picking and pushing food all over the plate and never finishing it? Eating too slow can lead to under eating which results in becoming underweight. For most adults, being a bit under weight is not a problem, but for growing children it can be. Picky eaters play with their food and eat very little at meal times. Only take on your plate what you think you will eat. It is better to ask for seconds than to waste food.

The Conscious Eater

Are you the **conscious eater**? The one who eats each mouthful slowly and chews each bite thoroughly while mixing the food well with saliva? When you feel satisfied, do you stop even if a little food remains on the plate?* This is the best way to eat. Weight issues are rare for this type of eater, unless poor food choices are made.

*Be careful in asking kids to clean their plate. While we do not want wasted food, eating more than your body needs can lead to overweight issues now and more serious health issues later in life.

Can food help the health of the mouth?

Yes, food can definitely help create a healthier mouth, especially healthier teeth. Food cannot be properly masticated – chewed into small bits – without healthy molars, which are the larger teeth at the back of the jaw. Many of the sugary, sticky foods like candy and gum cause them to be the first to decay. Toddlers who drink too much juice often have premature decaying of the teeth. While fresh squeezed, organic juice is far more nutritious than the concentrated, pasteurized counterpart, fruit juice is still full of fruit sugar – fructose – and too much can be harmful to young teeth. The best thing to drink for the health of the teeth is **pure water**.

Foods rich in **calcium** like spinach, broccoli and kale are great for teeth health. Dairy products like milk, cheese and yogurt are other sources of calcium, but dairy products are mucus forming and can pose problems for those with upper respiratory issues and allergies. If you choose to consume dairy products, the best by far is raw cow or goat milk and dairy products. However, there are many fresh vegetables high in calcium that will supply the needed amount of calcium. Calcium and teeth will be covered in greater detail with the skeletal and muscular systems in Unit 4.

Like all parts of the body, even our teeth need exercising. Try chewing hard crackers or toast (Zweiback, Melba), but not chewing gum. Gum does several harmful things to the teeth and mouth. It weakens and dilutes the normal digestive juices created to break down the food. A lifetime of chewing gum or even sucking mints may compromise digestion. When proper oral care is used, the mouth also is free of odor-causing bacteria.

Can food help the esophagus?

Yes, food can help create a healthier esophagus. Certain good food can help prevent health issues in the esophagus, like acid reflux and even esophageal cancer.

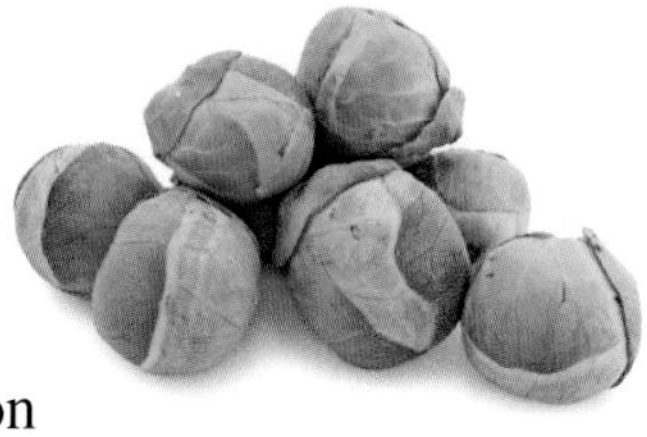

Esophageal Cancer

One of the more serious health conditions concerning the esophagus is cancer. One contributing factor, according to natural health experts may be the excessive consumption of soda pop, which contains high fructose corn syrup and carbonation. Several studies have shown that certain foods help decrease the risk of esophageal cancer. Among them are green vegetables, cruciferous vegetables, yellow vegetables, yellow fruit and vegetables and fruit high in carotene, vitamin C and vitamin E.[1] A diet high in fiber also has been shown to help reduce the risk of esophageal cancer.[2]

Cruciferous Vegetables

Broccoli, Brussels sprouts, cabbage, cauliflower, collard greens, kale, radishes, turnips, watercress

Heartburn/Acid Reflux

When a person has heartburn, or acid reflux, high-acid food particles and digestive juices from the stomach leak back into the esophagus causing discomfort and a burning sensation. Reflux disease, also known as gastroesophageal reflux disease or GERD, as well as heartburn and acid indigestion are becoming some of the most common health complaints of modern time. A 2006 medical review stated, "There is evidence that the prevalence of GERD has increased during the past two decades. If this trend continues, it could contribute to the more serious complications associated with GERD, such as esophageal adenocarcinoma (cancer)."[3]

The standard treatment for these conditions is proton-pump inhibitors drugs, known by the brand names Aciphex®, Nexium®, Prevacid®, Prilosec® and others. These pharmaceuticals work by inhibiting the generation of acid-ions known as protons. All of which potentially have some serious side effects.

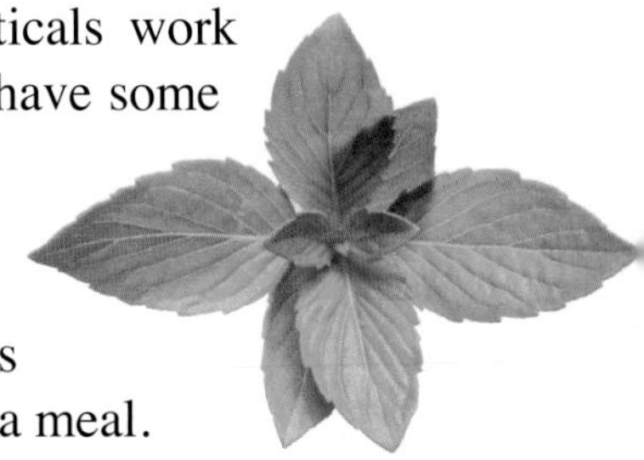

Peppermint is a plant and natural aid for esophageal issues without dangerous side effects. Have you ever wondered why some restaurants give out peppermint candies after you eat? This is not only to help with bad breath but to help with digestion after a meal.

God's word tells us we are to use plants for our medicine. Ezekiel 47: 12 states, "And by the river upon the bank thereof, on this side and on that side, shall grow all trees for meat… and the fruit thereof shall be for meat, and the leaf thereof for medicine."

1 "Diet and oral, pharyngeal and esophageal cancer" Chainani-Wu N, Nutr Cancer, 2002;44(2): 104-26.

2 "Fiber intake and the risk of oral pharyngeal and esophageal cancer" Soler M, Bosetti C, Franceschi S, Negri E, Zzmbon P, Talamini R, Conti E, La Vecchia C. IntJ Cancer. 2001 Feb 1;91(3):283-7.

3 "Time trends of gastroesophageal reflux disease: a systematic review" El-Serag HB, Clin Gastroenterol Hepatol. 2007 Jan;5(1):17-26.

Peppermint can be made into a tea (one teaspoon of fresh or dried peppermint leaves in eight ounces of water; steep six minutes, strain and drink) and can be served hot or iced. A favorite and fast acting way to use peppermint is the essential oil peppermint. Place one to two drops of therapeutic-grade peppermint essential oil[4] in a small amount of water, drink, and in minutes the discomfort can stop. CAUTION: Do not use peppermint oil if it is not labeled for use as a dietary supplement intended for oral consumption[4].

How can food help the stomach?

It may sound odd, but people with open stomach ulcers often find relief by taking **cayenne pepper** orally in capsules or by eating it raw. The ingredient capsicum found in hot peppers promotes mucus secretions that cover and protect ulcers.

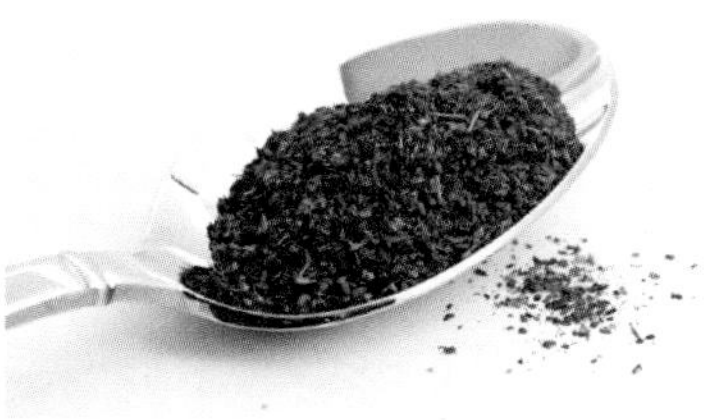

Many people with digestive complaints actually are not producing enough stomach acid – hydrochloric acid or HCI. A simple way to assist the body in proper HCI production is with soaked almonds.

Soaked almonds: Take one almond for each 10 pounds you weigh. Soak in a small amount of distilled water overnight in the refrigerator. In the morning, drain off excess water and eat. Soaking the almonds releases nitrogen, which, when consumed first thing in the morning, sets up proper HCI production for the day.

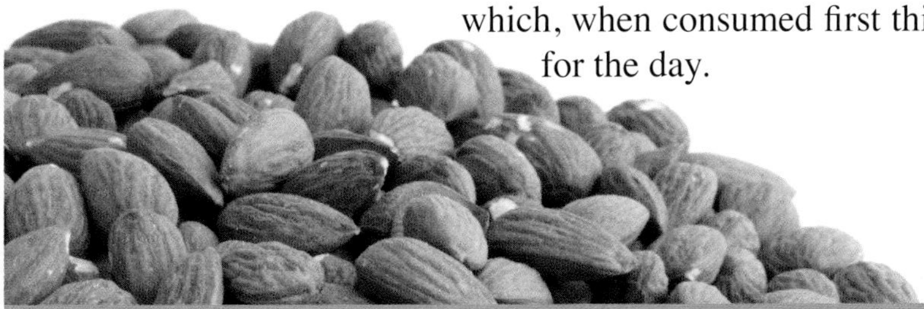

Good Eating Habits For The Digestive System

1. Keep meals simple and as nutritious as possible.

2. Eat regular meals, but only when hungry.

3. Do not consume ice cold drinks with meals. Drinking cold drinks, even water, can cause fatty foods to congeal in the stomach making them harder to digest. Sip on room temperature water or herb teas before, during or after meals. Drink the really cold drinks between meals. Liquids are important to activate digestive enzymes, but excess can also dilute them. Keep liquid intake to under eight ounces per meals. Foods that contain high amounts of water (fruits such as watermelon, honeydew, cantaloupe, grapes, and tomatoes) do not need additional water when eating.

4. Relax, eat slowly and chew food well. Do not eat when stressed or nervous. Stress causes digestive juices to shut down. Eating quickly interferes with the body telling the brain we are full and makes us overeat.

5. Avoid or reduce citrus with meals other than breakfast. Citrus fruits are digested quicker than many other foods and are regarded as cleansing foods rather than their vegetable counterparts which are thought of as nourishing foods. Citrus moves rapidly through the digestive track and can hasten a bowel movement.

6. Get plenty of fiber at each meal. Twenty-five to 30 grams of fiber is the recommended daily amount. See the fiber chart in Appendix K.

7. Keep sweets to a minimum. Sugars tend to ferment in the warm stomach and cause excess gas, bloating and indigestion.

4 See Appendix DD for the authors' supplement recommendations.

Acid/Alkaline Balance

No discussion of the digestive system would be complete without a word on the acid alkaline balance of the body. The food we eat, the toxins we breathe, emotional stress, and medication will all create an acid or alkaline pH in our body.

What is pH?

pH stands for potential of hydrogen and is the measure of the acidity or alkalinity of a solution.

The measurement is graded on a scale from 0 to 14 where 0 (or below) is the most acid and 14 is the highest alkaline. The number 7 on the scale is neutral.

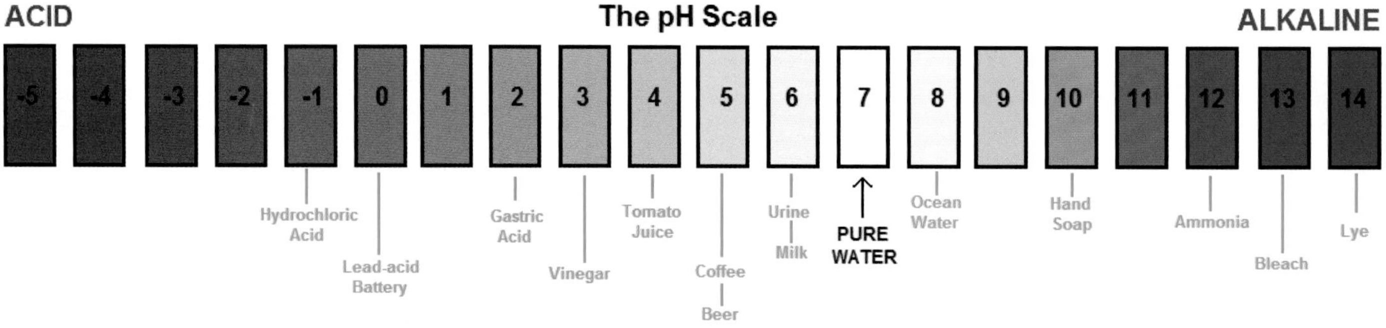

The body is 70 percent water, which allows for the transport of nutrients, oxygen and various chemicals to go from place-to-place and from cell-to-cell. This water will have either acid or alkaline properties as measured on a graduated scale. It is important to note that the pH of the body does not refer to the pH of the stomach, stomach acid or even the blood, but of the body's fluids – saliva and urine -- and tissues.

Is pH important?

Yes, the pH of the body is *very* important. In measuring the body's pH, the lower numbers mean the greater the acidity and less oxygen in the cells. The higher numbers mean the greater the alkalinity and more oxygen in the cells. Slightly alkaline bodies are healthy bodies, while acidic bodies are prone to sickness and disease.

What should the body's pH be?

The pH of 7.2 to 7.6 is the best to achieve.

All the body's regulatory systems - breathing, circulation, hormone production, etc. - aid in balancing the body's pH. By far, the single most contributing factor in achieving and maintaining balanced pH levels is our diets – the food we eat.

What happens when the body's pH is too acidic?

In America, largely due to the Standard American Diet (SAD) with its high-acid producing proteins, eggs, dairy, medications, etc. and its low consumption of alkalizing fresh fruits, vegetables and mineral-rich foods, acidosis is common. The body tries to compensate for the high acidity by using alkaline minerals - including calcium, magnesium, potassium and then sodium – from vital organs and bones to neutralize the acid even at their expense. High acid levels contribute to fatigue, the inability to repair damaged cells, excess mucus, the inability to detoxify and generally poor health. Eventually, it may lead to degenerative conditions, such as heart disease, cancer, diabetes and obesity. An acidic body also allows diseases including cancer and tumors to thrive.

When the body's acid load becomes too great, some of these acid particles remain in the blood. It is believed that these acids can scratch the artery and blood vessel walls. This triggers cholesterol to be produced to patch the damage, which then may result in narrowing of the arteries leading to heart disease. High acid in the blood and tissues also may be a contributing factor in some cancer development.

Symptoms of pH imbalance include acid reflux, indigestion, weight gain, difficulty losing weight, poor metabolism, mineral deficiencies, constipation, fatigue, brain fog, frequent urination, hypoglycemia, hormonal imbalances, sore muscles and many more.

Fun Fact

If the blood's pH reaches 6.9, which is only slightly acidic, it can induce coma and death. So the body will neutralize the blood at all costs even if it means having to leach calcium from bones causing them to become brittle.

Test the body's pH

The best way to test whether the body is maintaining a proper pH balance is through the urine. This is the most accurate way to test the overall pH of the body/blood. The kidneys are the organ responsible to balance the pH of the body/blood. If a person becomes too acidic, the kidneys will eliminate and remove acid through the urine.

Optimal testing should be done throughout a 24-hour period, and then the average calculated. The optimal urine pH is between 6 and 7. Below 6 is too acidic, and above 7 is too alkaline.

Testing saliva is a good indication of mineral reserves for alkalinity in the body. If saliva tests acidic, this may reveal a mineral deficiency based on the dietary intake of alkaline food.

It is simple to check the pH with urine and saliva pH test strips available through most health food stores and some pharmacies. The pH test strips container should include a pH chart with a colored grading scale and full instructions on how to use it. Many charts look like the one below.

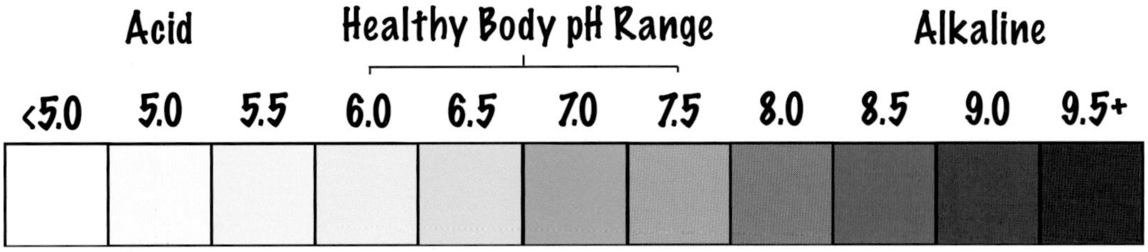

Does food affect pH?

Food definitely affects pH. When food has been digested and metabolized, the remaining chemical and metallic residues called ash, yield either acid or alkaline and cause the body fluids and tissues to become acid or alkaline. Appendix H includes a chart comparing foods and whether or not they are alkaline or acid once digested.

To maintain health, the diet should consist of 60 percent alkaline-forming foods and 40 percent acid-forming foods. To restore health, the diet should consist of 80 percent alkaline-forming foods and 20 percent acid-forming foods.

Although it might seem that citrus fruits would have an acidifying effect on the body, the citric acid they contain actually has an alkalinizing effect in the digestive system. A food's acid- or alkaline-forming tendency in the body has nothing to do with the actual pH of the food itself. For example, lemons are very acidic. However, after digestion and assimilation the metabolized product is alkaline; so lemons are alkaline forming in the body. Likewise, meat will test alkaline before digestion, but it leaves very acidic residue in the body. Nearly all animal products are very acid forming.

Serious acid imbalances can be addressed with alkaline promoting supplements, but the goal should be to change the diet to eat greater amounts of alkaline foods.

Acid/Alkaline Food Chart - Appendix H

We do not need to adhere strictly to the alkaline side of the chart. God made all foods to nourish and support the body, even some from the acid side have a bounty of minerals, amino acids and vitamins the body needs. A good percentage of the food we need comes from the alkaline side.

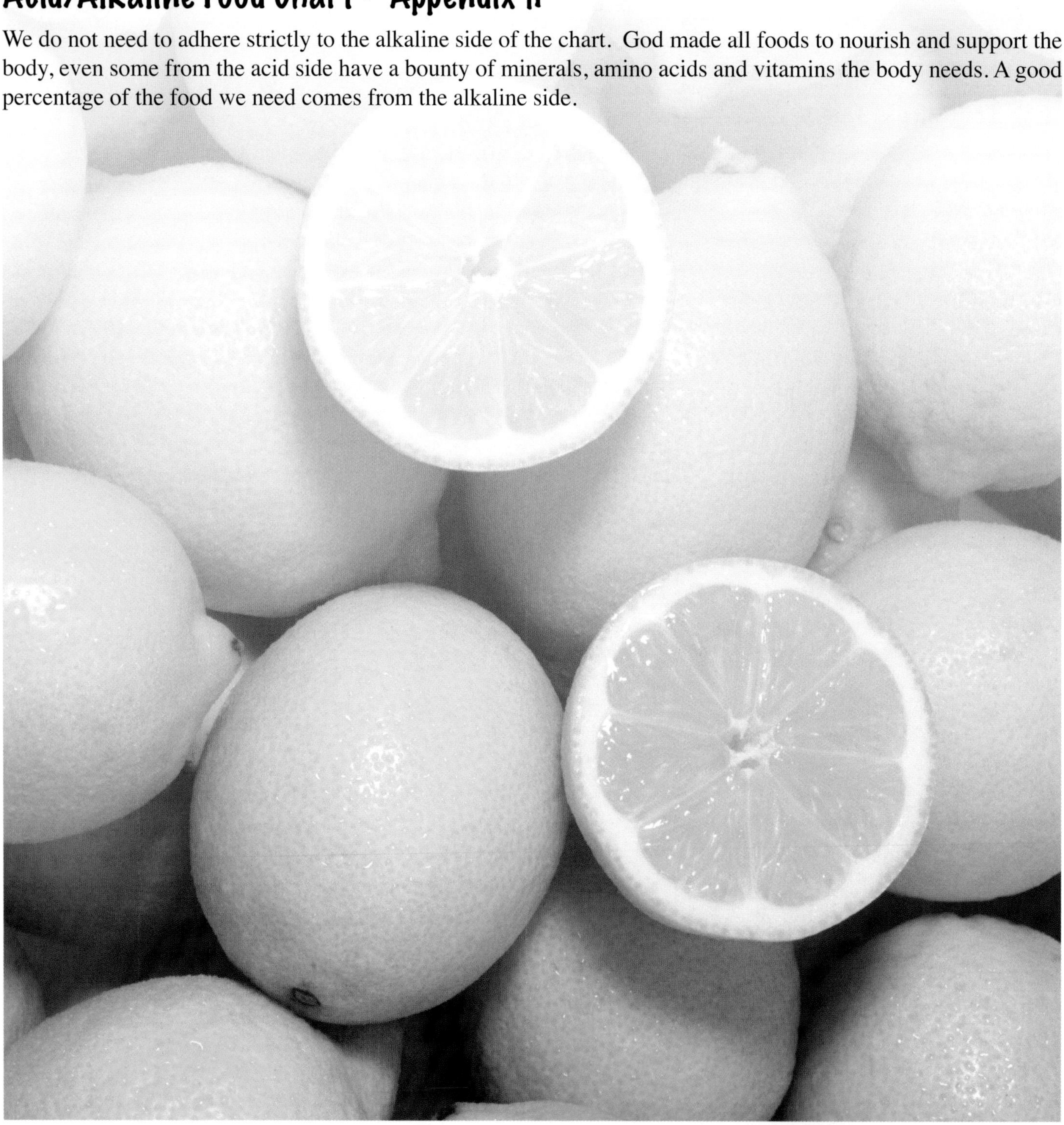

Water

"Jesus answered and said unto her, 'Whosoever drinketh of this water shall thirst again: But whosoever drinketh of the water that I shall give him shall never thirst; but the water that I shall give him shall be in him a well of water springing up into everlasting life.'"
John 4:13-14

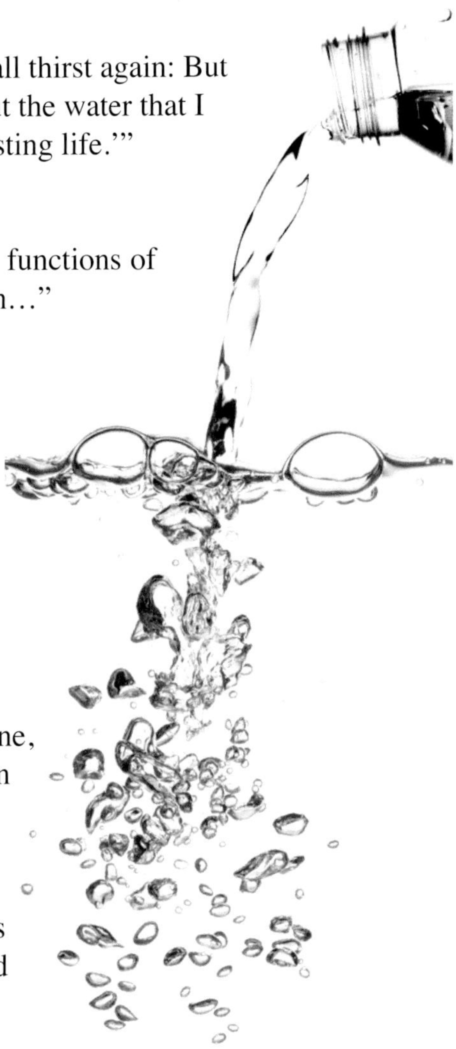

Water has so many purposes. The first reference in the Bible to one of the functions of water is in Genesis 2:10. "And a river went out of Eden to water the garden…"

Every living thing, including plants and animals, needs water.

What does water do for us?

Without water, we could not exist. Because the body is 70 percent water, it has an important role in nearly every process of our bodies.

Energy

Water is the main source of energy for the body. Within a cell membrane, there are tiny little pumps much like turbines at hydroelectric dams. In an effort for water to get into a cell, it turns the pumps, which creates energy – kind of like hydroelectric energy. When we drink water, it is free to move about and can generate energy at the cellular level. Water from fruits or vegetables binds to other nutrients and is not free to pass through the pumps to create energy. This is a reason why water itself needs to be consumed throughout the day.

Temperature Regulation

Water is essential for the body's cooling (sweat) and heating (electrical) systems. Because it changes temperature slowly, water acts as a good heat storing material. Water evaporates from body surfaces as sweat and cools the body. Throughout the day and night, sweat is constantly being released in barely noticeable amounts as the body regulates its temperature. The sweat increases and becomes more visible in hot, humid weather or during exercise.

Fun Fact

You can lose up to a pint of water a day just by unnoticeable sweating.

Blood Cell Transportation System

Water is the vehicle of transport for the circulation of blood cells. When the body is fully hydrated, the blood is 94 percent water.

Oxygen Transportation System

Water helps blood carry the oxygen we breathe in from the lungs to all the cells in the body. When water reaches a cell, it carries the oxygen into the cell and then takes the waste gases (carbon dioxide) out of the cell and to the lungs for disposal. There will be more on how this process works in Unit 3, regarding the respiratory system.

Nutrient Transportation System

Water is crucial for the delivery of nutrients to every cell in the body. Once nutrients are broken down from food in the digestive tract, water aids in transporting the nutrients to the liver and kidneys for filtering and then to all the cells in the body.

Hydrolysis is the loosening, dissolving, breaking or splitting by the participating action of water. It is necessary in the digestive system for breaking down nutrients into smaller particles. Without water, hydrolysis cannot take place. That is why we need to supply the body with water **before** we eat solid foods.

Fun Fact - Thirst pains can often be mistaken for hunger pains. Drink some water first to make sure you are not just dehydrated. This also will help you avoid overeating.

Waste Transportation System

After water carries nutrients to the cells, it then takes waste from the cells and sends it to the kidneys and liver to filter. Then, water is used to eliminate waste through sweating, urinating and defecating. Water in the colon helps move along waste. A lack of water – or dehydration -- can lead to constipation.

Joint and Organ Protection

Water lubricates, cushions and protects joints. It also protects the spinal cord, organs and other sensitive tissues. Water is the bulk material that fills empty spaces in the body.

What happens if we don't get enough water?

Through sweating (perspiration), urinating and even breathing (respiration), we are losing water constantly from our bodies. When we exercise or go outside on a hot day, we lose even more water. That is why we need to replenish water in our bodies by drinking it throughout the day.

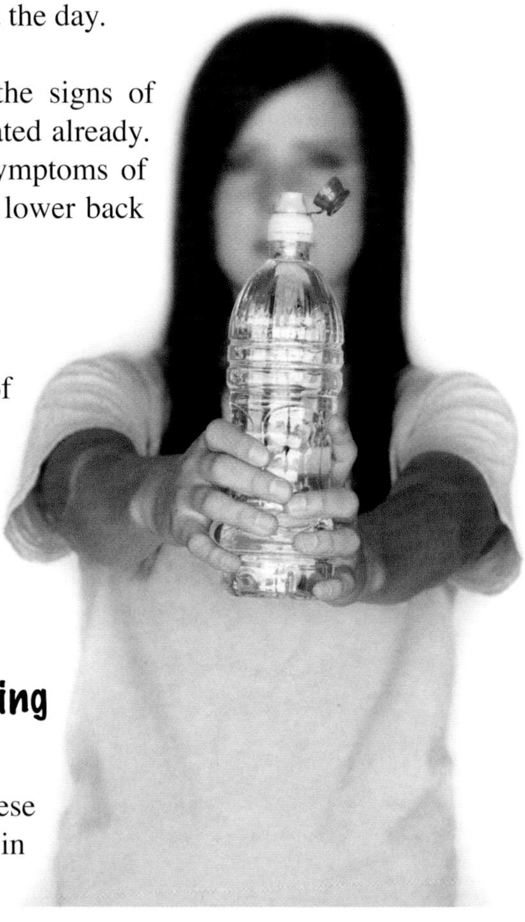

When we lost too much water, we become dehydrated. One of the signs of dehydration is thirst. By the time a person feels thirsty, he is dehydrated already. We all need good, clean, pure water to drink throughout the day. Symptoms of dehydration include reduced energy (fatigue), joint and muscle pains, lower back pain, headaches, fatigue and constipation.

How much water do we need?

Most people think that everyone needs eight glasses of eight ounces of water a day, for a total of 64 ounces. This is great for a 128 pound person. For a 60 pound child, drinking that much water would be a daunting task and may be more than is needed. For a grown male over six feet tall, this is too little water. Most nutritionists recommend that each person drink half his or her weight in ounces of pure water each day.

Can we get enough water just by eating food or drinking tea or other beverages?

No. Only 20 percent of your daily water intake should come from these sources. The rest should come from drinking half your body weight in ounces of pure water.

Water Dilemma

Water, water, everywhere, but not a drop to drink. This is an old saying, but how true it is today. Drinking pure water is a must for a healthy body, but which water do you pick - bottled, spring, distilled, reverse osmosis, mineral or purified? Should we buy from the store, have it delivered or install a home filtration unit?

Distilled water is generally tap or well water that has been steam distilled. Steam distillation is boiling water, trapping the steam and collecting the condensation into another vessel. This process destroys living organisms and allows for any contaminants to settle at the bottom of the boiling chamber. The resulting water contains no minerals and is completely pure. Distilled water is especially good for those with joint and arthritic issues, since the minerals that have collected in the joints over the years will slowly be grabbed by the distilled water. As long as a person consumes a diet rich in organic minerals, there is no need to be concerned over removing necessary nutrition from the body by drinking distilled water. It is considered by most health professionals to be the water of choice.

Reverse osmosis (RO) water is regarded as your second best water choice. A membrane in the reverse osmosis chamber filters out unwanted pathogens and hard minerals. The only draw back to home RO equipment may be in the cleaning process. Without frequent membrane cleaning, contaminants can make their way back into the water.

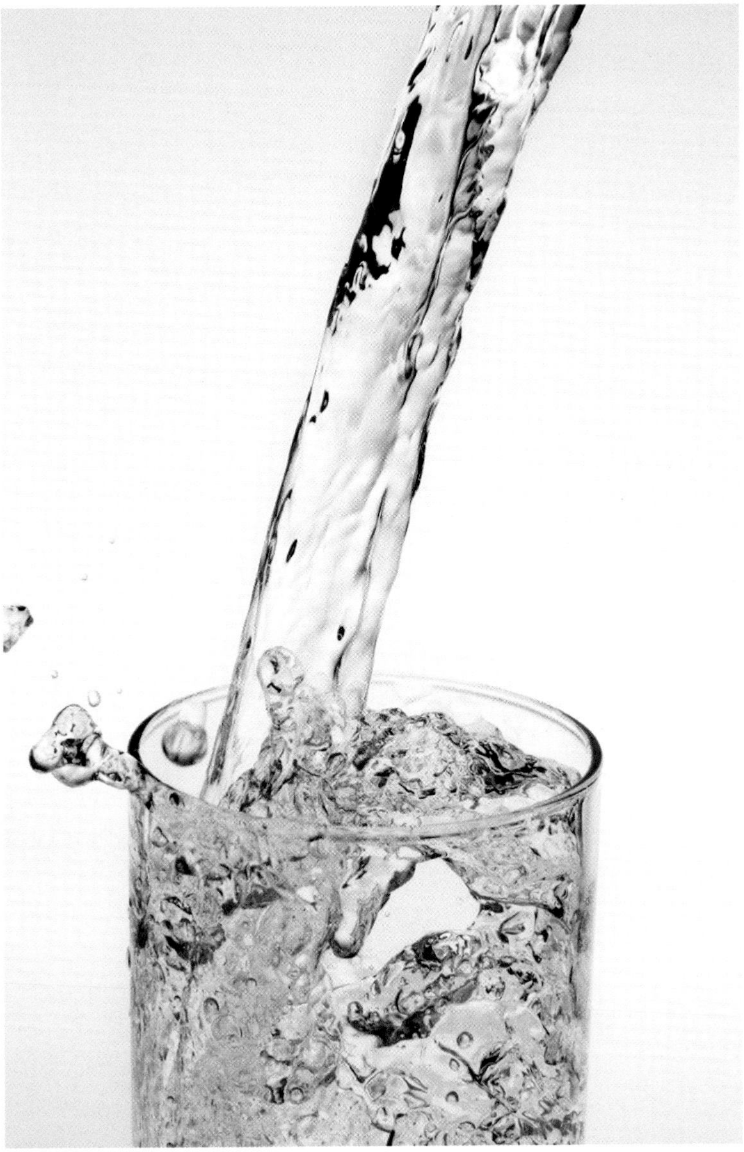

Spring water is water taken from a natural spring and bottled with no additional purification, unless specified on the label. Some spring water has been known to be simply purified tap water, and others have been found to contain bacteria because of not being purified.

Mineral water, which can sometimes be spring water, can be very healthy if from a good source. Mineral water is full of minerals, which the body may or may not fully absorb.

Purified water may be the most questionable. How is it purified? If the water is charcoal and/or carbon filtered, reverse osmosis and distilled, you can be sure that nothing harmful remains in the water. Most purified water is bought from the store in plastic containers, which have their own set of hazards.

Installing a home purification unit (pitcher style, faucet mount, whole house, under sink) can be well worth the cost. The main consideration for any purification system should be its ability to remove germs, chlorine and fluoride.

Unit 2 Chapter 2
Discussion Questions

1. I Corinthians 6:19 tells us that our bodies are the temple of the Holy Spirit. What does this mean?
2. Do you care for your body as the temple of the Holy Spirit?
3. What improvements can we make to take care of the bodies God has blessed us with?
4. Besides the food we eat, what other ways can we take care of our bodies?

Activities - plus the Green Apple Bean Salad "Power" Recipe and activities.

Elementary

1. This experiment will help you see how many times you need to chew a piece of food. Take a plastic baggie with a zipped closure and place a "bite" of cauliflower in the bag. With a meat cleaver or flat pounding device, pound gently on the cauliflower with the same pressure that you chew and count how many times you need to do this to turn it into a paste. This will equal the number of times you need to chew the cauliflower in your mouth. Would you need to chew a piece of chicken the same number of times?
2. At the beginning of the next family meal, tell everyone about the experiment in activity #1 and how many times to chew each bite and why it is important to do this.
3. Find out the definition of a cruciferous vegetable. Make a list of ten of these vegetables and put it on the refrigerator. Each time you eat one of the vegetables on the list, cross it off the list until you have tried each one.
4. Using the Acid Forming Chart in Appendix H, find all of the foods you have eaten in the past three days. Is this your typical diet? Is it more acidic or alkaline?
5. Prepare the Lemon/Lime pickles as outlined in the Additional Recipes section at the end of Unit 2, sample it and make note of the taste, texture, etc. Let them ferment for two weeks, and in the activity section of Chapter 4 of this unit, we will revisit them.
6. Using the Minerals chart in Appendix G, find the foods are high in calcium. If you eat a lot of dairy products, substitute one calcium-rich vegetable for one dairy product in your diet.
7. Conduct an experiment to taste test the quality of a) distilled, b) reverse osmosis c) spring water and d) tap or well water. Use separate containers for each and disposable paper cups for sampling and label these accordingly (A for distilled, B for reverse osmosis, etc.). Make a chart that records your findings. Label each column with each type of water, and use the rows to identify qualities of the water, such as flavor, color, smell, visible objects in the water, grit, etc. Each quality should be given a score of one to three, with one being bad, two being neutral and three being good. Have family members participate. Total the scores each type of water receives and determine a winner. Prepare a written or oral report with your findings and share it with your family as you drink the water that scored the highest in your experiment.

Secondary

Choose any from above plus

1. Study the preparation of foods and mealtime in the Bible. Expand your study to learn how foods were prepared in Biblical times and foods that were used. Prepare a Biblically correct meal for your family to enjoy.
2. Hydrochloric acid (HCI) can dissolve concrete, but does not damage the stomach. Why is this? Prepare a written or oral report on your findings.
3. Conduct an experiment to test how a plant reacts to a) distilled, b) reverse osmosis c) spring water and d) tap or well water. Get four small plants of the same variety in their own identical containers that support them appropriately. Label each type of water and each plant (A for distilled, B for reverse osmosis, etc.). Using a measuring device to give each the plant the same amount of water according to their daily need and make sure they receive necessary and equal amounts of sunlight.

Create a chart that allows you to record your observations each day. After four weeks, summarize your findings in a written or oral report.

4. Using the same premise from the previous activity, prepare two plants. Select the type of water that tested the best in the last experiment. Measure identical amounts of the water to give each plant, but microwave one in a glass container for 15 seconds before giving it to the plant. Create a chart that allows you to record your observations each day. At the end of two weeks, summarize your findings in a written or oral report.
5. Acquire pH test strips and create a chart with all of the members of your family. Encourage each person to test his or her acid/alkaline level (remember to test several times in a 24-hour period and take an average) and record findings on the chart. Modify your diets according to the test results. After implementing these changes for several days, retest the participants. Repeat. Some family members may need to try a more regimented diet or incorporate supplements to get results. Always consult a trusted health practitioner.

Additional Resources

Books:

1. "Healthy Digestion," part of the Storey Medical Herb Guides www.storeybooks.com or local bookstores.
2. "Good Digestion," part of the Alive Natural Health Guides sold in bookstores or through Nutri-Books to retailers for sale in their stores.
3. "101 Foods That Could Save Your Life," David Grotto, R.D., L.C.N., by Bantum Publishing 2007.
4. "Water For Health, For Healing, For Life: You're Not Sick, You're Thirsty!" by F. Batmanghelidj, Published by Warner Books, 2003.

Digestive System Power

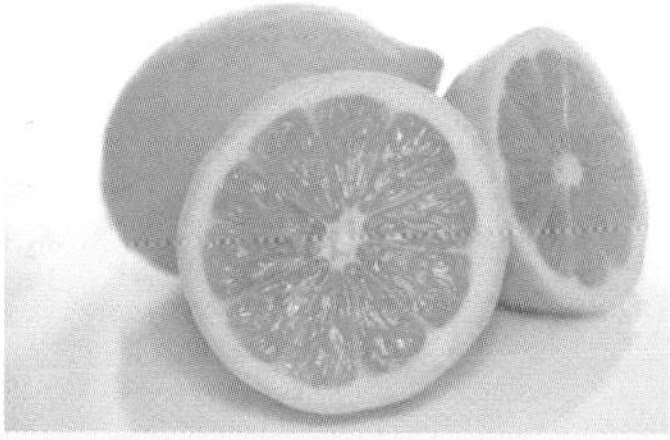

LEMONS

Although an acid in its natural state, once lemons or lemon juice enters the digestive system, they become a beneficial alkaline food.

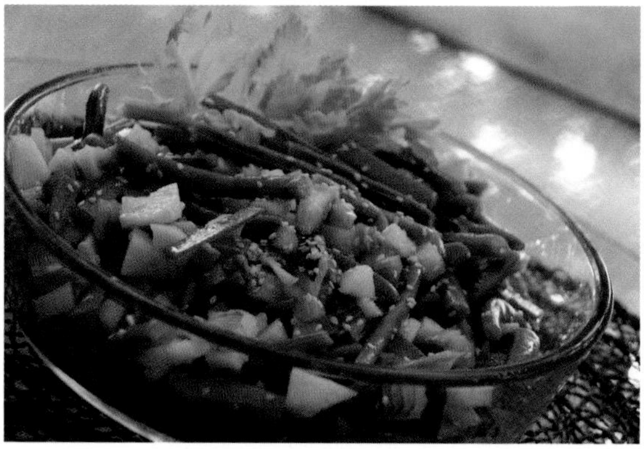

Green Apple Bean Salad

1 cup fresh, washed green beans, cut in half
2 large Granny Smith apples, peeled, cored and diced
3 large carrots, peeled and julienned
3 stalks celery, diced
2 Tbs. sesame seeds
¼ cup red onion, finely diced
3 to 4 Tbs. oil – select a new oil such as hazelnut or walnut oil
Juice from one lemon

Blanch green beans for two to three minutes and remove to a cold water bath. Once cooled, combine green beans, vegetables and sesame seeds in a large bowl with the lemon juice and oil. Spoon into bowls and enjoy.

Activities

Elementary

1. What does it mean to julienne when cooking? What is blanching?
2. Why is this variety of apple called Granny Smith?
3. Some people cry while cutting onions. Why is this?

Secondary

Choose any from above plus

1. What causes the lemon juice to change from an acid to alkaline? How does this affect your health? How can you test the acidity of something?
2. Create a homemade pH testing strips with the directions found in the Activity Guide.
3. As you help prepare a meal, set aside some ingredients to test with your ph testing kit. Compile your findings on a chart that lists the food and whether or not it tested acidic or alkaline.

Chapter 3

Enzymes

"He causeth the grass to grow for the cattle, and herb for the service of man: that he may bring forth food out of the earth." Psalm 104:14

What are enzymes?

Enzymes are catalysts that:

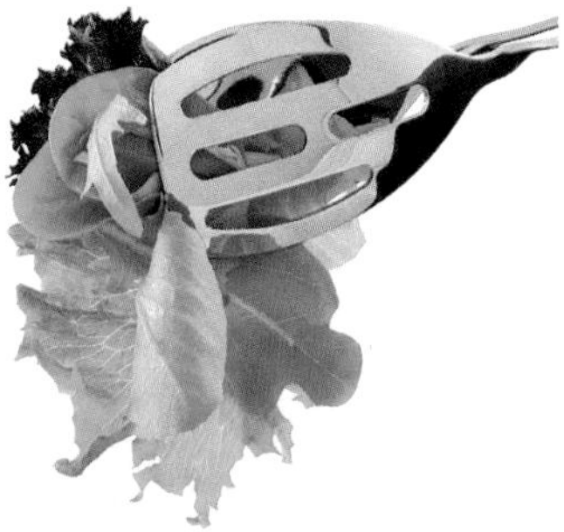

- cause a chemical reaction to happen faster – like digestion.
- are comprised of amino acids.
- are not alive, nor are they living cells.
- are sensitive to their surroundings and can become inactive or denatured.

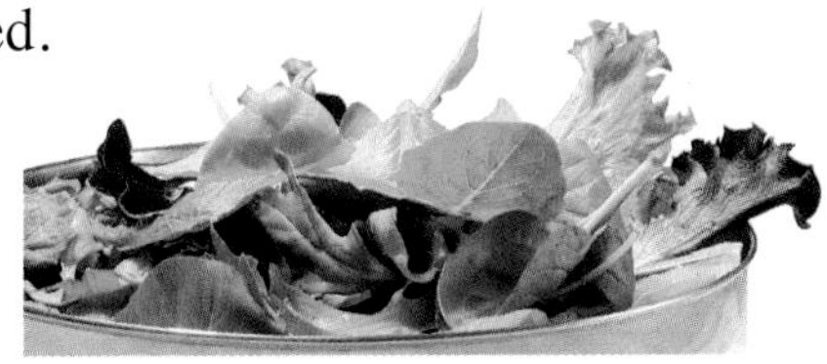

There are approximately 20,000 different enzymes found in the human cell. Combining with vitamins and minerals, enzymes form nearly 100,000 various chemicals that enable you to see, hear, think, feel, move and digest food.

How important are enzymes?

We cannot breathe without enzymes. They are the catalysts of biochemical reactions -- the formation, breakdown and rearranging of molecules – providing us with the energy and materials needed to live and function. Without enzymes, digestion of food in the body would occur too slowly for proper metabolism and food would stay in the digestive tract and ferment. This would cause bloating, gas and pain.

Energy exists in the food that we eat, but it must be unlocked and broken down before the cells in our bodies can absorb that energy. A random chemical process could take years to break down the food, whereas enzymes speed up the process so the cells get what they need.

Fun Fact

Magnesium is an important mineral in enzyme reactions. There are over 300 enzymatic reactions in a single human cell. None of which will occur without the presence of magnesium.

What do digestive enzymes do?

Enzymes perform many functions. They:

- break down proteins, fats, and carbohydrates to avoid fermentation in the gut.
- aid in proper digestion.
- replenish and preserve pools of other enzymes that perform countless metabolic functions in the body not associated with digestion.

Besides the digestive system, are other organ systems affected by enzymes?

Problems digesting food can cause the endocrine system to be overworked leading to health concerns such as hypoglycemia, diabetes and obesity. This can lead to over stimulation of digestive organs demanding more food than necessary that then may lead to weight imbalances. Eating more raw foods, which contain a rich supply of enzymes, takes stress off the endocrine glands.

What are the digestive enzymes and what do they break down?

There are four different digestive enzymes with specific assignments.

- **Protease** breaks down animal and plant based proteins.
- **Lipase** breaks down lipids, also called fats.
- **Amylase** breaks down carbohydrates, such as bread, pasta, rice and starchy vegetables.
- **Cellulase**, technically a form of amylase, breaks down cellulose, or the fiber in vegetables.

The digestive process would not be possible without these catalysts performing and completing necessary biological activity. This energy from the biological process is what enables the enzymes to break down proteins, fats and carbohydrates into their simplest components: amino acids, essential fats and sugars. Enzymes also assist in the extraction of vitamins and minerals. These beneficial components are delivered to the trillions of cells throughout the body, while those that are non-essential or toxic are carried out of the body. Without enzymes to carry out this process, you would die of malnutrition. For more information on specific enzymes, see Appendix CC.

The moment you pick an apple off a tree, the enzymes contained in the apple begin to break down the nutrients in it. If it is not eaten within a week or so, it will start to go bad. If it goes straight into your mouth, your digestive system will be aided by the naturally occurring enzymes found in that apple. The enzymes once instrumental in cellular biochemical reactions necessary for the growth of the apple will now contribute to the digestion of the apple in the upper portion of your stomach.

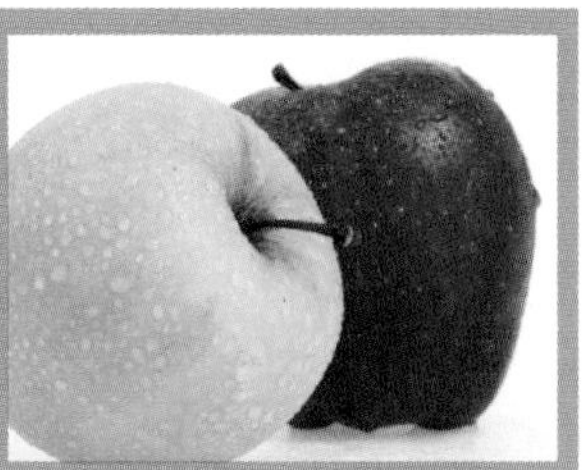

The soft portions – or bad spots -- on an apple reflect that the apple's enzymes have been released from the cells, and it is now quickly being digested. Soon, if it is not eaten, it will continue to digest itself, rot and eventually completely decompose.

When and where do the enzymes work in digestion?

Mouth

In the mouth, three different types of **amylase** are secreted to immediately begin digesting carbohydrates. The act of chewing breaks down and grinds the food into smaller pieces to be swallowed. When swallowed, the food travels down the esophagus to the mouth.

Stomach

The majority of the carbohydrate digestion occurs in the upper stomach (the pylorus) due to the amylase and saliva that was mixed with the food. Raw foods that have not been cooked or processed are the only foods that are partially digested in this part of the stomach. The food then enters the lower stomach (the fundus) where **pepsin** – a protease -- and **hydrochloric acid (HCl)** are secreted for protein digestion.

Small Intestine

Once the chyme enters the duodenum, **lipase** from the pancreas and **bile** from the gallbladder assist in fat digestion. Additional enzymes are added to finish digestion supplied by the pancreas.

Large Intestine

Once the chyme enters the large intestine, no more enzymes are released. However, the large intestine is where good bacteria, water and fiber perform specific functions, which will be discussed in detail later.

How do we get enzymes?

We are born with a reserve of enzymes that was given to us from our mothers. Additional enzymes come from uncooked, unprocessed, organic food that is needed to digest that particular food. Enzymes also are made from healthy bacteria in the colon. Other enzymes come from enzyme supplements, which are generally plant derived.

FUN FACT

Over 70 years of research shows zero reports of problems taking plant-based enzymes. Enzyme supplements also are safe for small children and pregnant or nursing mothers.

What food contains enzymes?

All whole, unprocessed, uncooked foods in their original created state – known as **raw** -- contain enzymes.

What happens to enzymes when food is cooked?

For the most part, once cooked, enzymes in food are inactivated or denatured. Enzymes are more heat sensitive than vitamins and are denatured or destroyed by cooking temperatures above 105° F, pasteurization, canning, and microwaving. Each plant enzyme does its work only at its own specific pH, temperature ranges and in the presence of moisture.

What foods can be eaten raw?

Fresh fruit and vegetables are the most common foods that may be eaten raw. A few exceptions such as broccoli, cabbage, cauliflower and Brussels sprouts contain compounds that may inhibit the function of the thyroid gland and should not be eaten raw in excess or frequently by those who have thyroid problems. They need to be lightly steamed.

Seeds, nuts, grains and beans have enzyme inhibitors that must be deactivated by soaking, cooking or sprouting to allow their enzymes to be released. Have you ever gotten constipated after eating a bunch of raw nuts? Soak them first, and see what happens.

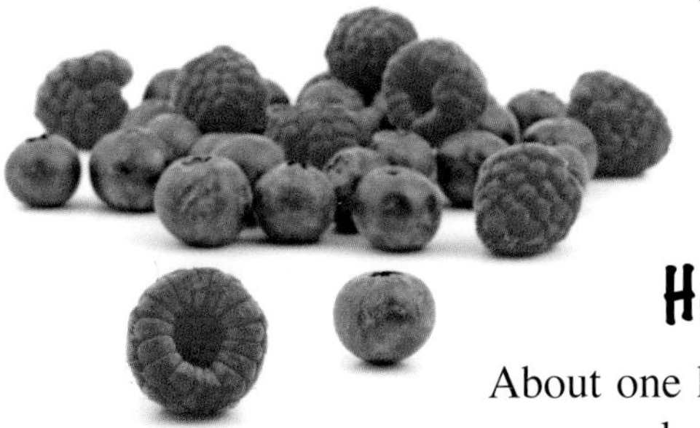

In general, meats, poultry and fish are not safe to eat raw and must be thoroughly cooked as they may contain harmful bacteria.

How much of my diet should be raw?

About one half of our diets should be raw. This gives us the sensation of being full sooner, and our overall vitality will increase. If a person is trying to regain better health, he can eat 75 percent raw. When eating cooked or processed foods, enzyme supplements may be necessary especially if a person is fighting a sickness, health concern or is older and has depleted enzyme reserves. Taking enzyme supplements should not be a substitute for healthy eating.

With eating so much raw food, wouldn't salads and fruit and vegetable trays get old?

From wonderful appetizers to delicious desserts, there are many wonderful Web sites and cookbooks with delicious, creative and diverse raw food recipes. In the recipe section for Unit 2, there are many great examples of tasty raw recipes as well.

Who should supplement enzymes?

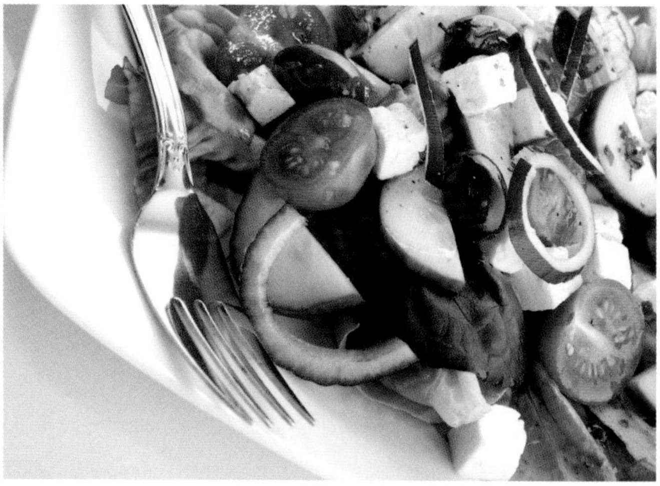

Those with a history of eating a poor diet or who have been fighting a long illness or health concern, your body may need help to reverse the depletion of enzymes. Physicians track certain enzyme levels in the blood to diagnose health problems. Liver function is monitored through enzyme levels. Kidney, heart and some concerns also are diagnosed according to enzyme levels. The following symptoms may suggest an enzyme deficiency: allergies, fatigue, bloating, gas, constipation, indigestion, irregular bowel movements, extreme mood swings after eating processed foods and sugars, or nausea and burping after eating greasy foods.

Causes of Enzyme Depletion

- Cooking at high temperatures (above 105° F) which denatures most enzymes.
- Chemicals, pesticides and herbicides that work by destroying enzymes in both plants and animals.
- Genetically engineered foods, which have little enzymes or none at all.
- Pasteurization or the heating of fruits, vegetables and dairy products to reduce potentially harmful bacteria.
- Irradiated food or exposing fresh foods, including meats to radiation to reduce potentially harmful pathogens.
- Microwaving, which uses directed microwave to alter food molecules, causing them to heat.
- Bovine growth hormone that are used in the dairy industry to cause cows to produce more milk.
- Unsaturated and hydrogenated fats – see Unit 1 for details.
- Fluoridated water, when fluoride is added to water to potentially fight tooth decay.

Enzyme Supplementation

A plant enzyme in supplemental form with a healthy diet of mostly raw foods may help reverse damage to the body. See Appendix CC for more information about choosing enzyme supplements.

What foods have no enzymes and should be avoided?

- Refined sugars - especially white sugar, fructose, corn syrup, sorbitol, mannitol and all synthetic sweeteners.
- Refined flours including white, unbleached, bleached and enriched.
- Synthetic fats - especially partially hydrogenated oils, margarines and vegetable shortening.
- Genetically Modified Organisms (GMO) unsaturated oils - soybean, canola, flaxseed, safflower, corn and fish oils.
- Homogenized, pasteurized, nonfat or acidophilus milk, and processed cheese.
- Commercial[1] nuts and seeds - oiled, sugared and salted.
- Drinks – commercial[1] sugared fruit juices, juice drinks and soft drinks.
- Canned coffee and decaffeinated coffee.
- All commercial[1] red meat and poultry that have added growth hormones and antibiotics and are not free range.
- Commercial[1] eggs or egg substitutes.
- Canned, precooked, microwaved and processed foods, fast food and junk food.

Fun Fact
Unless a food package says, non-GMO, it could be GMO. Manufacturers are not required to label their products either way.

What foods are good and are loaded with enzymes?

- Natural sweeteners - fruit juices, raw honey, organic maple syrup, molasses, barley malt, sucanat (organic sugar cane).
- Organic whole grains: best are heirloom (non-genetically altered) kamut, quinoa, amaranth, and spelt.
- Raw, unpasteurized, whole milk, cultured milk products; kefir, yogurt or buttermilk, and goat's milk; unprocessed cheese. Use in moderation because these are mucus forming.
- Butter, preferable raw (from raw cow's milk) and organic, extra virgin olive oil or coconut oil.
- Buy organic, free-range beef or poultry and fish from non-polluted waters.
- Raw juices; juice your own or buy raw, organic.
- Organic herbal teas.

Shopping Tip
First buy fresh, organic foods; the second best option is to buy fresh, non-organic foods; thirdly frozen foods; and lastly canned if that is the only food available.

The more live, enzyme-replete food that we eat, the healthier it will make our digestive systems and overall health.

---

1 The word commercial here has to do with foods prepared in large volumes by companies with no regard to organic, chemical-free and natural preparation standards.

Unit 2 Chapter 3
Discussion Questions

1. What is an enzyme?
2. What is the difference between an enzyme and bacteria?
3. How has refrigeration helped and/or hindered the quality of our food?
4. How does dehydrating food differ from cooked food? At what temperature should it be dehydrated?

Activities - plus the Quinoa Vegetable Risotto "Power" Recipe and activities.

Elementary

1. Take a fresh banana that still has a bit of green at the stem. Cut it in half and place one half in the refrigerator and the other on the counter. Watch each to see which one gets it's spots faster. What is the texture of the banana before spots and after it is full of spots?
2. Papaya is a fruit loaded with enzymes. In fact papaya enzymes are used in women's facial peels. See if you mom has some papaya or other plant-based enzyme peel that you can use on your arm to see this product digest the dead skin cells.
3. Color a picture of an enzyme and a bacteria.
4. Name the foods we know Jesus ate.

Secondary

Choose any from above plus

1. Write a paper on the difference between bacteria and enzymes.
2. Build a daily menu including breakfast lunch and dinner with 75 percent of the food choices raw and with at least 50 percent on the alkaline side. Be sure to plan in accordance with the **Nutrition 101: Choose Life!** Food Guide Pyramid in Appendix B. Also be sure to include proper amounts of magnesium, calcium and protein.
3. Read Matt. 9:17, Mark 2:22 and Luke 5:37-38. In this parable, what did Jesus say will happen to new wine put in old wineskins? Explain the literal meaning of this parable. Why would Jesus use this illustration to explain a spiritual truth?
4. What is fermentation?
5. To learn more about fermentation as eluded to in Jesus' parable, try the following experiment. You will need dried yeast, sugar, half a cup of warm water, a clear glass container, a towel and an empty insulated ice chest. Pour half a cup of warm water into a glass. Dissolve 1 teaspoon of sugar of the water. Then add 1 teaspoon of the dried yeast and mix it in well. Write down how it looks and smells. Set the glass in an area that is warm, but not hot. Then, place a towel around the glass and carefully set it in an insulated ice chest (also used to keep things warm). After five minutes, check the glass. What has changed? Check it again after another five minutes. Record your findings.

Additional Resources

Take your fermentation experiment further: http://www.brightminds.uq.edu.au/kidsactivities/thelab/fermentation/design_experiment.html

Book:

"Living Longer, The Magic of Enzymes & Nutrition" Dick Couey, Ph. D. and DicQie Fuller, Ph. D. Transformation Enzyme Company, 2005.

Digestive System Power

RAW VEGETABLES

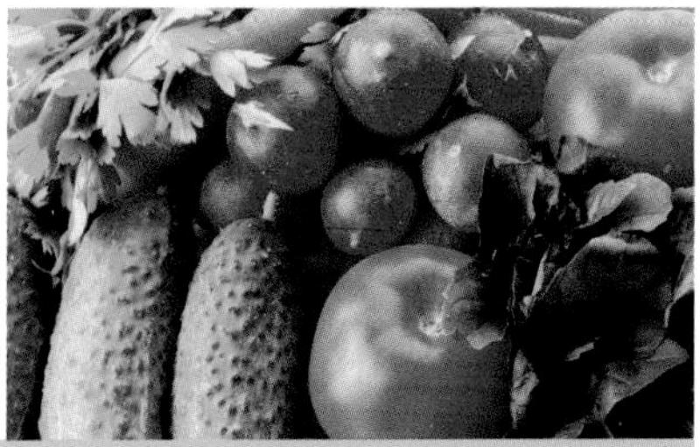

Raw vegetables are a great source of enzymes and fiber for great digestive health.

Quinoa Vegetable Risotto

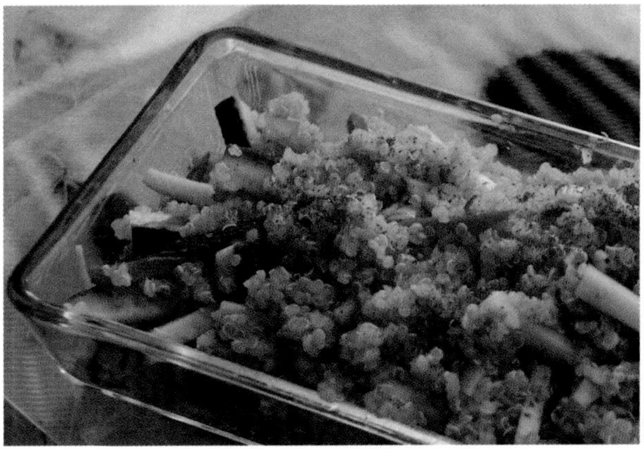

½ cup quinoa
1 cup water
1 large carrot, julienned
1 zucchini, julienned
2 cloves garlic, minced
¼ cup red onion, finely diced
½ Tbs. olive oil
Pinch of salt and cayenne pepper

Cook quinoa according to package directions: Bring one cup water with salt and quinoa to boiling. Turn heat to simmer for 15 minutes or until water is absorbed. Stir to fluff quinoa. Add vegetables, garlic, onion, olive oil and pepper. Press mixture into a small, square baking pan. This is generally not cooked any further. The vegetables will be warmed by the quinoa but still raw, so all the enzymes remain for good digestive health.

This dish goes well with fish or chicken.

Fun Fact

Risotto typically refers to an Italian dish of rice and vegetables heated in a broth. This recipe substitutes the easily digested, wheat-free, low gluten, high protein quinoa for traditional rice.

Activities

Elementary

1. What does the word raw mean?
2. Why is it important to eat raw fruits and vegetables?
3. Find out more about quinoa. What is it and how is it pronounced?
4. Using only the letters from the words of the ingredients in the recipe (quinoa, water, carrot, zucchini, garlic, onion and pepper) see if you can spell your first, middle and last name.
5. Find out where and how quinoas grow? What are the health benefits of it? Where can you buy quinoa? Tell your family about quinoa as you sample the recipe.
6. Use quinoa as a substitute for rice in another recipe and serve it as a side dish during dinner.

Secondary

Choose any from above plus

1. Prepare an oral or written report describing the difference between raw and cooked fruits and vegetables and how they impact digestion and elimination.
2. The history of quinoa involves its near extinction. Research how this happened and what caused quinoa to gain prominence again.
3. Search for other quinoa recipes online and prepare at one for breakfast, one for lunch and one for dinner over the course of a week.

Chapter 4

Elimination

"Try us out for ten days on a simple diet of vegetables and water. Then compare us with the young men who eat from the royal menu. Make your decision on the basis of what you see." Daniel 1:11

The final stage of digestion is the elimination of waste. Foods, devoid of nutrients through proper digestion, and fiber from these foods accumulate along the colon wall. When there is sufficient peristalsis – the wave like movement in the colon that propels this waste material (feces) along the colon – and the rectum is filled, the waste material is eliminated.

How many times per day should you eliminate waste?

Many people have only one bowel movement per day or worse, one per week. Ideally, a person should have a bowel movement after each meal or three per day. Having less than the two to three bowel movements per day results in inefficient cleansing of the colon and allows the waste matter to putrefy (rot) in the colon. This degrading matter leaches toxic gases and liquids back into the bloodstream. Poor elimination has been shown to contribute to many health conditions. In order for the entire digestive system to work properly, the process of elimination must work at optimum as well.

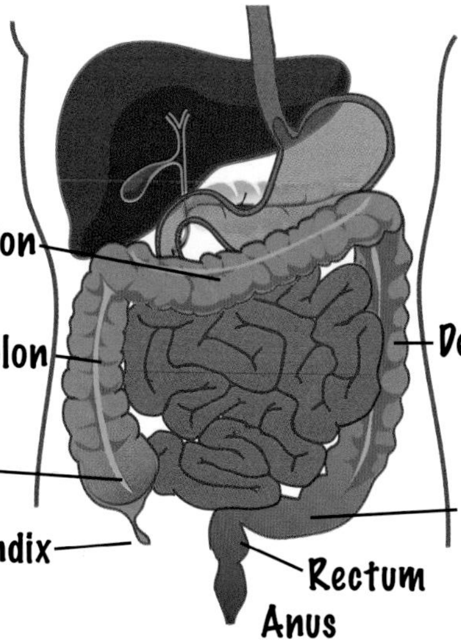

The two most important items in a person's diet that will contribute to proper elimination are **water** and **fiber**. If water intake is not sufficient the stool (eliminated feces) will be dry and hard to pass. Too little fiber in the diet and the stool will have no form. Too little of both and the colon is left without a scrub brush to keep itself clean.

What is constipation?

Constipation happens when elimination does not happen and food wastes block parts of the colon. This generally happens in the descending and sigmoid colon. Hemorrhoids often occur in people with constipation. Using an over-the-counter hemorrhoid relief ointment may provide temporary relief, but does not address the problem at its root. Good, wholesome, fresh food does not clog the colon; obstructions are formed by overcooked, mucus-forming, pasty foods.

How does water help the colon?

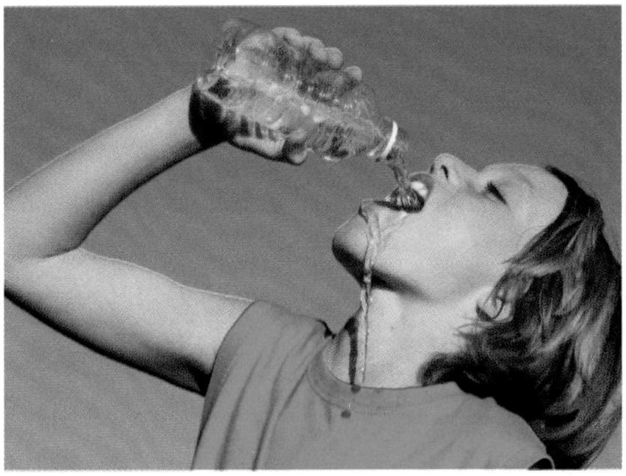

By the time digested food reaches the final stage of digestion in the colon, most of the nutrients have already been broken down and absorbed. At this stage, the digested food is called **feces** and includes fiber, indigestible waste and water. The water helps the feces move easily through the colon. Two-thirds of the water is actually absorbed at this final stage along with any remaining nutrients.

If enough water is not consumed, the waste material will have a hard time passing through the colon and constipation can occur. So, it is very important for a person to drink at least half of his body weight in ounces of pure water each day.

What is fiber and what does it do?

Fiber is the material in plants that are not digestible and move along the digestive tract soaking up water and making elimination of waste much easier.

There are two types of fiber.

1. **Soluble fiber** is soft, helps to soften the stool and absorbs waste like a sponge.
2. **Insoluble fiber** passes through the colon largely unchanged and adds bulk to stools, which in turns helps to stimulate bowel contractions and scours the colon like a scrub brush.

How much fiber do we need?

The average American's daily intake of fiber is about five to 14 grams per day. This may account for a significant number of health issues families face, such as constipation, diabetes (Type 2), obesity, some cancers and heart disease. The current recommendations from the National Academy of Sciences Institute of Medicine are to achieve an adequate intake of fiber based on your gender and age. This recommended amount is expected to meet or exceed the average amount needed to maintain a defined nutritional state of health.

On average, adults need **20 to 30 grams of fiber per day**. As a child's fiber recommendation has not been established, **15 to 20 grams** is a good amount for colon health. If a person is not used to consuming that much fiber, it may cause a bit of bloating, even cramping as the colon wakes up to being full of cleansing fiber. But it will soon pass. For a list of high fiber foods, see Appendix K.

Some helpful tips about adding fiber.

1. **Increase slowly:** The best way to begin is to figure out how much fiber is currently consumed each day. Once the number is known, slowly increase how much is eaten until the recommended amount is reached. Increasing too quickly can lead to gas, bloating, and/or diarrhea.

2. **Drink water:** Without enough pure, clean water in a high-fiber diet, constipation may result. The fiber will swell, peristalsis (the wave like motion of the intestines) will not ocurr, and bowel movements will be hard. Drink at least 16 ounces of pure water between meals.

3. **Don't add too much too quickly:** More is not always better, so fiber should be increased a little at a time. There is no limit on how much fiber can be consumed, and there are no reported problems with excess fiber intake. We should listen to our bodies and pay attention to how our health challenges and bowel movements are responding to fiber intake.

4. **Creative ways to add fiber to mealtime**

   a. Add flaxseeds, chia seeds, seeds, or nuts to salad, soup, cereal or yogurt.

   b. Keep fresh and frozen fruit such as peaches, blueberries, strawberries and raspberries to add to cereal, dessert, shakes or yogurt.

   c. Use pre-cut-up vegetables, stored in small baggies for snacks and to quickly add to a soup or salad.

d. Choose a whole grain cereal with a minimum of four grams of fiber in each serving. Eat it as a meal or alone as a snack.

e. Lentils, beans and peas go with everything. Add them in salad or soup or have them with meals or as snacks.

f. Select breads and pastas made from whole grain flour. The off-white color is easy to cover with a fresh tomato sauce until everyone is used to the color. Vegetable powders often are added to pasta for unique natural colors, which are great for summer pasta salads.

g. Have vegetables with meals whenever possible.

h. Use fruit with, or in between, meals. Set a minimum number of servings to have each day and be sure to reach it. Always go for the fruit with the skin and/or seeds for the fiber.

5. **Gas and bloating:** Taking an enzyme with specific starch and fiber components will greatly reduce bloating and gas from the extra fiber in the raw vegetables and/or beans and make eating much more pleasurable.

What is gas?

Gas is composed mainly of odorless chemicals -- hydrogen, nitrogen and carbon dioxide. About one in three people also produce methane, while the rest do not. Flatulence occurs when gas is released for two reasons: pockets of swallowed air from a person gulping his food or the toxin formation occurring inside the digestive tract from rotting of incompletely digested food. While releasing gas helps these toxins from entering the bloodstream, it may be a symptom of a larger issue.

Refined vs. Whole

Throughout **Nutrition 101: Choose Life!**, whole foods and refined foods are mentioned. By far the most refined foods are grains. This means bread, muffins, bagels, pancakes, waffles, tortillas, pasta and anything made from flour. Sugar also is highly refined. More information on that will be included in a later unit. When a grain is harvested, it can be stored for milling at a later date without going rancid, often for several years. Once commercially milled – ground into flour – the wheat germ and bran are removed. This removes most of the vitamins and minerals as well.

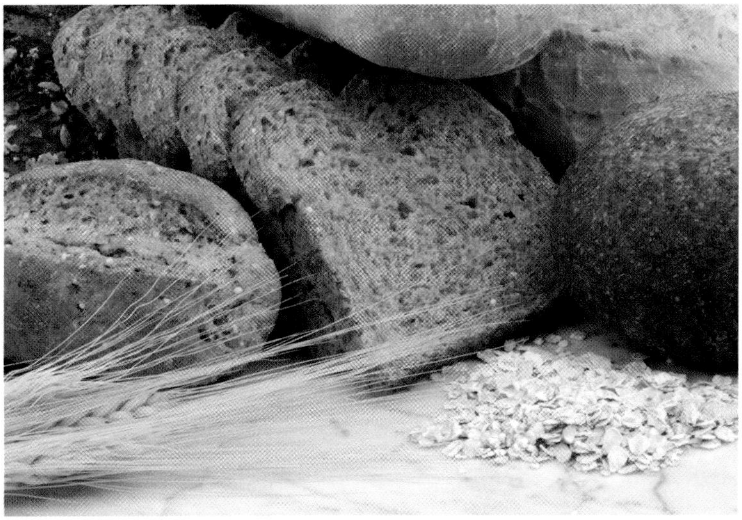

In the book "Eat to Live", Joel Fuhrman[1], links refined foods to the following health concerns: oral cavity cancer, stomach cancer, colorectal cancer, intestinal cancer, breast cancer, thyroid cancer, respiratory cancer, diabetes, heart disease and gallbladder disease.

God made the grains whole, and man has refined them for better taste and texture. However, the nutrient value has been removed leading us down a path of ill health.

1 "Eat to Live" Fuhrman, Joel. Little, Brown and Company Bachette Book Group USA. 2003.

Refined white flour used in breads and pasta are typically missing:

- 95 percent of the Vitamin E (contained in the wheat germ)
- 78 percent of the B6
- 78 percent of the fiber (colon and intestinal health)
- 72 percent of the magnesium
- 72 percent of the chromium (blood sugar control)
- 62 percent of the zinc (essential for immune system support)
- 50 percent of the folate

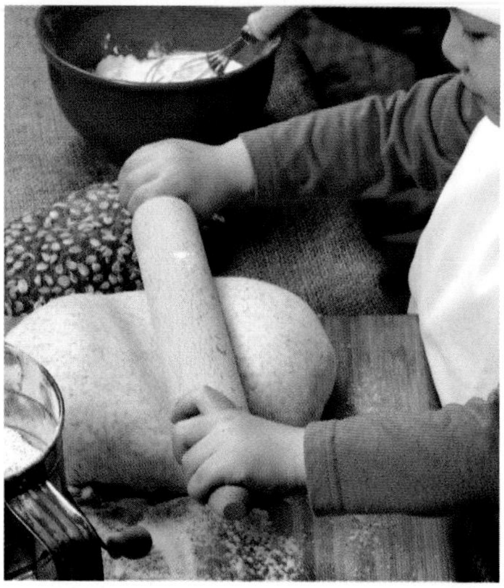

What remains is so depleted the United States government requires this flour be enriched with synthetic nutrients. One of the most important health skills a parent can teach his or her sons and daughters is to make homemade whole grain breads. See Appendix L on Baking with 100 percent Whole Grain.

Got good gut bacteria?

The colon contains millions, maybe billions of **friendly bacteria**. This good bacteria makes important B vitamins and vitamin K, some enzymes and further breaks down food into usable nutrients, from which the body creates its own natural antibiotics and fights off harmful bacteria.

Years of high sugar consumption disrupts this balance of bacteria, eventually leading to an over growth of the yeast strain candida albicans. Bacteria and yeast feed on sugar, especially allowing the candida to thrive. Eliminating daily sugar foods and only having a treat once per week is a good start. Consuming higher fiber foods, namely raw vegetables, will help the body to capture and remove some of the excess yeast. Consuming foods high in friendly bacteria such as miso, some yogurts and keifer help to re-establish the good bacteria. A great homemade gut bacterial balancer called Rejuvalac really helps as well. This recipe can be found in the Unit 2 Additional Recipes section.

Fun Fact

There are one million bacteria in a milliliter of fresh water and five nonillion bacteria on Earth. So, how many zeros are in a million and how many in a nonillion?

Antibiotics sabotage the colon's good bacteria. While they may do their job to kill off a harmful bacteria, most do not discriminate and kill off the good bacteria as well. Keeping the digestive system clean and in top working order will help boost the immune system, and the need for antibiotics will be reduced or eliminated. If you have taken an antibiotic within the past two years or have a colon health issue, supplementing with a good probiotic is a must to reestablish the beneficial bacteria, improve digestion and reduce yeast.

Probiotics can greatly help boost the immune system. In 2006, a double-blind study involving 248 children tested the effect of several super strains of bacteria, including *B lactis* HN019 and *L rhamnosus* HN001. The children were tested from November to May when they were most susceptible to colds and flu. After having been given proper probiotic supplementation, the number of sick days was reduced by almost 50 percent, and the need for antibiotics reduced by 80 percent.[2]

Those who are older also may want to supplement with a probiotic. A recent University of Reading study in the United Kingdom noted that levels of beneficial bacteria in the gut drop by 1,000 times by the age of 65.[2]

---

2 http://www.howaru.com/cms/connect/howaru/science+behind+howaru/

Cleansing

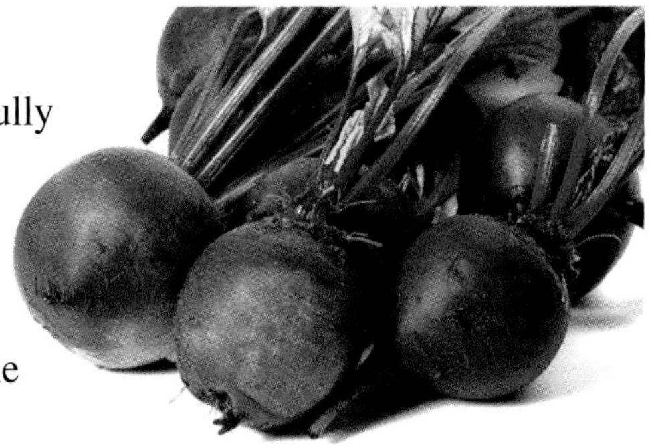

Naturally minded Christian health professionals believe the body is fearfully and wonderfully made by God and has the ability to heal itself, provided it is supplied with the nutrients it needs. Many believe that failure, at varying degrees, to eliminate waste is at the heart of all health issues. Cleaning the colon of years of impacted waste mater allows nutrients to be properly absorbed and waste material to leave the body before it has the chance to secrete toxins back into the body.

Because 70 to 80 percent of the immune system is in the digestive tract, it is imperative that we keep the digestive system clean and in top-notch working order. A clogged or sluggish colon means less nutrition for the body. Even persons switching to eating healthy raw foods, may not be absorbing the nutrients from the foods right away if their colon is clogged with built up debris from past poor eating habits.

Whenever you make a change to healthier eating habits, give your body time to adjust, cleanse and nourish.

One of the most common cancers in America is colon cancer with an estimated 150,000 or more new cases diagnosed yearly. Colorectal cancer can be chiefly related to constipation, resulting from inadequate water intake and low fiber consumption. We eat food, we extract the nutrients, and then eliminate the waste. It sounds simple. However, most Americans have one or less bowel movement per day, yet eat three to five times per day, putting them very behind on bowel movements.

Think about this. The normal amount of bowel movements should be at least two, preferably three. If a person has only one per day, then at the end of the week he is seven to fourteen behind. After a month, he is more than 28 behind. In a lifetime, Dr. Richard Schultze estimates most Americans store from 10 to 12 pounds of fecal waste in their colon and are 70,000 bowel movements behind schedule.[3] It is no wonder why digestive complaints are on the rise and why allergies and fatigue are rampant.

Allergies and respiratory issues almost always clear up when the digestive tract as a whole is cleaned through a process known as a colon cleanse. During the colon cleanse, no mucus-forming foods are consumed including milk, cheese, yogurt, sugar and ice cream. It's a small price to pay for robust, optimal health and is definitely worth it.

Colon Health Issues

According to Dr. Schultze, "Our lack of attention on good elimination and digestive health and our increased consumption of junk food has awarded Americans with the highest level of digestive disorders, bowel disease and colon cancer in the world.[4]"

Irritable Bowel Syndrome (IBS) often is signaled by bouts of constipation alternating with diarrhea. While the exact cause is not known, many experts believe it to be a stress-related issue. Children and adults with ongoing high stress levels can all fall victim to IBS. To avoid this, we should make sure our diets are the very best they can be and take time each day to relax and let the stress of the day melt away. We can take time alone to read, pray and, as the old saying goes, stop and smell the roses. Maybe take a soothing bath with therapeutic-grade essential oils in the water or diffused in the room. Also, peppermint tea can be very soothing to inflamed intestines. Everyone needs to unplug once in awhile; those who are suffering with IBS symptoms are long overdue.

---

3 American Botanical Pharmacy, Summer 2008 catalog, page 23, Natural Healing Publications, Marina Del Rey, CA
4 Dr. Schultze's News, March 2005, page 3, Natural Healing Publications, Marina Del Rey, CA

Diverticulitis is caused when harmful bacteria invade the pea-sized protrusions of the intestinal wall – called diverticula – resulting in infection and inflammation. This condition frequently appears in those suffering from constant constipation, and low fiber diets may be partially to blame. Without sufficient fiber to soften and bulk up the stool, they are harder to pass. This increased pressure to pass a stool causes pouches to form at weak points in the colons. Bacterial infection sets in and pain is the result. Adding raw garlic to salads, as toppings to vegetables or as a bread dip is a tasty way to normalize harmful gut bacteria. Garlic has long been regarded as anti-bad bacteria. It is important to slowly increase fiber and eat absolutely no junk food. During an acute attack, a soothing enema from lukewarm water and the juice of one lemon may provide relief. Therapeutic -grade essentials oils applied topically also have provided relief.[5]

Specific Digestive Disorders

Celiac
Colitis
IBS
Heartburn
Acid reflux
Diverticulitis
Gall stones
Hemorrhoids
Ulcers
Leaky gut
Crohn's
Constipation
Cramping
Diarrhea

Ulcerative colitis is a condition in which the mucus membranes lining the colon become inflamed and develop ulcers, resulting in bloody diarrhea, bloating, gas and at times hard stools. This can lead to diverticulitis. Keeping a food journal to see if there is a particular offending food may cut down on acute attacks. A person with this condition should increase plant source proteins, lightly steam vegetables, lower carbohydrate intake and eliminate all fats. Fruit is very cleansing and can trigger a bowel movement; eating fruit between meals when there is still some food residue from the past meal is helpful. Iron loss can be a problem with this group of people; eating higher iron foods, such as beets, dark green leafy foods and spinach also is beneficial. See the mineral chart in Appendix G for a complete list of foods containing iron.

Diarrhea is when the body produces extra soft stools more than four times a day (except if doing a cleanse). Dr. John Christopher said, "… diarrhea is simply a bad condition in which the intestinal tract has become badly clogged, so that all the fecal solids are being held back and only the eliminative liquids are getting through.[6]" So much mucus forming sludge lines the colon that everything eaten just slides on through. If diarrhea is a daily occurrence, increase your fiber and change your diet.

Pregnant women and infants often suffer from nausea, upset stomach, constipation and diarrhea. The book "Gentle Babies: Essential Oils and Natural Remedies for Pregnancy, Childbirth and Infant Care" by Debra Raybern provides natural solutions to these concerns.[7]

Choosing Supplements

Because the health of the colon just may be the single most important factor in your health and well being, in addition to the food suggestions and recipes in this study, see a list of colon cleansing products in Appendix DD.

Quick constipation relief may be found by drinking a large glass of warm, **lemon water** every 10 minutes for half an hour upon rising. Eating unprocessed **prunes** or **figs** can be beneficial too. Stomach crunches and abdominal exercises also may help.

Slippery elm bark is an herb the U.S. Food and Drug Administration has established as safe for use with digestive complaints. In capsules, prepared like gruel or added to a hot cereal like oatmeal, slippery elm bark is very soothing to a damaged colon. It is a gentle, non-habit forming laxative.

5 See Appendix DD for authors' recommendations.
6 "Herbal Home Health Care" Dr. John Christopher. Christopher Publications, 1976.
7 "Gentle Babies: Essential Oils and Natural Remedies for Pregnancy, Childbirth and Infant Care" Debra Raybern, N.D., M.H., C.N.C., I.C.A., Growing Healthy Homes LLC, © 2008. www.GrowingHealthyHomes.com.

There is much debate over whether or not certain herbs that promote a laxative effect are actually habit forming. If a person is constipated, the occasional use of an herbal, natural laxative will not prove harmful. As they vary in strength from mild to dynamite, one may have to experiment, start slow and build up until the desired effect is achieved. Remember, taking an herbal laxative is not license to continue poor eating habits. It can be likened to a man with a broken leg on crutches. Once the leg is healed, he can throw the crutches away.

"In my nearly 20 years of helping people, I have yet to see any of the laxative herbs – cascara sagrada, senna or others – become habit forming when used as directed while a person is transitioning to a healthier colon friendly diet that then no longer requires laxative assisting herbs." Debra Raybern, N.D.

Probiotic Supplementation

Consumer Reports showed that less than one-tenth of one percent (0.01 percent) of the bacteria in a leading probiotic yogurt reached the intestines alive. For this reason, it is vital that probiotics include cultures that are resistant to stomach and bile acids.

From millions, to billions to trillions of strains of good bacteria - or gut flora -- probiotic supplement manufacturers all want you to think theirs is the best. A probiotic supplement can be as simple as acidophilus found in yogurt or capsules taken orally. Since there are multiple strains of good gut flora, the wise and educated consumer will choose a product based on a variety of bacteria, their particular health challenge and the ability of that bacteria to actually make it past the high acid environment of the stomach and implant a productive colony in the colon, thus edging out the bad bacteria and overgrown yeast permanently.

When looking for a probiotic supplement, it should have:

- Active and viable cultures that are not subject to heat during preparation.
- Clinically proven strains at the proper amounts.
- Strains proven to adhere and colonize in the intestines.
- Super strains proven to boost immunity, improve nutrient absorption and relieve bowel distress.

Beware of taking a probiotic that recommends eight, 10, 12 or more daily; typically two to four specifically formulated capsules will do. The goal is for these super strains of bacteria to adhere to the colon wall and promote the development of good bacteria colonies.[8]

Many people with chronic colon health problems who may have impaired ability to assimilate nutrients from tablets or capsules can improve their situation by consuming freshly prepared vegetable juices. In selecting supplements, choose whole-food vitamins and minerals.

Good Colon Foods

apples, pears, beets, bananas, dried peas, okra, carrots, cabbage, barley, legumes, asparagus, figs, grapes, berries, brown rice, wheat bran, rice bran, green leafy vegetables, garlic, flax seed, chia seed, psyllium husk, aloe vera juice, green drinks or juice

Bad Colon Foods

sugar, refined white flour, excess meat, sodas, dairy, fats, spicy foods to excess, salt, coffee, drugs, alcohol, over-the-counter and prescription drugs

8 See Appendix DD for the authors' supplement recommendations.

Unit 2 Chapter 4
Discussion Questions

1. Can you think of a Bible story where long-term grain storage is mentioned?
2. What are some of the good that can cause digestive concerns? How many of these does your family consume?
3. What does it mean to supplement your diet?

Activities - plus the Spice Cookies "Power" Recipe and activities.

Elementary

1. If you made the Lemon/Lime Pickles in Chapter 2 and if it has been two weeks since you made them, try them now and compare the taste. Do they taste different? Do they taste better?
2. Using a piece of poster board, make a chart and have each member of the family place a star for each time they have a bowel movement daily. The person with the most stars at the end of the week will most likely be the healthiest. If you do not have at least 12 stars, make a list of five high fiber foods you will begin eating to increase your number of stars. When you reach 14 stars, make some Spice Cookies from the "Power" Recipe for this chapter to celebrate.
3. Find out how much each person in your family weighs and figure how much water in ounces they should drink each day.
4. Track how much water you drink each day for a week.
5. Track the fiber-rich foods you eat. Add a new one to your diet each week.

Secondary

Choose any from above plus

1. Take long balloons, equaling 30 feet, and fill with dry sand, rice, etc so that the total weight is 15 pounds. Wind the filled balloon on the body poster you made in Chapter 1 to see just how much waste matter can reside in your colon if not properly digested.
2. Create a menu of fiber-rich foods for a daily total of 20 grams. Only half of the fiber may come from grains, and there must be variety.
3. Beans are largely regarded as causing gas. Research why. Are there other foods that you enjoy that cause gas? Research these as well.
4. Read Ezekiel 4. What whole grains are listed?

Additional Resources

Web site:

http://www.howaru.com/cms/connect/howaru/howaru%20and%20your%20body/

Book:

"Inner Transformations Using Essential Oils: Powerful Cleansing Protocols for Increase Energy and Better Health" Dr. LeAnne Deardeuff, DC and Dr. David Deardeuff, DC.

Elimination Power

OATS

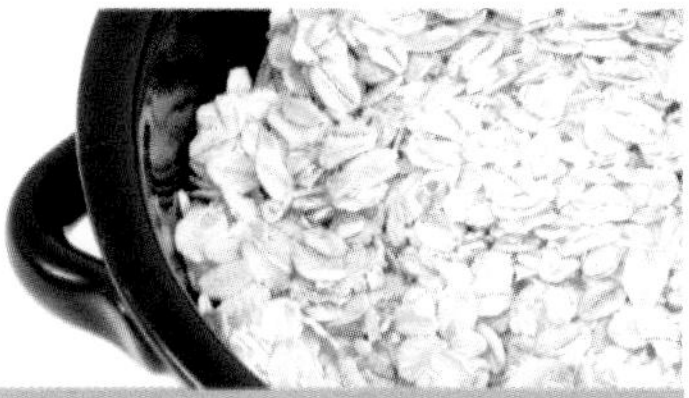

Oats are a great source of fiber for good digestive health.

Spice Cookies

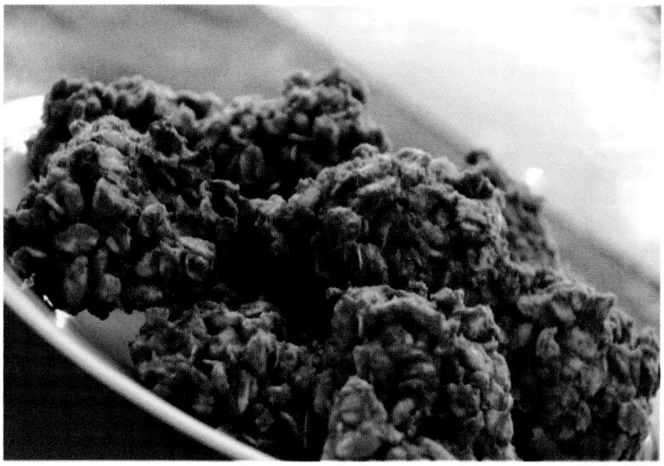

1 cup fresh milled whole wheat flour
1 cup fresh rolled oats
1 cup crispy organic rice cereal
½ tsp. baking soda
½ tsp. cream of tartar
1 tsp. cinnamon
¼ tsp. nutmeg
½ tsp. ground allspice
½ cup honey
½ cup apple sauce
1 tsp. vanilla
2 ½ ounces prune puree or one jar of prune baby food
½ cup raisins or chopped dates

Preheat oven to 350° F. In a large bowl, combine flour, oats, cereal, baking soda, cream of tartar, cinnamon, allspice and nutmeg and mix well. In a medium saucepan, combine honey, applesauce and prune puree. Bring to a boil over medium heat and simmer for one minute. Remove from heat and add the vanilla and raisins. Gently stir into cereal mixture. Drop batter by the teaspoonful onto a non-stick cookie sheet. Bake for 12 minutes. Cookies may appear undercooked, but they will get firmer as they cool. After five minutes remove from cookie sheet.

Activities

Elementary

1. How much water should you drink each day?
2. How much fiber should you consume each day?
3. Most cookies have sugar, but these do not. What makes them sweet?
4. How much water and fiber should each of your parents consume each day?
5. Using your favorite cookie recipe, modify it with some of the healthier alternatives in this recipe for a treat that is better for your body.

Secondary

Choose any from above plus

1. Complete the first and second questions in the Elementary section.
2. Calculate how much water and fiber each member of your family should consume each day.
3. Create a chart with the names of each family member and the amount of water and fiber each person should consume daily. Have each member of the family record his or her water and fiber consumption for the day for a month. At the conclusion of the month, observe how each family member did and ask each person if he or she noticed an improvement in health.

Unit 2 Additional Recipes

Use organic ingredients when possible.

Lemon/Lime Pickles (Chapter 2 Activity)

Did your mouth pucker when you read the activity's title? Well, wait until you taste them! Lemon or lime pickles are digestive enhancing pickles from India. Forget any notion you have concerning bread and butter or dill varieties, these have a distinctively bitter taste that stimulates the saliva and lets those digestive juices start flowing.

Today as people hurry here and there, many are probably guilty of eating the chomp-and-swallow way. By eating this way a person fails to masticate his or her food into small particles, and not enough saliva is mixed with the food. Eating just a small sliver of a lemon or lime pickle increases the saliva dramatically.

At first the taste is very foreign, but as you continue to eat them on a daily basis, you will come to like this unusual fruity preparation. They are extremely easy to prepare – just slice and stir. No cooking necessary.

Thanks to Debra Raybern's friends from the Montgomery Herb Growers Group for this sensational recipe.

Ingredients

6 to 8 washed lemons or limes, well dried
1 1/2 Tbs. pickling or sea salt
1 tsp. cayenne pepper powder
1 tsp. roasted fenugreek seed powder
1/2 tsp. turmeric powder
2 tsp. organic raw sugar

Pint or quart canning jars with plastic lids or a piece of sterilized muslin and a rubber band.

Preparation

Slice cleaned lemons and/or limes into eight pieces and place in a mixing bowl. Add salt, cayenne, fenugreek, turmeric and sugar. Stir all the ingredients together. Spoon into clean jars, about two thirds full. Close the jar with a plastic lid or cut a piece of muslin and cover using the rubber band to secure. Keep in a sunny location and turn jar daily to keep the spices mixed. Leave for two weeks.

The limes or lemons will begin to turn brown and most of the pulp will dissolve a few months. These never spoil and just keep getting better as they age.

Cut one of the eighth pieces of pickle into four additional pieces. One of these small pieces is what you eat, chewing slowly. You may have a second piece during the meal if desired. Jars of both lime and lemon pickles are ready to eat. No refrigeration is needed.

The **fenugreek seeds** are used for their culinary and medicinal value, and the extract is used to flavor damaged hay and is enjoyed by cattle. In India, its culinary virtues make it an important ingredient in curry powders. Today fenugreek seeds are used to provide a maple flavoring to confectionaries.

You can roast the fenugreek seed in a heavy skillet with 1 teaspoon of olive oil. They also may be roasted dry. An old herbal remedy for menstrual cramping was to swallow six fenugreek seeds with a little buttermilk and the cramping would stop in just a few minutes. In addition, they have been shown to balance blood sugar levels. The leaves of the fenugreek herb may be eaten in salads. Today many remedies for lung healing and cough expectorant formulae contain fenugreek. The seeds are rich in fiber and fixed oils. They contain choline and vitamin A. If your seeds ever smell like fish, they have turned rancid and should be thrown out.

Chopped Lettuce Salad with Mexically Topping

3 to 4 leaves of leaf lettuce (green leaf, Romaine, Red leaf, etc.)
¼ head of Iceburg lettuce

Topping:

½ fresh or frozen/thawed kernel corn
½ cup rinsed and drained black beans (may substitute garbanzos)
½ cup diced tomatoes
¼ cup finely chopped red onion
¼ cup shredded carrots
2 Tbs. fine chopped cilantro
2 Tbs. organic or homemade salsa

Chop the lettuces very fine and place a mound onto serving plates for each person. Mix the topping well and place it upon each mound of lettuce.

Raw Shredded Vegetable Salad

Yellow squash
Cucumber
Zucchini
Red radish
Carrots
Head of Romaine or Red Leaf Lettuce, washed and torn into small pieces

Shred the vegetables with a vegetable shredder or thin slicer and place in a bowl. Toss with one tablespoon olive oil and one teaspoon vinegar or two tablespoons Italian dressing. Place about ½ to one cup lettuce on the plate and top with the shredded vegetables.

Vegetarian Shepherds Pie

Topping:
2 Russet potatoes or 2 sweet potatoes
3 cloves fresh garlic, minced
½ cup kefir or buttermilk or non-fat, plain yogurt

Filling:
1 cup diced or mini carrots
¼ cup sliced celery
½ cup diced onion
1 cup zucchini, sliced
1 cup yellow squash, sliced
1 cup cauliflower pieces
1 cup broccoli pieces
1 Roma tomato, diced
1 cup eggplant, diced
2 Tbs. olive oil
¼ cup water
½ Tbs. herbal seasoning mix of your choice (Herbmare, Spike, etc.)

Wash and cook the potatoes in water until soft. Strain. Let cool slightly and remove some of the peeling. Combine with the minced garlic and kefir, milk or yogurt and mash.

Place vegetable filling (uncooked) in an oven safe baking dish. Spoon on the potato topping and spread to cover vegetables. Cook in a 375° F oven for 30 to 45 minutes or until potatoes begin to brown. Vegetables will be slightly crunchy. If you need them cooked a longer, precook the vegetables in the oven, covered for 30 minutes. Then, remove from oven, add the potato topping and return to oven for browning.

Digestive Soup

3 chopped carrots
3 stalks chopped celery
1 onion, chopped
1 Tbs. grated ginger
3 garlic cloves, minced
¼ cup miso (miso contains beneficial gut flora)

Cook the vegetables in one quart water or vegetable broth. In the last five minutes, add the miso.

Rejuvalac

½ gallon Mason Jar
2 cups whole wheat berries (soft wheat preferred, but not required)
½ gallon purified water

Combine wheat and water in a glass jar with cheesecloth lid fastened by a rubber band or the jar lid rim. Let sit in the refrigerator for 10 to 15 hours. Remove and strain off the water and discard the water. Do not rinse the wheat berries.

Return the wheat berries to the jar, then allow to sprout for two days on countertop, not the refrigerator. Keep covered with the cheesecloth and do not rinse. When white sprout tails begin to show, add six cups purified water, cover jar with cheesecloth, put in a warm place where it can be exposed to at least 70° temperature for 2 days.

Then pour off liquid Rejuvelac into another jar. Cover and refrigerate; it will keep for several days. Then leftover wheat berries can be composted, or thrown to the birds. This is to be consumed by the tablespoonful and supplies the body with excellent pre-biotic cultures to aid in gut health. Rejuvelac should be served at room temperature.

Hot Blender Raw Soup

Eating more raw foods may be easy in the hot summer months, but harder in the cold winter months. This easy soup makes it easy to eat raw and still have a satisfying warm soup.

Warm one quart of vegetable or chicken broth on the stove until very hot. While heating, slice or dice two cups raw vegetables into very small pieces. These can include carrots, yellow and zucchini squash, green beans, spinach, etc. Add the hot broth to a blender with the chopped vegetables and whiz until pureed. For added texture you may add in at the final 30 seconds of blending some precooked rice or noodles. The addition of spices – Italian or Mexican – will change up the flavor to accompany any entree.

Whole Wheat Cinnamon Rolls

2 tsp. active dry yeast (SAF brand is recommended.)
2 cups warm water
6 ½ to 7 cups finely ground whole white wheat or store-bought organic bread whole wheat flour
2 Tbs. honey
2 Tbs. olive oil
¼ tsp. salt

butter
organic brown sugar
organic cinnamon
raisins

Combine the water, oil, salt, honey and three cups of the flour in a mixing bowl. Set on medium speed and mix for one minute. Add yeast, mix one minute and let stand one minute. Begin mixing and add the remaining flour one cup at a time. When the sides of the bowl are clean, stop adding flour. (Some mixers do not perform as the Bosch Universal, for which this recipe was prepared.) Do not exceed the seven cups of flour. Knead (mix) for a total of 10 minutes. Remove from the bowl onto an oiled, not floured surface. Using a rolling pin, roll out the dough to a large rectangle. Spread with a little butter, organic brown sugar, cinnamon and raisins. Roll it up to form a long roll and lightly mark with a knife into 12 rolls. Use dental floss to slide under the dough and cross over to cut. This avoids pressing down the dough. Place in a greased baking dish and bake for 25 to 30 minutes at 350° F.

Unit 3

The Respiratory, Olfactory, Auditory and Visual Systems

We hope and pray learning about nutrition and its impact on our health these past two units has been a delicious and nutritious experience. As we enter the halfway point of this health program and food adventure, participants should be experiencing improved health. We will now learn about the respiratory, olfactory, visual and auditory systems.

For some families, after completing the chapter on the respiratory system, the information learned and implemented will do way more than enhance the quality of life. The millions affected by allergies, asthma or other respiratory conditions may be able to reduce or even eliminate the use of prescription medicines and breathe easy.

After studying the olfactory chapter, the nose may look a bit different. No longer will it just be a pointy or flat or rounded protrusion in the middle of the face, but an awesome creation that is capable of distinguishing scents, enhancing taste and unlocking memories.

Sometimes when we listen to a recording of our voices, it doesn't sound right. A person might say, "That isn't me!" But it is, and it does sound like her – at least the way everyone else is accustomed to hearing her voice. The reason the voice does not sound the same to her on tape as it does when she hears herself is because of the two sets of ears she has. That's right. Not because she has two ears; rather because she – and we – have two sets of ears. They are called the outer ear and inner ear. The outer ear is the portion we can all see, and the inner ear is comprised of the boney parts inside the head. We'll learn more about the parts of the ear in Chapter 3 of this unit.

When a person speaks, he gets some sound through the outer ear, but most of the sound comes through the inner ear. That is why if he plugs his ear and speaks, he will notice the sound is louder because he is stopping up the outer ear. The Bible has something very important to say about the way we hear: In Romans 10:7, the apostle Paul wrote, "Faith cometh by hearing and hearing by the word of God." God designed our bodies in such a way that the words we speak are picked up by the inner ear and go directly to the human spirit and build our faith.

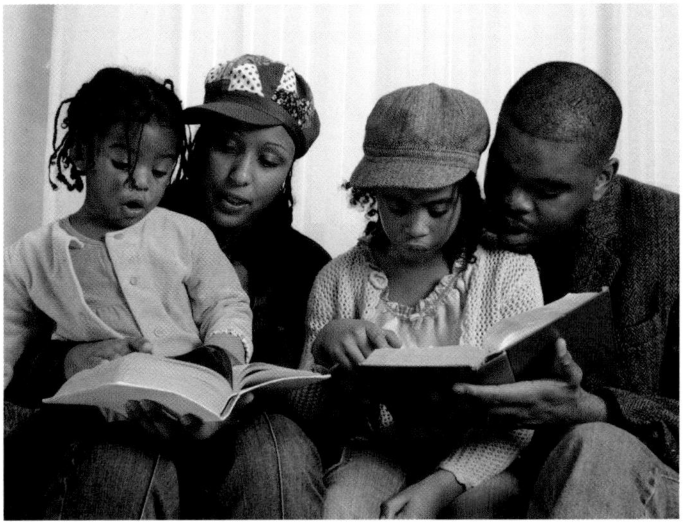

So how can we be doers of the word, not hearers only? We've learned about making good food choices, but it is important that our actions align with our words and the word of God. Hebrews 4:12 says "For the word of God is quick, and powerful, and sharper than any two edged sword, piercing even to the dividing asunder of soul and spirit, and of the joints and marrow, and is a discerner of the thoughts and intents of the heart." Has this program been challenging? Sometimes the old habits or our bodies or minds try to fight the healthy changes that we implement. As we make a physical transformation, we must align our words and actions. Speak His word and ask Him to help you make healthy choices. Read His word and see what the Bible can teach you about speaking it.

Chapter 1

The Respiratory System

"And the Lord God formed man of the dust of the ground, and breathed into his nostrils the breath of life; and man became a living soul." Genesis 2:7

Breathe in … breathe out … breathe in … breathe out. The function of our lungs is to expand, drawing in air full of life-giving oxygen, and then contract, expelling carbon dioxide. We could live for weeks without food, days without water, but only a matter of minutes without air. Whether we are sleeping or awake, we do not have to think about breathing. It is so vital to life that God created it to happen automatically.

Respiration is the process of the lungs expanding and contracting, which we know as breathing. It takes place about 12 times per minute. When we exercise or perform other vigorous activity, the rate can increase to 80 times per minute. Considering all the organs in the body, only the heart works harder than the lungs.

Each day you breathe about 20,000 times. By age 70 you have taken at least 600 million breaths.

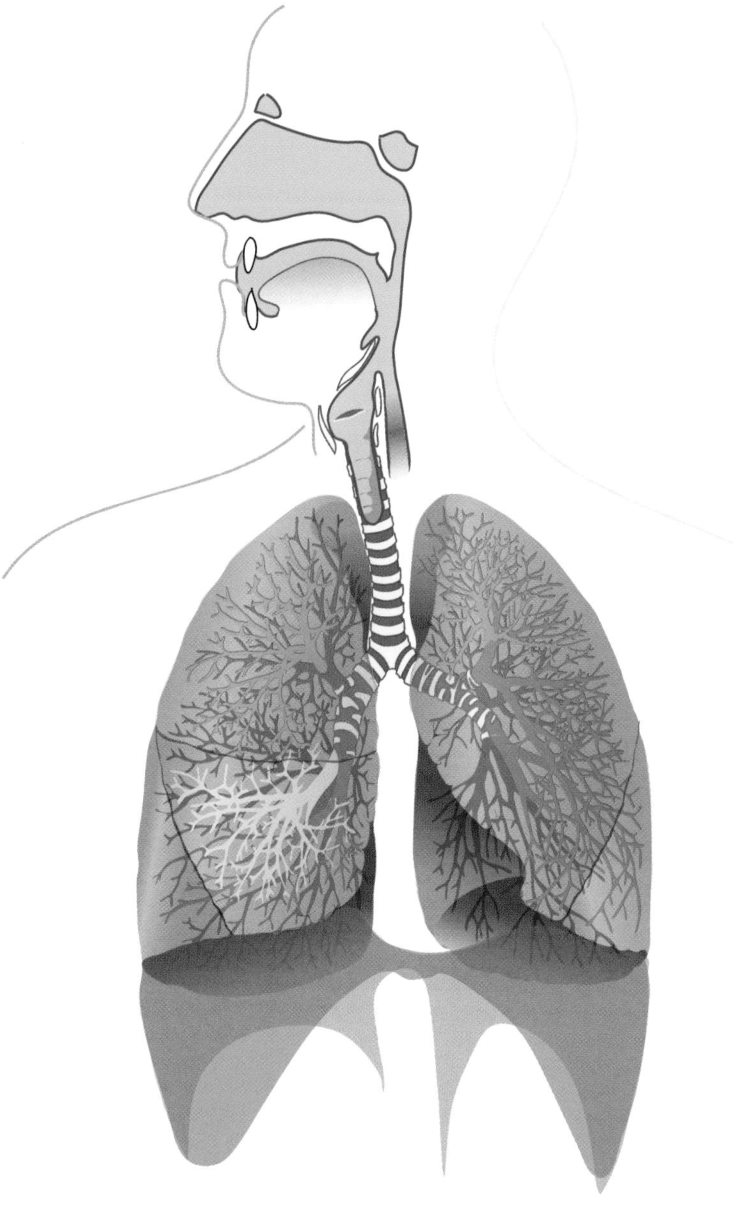

Because of our respiratory system, every cell in our bodies get oxygen, which is essential for them to live and function. Without the oxygen, the cells would die, and we would die. Our respiratory system refreshes our cells by eliminating waste gases known as carbon dioxide, which is a by-product of the energy-making process of the body. If these gases stayed in our bodies, we would die.

The air we breathe is vital to the health of our bodies. Oxygen makes up about one-fifth of the air, while nitrogen makes up the rest. Microscopic amounts of bacteria, mold, dust, toxins, pollen and viruses also are found in the air. As these microorganisms are inhaled, they can lead to respiratory infections and cause lung inflammation and tissue damage. So the quality of the air we breathe also is vital to the health of our bodies.

Nutrition plays an important role in the function of the respiratory system. But to understand how food affects our respiratory systems, we must first understand how it works.

Fun Fact

While most people can only hold their breath less than a minute, swimmers can hold their breath up to a couple of minutes.
David Blaine recently set the world record by holding his breath for 17 minutes 4.4 seconds.
Don't try this at home without adult supervision!

What are the parts of the Respiratory System and what do they do?

The respiratory tract is divided into two sections, the upper respiratory tract and the lower respiratory tract. The upper respiratory tract includes the nasal cavity, pharynx and larynx. The lower respiratory tract includes the trachea, bronchi and lungs.

Nasal Cavity

The nasal passage or **nasal cavity** includes the nose and the space directly behind the nose. When we breathe, we inhale air through our noses or our mouth or a combination of both. Ideally, we should breathe through our noses. Tiny hairs in the nose called **cilia** trap and filter unwanted particles. Sticky mucus lines the nasal passages and catches these particles and even many germs before they can enter too far into the respiratory system. The mucus also warms and moistens the air. Warming the air during extremely cold weather is very important. Otherwise, super cold air would damage the lining of the lungs.

Pharynx

The **pharynx** is part of the digestive system and the respiratory system. It is the part of the neck and throat that lies behind the nasal cavity and mouth and just above the esophagus and trachea (or windpipe). Both food and air pass through this space. If food or liquid passes through the pharynx, a flap called the **epiglottis** closes over the trachea so the food doesn't go into the lungs. If air passes through the pharynx, the epiglottis stays open and the air is directed down through the trachea.

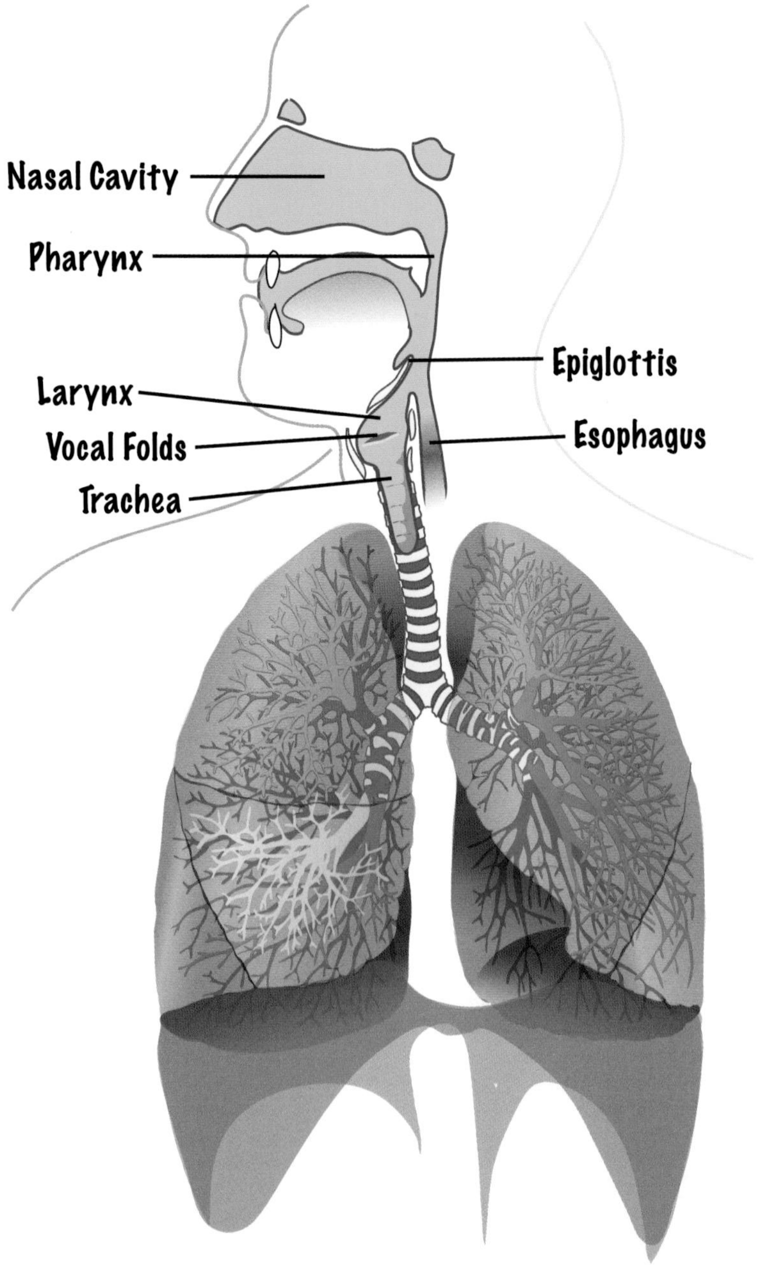

Larynx

The **larynx** is a short tube that lies just below where the esophagus and trachea split and at the top of the trachea. Also known as the **voicebox**, the larynx houses the vocal cords, or **vocal folds**, which vibrate to produce sound. If food or ingested material gets past the epiglottis, it stimulates the larynx to create a coughing reflex to protect the lungs.

Trachea

The **trachea** also is known as the **windpipe**. It is lined with stiff rings of cartilage to keep it open and measures approximately 13 centimeters in length, with half its length in the neck and the other half in the chest. The lower end of the trachea divides into two tubes called **bronchi** that carry air into the lungs. The trachea also is lined with **cilia**, which filters air and keeps fluids and foreign particles from going into the lungs.

Bronchi

The **bronchi** are two air tubes that branch off the trachea and carry air directly into the lungs. One bronchus goes into the right lung and the other into the left lung. Each bronchus divides into smaller tubes called **bronchioles**.

Fun Fact
The network of alveoli, bronchioles and bronchi is known as the bronchial tree.

At the end of the bronchioles are the **alveoli.** The alveoli are tiny, stretchy air sacs where gas exchange occurs with the blood. These sacs blow up like tiny balloons during inhalation. In a process called **diffusion**, oxygen from the air passes through the walls of the alveoli to the blood through blood vessels, also known as **capillaries**, lining the alveolar walls while carbon dioxide is exchanged. The alveoli contain white blood cells (macrophages) that ingest and destroy the airborne bacteria, fungi, viruses and other microorganisms that are inhaled. The process of filtering out contaminants can be thwarted by the inhalation of substances such as gases, fumes, chemicals or mineral dust. These pollutants increase immune response, which increases inflammation to the lungs, the heart and arteries. Anything inhaled enters the bloodstream within seconds. For these reasons we need to pay more attention to the air in our homes, vehicles, offices and environment. Inhaled irritants also include perfumes, fragrances in soaps, detergents, air fresheners and household cleaning agents.

Lungs

As the largest organ inside the body, the our **lungs** contain about 300 to 400 million alveoli and elastic tissues that allow the lungs to inflate and deflate without loosing their shape or collapsing. The lungs, along with all the elastic tissues, are encased by a thin lining called **pleura**.

Fun Fact
Your lungs contain almost 1,500 miles of airways!

The lungs and respiratory system allow oxygen in the air to be taken into the body during inhalation, while enabling the body to get rid of carbon dioxide during exhalation. **Carbon dioxide** is the waste gas produced when carbon is combined with oxygen as part of the energy-making processes of the body.

The **hemoglobin** in red blood cells in the capillaries is responsible for picking up the oxygen and carrying this oxygen to the cells that need it. They then pick up carbon dioxide, which is transported back through the bronchi and trachea for exhalation.

Virtually all the body's blood travels through the lungs every minute.

The lungs add and remove many chemical messengers from the blood as it flows through the **pulmonary capillary bed**, a network of blood vessels that supply an organ. The oxygen-rich blood flows back to the heart, which pumps it through the arteries to oxygen-hungry

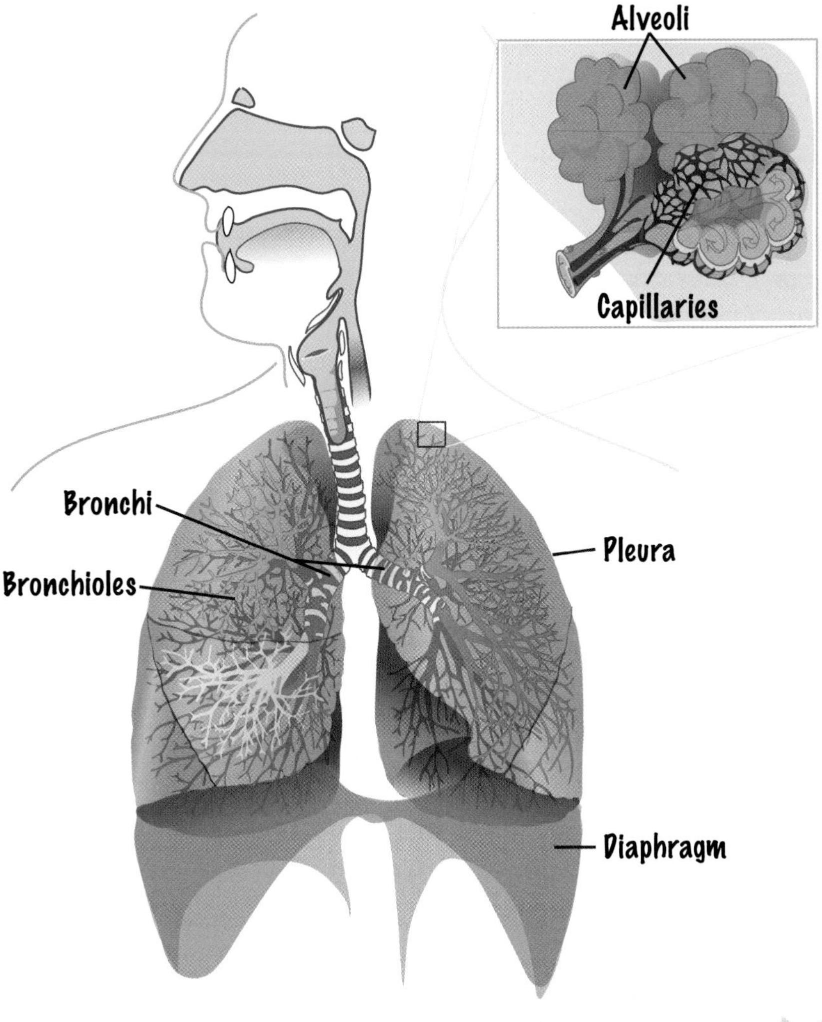

tissues throughout the body. In the tiny capillaries of the body tissues, oxygen is freed from the hemoglobin and moves into the cells. Blood rich in carbon dioxide then returns to the heart via the veins. From the heart, this blood is pumped to the lungs, where carbon dioxide passes into the alveoli to be exhaled. This process will be discussed further in the Cardiovascular Unit.

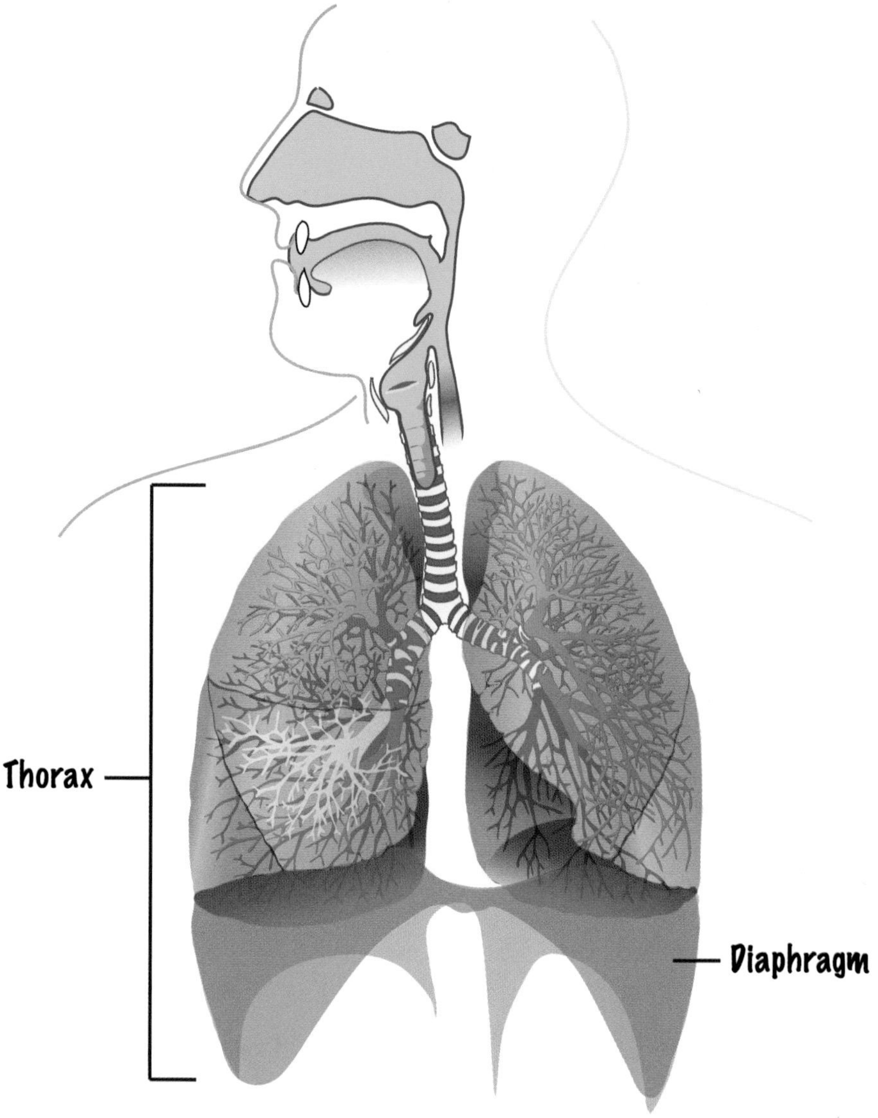

Diaphragm

The **diaphragm** is the dome-shaped muscle at the bottom of the lungs where breathing begins. As we inhale, the diaphragm contracts while flattening out and pulling downward. This movement enlarges the space where the lungs sit in the abdomen so that air can be pulled into the lungs. When we exhale, the diaphragm expands while reducing the space for the lungs and forcing air out. The diaphragm is the main muscle involved in breathing and separates the chest from the abdomen.

Enclosed in the rib cage is the chest cavity or **thorax**. This is an airtight box that houses the bronchial tree, lungs, heart, and other structures. The top and sides of the thorax are formed by the ribs and attached muscles, and the bottom is formed by the diaphragm. The chest walls form a protective cage around the lungs and other contents of the chest cavity.

Have you ever had the hiccups?

Hiccups are the sudden movement of the diaphragm. This action is completely involuntary. A person has no control over hiccups. Many causes are listed for hiccups: eating too fast, getting irritated and even a substance in the blood have been implicated. Are there any cures? Everything from sipping water, holding your breath, breathing into a paper bag and eating a spoonful of sugar have all been tried to put a stop to this nuisance. Usually, you'll just have to wait, and they will subside on their own.

Fun Fact

Charles Osborn was recorded by the *Guinness World Book of Records* with the longest attack of hiccups. The hiccups started in 1922 at a rate of 40 times per minute, slowed to 20 hiccups per minute and lasted 68 years while eventually stopping on June 5, 1990, for an estimated total of 430 million times.

How do you breathe? Deep or shallow?

Oxygen is vital to good health. Shallow breathing starves the body of oxygen. When only ¼ to ½ of the lungs is used to breathe, cells cannot function properly. Without sufficient oxygen, the body cannot even utilize food that is eaten, no matter how nourishing it may be.

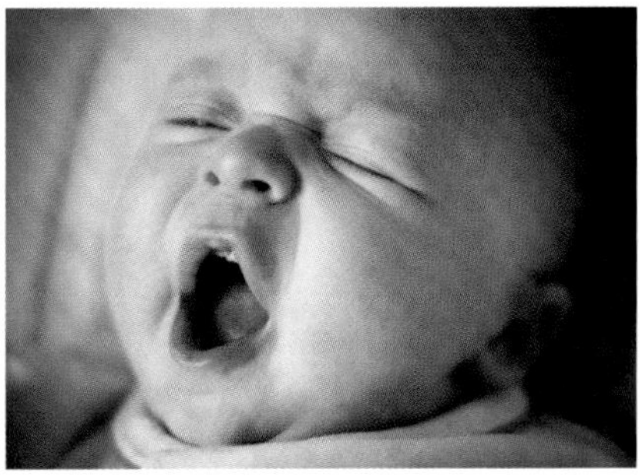

Yawning

When you are sleepy you may yawn. Do you know why? When you begin to get sleepy, respiration begins to slow down resulting in a little less oxygen being inhaled into the lungs. This causes an oxygen shortage. When the brain senses this, it sends a message to the lungs that causes a deep long breath called a Y-A-W-N.

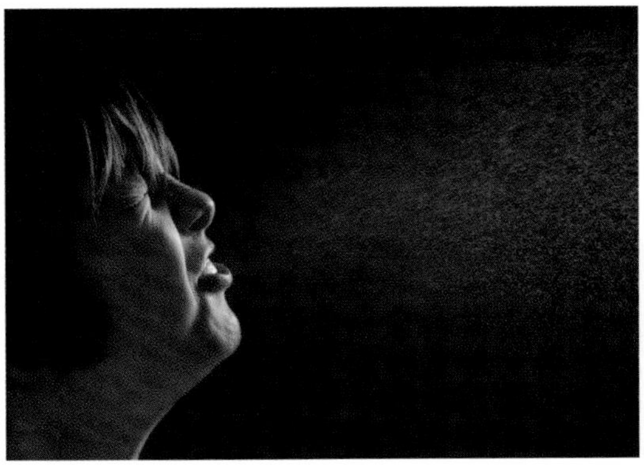

Sneezing

Sneezing is actually a cough in the upper respiratory system. It is the body's way of removing an irritant from the mucus membranes of the nose. These could be pollen, mold, dust and powders. Sometimes even a cold blast of air can cause a person to sneeze.

Fun Facts

A sneeze can blast out of your nose at a speed greater than 100 mph!
When you sneeze, all bodily functions stop, even your heart!
The average cough comes out of the mouth at 60 mph.

Coughing

Coughing happens in the lower respiratory tract in the lungs. Just as with sneezing, a cough is the body's way to remove an inhaled irritant. A cough also can be the body ridding itself of germs and accumulated mucus.

Problems of the Lungs and Respiratory System

The respiratory system is susceptible to a number of diseases, and the lungs are prone to a wide range of disorders caused by pollutants in the air. Health concerns of the lungs include allergies, asthma, cancer, colds, COPD, coughs, emphysema and whooping cough. Although some respiratory diseases may not be prevented, many chronic lung and respiratory illnesses can be prevented by avoiding smoking, staying away from pollutants and irritants, and practicing good hygiene. This includes washing hands often to control the spread of germs[1]. Some of the most common problems of the respiratory system are:

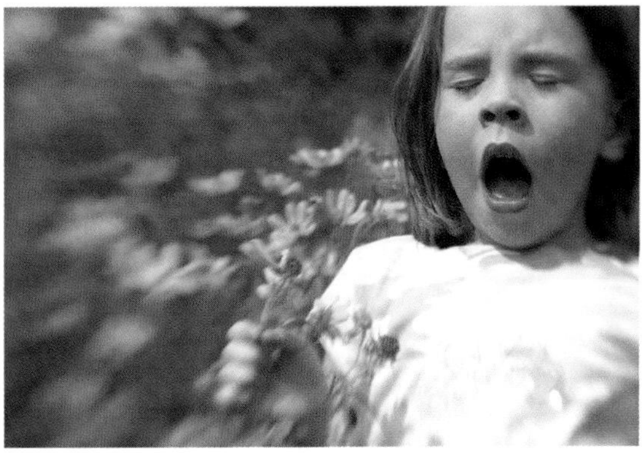

Allergies are really just an over reaction of the body's immune system to what is otherwise a normally harmless substances like mold, dust, pollen and animal dander. The body responds as if these substances were invaders wanting to do harm. The body sends out a barrage of antibodies to attack, which in turn triggers a cascade of inflammatory responses. This inflammation constricts airways and nasal passages making it hard to breathe. The cough is the body trying to expel the invader. Sniffing, sneezing, coughing, watery eyes and post nasal drip are all symptoms of allergies.

---

1 Be sure to wash hands with a pure hand soap. Many of the "antibacterial" hand soaps contain triclosan which can turn into the deadly poison dioxin when exposed to excessive heat or sunlight. ("Green This!" by Deirdre Imus. Simon & Schuster. 2007.)

Asthma affects more than 20 million people in the United States and is the number one reason that children miss school.[2] Asthma is chronic inflammatory lung disease that causes the airways to tighten and narrow. Often triggered by irritants in the air such as cigarette smoke, asthma episodes involve contraction and swelling of the muscles lining the tiny airways. The resulting narrowing of the airways prevents air from flowing properly, causing wheezing and difficulty breathing, sometimes to the point of being life-threatening. Controlling asthma usually involves avoiding asthma triggers, including chemical and airborne irritants. For more information about asthma and nutrition, see Appendix Q.

Respiratory syncytial virus (RSV) affects mostly infants and young children, and can cause wheezing and serious difficulty breathing.

Chronic obstructive pulmonary disease (COPD) is a term that describes two lung diseases: emphysema and chronic bronchitis. Emphysema is most often caused from long-term smoking. In emphysema, the lungs produce an excessive amount of mucus and the alveoli become damaged. It becomes difficult to breathe and get enough oxygen into the blood. In **bronchitis**, a common disease of adults and adolescents, the membranes lining the larger bronchial tubes become inflamed and an excessive amount of mucus is produced. A bad cough is developed as the body tries to get rid of the mucus. Cigarette smoke is a major cause of chronic bronchitis in teens.

The **common cold** is caused by over 200 different viruses, which result in inflammation in the upper respiratory tract. It is the most common respiratory infection. Symptoms may include a mild fever, cough, headache, runny nose, sneezing and sore throat.

A **cough** is actually a symptom of an illness, not an illness itself. There are many different types of coughs and many different causes, ranging from not-so-serious to life-threatening. Some of the more common causes affecting children are the common cold, asthma, sinusitis, seasonal allergies, croup and pneumonia. Among the most serious causes of cough are tuberculosis (TB) and whooping cough (pertussis).

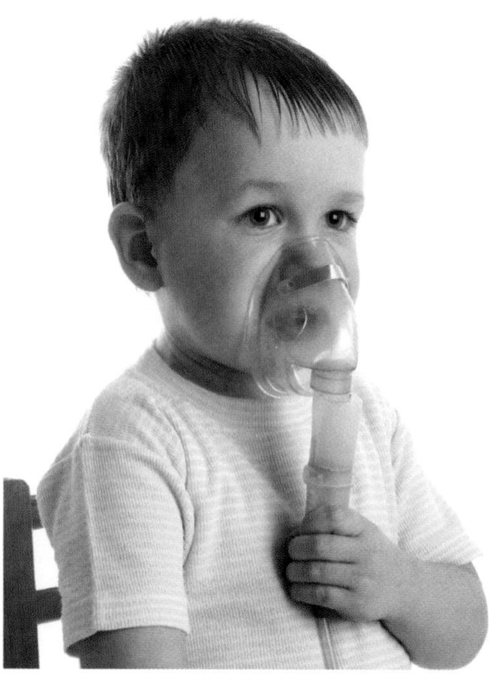

Affecting more than 30,000 children and young adults in the United States, **cystic fibrosis (CF)** is the most common inherited disease affecting the lungs. Affecting primarily the respiratory and digestive systems, CF causes mucus in the body to be abnormally thick and sticky. The mucus can clog the airways in the lungs and make a person more vulnerable to bacterial infections.

Caused by an abnormal growth of cells in the lungs usually due to smoking cigarettes, **lung cancer** is a leading cause of death in the United States. It starts in the lining of the bronchi and takes a long time to develop. Symptoms include a persistent cough that may expel blood and produce chest pain, hoarseness and shortness of breath. Exposure to radon gas, a gas that occurs in soil and rocks, also may be a cause of lung cancer. Radon is more likely to occur in certain parts of the United States. Radon levels in the home are detected by purchasing a radon kit at a local home supply or hardware store. Refer to Appendix W for more cancer information.

2 American Academy of Allergy Asthma and Immunology http://www.aaaai.org/media/resources/media_kit/asthma_statistics.stm

Pneumonia is inflammation of the lungs caused by bacterial or viral infection. It causes fever and inflammation of lung tissue and makes breathing difficult because the lungs have to work harder to transfer oxygen into the bloodstream and remove carbon dioxide from the blood. Common causes of pneumonia are the influenza virus or infection from the bacterium *Streptococcus pneumoniae*.

Pulmonary hypertension is the condition when the blood pressure in the arteries of the lungs is abnormally high. This means the heart has to work harder to pump blood against the high pressure. Pulmonary hypertension may occur in children because of a heart defect present at birth or because of a health condition such as HIV infection.

How does food affect the Respiratory System?

Good nutrients for the respiratory system include Vitamin A and C, magnesium, zinc and antioxidants.

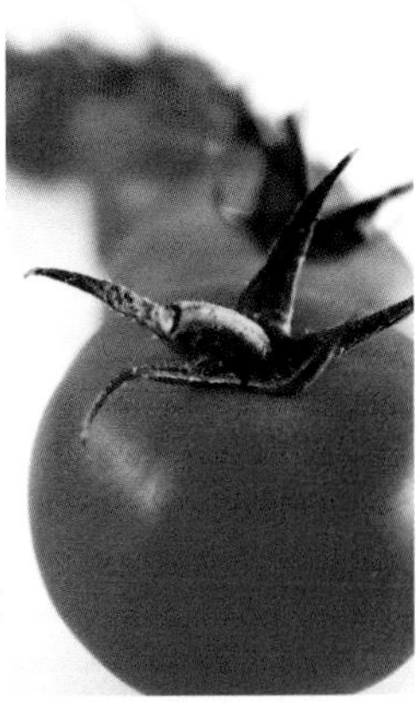

Vitamin A is good for respiratory health, since it is instrumental for the growth and development of tissues lining the lungs. Recent research also suggests that Vitamin A protects the lungs from the damaging effects of smoking.

Vitamin C boosts the immune system and is often suggested as a nutritional supplement along with **zinc** to help bring relief to allergy sufferers.[3]

Beta-cryptoxanthin, a powerful carotenoid antioxidant, has been found to be especially protective in lung health and is found in abundance in winter squash. Increasing the intake of beta-cryptoxanthan foods has a significant effect on reducing the risk of developing lung cancer.

Beta-cryptoxanthin Foods

Cilantro, citrus fruits, oranges, papaya, red bell peppers, watermelon, and winter squash

Magnesium is a nerve and muscle relaxer which can help open bronchial passages in the lungs.

Magnesium Rich Foods

Broccoli, pumpkin seeds, spinach, summer squash, and Swiss chard

Lycopene, which is available naturally in **tomatoes**, has been shown to be beneficial to persons with exercise-induced asthma.

Bad Foods for the Respiratory System

Some foods may cause excess mucus in the respiratory tract. These include dairy products, sugar, bananas, chocolate and refined, fried and junk foods.

Dairy

Dairy is mucus forming. Dairy products made from pasteurized cow's milk are very mucus forming. This includes milk, ice cream, cheese, sour cream and yogurt. It will take about three months of absolutely no dairy to completely cleanse the lungs of mucus and therefore show positive results in asthma-related symptoms, but the person will begin to realize relief much sooner. Lemon, anise and fennel are foods known to reduce bronchial mucus. Eating a more alkaline diet also is helpful.

What about calcium intake? Milk is not the best choice. It is possible to get the calcium needed without dairy products, contrary to the statements by the milk and dairy industry.

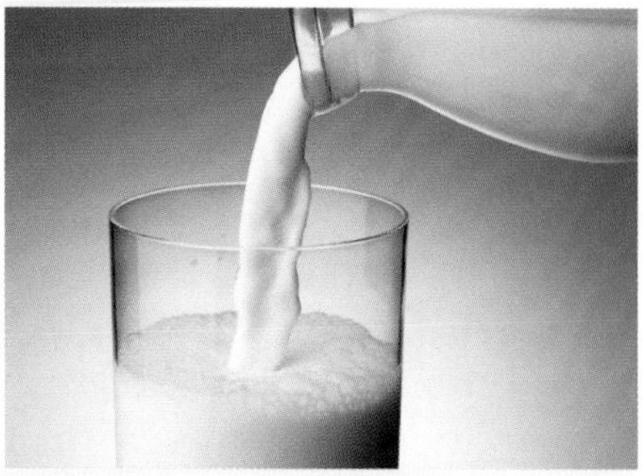

Many vegetables even contain calcium, particularly green leafy vegetables like spinach, turnip greens, mustard greens and collard greens. Nuts are an amazing powerhouse of usable calcium.

One cup of sesame seeds gives 2,200 mg of calcium. In contrast, one cup of whole milk delivers just 288 mg. Sesame seeds can be used as nut butter, sprinkled over vegetables, ground and used in casseroles. The uses are endless and with such a mild taste, everyone is sure to enjoy them.

Sugar

Sugar suppresses the immune system function and is very acid (inflammatory) and mucus forming. Don't just switch to raw sugar, maple syrup, agave or honey; instead curb a sweet tooth with fresh fruit (see the recommended fruit servings in Appendix B: **Nutrition 101: Choose Life!** Food Guide Pyramid). An occasional treat is not the offender, but the problem is daily consumption of sugar from food and drink.

Cleansing

The inside of the body can be cleansed by doing various cleansing routines to help remove the old toxic buildup.[3] Enzymes are great at cleaning up undigested proteins that can cause inflammation. (See Appendix CC for enzyme information.) A good Omega-3 supplement can fight inflammation further.[3] Increase your raw food consumption to at lease 60 percent raw and 40 percent cooked.

Food in general should be made from scratch using only whole food ingredients. Fresh, raw or lightly steamed fruits and vegetables are more beneficial than when processed or cooked.

Good Food for the Respiratory System

Apples, carrots, citrus fruit, garlic, lemons, limes, onions, papaya, spinach, tomatoes

Bad Food and Items for the Respiratory System

Alcohol, artificial colors and flavors, artificial sweeteners, caffeine, cakes, candy, dairy products, fried foods, red meat, household chemical cleaners, artificial room air fresheners

Household Toxins

Keeping the home free of chemical toxins and irritants can greatly improve home air quality, which results in a better environment for those with respiratory concerns including asthma and allergies. We do not have to forfeit quality and germ-fighting ability by replacing toxic household cleaners for safer, toxic-free cleaners.

Some common household items can be used when cleaning the kitchen, bath, flooring and carpets. Borax, baking soda, cornstarch, white vinegar, distilled water and a supply of a few specific essential oils[3] can keep the home clean, green and toxin free. Essential oils used in cleaning include: lemon, lavender, thyme, rosemary and cedarwood.

3 See Appendix DD for authors' supplement recommendations.

Environmental Changes for Respiratory Health

1. Carpets, upholstery in furniture, drapes and curtains, bedding and mattresses all harbor dust and dust mites. Cleaning carpets two to three times per year and vacuuming with an advanced HEPA (high efficiency particulate air) or water filtration cleaner will dramatically cut down on the number of allergens floating within a home.
2. Dust with a slightly damp cloth (see dusting formula below), so that dust does not just float around to land somewhere else.
3. Air conditioning filters should be changed regularly and upgraded to allergen trapping models.
4. Mattresses should be covered with dust mite protective covers. Stay away from foam mattresses or pads as they breakdown over time and emit small particles of chemical foam into the air. Replace mattresses over ten years old.
5. No smoking for anyone in an asthmatic household.
6. Use chemical-free products throughout the home for cleaning, bathing, skin care etc.
7. Change out landscaping for non-pollinating plants and shrubs.
8. Deep clean closets and shelving at least twice per year, as dust can collect, especially on books.
9. Clean the air in the home by diffusing therapeutic-grade essential oils. Please do not think that the air fresheners bought at the store have anything but detrimental effects with allergies as they contain many synthetic and even toxic substances.

Dusting Recipe 1

2 drops Young Living thyme essential oil[4]
4 drops Young Living lemon essential oil
1-2 Tbs. olive oil, or walnut oil

Combine in a small spray bottle, spray cloth and dust.

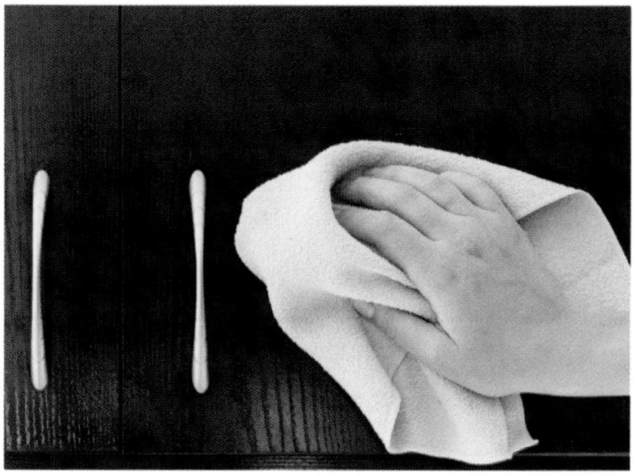

Dusting Recipe 2 - more of a cleaner and duster combo

½ cup Young Living Bath and Shower gel base, unscented
3/4 cup water
5 drop Young Living orange essential oil
20 drops Young Living cedarwood essential oils

Combine in a spray bottle. It works great for kitchen cabinets, tables, bookcases, etc.

---

4 Use only Young Living® therapeutic-grade essential oils which are completely unadulterated and have antiseptic properties. Unlike essential oils found in health food stores, Young Living® essential oils may be ingested, applies topically and inhaled for therapeutic purposes.

Unit 3 Chapter 1
Discussion Questions

1. What does inhale mean? What does exhale mean? Demonstrate.
2. How long can you safely hold your breath? Have your mom or dad time you.
3. What kind of air is in a balloon that you blow up? Oxygen? Carbon Dioxide?
4. God made plants for us for so many reasons. Can you name some of the reasons?
5. Find two scriptures in the Bible that tell why God gave us plants.

Activities - plus the No Dairy No Chocolate "Chocolate" Pudding "Power" Recipe and activities.

Elementary

1. Name three professions you think require good lung function.
2. Name three professions that deal with the lungs or the air we breathe.
3. Count how many breaths you take while in a rest in mode. Now count your breaths after running in place for 30 seconds, and one minute. CAUTION: Make sure your children are fit enough to perform this task.
4. Using a tape measure, stretch it around the chest and see how many inches it measures when you inhale verses exhale.
5. Look at a map, find New York City, and then using the map key find a location 1,500 miles away from it. Then, measure 1,500 miles away from your home.
6. Go to http://www.vtaide.com/png/assess.htm, and take the respiratory quiz at the bottom of the page.

Secondary

Choose any from above plus

1. Considering that you breathe about 20,000 times a day, calculate how many times you have breathed in your life.
2. Choose a food that you have never tried that is rich in beta-cryptoxanthin. If you have tried them all, choose your favorite if it is in season.
3. Choose a food that you have never tried that is rich in magnesium. If you have tried them all, choose your favorite if it is in season.
4. Make the Super Tonic recipe from the "Additional Recipes" section for Unit 3. Follow the directions and then try it in two weeks. What do you think of the taste? How did it make you feel? Try it each day for a few weeks and keep a log of how it makes you feel.

Additional Resources

Books:

1. "Super Power Breathing for Super Energy" Paul C. & Patricia Bragg, Health Science, 1999.
2. "The Naturally Clean Home" Storey Books, 1999.
3. "Clean and Green" Diedra Imas, 2007.

Web sites:

1. http://www.imcpl.org/kids/guides/health/respiratorysystem.html
2. http://yucky.discovery.com/flash/body/pg000138.html

Respiratory System Power

Blue Agave Carob Avocados

Raw Blue Agave Nectar is a wonderful alternative to mucus forming sugar. Plus, it is low glycemic. See the Glycemic Index Chart in Unit 5.

Carob is a great alternative to chocolate in that it contains no caffeine, which can cause excess mucus.

In this recipe, avocados provide the smooth, creamy texture in place of mucus forming cream and milk found in traditional puddings. Plus, it has healthy brain power fat.

No Dairy No Chocolate "Chocolate" Pudding

Your family will never guess that the main ingredient in this dairy-free recipe is avocados. Your respiratory system and brain will thank you for it.

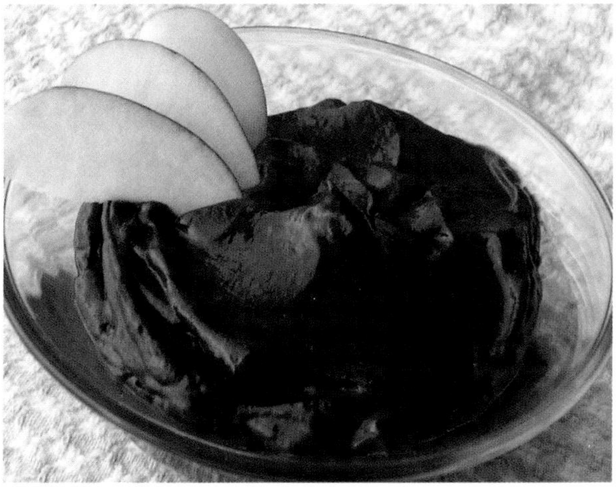

2 small ripe avocados
½ to ¾ cup Blue Agave Nectar
¼ cup carob powder
2 Tbs. coconut milk or rice milk
1 Tbs. organic vanilla extract
Pinch of sea salt
Pinch of cinnamon (optional)

Make sure the avocados are ripe, as unripened avocados will change the flavor. Place ingredients in a high-power blender or food processor and blend on high until smooth. Chill until serving. Double the recipe for an amazing icing or pie filling. Makes about two cups.

Activities

Elementary

1. Before making this recipe, write down what you think this will taste like. After you try the pudding, compare it to what you thought it would be like. How is it different from other puddings that you've had?
2. What does it mean for fruit to be ripe? Why would the flavor change if the fruit was not ripe?
3. Research more about carob powder. What are its nutritional values versus cocoa?
4. At the grocery store, look at the ingredients list of a regular package of pudding. What type of sugar is listed? What type of dairy is listed? Are there any other ingredients you should avoid based on the list of bad foods for the respiratory system in Unit 3 Chapter 1?

Secondary

Choose any from above plus

1. Why does this recipe call for coconut milk? What other non-dairy substitutions would work?
2. How can you incorporate non-dairy substitutes in other recipes?
3. At the grocery store, check the salt packaging for the ingredients. What do they contain besides salt? Write down any additional ingredients that you have never heard of and find out what it is and why it is included. Determine whether or not it is good or bad for you.

Chapter 2

The Olfactory System and The Nose

"And he shall take of it his handful, of the flour of the meat offering, and of the oil thereof, and all the frankincense which is upon the meat offering, and shall burn it upon the altar for a sweet savour, even the memorial of it, unto the Lord." Leviticus 6:15

Bread baking in the oven. The fresh air after the rain. Fresh towels from the laundry. Many scents, or odors, fill our lives every day. Odors can alert us to danger, as in the case of smoke. They can give us pleasure and enhance mealtime as we smell the various aromas of our food. In fact, the flavor we describe from food actually comes from the food odor molecules wafting up the nose.

When we breathe, we can feel the lungs expand and contract. This action is observed as the chest moves in and out. What we do not notice is what goes on in the nose before air or odors (good or bad) arrive in the lungs. The act of smelling, or the sense of smell, is called **olfaction** and involves the detection and perception of chemicals floating in the air.

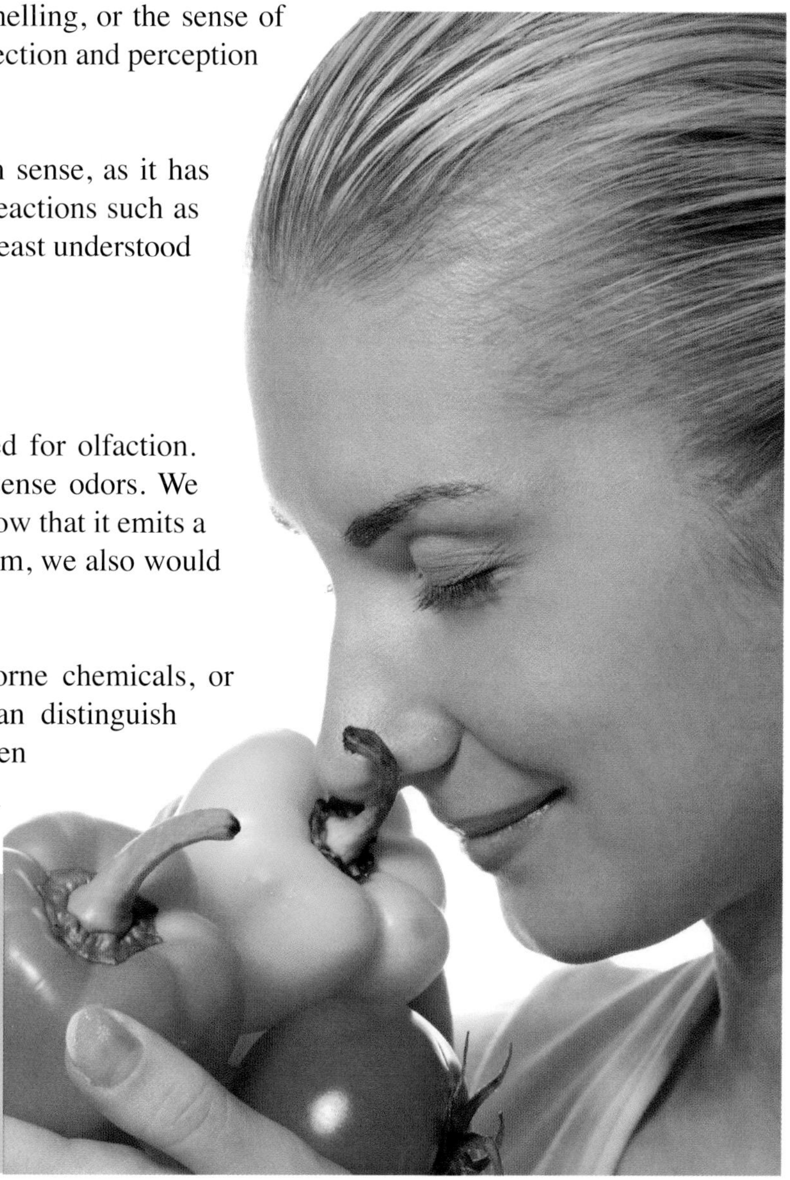

The sense of smell is the most powerful human sense, as it has a direct trigger to the brain and evokes instant reactions such as memory recall and emotions. However, it is the least understood of the five senses.

What is the Olfactory System?

The olfactory system is the sensory system used for olfaction. Without it, we would only breathe and never sense odors. We would see a beautiful rose, but you would not know that it emits a wonderful fragrance. Without the olfactory system, we also would not taste our food.

The olfactory system allows us to detect airborne chemicals, or odors, and identify what they are. Humans can distinguish approximately 10,000 odors or substances even in concentrations as low as a few parts per billion.

Fun Fact

Humans are very sensitive to the smell of bell peppers. It is detected even when mixed with air at only 0.5 parts per million.

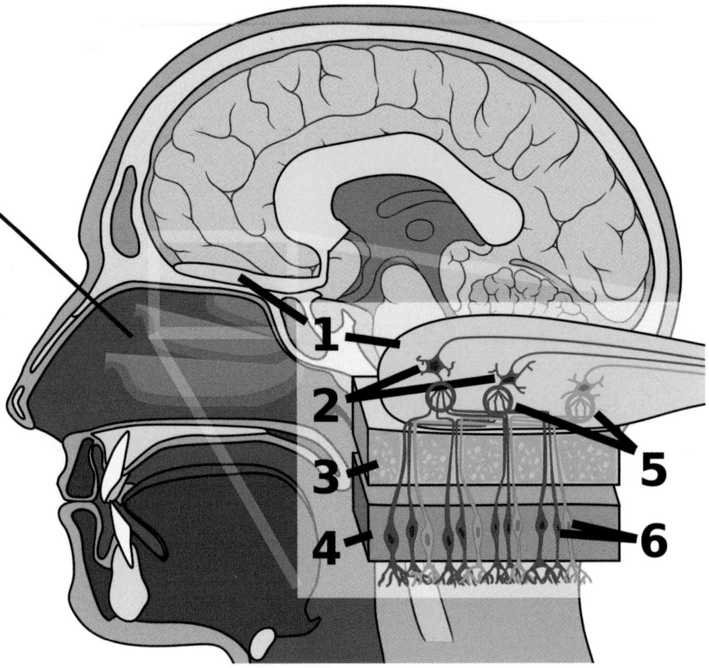

What are the parts of the Olfactory System and how do they help you smell?

To best understand the parts of the olfactory system and how they work, let's follow the scent of an apple.

After biting into an apple or smelling an apple pie cooking in the oven, the chemical molecules in the air that were released from the apple enter the **nose**. These chemical molecules are called **odors.**

Once inside the nose, the molecules from the odors travel to the top of the nasal cavity and lock onto receptor cells in the **cilia**. The cilia are bundles of six to eight hairs that extend from some 10 million olfactory nerve cells. These nerve cells or **olfactory receptors** make up a membrane called the **olfactory epithelium**. The olfactory receptors in the epithelium can detect new odors even in the midst of an environment full of common odors.

Fun Fact

A human has about 40 million olfactory receptors, while a German Shepherd dog has about two billion olfactory receptors.

The olfactory receptors are connected to **neurons** that turn the odor molecules into electrical signals. The signals are sent through the **olfactory nerve** to the **olfactory bulb**, which is located about seven centimeters up the nose and belongs to the central nervous system.

Inside the olfactory bulb are **axons** that form to create **glomeruli** (singular glomerulus), which send the signal to **mitral cells** that are connected to various parts of the brain such as the **olfactory cortex**, the **hippocampus**, **amygdala** and **hypothalamus,** which make up the limbic system of the brain.

Fun Facts

One result of the human genome project (HUGO) was the discovery of 1,000 odor receptors. More receptors are dedicated to the sense of smell than the other senses. This large number of receptors provides a system for discriminating between as many different odors as possible.

In 2004, Linda B. Buck and Richard Axel won the Nobel Prize in Physiology or Medicine for their work on olfactory receptors.

The olfactory nerve, olfactory bulb and brain are collectively known as the rhinencephalon.

The **limbic system** of the brain is directly connected to the parts of the brain that control heart rate, breathing, blood pressure, stress, memory and hormone levels. Feelings of joy, anxiety, fear, anger and depression all emanate from this region. Specifically, the amygdala is a very important center for storing and releasing trauma memories.

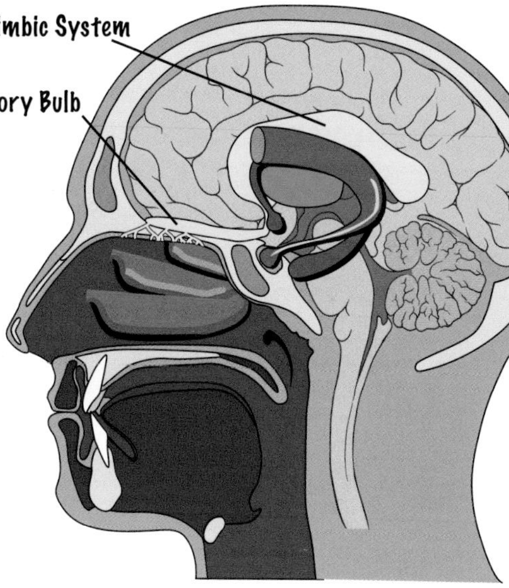

The sense of smell is the only one of the five senses directly liked to the limbic lobe of the brain – the emotional control center.

So the apple smell is sent by means of electrical impulses from cilia to the olfactory bulb, then to the amygdala and then to the limbic region of the brain. Scientists do not know what actually causes these receptors to react. Some guess it is the odor's chemical markers, its size, shape or maybe its electrical frequency.

Smelling

When we wake to the smell of fresh baking bread, we breathe deeply and draw the odor molecules up to the top of the nasal cavity. Several types of molecules are present and each fits into a slot on an olfactory receptor that accommodates only that particular molecule. As soon as these molecules stick to their receptors, intracellular enzymes and substrates quickly cause each cell to produce an electrical signal. This signal flashes through the axon of each olfactory sensory neuron and onto cells in the olfactory bulb. From there the message from each cell goes to the olfactory cortex. This is when we have the "ahhh" sensation, realizing there will be fresh bread for breakfast.

One way to realize the connection between our sense of smell and memory is from previous experiences. Hot cocoa can smell wonderful, but not to the person who was sick and vomited their hot cocoa, causing him to be repulsed at the smell of it afterward and never want it again.

Smelling certain scents, such as therapeutic-grade essential oils, can have a profound effect on our emotional and physical health. Some scents are invigorating, while others are calming. The science of how various aromas affect the body is called **aromatherapy**.

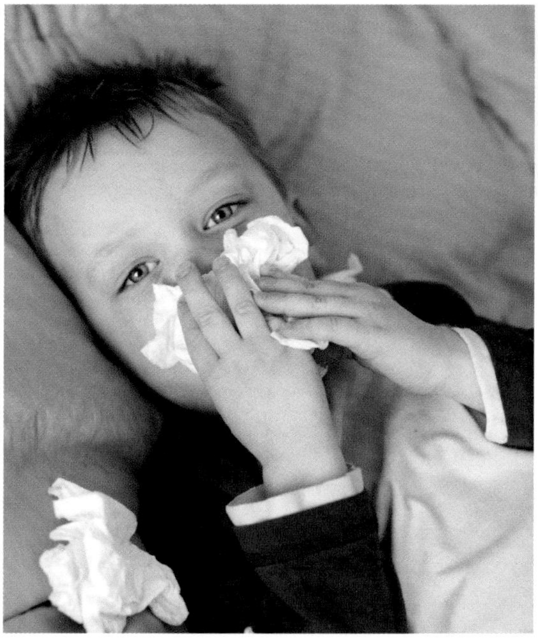

Smelling certain odors will almost always bring up memories. Roses remind you of the time your dad gave your mom roses for their anniversary. Burnt toast reminds you of the picnic when the hot dogs caught fire.

Why can't we taste our food when our noses are stuffy?

Seventy to seventy-five percent of what we taste when we eat is actually perceived by the olfactory system. Taste buds can only detect bitter, salty, sweet and sour flavors. When we are chewing food, some of the odor molecules travel to the back of the mouth and up into the nasal cavity to the olfactory receptors. When the olfactory receptors are covered with thick, excess mucus, they are not able to detect the odor molecules. Thus, we do not taste our food.

How does food affect the Olfactory System?

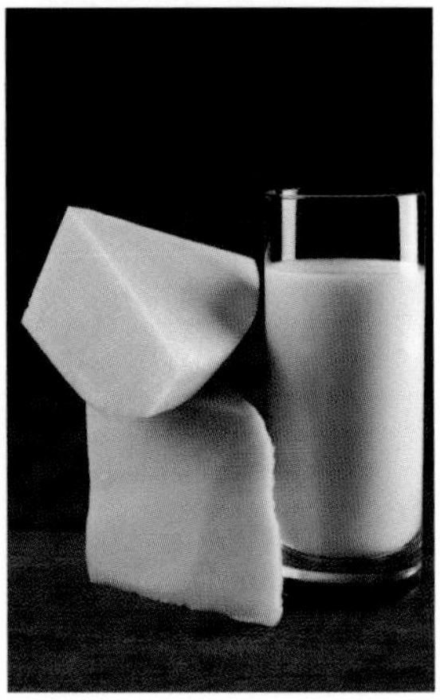

Many of the health conditions that affect the respiratory system also affect the olfactory system. As excess mucus blocks the nasal passages and creates nasal congestion, the odor molecules cannot reach the olfactory system or limbic regions, which can keep a person from smelling anything. Colds, viruses, sinus infections and allergies are some of the more common health issues with symptoms of excess mucus that hinder the olfactory system.

Dairy

Almost all dairy is mucus forming. Dairy products made from cow's milk are very mucus forming. This includes milk, ice cream, cheese, sour cream and yogurt. Eliminating them from the diet for a period of time can help reduce the mucus in the nasal cavity. See Appendix O for more detailed dairy information.

Sugar

Sugar suppresses the immune system function and is very acid (inflammatory) and mucus forming. Don't just switch to raw sugar, maple syrup, agave or honey; instead curb your sweet tooth with fresh fruit. An occasional treat is not the offender, but the problem is daily consumption of sugar from food and drink. See Appendix P for a list of natural sugar substitutes. Lemon, anise and fennel are foods known to reduce mucus. Eating a more alkaline diet also is helpful.

The Loss of Smell

The sense of smell is lost when disorders prevent air from reaching the olfactory receptors in the nose. The loss of smell can be temporary as in the case when someone has nasal congestion. This is not serious and will return as soon as the cold or congestion has subsided.

In some people their loss of smell may be due to allergies, asthma or health concerns such as nerve damage, nasal polyps, head trauma, Alzheimer's, medications and tumors. Some loss of smell occurs with age, and in most cases with no apparent cause, no treatment is recommended.

Fun Fact - People who have lost their sense of smell often have difficulty distinguishing between salty, bitter, sugar and sour tastes as well.

Olfactory Research

A few research projects dealing with the sense of smell have made some outstanding discoveries.

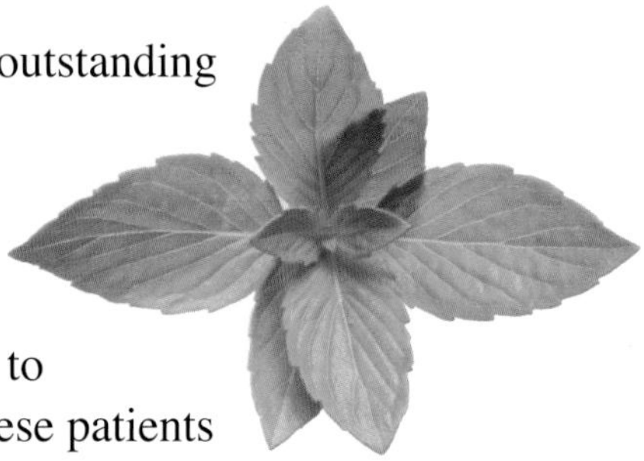

- **Peppermint** diffused into the air was shown to increase attention and attentiveness.[1]
- Patients undergoing an MRI scan, which can be stressful, were exposed to bursts of a **vanilla** scent while in the MRI tube, and 63 percent of these patients had less anxiety.[2]

---

1 Joel S. Warm, Ph. D., William Dember, Ph. D. and Raja Parasuraman, Ph. D. http://www.scenttechnologies.com/research/en/

2 Memorial Sloane-Kettering Cancer Centre, William Redd, Ph. D. and Sharon Manne, Ph. D. http://www.scenttechnologies.com/research/en/

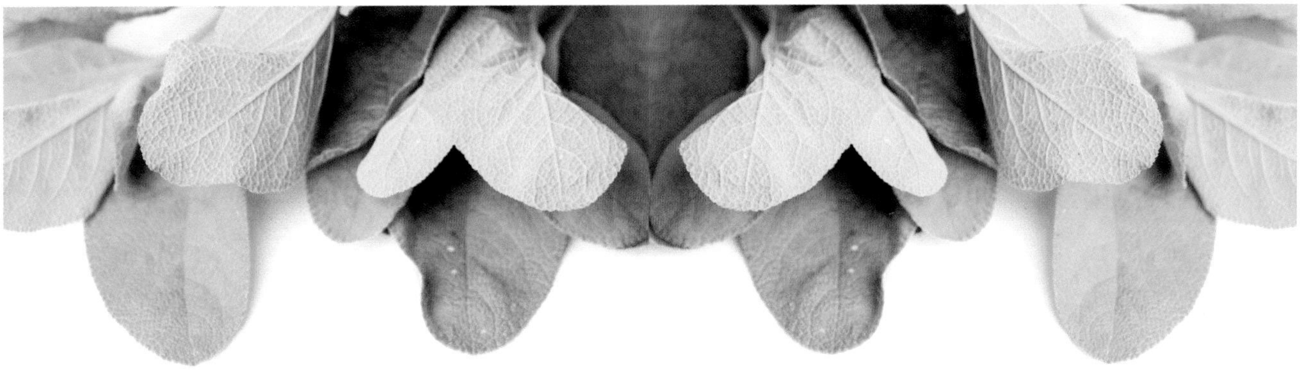

- In a large clinical study, Alan Hirsch, M.D., used fragrances, including **peppermint** to trigger significant weight loss in patients who had been unsuccessful in any type of weight management program.[3]

Herbs for Improving the Sense of Smell

If there are no obvious reasons a person has lost their sense of smell, it may be partially or fully restored using herbs and spices. The most widely recommended is **basil**. Others include **peppermint** and **thyme**.

Household and Personal Care Toxins

Synthetic fragrances in perfumes, cosmetics, body care products and cleaning agents have been known to cause widespread damage to the brain and spinal cord of animals. For the health of the olfactory system and the body's general health, use pure, effective personal care products preferably made with therapeutic-grade essential oils that contain no synthetic fragrances or ingredients.

The toxins in household cleaners are not only harmful to the olfactory system, they are very harmful to the nervous system and respiratory systems as well. Replace household toxic cleaners with safer, all natural cleaners. White vinegar, baking soda, pure grain alcohol or ordinary pure soap will clean without adding to the toxic soup in your home. Thieves Household Cleaner[4] can be used for everything in the home from floors, cabinets and counter tops, the bathroom from sink to toilet, in the laundry, and for walls and windows. It is safer to use than most so-called natural cleaners, and in addition to cleaning things naturally, it kills harmful germs as well.

Reduce airborne contaminants in the home that irritate the nasal passages and sinuses by regularly dusting with one of the dusting recipes from Chapter 1 and cleaning the air by diffusing with therapeutic-grade essential oils.[4]

Be Label Readers!

Watch out for the term "fragrance" in the ingredients list in personal care and household cleaning products. "Fragrances" are synthetically made and can irritate tissue in the nasal passages and bronchial tubes.

3 "Inhalation of Odorants for Weight Reduction" Hirsh, AR, Int J Obex, 1994, page 306

4 See Appendix DD for authors' product recommendations.

Unit 3 Chapter 2
Discussion Questions

1. Have you ever smelled an odor that triggered a memory of long ago? What was the memory?
2. What smell do you not like? Why do you not like it?
3. Find a Bible verse related to odors or smells.
4. Have you ever smelled something that made it harder to breathe? What smells help you breathe?

Activities - plus the Basil and Garlic Pesto "Power" Recipe and activities.

Elementary

1. Find five strongly scented items. Blindfold someone and have them smell each item and guess what it is. Try this with several people and different objects and see who has the best sense of smell. (Try perfume, essential oils[5], onion, tuna fish, bell peppers, cheese, coffee grounds, etc.) Do not choose chemicals as they can pose a hazard when inhaled.
2. Choose one favorite smell that represents each of the four seasons and write a poem or short story that includes the season, the item that you like and why you like the smell.
3. While at the grocery store, take a notepad and write down all of the smells that you experience. Were they good or bad?
4. Research which animals are known for their sense of smell. If possible, find an animal trainer in your area that will allow you to see the animal smelling in action. For example, you may contact the police department's canine unit or a zoologist.

Secondary

Choose any from above plus

1. Prepare two separate meals on different days. Make one meal with several strongly scented foods or spices and make the second meal with little to no smell. Take a poll to see which meal was most enjoyed.
2. Over the next week, keep a journal of various strong smells you encounter. How do they make you feel?
3. Some scientists say that when you eat an excessive amount of foods with very strong scents such as garlic, the odor molecules from those foods can travel through your body and be released through your sweat glands making you smell like garlic. If you are brave and would like to test this theory, make the Basil and Garlic Pesto "Power" recipe, but instead, make it with 12 cloves of garlic and eat that once a day for 3 days consecutively. You can also do this with the garlic recipes in the "Additional Recipes" section. Just triple or quadruple the amount of garlic in the recipe. A few hours after the meal on the 3rd day, do jumping jacks or run in place for 10 minutes or at least long enough to break a sweat. Find a family member with the best sense of smell. Have them smell your arm to see if they can smell the garlic. If not, you might want to try eating the recipe for two more days and then try it again. What were you findings?

Additional Resources

Books

1. "The Naturally Clean Home," Storey Books, 1999.
2. "Clean and Green" by Diedra Imas, 2007.

---

5 If using essential oils, even for inhalation, please use only Young Living with their guaranteed potency, purity and quality from seed through harvest to distilling and bottling, no harm will come from smelling.

Smelling Power

Basil

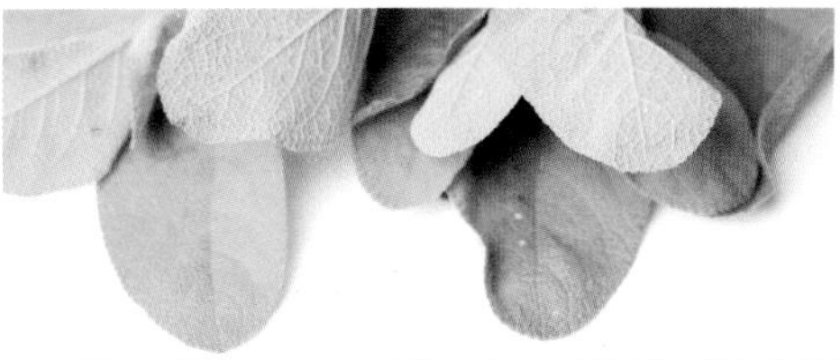

Basil can help improve the sense of smell. It also contains calcium, antioxidant flavonoids, iron, potassium, magnesium, fiber, vitamins A, C and K and manganese.

Basil and Garlic Pesto

This is a fresh way to enliven an old favorite. Modify this recipe to make it your own.

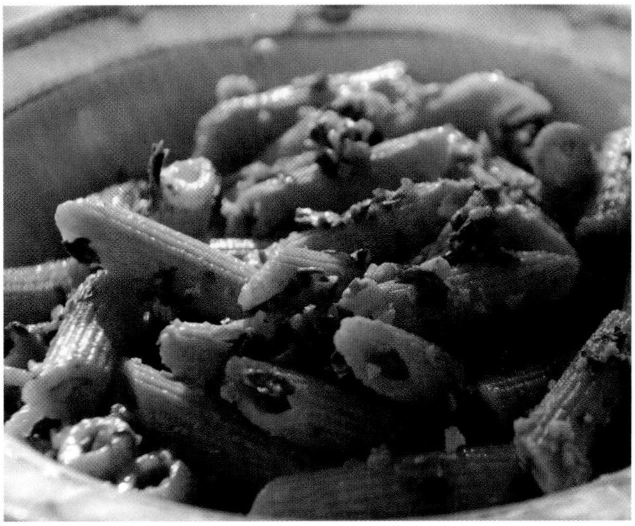

2 cups firmly packed fresh basil leaves
½ cup chopped walnuts and/or pine nuts
¼ cup extra virgin olive oil
4 cloves of garlic peeled and quartered
¼ tsp. sea salt
Pepper

Remove the basil leaves from the stalks and wash and dry them. Place all ingredients in a blender or food processor and blend until nearly smooth, stopping and scraping sides as necessary. Add pepper to taste. Toss with warm whole grain pasta or spread on Italian bread. Any leftover pesto can be refrigerated for one to two days or frozen for up to three months. Makes six side-dish servings.

Activities

Elementary

1. Basil is an herb. What is an herb?
2. Smell the basil leaves and compare them to dried basil. What are the differences?
3. If you are making this recipe for 10 people, how many times would you increase the recipe? For 30?

Secondary

Choose any from above plus

1. How does basil grow?
2. Buy a small basil plant and grow it. Use the basil leaves for the Basil and Garlic Pesto recipe.
3. Research to find the medicinal purposes for basil.
4. If using a dried herb, will it take more or less in the recipe? Why is this?

Chapter 3

The Auditory System and the Ears

"So then faith cometh by hearing, and hearing by the word of God." Romans 10:17
"He that hath ears to hear, let him hear." Matthew 11:15

Shhh! Did you hear that? Sound can alert us to danger, such as the honk of a car horn or train whistle, or put us to sleep as soft music or a mother's lullaby. Some people take the sense of hearing for granted -- that is until it becomes impaired, even if temporarily due to a common cold or ear infection.

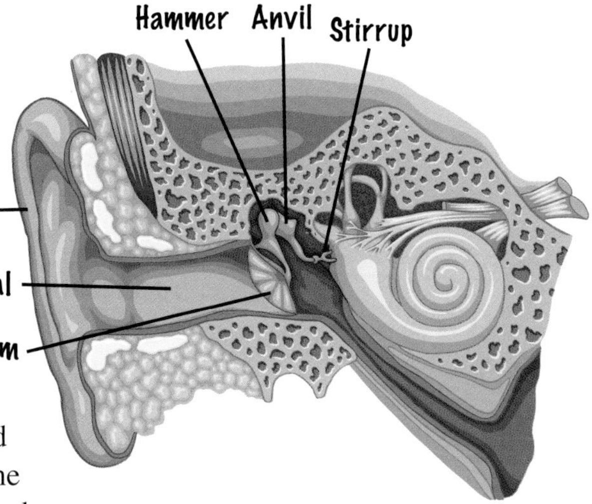

What is sound?

Sound is vibrations composed of frequencies that move through air, water and even solid objects.

What is hearing?

Hearing is one of the five senses. It also is known scientifically as **audition** and is the ability to perceive sound by detecting vibrations with the ear. The inability to detect vibrations with the ear is called **deafness**. The loudness of sound is the force of sound waves against the ear and is measured in decibels (dB). The louder a sound, the more decibels it is. Humans can hear sounds in a range from 20 to 20,000 dB. A dog can hear sounds from 60 to 45,000 dB.

What are the parts of the ear and how do they work?

The ear is part of the **auditory system** and is a sense organ that collects sound, processes it and send sound signals to the brain. It also plays an important role in the sense of balance and body position. There are three main parts to the ear: the outer ear, the middle ear and the inner ear.

Outer Ear

The part of the ear that people can see is the outer ear, which is called the **pinna** or **auricle**. Its job is to collect sounds and send them through the ear canal. The **ear canal** is where earwax is produced. **Earwax**, or cerumen, contains chemicals that fight off germs that could infect the ear canal. It also traps dust and other foreign matter that floats in the air keeping it from going into the ear and causing problems.

Middle Ear

Once sound waves are collected and sent through the ear canal, they arrive at the middle ear. The middle ear is where sound waves are converted into vibrations and then sent to the inner ear. The **eardrum**, or tympanic membrane, separates the outer ear from the middle ear. When sound waves reach the eardrum, the eardrum vibrates. The vibrations cause very tiny bones called ossicles to move. The **ossicles** are the three tiniest bones in the body. The eardrum is connected to the malleus, or **hammer**, and the malleus is connected to the incus, or **anvil**, and the incus is connected to the stapes, or **stirrup**. When the eardrum vibrates, the sound moves through the hammer, then the anvil, next to the stirrup and into the inner ear.

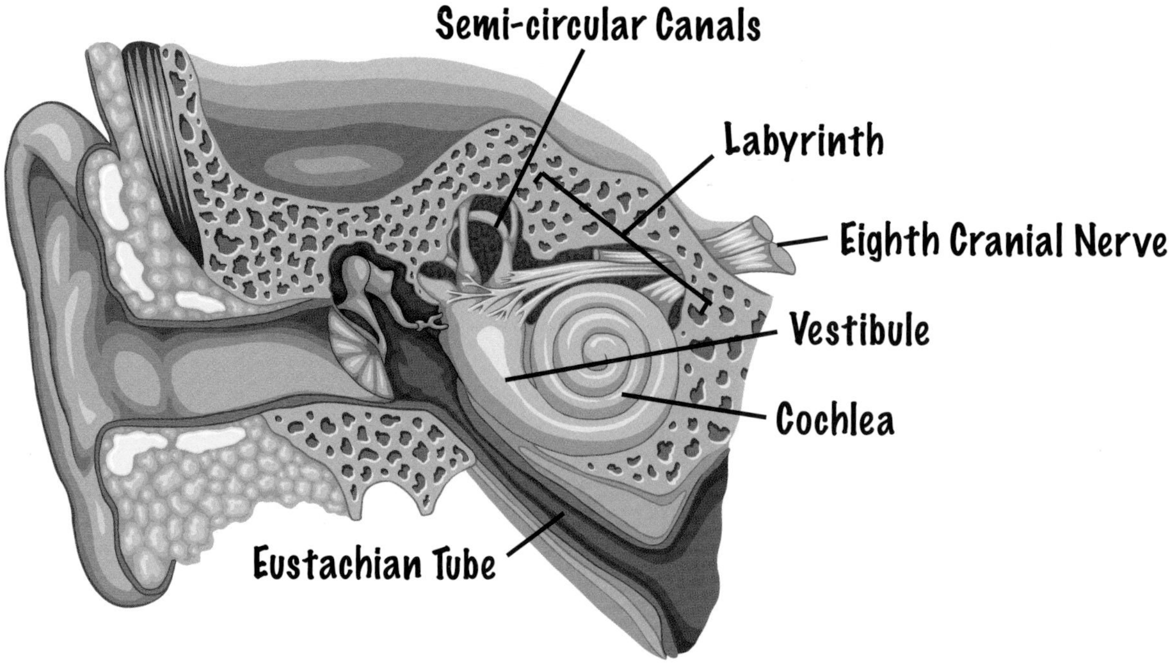

The **Eustachian tube** also is located in the middle ear. It is a narrow tube that runs from the middle ear down to the back of the pharynx and usually is collapsed. As the air in the middle ear is contained and not open to the air in the atmosphere like the outer ear, the Eustachian tube helps to equalize pressure by gaping open during swallowing and positive pressure. The popping noise heard when in an ascending airplane is the Eustachian tube opening up to equalize air pressure for the middle ear.

Inner Ear

From the stirrup, sound moves into the inner ear, which is the hardest bone in the body. Part of the inner ear is the cochlea. The **cochlea** is a small curled tube which is filled with liquid. When the ossicles vibrate, the liquid is set into motion. The cochlea is lined with tiny cells covered in very tiny hairs. When the liquid moves, it moves the hairs which create nerve signals that are sent along the **eighth cranial nerve** to both sides of the brain stem and then up to the auditory portion of the cerebral cortex called the temporal lobe.

The **temporal lobe** processes the sound signals and identifies them. This is when we are able to perceive low or high pitches of a song or when we distinguish a mother's voice from a father's voice.

The sense of balanced also is perceived in the inner ear. Within the inner ear is the **labyrinth** which is a system of fluid passages. It includes the cochlea, which is part of the auditory system, and the **vestibule** and **semi-circular canals**, which are part of the vestibular system. The **vestibular system** gives us our sense of balance and our sense of spatial orientation. It helps us stay upright in a rocking boat and helps us to know if we are upright or upside down.

Fun Fact

You get dizzy after spinning around because when you spin, fluid in the semi-circular canals starts to move. After you stop spinning, the fluid is still moving, so your brain thinks you are still spinning.

What is hearing loss or hearing impairment?

Hearing loss can come on suddenly or gradually. The extent of the loss will impact how well you hear. Some hearing loss is temporary and mild, while other cases are severe and permanent. Gradual hearing loss affects people of all ages and is considered the third most chronic health concern of older Americans affecting up to 40 percent of people age 65 and older and up to 80 percent of people older than 85. You may have a grandparent with some form of hearing loss. In older adults the hearing loss is often so gradual that it is usually a friend or family member who brings this condition to their attention. Younger people with profound hearing loss will generally learn sign language in order to communicate with the world. In adults, the most common causes of hearing loss are noise and aging.

Word Power

Chronic

Pronunciation: \krä-nik\

Function: *adjective*

Etymology: French *chronique,* from Greek *chronikos* of time, from *chronos*

Date: 1601

1 a**:** marked by long duration or frequent recurrence **:** not acute <*chronic* indigestion> <*chronic* experiments> b**:** suffering from a chronic disease <the special needs of *chronic* patients>

2 a**:** always present or encountered ; *especially* **:** constantly vexing, weakening, or troubling <*chronic* petty warfare> b**:** being such habitually <a *chronic* grumbler>

Noise-induced hearing loss can affect people of all ages and most often develops gradually over many years. Over long periods of time, excessive work noise, listening to very loud music, even loud noises from the lawn mower, power tools, heavy equipment, etc. can lead to hearing loss. Loud noises, especially high pitched sounds destroy hair cells in the inner ear causing sensorineural – nerve related – hearing loss.

Age-related hearing loss is known as presbycusis. As we age, changes occur in the middle ear that causes gradual but steady hearing loss. The damage is usually attributed to the nerves.

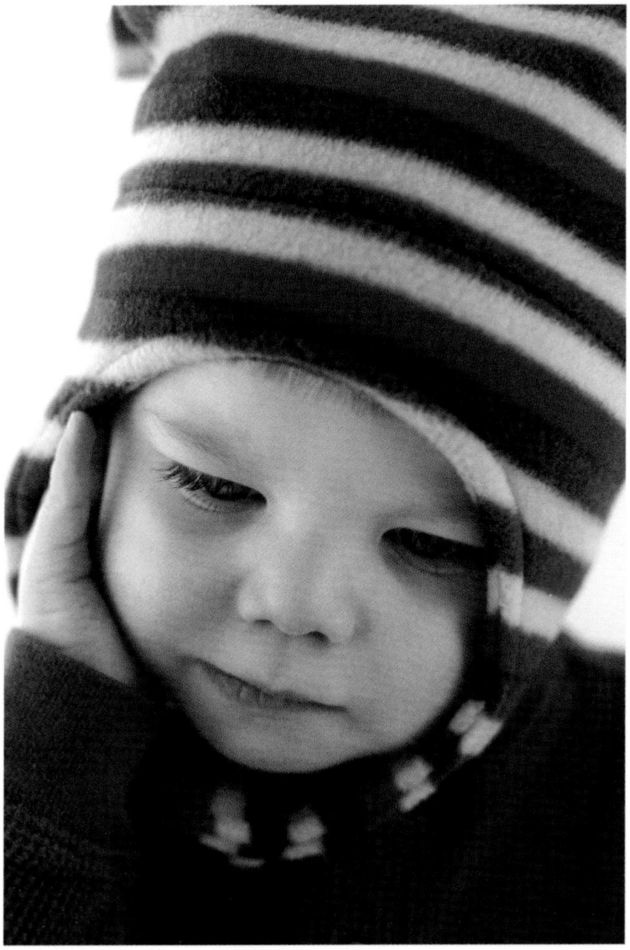

Other causes of hearing loss include earwax buildup, an object lodged in the ear, injury to the ear or head, ear infection, a ruptured eardrum and repeated, untreated ear infections. Most of these causes can be treated with hearing loss restored. For many people suffering from hearing loss, mechanical devises such as hearing aids will help with hearing.

People who smoke are twice more likely to lose their hearing than non-smokers. The ears are nourished by the blood supply and smoking constricts blood vessels.

Ear Infections

Ear infections are caused when germs get passed the Eustachian tube and into the middle ear. The middle ear fills with fluid, or puss, which contains germ fighting cells. When the fluid builds up, it causes pain in the ear.

Children under the age of three are more likely to develop ear infections as their Eustachian tubes are much shorter and are not as able to keep excess fluid and germs from entering the middle ear. Many times, the germs and fluid are from colds or other infections that have not drained or been eliminated from the body properly.

Bad Foods for Hearing

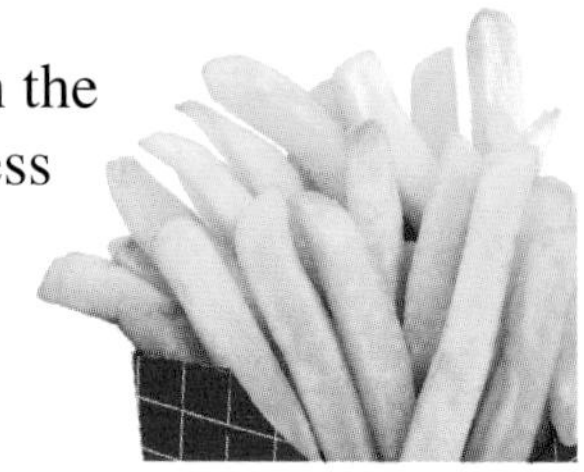

Refined foods, junk foods, caffeine, sugar, saturated fats, salt (can cause fluid retention in the ears resulting in tinnitus, which is a ringing in the ears), and excess dairy (can cause excess mucus buildup). Heavy metals such as mercury, aluminum and lead have been shown to impair circulation and cause nerve damage. A vast number of other commonly used drugs and chemicals can also affect hearing quality (clarity).

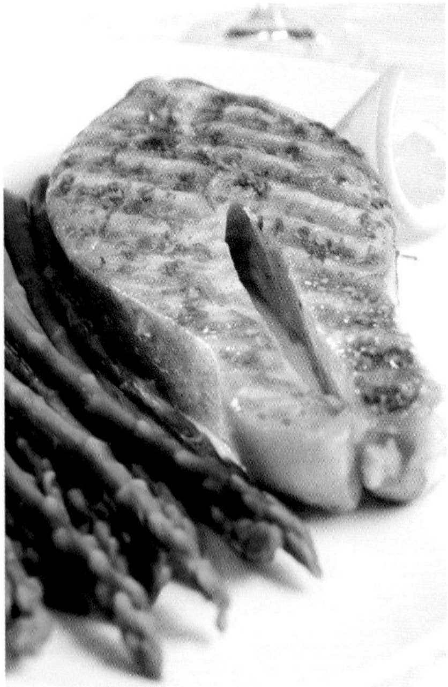

Good Foods for Hearing

Fresh fruit and vegetables, cold water fish rich in Omega-3 fatty acids (see Unit 1 Chapter 2), whole grains, seeds and nuts.

Herbs for Hearing Support

Ginkgo biloba, periwinkle (vinpocetine) and butchers broom can help hearing disorders by improving nerve function and blood supply. They also can protect against drug or free radical damage.[1]

Supplements for Hearing Support

Antioxidants support nerves and generate energy-producing mitochondria in the hair cells of the cochlea. Antioxidants are found in foods rich in vitamins A and E[2] and alpha-lipoic acid[3]. See Appendix F for a list of foods high in vitamins A and E.

Supplementing with the following also may be beneficial: **vitamin B1** (thiamine), **B2** (riboflavin), **B3** (niacin), **B6** (pyridoxine), **B9** (folic acid), **B12** (methylcobalamin), **magnesium**, **zinc**, **acetyl l-carnitine** and **n-acetylcysteine**.

Food Rich in Alpha Lipoic Acid

Organ meats such as liver, spinach, broccoli and potatoes

1 Presse Med, 1986; 15: 1559-61; Acta Pharm Hung, 1996; 66: 213-24; Otolaryngol Pol, 1990; 44: 122-9
2 Acta Vitaminol Enzymol, 1985; 7 Suppl: 85-92
3 Am J Otol, 2000; 21: 161-7; Acta Otolaryngol, 2000; 120: 596-9

Unit 3 Chapter 3 Discussion Questions

1. What sounds do you hear when you first wake up in the morning? What sounds do you hear only at night?
2. What are your top five favorite sounds? What are the worst?
3. In what ways can we protect our ears?
4. Can you remember a time when you both heard and felt a sound?

Activities - plus the Spinach Salad "Power" Recipe and activities.

Elementary

1. Blindfold a member of the family and have other members of the family try to disguise their voices. See if the person who is blindfolded can tell who is speaking.
2. Sound is composed of frequencies. How are frequencies measured?
3. Why can dogs hear sounds that humans can't, such as a dog whistle?
4. People who are deaf speak using sign language. Michigan State University has an American Sign Language Browser (http://commtechlab.msu.edu/sites/aslweb/browser.htm) that allows you to look up words and see a person using the sign for that word. Choose three foods that are good for hearing and learn the sign for each.
5. Refer to Appendix F and find one new food rich in Vitamin A that you have never tried and one new food rich in vitamin E. Try each one during a meal. What did you think of the taste? Did you like them?
6. Memorize Proverbs 28:9: "He that turneth away his ear from hearing the law, even his prayer shall be abomination."

Secondary

Choose any from above plus

1. Heavy metals such as mercury, aluminum and lead are known to cause hearing impairments. How are these metals used in your environment? What can you do to remove or replace them?
2. Using the Michigan State University American Sign Language Browser (http://commtechlab.msu.edu/sites/aslweb/browser.htm), learn to sign the following words and phrases: breakfast, lunch, dinner, please, thank you and you are welcome.
3. For whom was the Eustachian tube named and why? How was this person instrumental?
4. Using Appendix F, find a food rich in Vitamin A, a food rich in Vitamin E and a food rich in alpha linoic acid. See if you can create a recipe using all three foods and prepare it for your family at meal time.
5. Memorize James 1:22-23: "But be ye doers of the word, and not hearers only, deceiving your own selves. For if any be a hearer of the word, and not a doer, he is like unto a man beholding his natural face in a glass"
6. What does this Scripture mean to you?

Additional Resources

Web sites:

1. http://faculty.washington.edu/chudler/chsense.html
2. http://faculty.washington.edu/chudler/chhearing.html
3. http://faculty.washington.edu/chudler/bigear.html
4. http://kidshealth.org/kid/htbw/ears.html
5. http://kidshealth.org/kid/word/

Hearing Power

Spinach

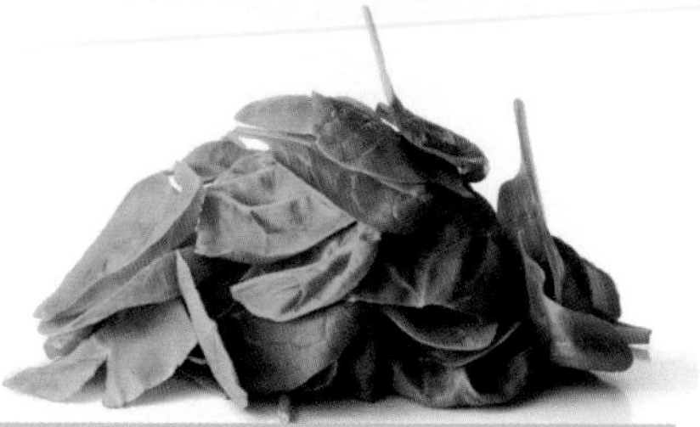

Spinach is an excellent source of vitamins A, B1, B2, B3, B6, C, E, K and folate which all support hearing and overall health. It also is high in calcium, iron, fiber, Omega-3 fatty acid, magnesium and many other nutrients.

Spinach Salad

The "Power" ingredients in this recipe are the raw vegetables, which are packed with vitamins that support hearing. Served this immediately or cold as leftovers. Larger families will need to double or triple the recipe.

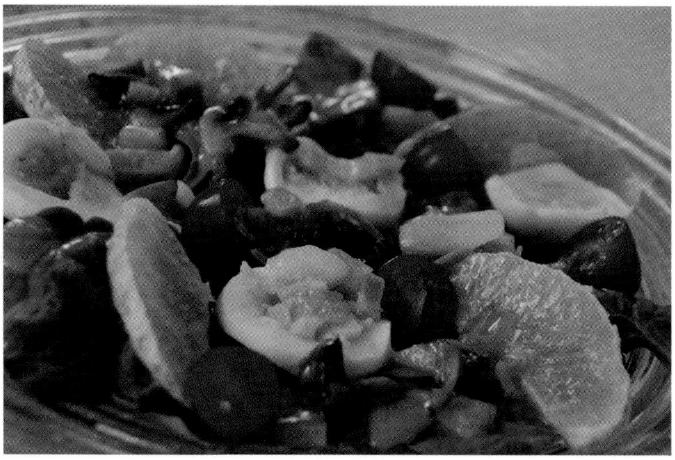

2 cups fresh washed spinach
1 hard boiled egg, sliced
1 small orange, peeled and sectioned
1 handful of cherry tomatoes

Combine these ingredients and set aside.

2 button mushrooms, sliced thin
¼ of a red onion, finely chopped

If desired, lightly sauté the mushrooms and onions in olive oil or coconut oil. Drain and set aside.

Dressing (This makes the salad warm and should be added before serving.)
2 Tbs. organic honey mustard dressing or 1 Tbs. dry mustard
1 Tbs. Blue Agave Nectar
1 Tbs. olive oil or coconut oil, blended

Mix together with the freshly sautéed mushrooms and onions and then add to the spinach mixture. Yields two servings.

Activities

Elementary

1. Go to the Vitamins and Minerals Appendix F and G and find spinach. What vitamins and minerals does raw spinach contain?
2. Mushrooms are classified as a fungus. What is fungus?
3. This recipe calls for red onions. What other kinds of onions have you eaten? What kinds of onions are offered at your local store or market?

Secondary

Choose any from above plus

1. When washing the mushrooms, it is important not to rinse them in water. Rather wiping them with a damp cloth is the preferred method of cleaning. Why is this?
2. What other fresh, raw ingredients could you add to this to support respiratory and eye health?
3. Tomatoes are good for heart health. What are some similarities between tomatoes and the heart?

Chapter 4

The Visual System and The Eyes

"The eyes of the Lord are in every place, beholding the evil and the good." Proverbs 15:3
"Let us find grace in the sight of my Lord," Genesis 47:25

Rainbows. Mountains. Waves crashing against the shore. A baby's precious face. These are all beautiful things God created that we love to see. But our eyes do more for us than just allow us to gaze upon God's creation. They help us find each other in a noisy crowd, watch for danger as we cross the street and drive a vehicle. Our eyes also help us communicate with others as we watch their body language and facial expressions.

Psalm 101:31 says "I will set no wicked thing before my eyes." A person who is very visual remembers nearly everything he or she sees. We should be careful to look at only those things that are good for the body, soul and spirit – including food. Supporting eye health through nutrition isn't just useful to maintain good vision, drive a car, read a book and play sports. According to Matthew 6:22-23 "eyes are the window to the soul." Often, people say they can tell if a person is truthful by looking into the eyes. Many health professionals can see the state of a person's physical health by looking at certain components of the eye that literally reflect nutritional status. To ensure a lifetime of viewing the wondrous creations of God, we must take care of our eyes. To understand how nutrition can support the eyes, we must first know how the eyes work.

What is sight?

The ability to interpret information from visible light reaching the eyes is known as **visual perception**, **sight** or **vision**. Because of visual perception, we don't just see light. We are able to see objects and know what they are. We are able to see an apple sitting on the table and know what it is and that it is red, round, shiny and an arm's reach away. Because of the sense of sight, we can perceive distance and distinguish between familiar and unknown objects. The sense of sight is the most complex of all the senses.

Fun Facts

Most people blink every two to ten seconds. Melanin is what gives color to the iris. People with blue eyes have less melanin than people with brown eyes.

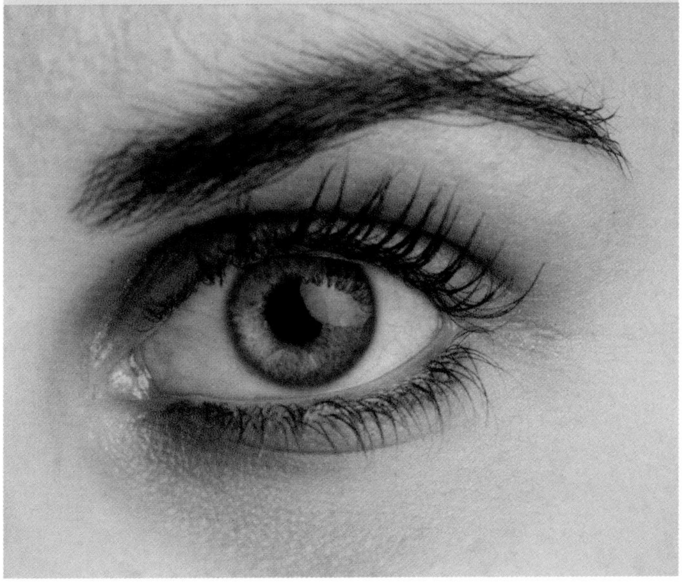

What are the parts of the eye and what do they do?

The eyeball is about the size of a ping pong ball and sits in the hollow eye socket of the skull. The eye lashes and eyebrows protect the eyes from dust and other flying debris. The eyelid also protects the front part of the eye by closing, or blinking, and spreading a thin, invisible layer of moisture called **tears** across the front of the eye. The tears are produced by the **lacrimal glands**, which are located in the upper outer corner of the eye socket. Once the tears have moistened the front of the eyeball, canals in the eyelids send the tears to the **lacrimal sacs**, which are located in the lower inner corner of the eye socket. The remaining tears then exit through a passage that leads to the nose.

The eyeball is formed by three different layers:

1. The outer layer is called the **sclera** and is white and covers most of the eye. It is attached at the front to the clear surface called the **cornea**.

2. The middle layer is called **choroid**, which contains the blood vessels that supply oxygen and nutrients to the retina.

3. The inner layer is the **retina**, which is soft, light-sensitive and part of the nervous system. It is connected to the **optic nerve,** which sends optical signals to the brain.

In the middle of the eyeball is a jelly-like matter called the **vitreous humor**. It helps direct light to the back of the eye and keeps the circular shape of the eyeball.

The **cornea** is a clear layer in the front of the eye. The clear fluid right behind the cornea is called the **aqueous humor**. Together they form an outer lens that helps to bend or **refract** light as the light enters the eye.

The circular membrane behind the cornea that actually gives us the color of our eyes is the iris. The **iris** is held into place by small muscles that help it control the amount of light that enters into the eye. The little black circle inside the iris is called the **pupil**, which opens and closes like a camera shutter to let the right amount of light into the eye. The pupil gets bigger when there is low light and smaller when there is bright light.

The **lens** sits right behind the iris and focuses the light to form sharp images that are then directed through the vitreous humor to the back of the eyeball onto the retina. The muscles that help the lens to focus on images are called the **ciliary body**. They flatten or contract the lens to focus on objects at different distances away. Many people over the age of 45 often need glasses to help them see clearer because their lenses have become less elastic.

At the back of the eye in the retina are millions of light receptors called rods and cones. There are about 120 million **rods,** which are very sensitive to light and allow us to see in dim light and detect shades of gray, but not color. There are six million **cones** that allow us see in bright light and detect color and detail. A small, specialized area on the retina of mainly cones and a few rods is called the **macula.** When looking directly at an object, the macula helps our eyes see fined details.

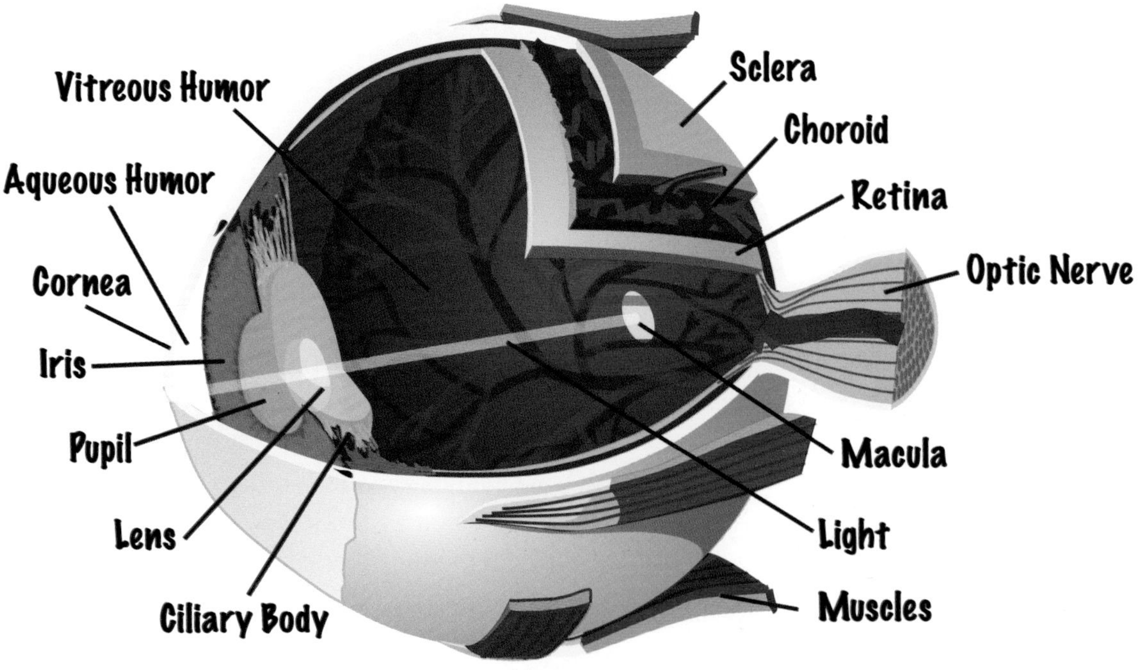

How do the eyes work?

When we look at an object like an apple, light is reflected off the apple and into our eye through the cornea which refracts the light. The light then goes through the pupil and then through the lens where it is focused onto the retina in the back of the eye. Once on the retina, the image of the apple is actually upside down. The rods and cones help to detect the color and any details and send the nerve signals through the **optic nerve** to the brain. The part of the brain that processes the visual signals and interprets the messages is called the **visual cortex**, which is at the back of the brain in the **occipital lobe**. At this point, the visual cortex recognizes the visual input and turns the image of the apple right-side-up.

Some animals like chameleons use both their eyes separately to see objects. However, humans use both their eyes together, which is called **binocular vision**. Through binocular vision, an object is seen slightly different through each eye because of the difference in distance from each eye. The brain takes both of these slightly different images to create a single, three-dimensional image and then judges the distance of the object based on the degree of difference in the images. The ability to sense distance is called **depth perception**.

Word Power

Optical

Pronunciation: \äp-ti-kəl\

Function: *adjective*

Date: 1570

1**:** of or relating to the science of **optics**2 a**:** of or relating to vision **:** VISUAL B**:** VISIBLE 1 <*optical* wavelength> c**:** of, relating to, or being objects that emit light in the visible range of frequencies <an *optical* galaxy> d**:** using the properties of light to aid vision <an *optical* instrument>3 a**:** of, relating to, or utilizing light especially instead of other forms of energy <*optical* microscopy> b**:** involving the use of light-sensitive devices to acquire information for a computer <*optical* character recognition>4**:** of or relating to optical art

All of the parts of the eyes and the parts of the brain that help with visual perception together is called the **visual system**. Because there are so many complex, fine tuned aspects to the visual system, it is so very easy for things to go wrong. Good nutrition is vital to help all of the components of sight to work properly.

Fun Fact

If you only had one eye, everything would appear two-dimensional. This effect does not work when only closing one eye.

Fun Fact

Everyone has a dominant eye. To find the dominant eye, point with your finger to an object far away from you. Focus on that object. Then, close the right eye and then the left eye. The dominant eye will perceive your finger directly at the object while the non-dominant eye will perceive the finger to one side of the object.

Eyesight Health Issues

Some people have misshapen lenses that keep them from focusing on objects located near or far away, which is called nearsightedness and farsightedness. To correct these eye issues, glasses are needed to further help with focusing.

Most people will occasionally experience some sort of temporary eye problems, such as itchiness, fatigue, twitching, dryness and blurriness. These conditions are quite annoying, but are usually short lived and go away without any permanent loss of sight. Some causes of temporary ear problems are caffeine, stress and fatigue.

The most common health related eye concerns in young people are pink eye (also known as conjunctivitis), a sty or an object in the eye. Keeping your hands washed may help stop the spread of bacteria or viruses responsible for most cases of **pink eye**. The membrane covering the whites of the eyes and the inner part of the eyelids is called the conjunctiva. This membrane reacts to a wide range of bacteria, viruses, allergens, irritants, and toxic agents. Once infected, the eye gets red and inflamed as if it has a cold. Pink eye causes the eye to produce a watery discharge and can even causing the eye to swell shut. Viral and bacterial forms of conjunctivitis are common in childhood, but they can occur in people of any age.

A **sty** is an acute infection or inflammation of one of the secretory glands of the eyelids blocking the gland. When the gland is blocked, the oil produced by the gland occasionally backs up and extrudes through the wall of the gland, forming a lump, which can appear white or red much like a pimple and sometimes can be painful. This may be caused by a particle of dirt, dust or bacteria. The lump can be visible or grow inward. The sty goes away when the blockage of the gland is resolved.

If an object is lodged in the eye, it may require an eye specialist – an ophthalmologist – for safe removal. This is one main reason to always wear protective eye goggles when playing sports, doing wood work, etc.

Word Power

Ocular

Pronunciation: \ä-kyə-lər\
Function: adjective
Etymology: Late Latin ocularis of eyes, from Latin oculus eye
Date: circa 1575
1 a: done or perceived by the eye <ocular inspection> b: based on what has been seen <ocular testimony>2 a: of or relating to the eye <ocular muscles> b: resembling an eye in form or function

As we age, many things can go wrong with our vision. Ultraviolet (UVA) light from the sun can damage the lens and cornea. Long hours spent in front of a computer can make your eyes tired, causing blurry vision. Wind, dust, chlorine fumes, automobile fumes, freezing temperatures and physical injury are examples of other threats to good vision. Age related loss of sight is common among people age 55 or older. Eye problems include: cataracts, glaucoma, macular degeneration and presbyopia.

Cataracts are the leading cause of visual loss in adults age 55 or older and the leading cause of blindness in the world. Cataracts are the clouding of the lens by accumulated dead cells in the eyes.

Glaucoma is a group of diseases that cause damage to the optic nerve. The optic nerve is damaged when the too much fluid in the eye causes pressure, or intraocular pressure. Causes may include trauma, genetic disorders and low blood flow to the optic nerve.

Presbyopia is the inability to focus on objects that are close. This condition is usually age related and occurs in people 40 years old and older due to the lens losing its flexibility and ability to focus on close objects.

Age-related Macular Degeneration, or AMD, is the leading cause of blindness in the United States and affects the macula, which is the area of the retina responsible for sharp, central vision. AMD causes objects to become blurred and distorted as cellular debris collects on the macula. In some cases, the retina becomes so deprived of oxygen that it signals new blood vessels to form in the area. These new blood vessels are very weak and can leak fluid and blood into the retina.

There are many safe, effective all-natural alternatives to many eye concerns.

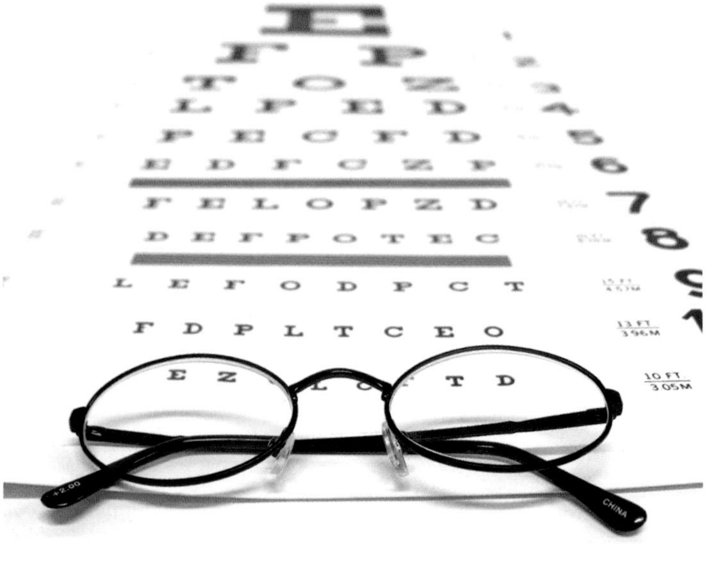

Nutrition for Healthy Eyesight

Based on information provided by the U.S. National Eye Institute, results of nutrition and eye health food studies have shown that consuming certain foods provide nutrition for the eyes and support good eye health.

Healthy vision is related to the health of the individual parts of the eye - the cornea, iris, macula, lens, optic nerve, pupil, retina and the vitreous humor. Nutritional support is one of the ways good vision can be supported even as we age. Nutrients for healthy eye support include: antioxidants, bioflavonoids, DHA, lutein and zeaxanthin.

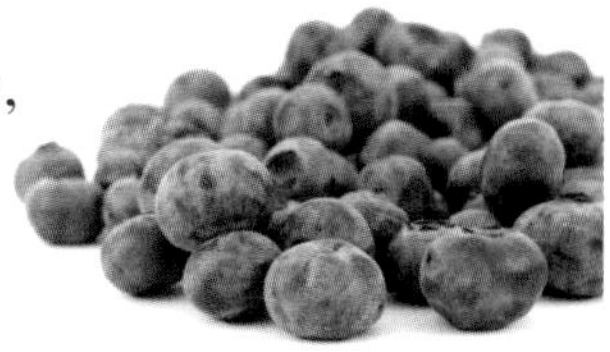

Antioxidants are powerful nutrients that can help prevent macular degeneration, one of the leading causes of blindness in the elderly. Berries, cherries, pomegranates and NingXia wolfberries are rich in antioxidants. Berries and cherries are concentrated with bioflavonoids that can strengthen small blood vessels supplying the eyes and brain tissue with oxygen and nutrients. Eating blueberries has been associated with the reduction of eye fatigue.

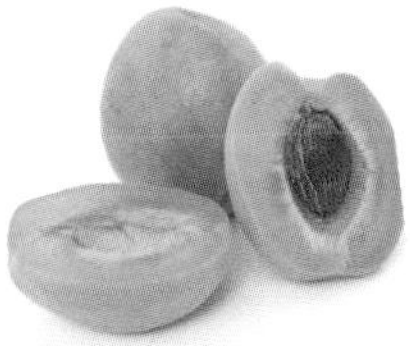

Beta-carotene is converted as needed by the body to **vitamin A**, an important antioxidant that resists oxidative stress damage to cells and tissues, including the eye lenses. If there is a severe vitamin A deficiency, then night blindness can occur. Vitamin A is needed to form the retinal, which is a light sensitive molecule found in the receptor cells of the retina. A deficiency may not allow enough light to permit proper vision. Apricots are rich in nutrients, such as beta-carotene and **lycopene,** that help promote good vision. Continued oxidative stress may result in the development of cataracts or damage the blood supply to the eyes and lead to macular degeneration.

Bilberries grow on small bushes and were used by British pilots to improve their night vision. Bilberry seems to improve eye health by increasing the blood supply to the eyes. The substance in bilberry that nourishes eye tissue is called **anthocyanosides.** Fresh bilberries and bilberry jams are tasty sources of this vision nutrition food. Bilberry also is sold in most health food stores in capsules.

DHA (docosahexaenoic acid – see the Brain Unit,) is a fatty acid found in the retina of the eye and can reverse some of the degenerative damage that comes with macular degeneration. DHA is one of the best sources for clear eyesight and eye health. Small fish – salmon, tuna, cod, haddock as well as sardines -- are some of the best food sources of DHA. Supplements containing DHA were discussed in Unit One.

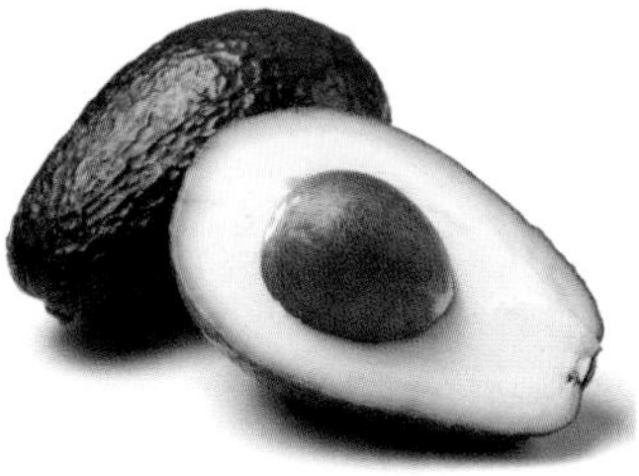

Lutein is an antioxidant that can help prevent free radical damage specific to problems with the lenses, retina, optic nerves and visual cortex. Lutein-rich foods include kale, collard greens, spinach, broccoli, Brussels sprouts, avocado, NingXia wolfberries[1] and organic egg yolks. It's important to note that lutein is a fat-soluble nutrient, so is best absorbed into the blood in the presence of healthy fats. It best to eat green, leafy vegetables with foods that are rich in healthy fats like avocado, olives, raw nuts, olive oil, coconut oil, organic eggs and organic butter.

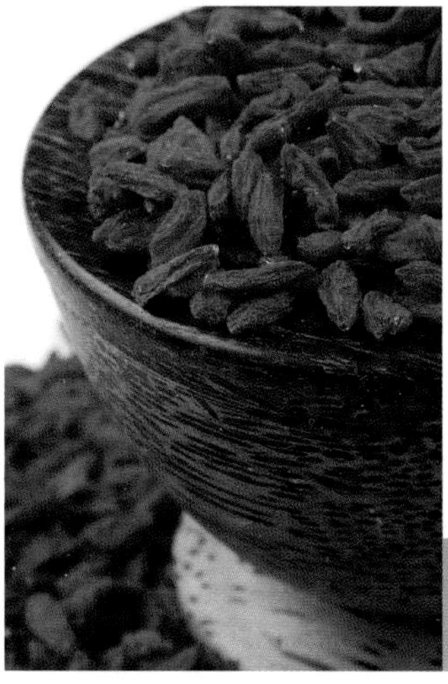

Zeaxanthin is a carotenoid nutrient. The highest source of zeaxanthin is red bell peppers, with the second best source the whole NingXia wolfberry[1]. Other food sources include broccoli, collard greens, green peas, romaine lettuce, spinach, turnip greens and zucchini.

Fun Fact - According to the National Eye Institute, persons with diets high in lutein and zeaxanthin were also less likely to need cataract surgery.

1 See Appendix DD for authors' supplement recommendations.

More good nutrients for the eyes include:

Alpha Lipoic Acid – ALA improves the performance of other antioxidants in the body.

L-Taurine – Helps protect the eyes from UV light and helps strengthen the retinal cells.

Lycopene – A strong antioxidant found in tomatoes.

N-Acetyl Cysteine – Helps protect the eyes from damage by UV light and strengthens the immune system.

Quercetin – A strong antioxidant that helps maintain lens transparency.

Vitamin C – Helps the body resist damage by oxidation or damage from long-term exposure to oxygen and light.

Zinc – Helps support macular and retina health; levels of zinc are definitely related to eye health.

Bad Eyesight Foods

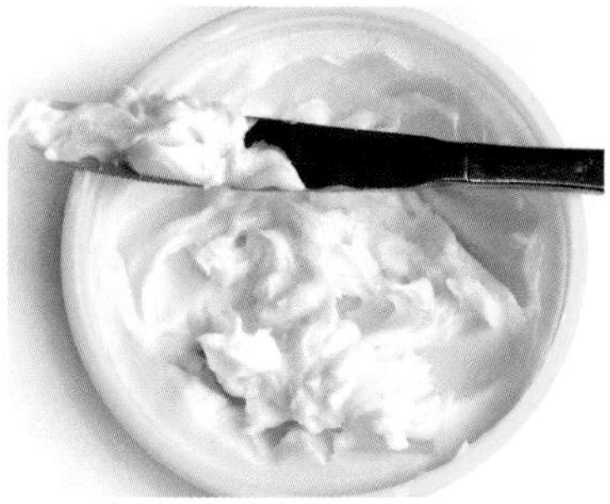

Trans fatty acids can cause direct damage to the blood vessels that supply your eyes and brain. The easiest way to identify foods that contain trans fats is to look for hydrogenated or partially hydrogenated oil on food labels. It doesn't matter which oil it is - soy, corn, palm, safflower or sunflower - all hydrogenated and partially hydrogenated oils come with trans fatty acids. We should stay away from all brands of margarine and spreads made from vegetable oils, commercially baked goods like donuts, pastries and cookies, and fried foods like French fries, tempura, fried fish and fried chicken.

Processed foods such as white rice, pasta and bread may worsen eyesight, especially as a person ages. These types of foods - carbohydrates with a high glycemic index - can cause age-related macular degeneration (AMD). Researchers from Tufts University have discovered that people whose diets are high in processed foods are much more likely to develop AMD.[2] High-glycemic foods cause a faster rise and fall in blood sugar levels and are associated with an increased risk of diabetes. The Tufts researchers analyzed data on 4,099 people who were participating in an eye-health study. They estimated that up to 20 percent of cases of AMD could have been prevented had the patients eaten far less processed foods. Even a simple dietary change of replacing white bread with whole grain bread could have reduced the risk.

2 American Journal of Clinical Nutrition, 2007; 86: 180-8

Unit 3 Chapter 4 Discussion Questions

1. How do you protect your eyes?
2. What did you learn in this chapter about your eyes that you did not know?
3. What foods are you going to eliminate from your diet because they are bad for your eyes?
4. What does this Scripture mean to you? "But as it is written, eye hath not seen, nor ear heard, neither have entered into the heart of man, the things which God hath prepared for them that love him." 1 Corinthians 2:9

Activities - plus the Fresh Carrot and Fruit Juice or Smoothie "Power" Recipe and activities.

Elementary

1. Have an adult blindfold you and help you with your usual tasks over the course of an hour. Was it hard or easy? Why?
2. Count all of the members in your immediate family. Now count the members of your family that wear glasses or contact lens. What is the percentage of people in your family that wear corrective lenses?
3. With an adult's help and supervision, shine a flashlight into his or her eyes. At what point does the iris open and close?
4. Help prepare a meal for your family that includes good foods for their eyes.
5. Using the melody of your favorite song, write new words for the song to describe the beautiful things you see each day.

Secondary

Choose any from above plus

1. Complete question two above. Interview the members of the family who use corrective lenses to find out how long they have worn them and whether they are near- or far-sighted. What can you learn about your families' eye health from this data?
2. Decreased blood supply to the eyes is dangerous. Smoking is one example of a choice that causes decreased blood supply. What are the dangers smoking presents to your respiratory system?
3. What is ophthalmology? What is optometry? What is the difference between an ophthalmologist and an optometrist?
4. Read Proverbs 29:18: "Where there is no vision, the people perish: but he that keepeth the law, happy is he." What is the difference between sight and the meaning of vision in this Scripture? What are other meanings of vision? Explain your findings during a family meal.

Additional Resources

Web sites:

1. http://faculty.washington.edu/chudler/chvision.html
2. http://www.nei.nih.gov/education/visionschool/index.asp
3. http://colormatters.com/kids/eye.html

Vision Power

Carrots

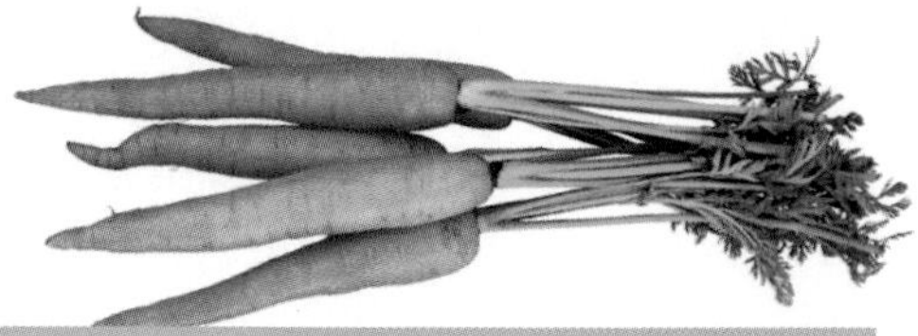

Carrots are an excellent source of vision promoting vitamin A, alpha-carotene and beta-carotene.

Fresh Carrot and Fruit Juice or Smoothie

Try the following as a breakfast drink or anytime snack. The smoothie is made in a blender, and the juice is best prepared in a juicing machine. Those who prefer juice, but do not have a juicing machine can purchase organic juices at the store. Please note that these products often contain sugar and preservatives.

Juice

2 fresh carrots
Any one or combination of fruits listed below

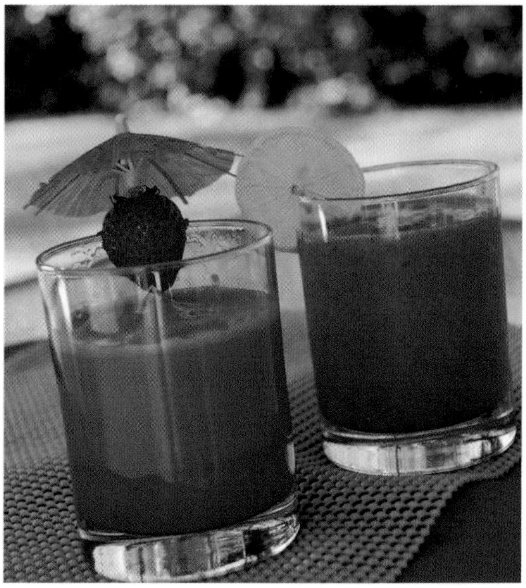

Smoothie

Juice of 2 fresh carrots or 2 oz. store bought carrot juice
Any one or combination of fruits listed below
1 banana
1 cup of ice
Blue Agave Nectar to taste
and any of the following:

3 apples	3 kiwis	1 pineapple
6 apricots	1 coconut	2 plums
1 handful of berries	2 mangoes	1 fig
1 quarter of a cantaloupe	1 papaya	1 quarter of a watermelon
1 lemon or lime	2 peaches	
8 strawberries	2 pears	

Juicing directions: (Yields about 8 ounces.) Wash and prepare the carrots and fruit per the juicer manufacturer's directions. Juice the carrots and then juice the selected fruit. Experiment with various combinations and amounts to obtain the desired taste. The pulp can be used for other recipes or put in a composting bin.

Blender directions: (Yields about 16 ounces.) Blend the carrot juice, desired fruit and ice.

Activities

Elementary

1. Have an adult help you cut a carrot in half to expose the rounded interior of the vegetable. What do you notice? How does it remind you of a human eye?
2. Identify which fruit listed above also is high in eye health properties.
3. What does a juicing machine do? What does a blender do?

Secondary

Choose any from above plus

1. What are some of the problems associated with buying processed juice?
2. What are some uses for pulp from the juicer?
3. If your family is interested in obtaining a juicing machine, research which products on the market best suit your needs and find a good deal.
4. After you make your juice or smoothie, research to find out how much vitamin A is in it.

Unit 3 Additional Recipes

Use organic ingredients when possible.

Super Tonic (Chapter 1 Activity)

This recipe has been around for many, many years and has been helping people just as long and is a very inexpensive all natural remedy to everyday ailments. The ingredients give a general sense as to why:

Cayenne – good for circulatory issues, cold hands, cold feet, the heart, blood pressure.
Ginger – works on small vessel and capillary circulation, good for digestive issues.
Onion – may make you cry, but great to combat a cough and other respiratory issues.
Garlic – hard to beat for as a natural antibiotic and aids in a healthy heart as well.
Horseradish – sinus problems run for cover, good upper body circulation, really opens up the sinuses.
Apple cider vinegar – use the real unfiltered Bragg's, Hain or Spectrum brands that are not distilled, we know this type of apple cider vinegar is alkalizing, good for digestive stress and helps with circulation.

To make Super Tonic, combine equal parts (Depending on the size of your blender, you can use one cup as a part.) of the following ingredients:

Fresh hot cayenne or habanero peppers
Peeled sliced ginger
Peeled chunked horseradish
Peeled chopped onion
Peeled garlic
One quart of apple cider vinegar

Pour into a blender and whiz on high for two to three minutes. Do not stand with your nose over the blender when taking the lid off, as it has been known to make people faint. After removing the lid, let it stand for a few minutes, then pour into a large wide mouth jar. Label it with the date. Seal tightly and shake twice per day for two weeks. Strain and bottle the liquid. The pulp may be discarded, or if you are brave enough you can use as a hot salsa dip.

Store in the refrigerator, but you may keep some in a small bottle on the table to use with olive oil as a salad dressing. Suggested use is one dropper full in eight ounces of water daily. You can use up to six droppers full per day if a bad cold or sinus infection has you down. Taken daily people report fewer colds and coughs, better blood pressure reading and overall better vitality. Used as a condiment, your family will never know they are taking their daily tonic.

Garlic Rosemary Pesto

Get creative with the following recipe by accompanying it with toasted bread, raw or steamed vegetables, rice or pasta.

1 large garlic bulb (not elephant garlic), minced
½ cup olive oil
¼ tsp. chopped, dried rosemary

Mix the ingredients and serve immediately.

Garlic Bread Dip

¼ cup extra virgin olive oil
2 Tbs. fresh minced garlic
1 tsp. course dried peppers

Spoon over warmed whole wheat French bread.

Onion and Garlic Poultice

This is actually a natural home remedy for chest congestion.

1 white onion, diced
Extra virgin olive oil
½ Tbs. minced garlic

Bake diced onion in a shallow glass pan at 300° F for 30 minutes or until the onion begins to become clear and slimy. Remove from oven. Rub a few drops of olive oil to the chest. Apply the warm - not hot - onion to the chest. Sprinkle the minced garlic over the chest. Cover it with plastic wrap, an old cloth and secure it with an ace bandage wrap. Let it sit for at least half an hour.

"When my son, Joshua, was a little over a year old, he had been up all night with severe chest congestion. As suggested by Debra Raybern, I applied the Onion and Garlic Poultice. In about 30 minutes, the congestion started to break up, and he began to have very productive coughs. I did it again about four hours later and by the time he went to bed that evening, his chest was totally clear." - Sera Johnson

Fun Fact - Along with vitamin C, garlic contains allicin, which is a sulfur compound that has anti-bacterial and anti-viral properties.

Veggie Tacos

Set out ingredients in separate bowls for a buffet style meal.

Soft or crispy taco shells, warmed (non-GMO, organic corn or whole wheat tortillas)
1 zucchini, julienned
1 yellow squash, julienned
¼ onion, diced
1 small tomato, diced
1 cup shredded lettuce
2 avocados, sliced
1 cup cooked brown or white rice

Grape Nest Salad

Adding fruit to this salad makes for a sweet combination.

2 Tbs. sesame seeds
¼ head small red cabbage
¼ head small green cabbage

1 Tbs. chopped scallion or chives
3 Tbs. olive or flax oil
1 Tbs. fresh lime juice
1 cup mixed red and green grapes, halved
Prepare above ingredients and combine in a large bowl. Chill before serving.

Sweet Apple Slices

2 cups almonds
1 tsp. Blue Agave Nectar
Oats
2 apples

Blend almonds and blue agave until desired consistency. On a baking sheet, toast oats at 275° for 10 minutes. Core and quarter the apples. Spread the nut butter on the apple slices and top with the oats or sprinkle the oats in the butter and dip the slices in the mixture. For a variation, use sesame seeds rather than oats.

Carrot Apricot Muffins

2 cups organic whole wheat flour
¾ cup Blue Agave Nectar
1 tsp. baking power (aluminum free)
1 tsp. sea salt
2 large eggs
½ cup butter, softened (Additional butter needed to coat muffin pans.)
½ cup organic buttermilk
2 tsp. of freshly squeezed orange juice or 2 drops of Young Living orange essential oil
½ cup of chopped apricots
1 ½ cups of grated carrots
½ cup chopped walnuts or almonds

Preheat the oven to 400° F. Generously coat a 12-cup muffin pan with butter or line it with paper muffin cups. Set the pan aside. Mix the flour, blue agave, baking powder, and salt in a large bowl.

In a separate large bowl, beat the eggs. Beat in the butter, buttermilk, and orange-juice or oil. Slowly add the flour mixture, stirring lightly and briefly, until just combined. (Avoid over mixing the batter, as this makes muffins dense and tough.)

Add the apricots to the flour mixture. Stir in the carrots and nuts until the ingredients are just combined.
Ladle the batter into the prepared muffin pan, filling each cup no more than three-quarters full. Bake the muffins until a toothpick inserted near their centers comes out clean, 20 to 25 minutes. Cool for 10 minutes on a wire rack before serving.

Carrot and Wheat Berry Salad

Yield: 8 servings (serving size: about 2/3 cup)
Ingredients

- 1/2 cup uncooked wheat berries (hard winter wheat)
- 1 1/2 tsp. sea salt, divided
- 2 pounds carrots, chopped
- 1/2 cup fresh lemon juice
- 2 tsp. ground cumin
- 2 tsp. paprika
- 1/4 teaspoon ground red pepper
- 2 garlic cloves, minced
- 1/3 cup golden raisins
- 2 Tbs. extra virgin olive oil
- 3 Tbs. chopped fresh parsley
- 2 Tbs. chopped fresh cilantro

Place wheat berries and 1/2 teaspoon salt in a medium saucepan; cover with water to 2 inches above wheat berries. Bring to a boil. Reduce heat; cook, uncovered, 50 minutes or until the wheat berries are tender. Drain.
Cook half of carrots in a large pot of boiling water 2 minutes or until crisp-tender. Remove with a slotted spoon. Rinse with cold water, and drain. Repeat procedure with remaining carrots. Combine carrots and wheat berries in a large bowl; add 1 teaspoon salt, juice, cumin, paprika, pepper, and garlic. Stir in the raisins and oil, and toss well to combine. Cover and refrigerate 1 hour or until chilled. Sprinkle with the parsley and cilantro.

Unit 4

The Skeletal and Muscular Systems

What makes a person different from say a worm or bacteria? A part of the answer lies in the study of the bones and muscles and the covering God gave human bodies. Standing tall, moving, walking, running and reaching; as opposed to slithering and sliding on the ground, these are just some of the ways God made human bodies different from His other creations. Fish have scales, dogs have fur, birds have feathers; humans have skin, hair, bone and muscles. Most animals have some sort of claw, while men and women have nails. In this amazing unit, we will learn how to fortify our bodies and keep our temples, not only worthy of the spirit's dwelling place, but an example of health.

It was said of Jesus in Luke 2:52, "that he grew in wisdom and stature." Stature is defined as ones physical appearance and condition. There are many examples of heralded physical performance in the Bible, can you name some? Sampson, Daniel, Paul, Moses and others have biblical accounts of physical performance beyond the norm. Be sure to read about these men of the Bible, and if it is recorded, list what they ate.

Some medical professionals have begun to study the link to our physical wellbeing and our thoughts, words and spiritual health. While we will look into the spiritual connection to our health in Unit 6, we know that the Bible tells us we have a body, a mind and a spirit and the health of one affects the others. Below are some examples concerning that which we are about to study. The following are scriptures to keep in mind with each chapter:

"There is no soundness in my flesh because of thine anger; neither is there any rest in my bones because of my sin." Psalm 38:3

"A merry heart doeth good like a medicine: but a broken spirit drieth the bones." Proverbs 17:22

"Pleasant words are as an honeycomb, sweet to the soul and health to the bones." Proverbs 16:24

"This I say then, Walk in the Spirit, and ye shall not fulfill the lust of the flesh." Galatians 5:16

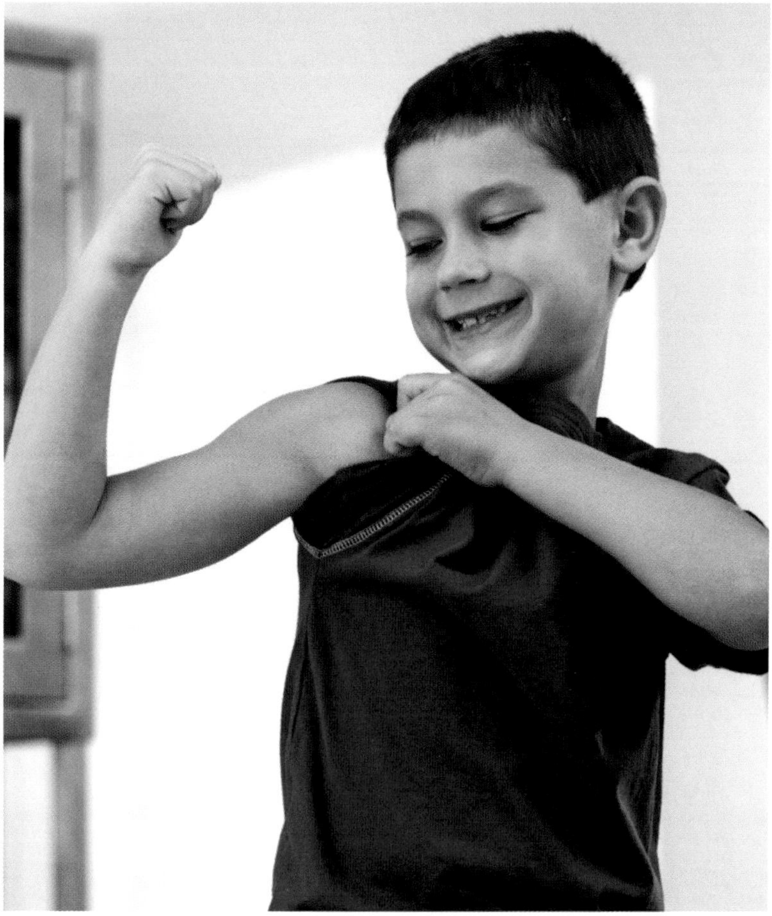

Chapter 1

The Skeletal System

"Thou hast clothed me with skin and flesh, and hast fenced me with bones and sinews." Job 10:11

What makes us stand up tall and not fall over like limp spaghetti? **Bones**. An adult has 206 bones in the body, but is born with 300 bones. Some of the bones in a baby's body are made entirely of a special material called **cartilage,** while other bones are only partially cartilage. This cartilage is soft and flexible, and as a person grows, the cartilage is slowly replaced by bone.

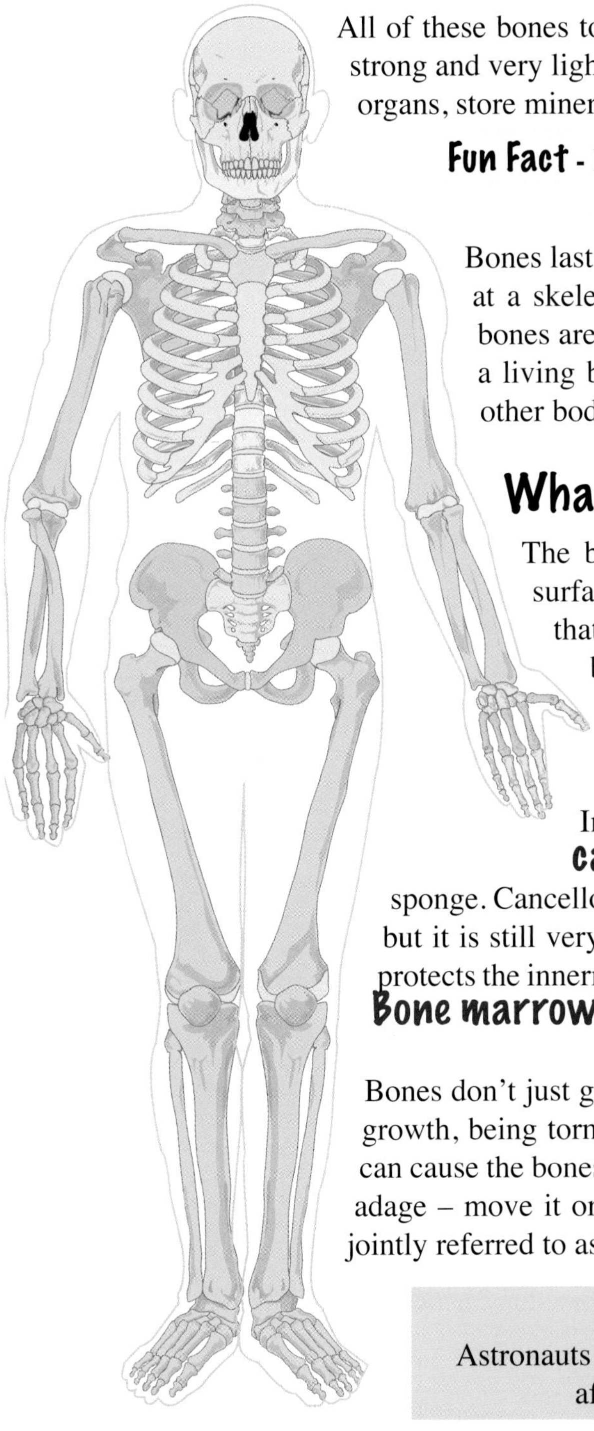

All of these bones together make up the skeletal system, or skeleton, that is both very strong and very light. In addition to supporting the body's shape, bones protect internal organs, store minerals and manufacture red blood cells.

Fun Fact - Human bones are able to withstand thousands of pounds of force per square inch.

Bones last more than a lifetime; they remain long after a person dies. Looking at a skeleton in a museum or science class, most people would think that bones are dry, crumbly and just for structure. However, when they are inside a living body they are very much alive, growing and changing like all the other body parts.

What makes up the bones?

The bones are made of the strongest material in the body. The outer surface of bone is called the **periosteum**. It is a thin, dense membrane that contains nerves and blood vessels that bring nourishment to the bone. The second layer is made up of very smooth, hard bone called **compact bone**. This is the part most commonly seen on a skeleton.

Fun Fact

Every second, bone marrow produces two million red blood cells.

Inside the compact bone are many layers of **cancellous bone**, which looks sort of like a sponge. Cancellous bone is not quite as hard as compact bone, but it is still very strong. In many bones, the cancellous bone protects the innermost part of the bone, called the bone marrow. **Bone marrow** is like a thick jelly, and its job is to make blood cells.

Bones don't just grow to a certain size and then stop. Bones are in a constant state of growth, being torn down and rebuilt over and over again. Long periods of inactivity can cause the bones to reduce their mass, leading to loss of strength and flexibility. The adage – move it or loose it – is true about our entire skeletal and muscular systems, jointly referred to as the **musculoskeletal system**.

Fun Fact

Astronauts suffer bone loss after long periods in space, but quickly regain it after returning to earth and performing vigorous activity.

Spine

The ring shaped **vertebrae** of the spine protect the spinal cord, a large bundle of nerves that sends information from the brain to the rest of the body. The spine lets us twist and bend, and it holds the body upright.

In between each vertebra – the name for just one of the vertebrae – are small **disks** made of cartilage. These disks keep the vertebrae from rubbing against one another, and they also act as the spine's natural shock absorbers. When an athlete jumps in the air, or twists while slamming a dunk, the disks give his vertebrae needed cushioning.

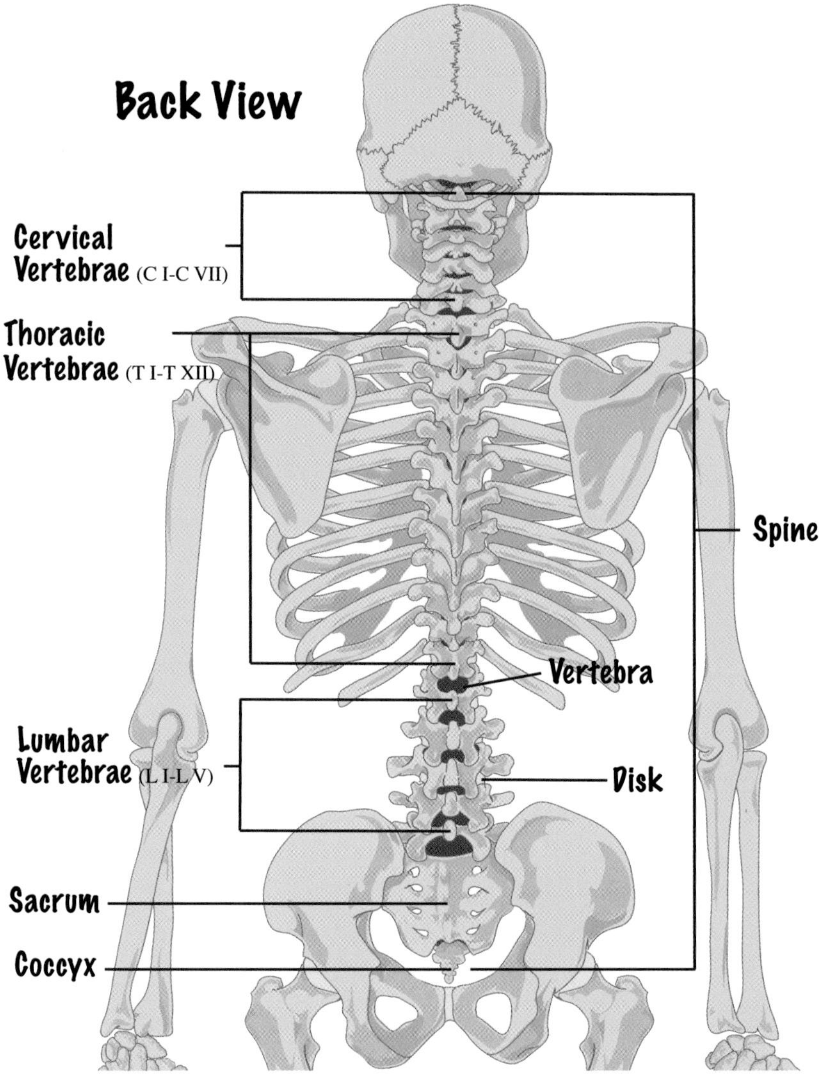

Problems to the disks can lead to back problems. When disks become flattened or dislodged, the vertebrae will touch causing pain. Back pain is one of the most common health concerns of Americans.

There are different types of vertebrae in the spine and each does a different kind of job:

The first seven vertebrae at the top are called the **cervical** vertebrae. These bones are in the back of the neck, just below the brain, and support the head and neck.

Below the cervical vertebrae are the **thoracic** vertebrae, and there are 12 in all. They anchor the ribs in place.

Below the thoracic vertebrae are five **lumbar** vertebrae. Beneath the lumbar vertebrae is the **sacrum**, which is made up of five vertebrae that are fused together to form one single bone.

Finally, all the way at the bottom of the spine is the **coccyx,** which is one bone made of four fused vertebrae. The bottom sections of the spine are important when it comes to bearing weight and providing a good center of gravity. So when a person picks up a heavy backpack, the lumbar vertebrae, sacrum and coccyx gives him the power. When a child dances, skips and even walks, these parts help keep her balanced.

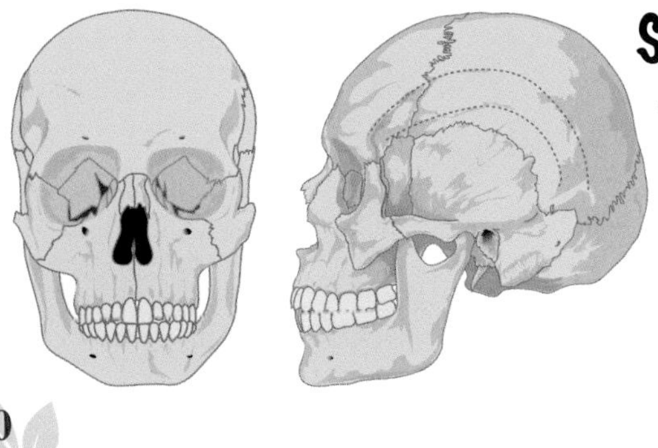

Skull

The skull actually is made up of different bones. Some protect the brain, while others make up the structure of the face. Touch beneath the eyes to feel the ridge of the bone that forms the hole where the eye sits.

The Smallest Bones

Thin tiny bones in the middle ear helps humans to hear over 40,000 distinct sounds. These bones are called the **hammer**, **anvil** and **stirrup**. See the ear illustration in Unit 3 Chapter 3. Another bone in the neck called the **hyoid** bone enables us to speak. The hyoid bone is the only bone in the body not attached to another bone, but instead floats freely in soft tissue.

Ribs

The **ribs** keep the heart, lungs and liver safe. Ribs act like a cage of bones around the chest. It's easy to feel the bottom of this cage by running the fingers along the sides and front of the body, a few inches below the heart. Inhaling deeply will make it easier to feel the ribs. Some people can even see a few of their ribs right through their skin.

Ribs come in pairs, and the left and right sides of each pair are exactly the same. Most people have 12 pairs of ribs, but some people are born with one or more extra ribs, and some people might have one pair less.

"And the Lord God caused a deep sleep to fall upon Adam, and he slept: and he took one of his ribs, and closed up the flesh instead thereof; And the rib, which the Lord God had taken from man, made he a woman, and brought her unto the man. And Adam said, This is now bone of my bones, and flesh of my flesh: she shall be called Woman, because she was taken out of Man." – Genesis 2:21-23

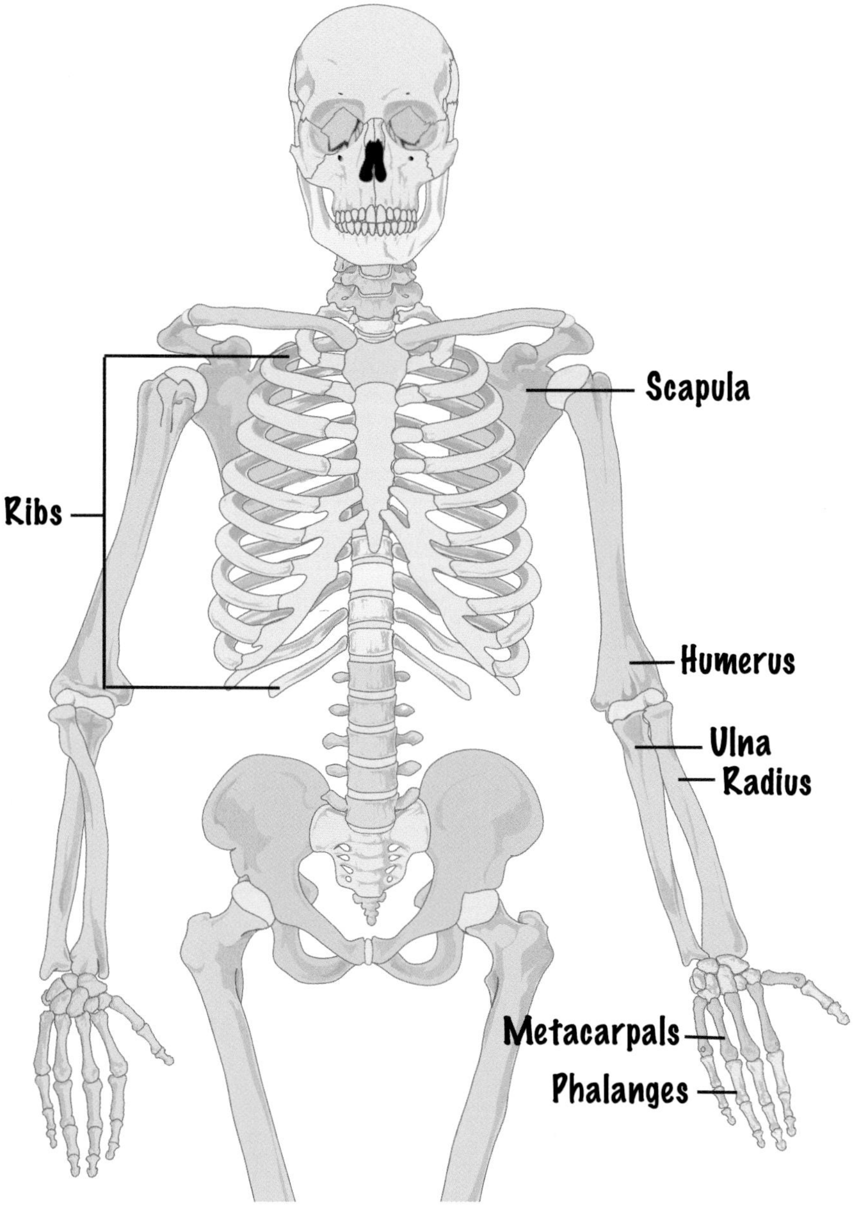

Arms and Hands

Swinging a bat, picking up toys, writing or typing – all these tasks uses the bones in the fingers, hand, wrist and arm. The arms are attached to the shoulder blades called **scapula**. The arms have three bones: the **humerus**, which is above the elbow, and the **radius** and **ulna**, which are below the elbow. Each of bones is wider at the ends and skinnier in the middle, to help give it strength where it meets another bone. At the end of the radius and ulna are eight smaller bones that make up the wrist.

The center part of the hand is made up of five separate bones called **metacarpals**. Each finger on the hand has three bones called **phalanges**, except for the thumb, which has two. There is a grand total of 54 bones that make up the arm and hands.

Legs

Jumping rope, walking, running or climbing a tree – not without the legs and feet. The legs are attached to a circular group of bones called the **pelvis.** The pelvis is a bowl-shaped structure that supports the spine. It is made up of the two large hip bones in front, and behind are the sacrum and the coccyx. The pelvis acts as a tough ring of protection around parts of the digestive system, the urinary system and the reproductive system.

The leg bones are the largest and strongest bones in the body. The **femur** bone extends from the pelvis to the knee and is the longest bone in the body. Protecting the knee is a triangular bone called the **patella**. Below the knee are two bones: the **tibia** and **fibula**. Just like the three bones in the arm, the three bones in the leg are wider at the ends than in the middle to give them strength.

The ankle is where the lower leg bones connect to a large bone in the foot called the **talus**. Next to the talus are six other bones which are all **tarsal** bones. The main part of the foot has five bones called **metatarsals**. Each toe has three tiny bones called **phalanges**, except for the big toe, which has just two. This brings the bone total in both feet and the ankles to 52, two less than the hands.

One important function of the feet people rarely consider is balance. Without all the bones, joints and muscles of the foot working together, it would be impossible to balance properly. This near flat, wide arrangement helps each of us stay upright.

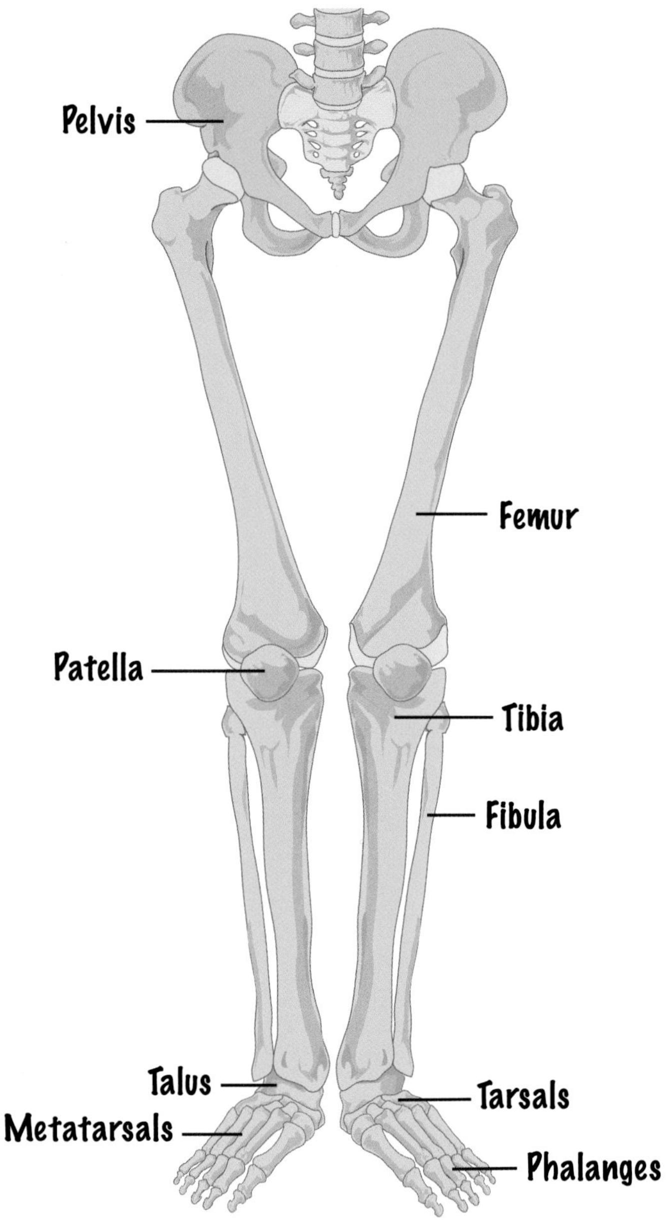

Bone Mass

Bones are the framework for a growing body. Bone is living tissue that changes constantly, with bits of old bone being removed and replaced by new bone. Think of bone as a bank account, where bone tissue is both deposited and withdrawn. During childhood and adolescence, much more bone is deposited than withdrawn as the skeleton grows in both size and density. The bone generally reaches its maximum size between age 18 to 20. Even though it is no longer growing in size, it still is living tissue constantly being used and replaced.

For most people, the amount of bone tissue in the skeleton, known as **bone mass**, peaks by the late 20s. At that point, bones have reached their maximum strength and density. Up to 90 percent of peak bone mass is acquired by age 18 in girls and age 20 in boys, which makes youth the best time for your kids to invest in their bones.

> "Building your children's 'bone bank' account is a lot like saving for their education: The more they can put away when they're young, the longer it should last as they get older."
> - National Institute of Health Web site

Health Issues of the Skeletal System

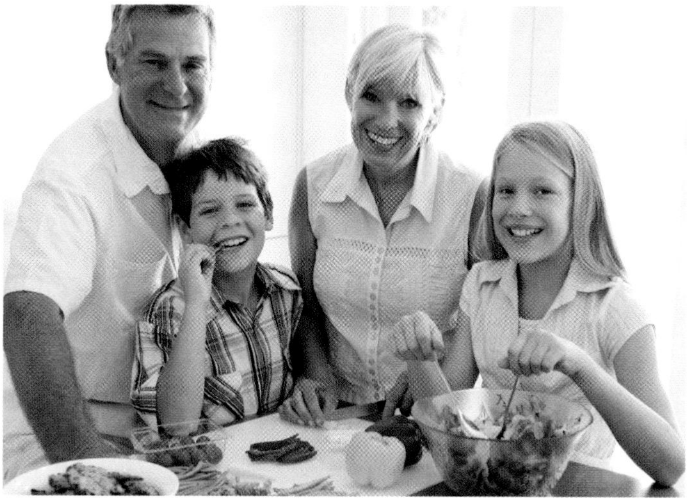

Diseases of the skeletal and muscular systems often are lumped together. The most common is arthritis, a condition that affects the joints. Health concerns like bursitis and fibromyalgia affect the muscles, and cancer affects the bones themselves.

Osteoporosis

According to the National Osteoporosis Foundation, roughly 55 percent of Americans, mostly women, are at risk of developing the brittle-bone disease, which leaves bones dry, weak and more likely to fracture.

For a lifetime of good skeletal heath, a person should eat a healthy diet, engage in moderate exercise (more about exercise in Chapter 4) and heed the words of Proverbs 17:22, "A merry heart doeth good like a medicine: but a broken spirit drieth the bones." We must have the mind of Christ, as stated in I Corinthians 2:16, and do not become bitter with life, God or other people.

What are minerals?

Minerals play a very important role in the health of the skeletal system. They are the building blocks of bones and can be found in many different good foods. Minerals are inorganic elements that naturally occur in the earth and in rocks. Unlike vitamins that are organic and can be destroyed by cooking, processing, oxidation or high heat, minerals always retain their chemical identity. Minerals are taken up by plants into forms that the human body can assimilate. The primary role of minerals in the body is the structural composition of the skeletal system. They also maintain body fluid composition and are essential to protein and enzymatic reactions. Keeping minerals in balance in every organ in the human body may be the key to maintaining optimal health.

Which minerals are most important to the Skeletal System?

Calcium, the mineral most abundant in healthy bones, helps maintain good bone health, supports nerve function and muscle health, and clots blood. Bones are formed through bone mineralization which uses calcium and phosphorus to join and form calcium phosphate, a main component of hydroxyapatite that gives structure to bones.

Calcium cannot be made by the body, and must be acquired through food. While many people believe milk to be the best food source of calcium, as discussed in the Respiratory Unit, this is not true. Green leafy vegetables, seeds and nuts are some of the best foods rich in calcium. For a list of calcium rich foods, see Appendix N.

If a person's dietary intake is insufficient to maintain other calcium dependant functions of the body, the body will draw calcium out of the bones, which after time will lead to **osteoporosis**. Highly acidic foods and foods containing excessive amounts of phosphorus also leach calcium from the bones.

Foods that leach calcium from the body include: caffeine, which inhibits calcium absorption, (teas, coffee, carbonated beverages), white refined sugar, phosphates found in soda drinks and excessive protein consumption.

While eating calcium rich food is the best way to get calcium, supplementation is also an option. Generally, it is recommended that calcium supplements be taken in separate doses. This is because 500 milligrams is all the body can absorb at one time.

Magnesium is another mineral that cannot be made by the body and a substantial amount from food sources should be consumed daily. Called a macronutrient, due to the large supplemented amounts necessary each day, magnesium is a relaxing mineral as well. In addition to relaxing nerves and muscles, it aids in the maintenance of strong bones and keeps the blood circulating. Unit 2 introduced magnesium as is an important mineral for proper acid/alkaline balance. Deficiencies may include headaches, muscle weakness, tremors, spasms, imbalanced blood sugar levels and elevated blood pressure.

Some of the best sources include Swiss chard, spinach, pumpkin seeds, green beans, sunflower seeds, sesame seeds, salmon and black beans.

Phosphorus is a mineral that likes to work with calcium, vitamin B6, manganese, iron and sodium. Phosphorus is toxic in high amounts, such as how it is often consumed in soda drinks. The results of toxicity include loss of calcium and brittle bones. Deficiencies include fatigue, irritability, bone pain, weakness, skin sensitivity and decreased appetite.

A study at Tufts University conducted on several thousand men and women, found that women who habitually drank caffeinated and non-caffeinated cola-based sodas, which contain phosphoric acid, "had almost four percent lower bone mineral density in the hip, even though researchers controlled their calcium and vitamin D intake." Despite phosphorus being an important bone mineral, disproportionate amounts could lead to bone loss.[1]

Some of the best food sources include millet (a cereal grain), cashews, sesame seeds, chicken, lima beans, asparagus, broccoli, legumes and dried fruits.

Often associated with lowered immune response, **zinc** is a mineral that also can help balance blood sugar levels, stabilize metabolism and support the sense of smell and taste. Lack of zinc can be seen in frequent colds and infections, depression, lack of appetite and in small children – failure to thrive and grow. Thin, peeling nails may be a sign of lowered zinc intake.

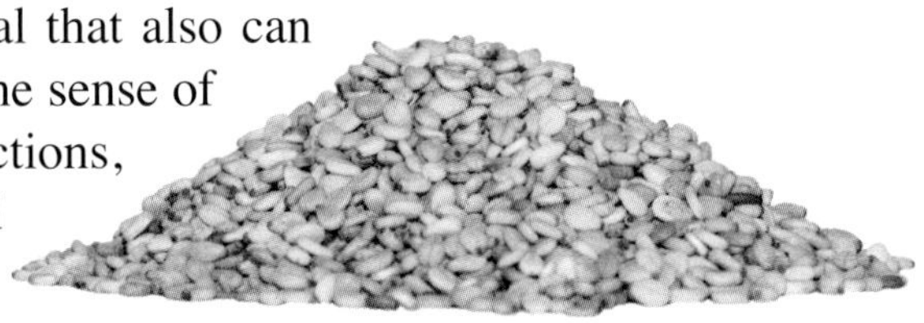

Zinc is found in grass-fed beef, sesame seeds, green peas, whole grains, pumpkin seeds, lima beans and fish.

Despite being needed by the body in trace amounts, **copper** plays an important role in health. It is an essential mineral, preserving the nerves' myelin sheath, helping the body utilize iron, maintaining the health of the bones and connective tissue, and acting as an antioxidant by reducing free-radical damage. But in recent years, due to high copper concentrations in drinking water, nutritionists are becoming concerned with copper toxicity. In pregnant women, high levels of copper in the body after birth have been linked to postpartum depression.

Foods with copper include nuts, seeds and vegetables. Eating a variety of foods containing copper should not be a concern.

Boron is a trace mineral that has been linked to bone health. According to Alexander G. Schauss, Ph.D of AIBR Life Sciences Division, boron has been found to be essential to human health and behavior.[2] Its importance to human health did not become apparent to scientists until the mid-1980's. Today it has been scientifically demonstrated that boron is important to brain function, especially in enhancing memory, cognitive function and hand-eye coordination. The highest concentrations of boron are found in the drinking water and soil of some of the driest climate areas in the world.

---

1 http://www.project-aware.org/Health/Osteo/osteo-bonehealth2.shtml

2 "Minerals, Trace Elements and Human Health" Life Sciences Press: Tacoma, (WA), 1996.

Evidence continues to mount that boron may reduce either the symptoms or incidence of arthritis. Although the connection between arthritis and boron was first discovered in sheep and chickens, researchers have found a curious association between the amount of boron in the soil and drinking water, and the incidence of arthritis in a population. For example, in the most arid areas of the world, the incidence of arthritis tends to be dramatically lower than in the rain-laden areas. Arid areas have been found to have the highest concentrations of boron in the drinking water and soil. This is most interesting since it is well known that boron can get more readily leached out of the soil in wet climates.

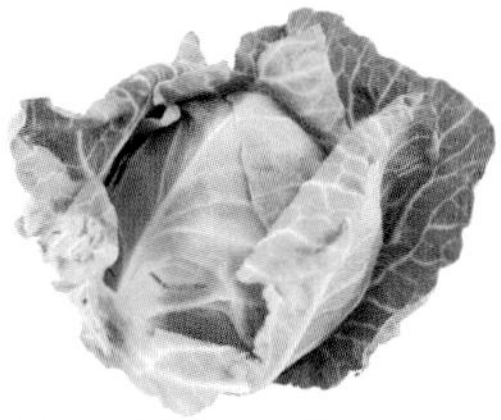

Making sure the diet has adequate levels of boron may ensure calcium and other bone building nutrients are able to assist in proper bone development and health. No recommended daily allowance (RDA) has been established for boron in humans at this time.

The best food source of boron is raw cabbage. Other sources are green leafy vegetables and nuts.

Collagen is an insoluble protein that acts as scaffolding to provide strength and rigidity to bones.

One of the best sources of collagen is unprocessed chicken broth.

Manganese is a trace mineral that assists in enzyme reactions in the body. It assists the body in the utilization of biotin, vitamin B1, vitamin C and choline. In addition, manganese activates the enzymes that are important in bone formation and is believed to be beneficial in the production of the hormone thyroxine for thyroid support.

The best food sources are pineapple, raspberries, brown rice, garbanzo beans, oats and flaxseeds.

Vitamin D is a fat-soluble vitamin that helps the body absorb calcium, regulates the growth and activity of cells and can help prevent excessive inflammatory immune related activity.

There are two types of vitamin D: ergosterol, the basic building block of vitamin D in plants; and cholesterol, the basic building block of vitamin D in humans. Ironically, there has been a vigorous campaign in the U.S. to lower cholesterol while osteoporosis has increased among Americans.

When sunlight hits the lead of a plant, ergosterol is converted into vitamin D2. In the same way, when sunlight hits the cells in our skin, cholesterol is converted into cholecalciferol, or vitamin D3. Vitamin D is measured in international units (IU). Current RDA guidelines (1997) suggest 400 IU daily for adults, yet many people actually need up to 1,000 IU for optimal bone health. Severe vitamin D deficiency in children is called rickets. Cod liver oil, which is rich in vitamin D, was once often recommended to children.

The healthiest sources of Vitamin D include: tuna, sardines, eggs and moderate sunlight.

Fun Fact

One cup of low fat fortified milk provides 97 international units (IU) of Vitamin D. One egg provides 22 IU. Four ounces of sardines provides 250 IU.

Good Foods for Bones

Black pepper, cabbage, fish oils, parsley, onions, garlic, kale, broccoli, turnip greens, millet, cashews, low-fat dairy and cheese (in moderation especially if respiratory issues are a concern), grass-fed beef, sesame seeds, green peas, whole grains, pumpkin seeds, lima beans, Swiss chard, spinach and legumes

Bad Food for Bones

Sodas, sugar and excessive red meat (high phosphorus)

Teeth

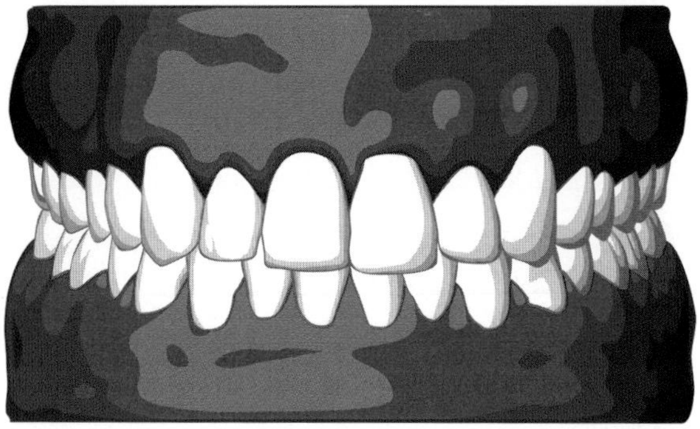

Think about the photos of skulls or those exhibited at museums. Even though they were unearthed 300, 500 or more years ago, they still have teeth. Often we see photos or video footage of people in countries where we think poor health, sanitary and food condition exist, but one thing many have in common is white, bright healthy teeth. Then why do so many people today have their teeth extracted, capped, crowned, straightened, filled and even replaced? What is wrong with our diets and lifestyles today that is proving to be harmful to our teeth?

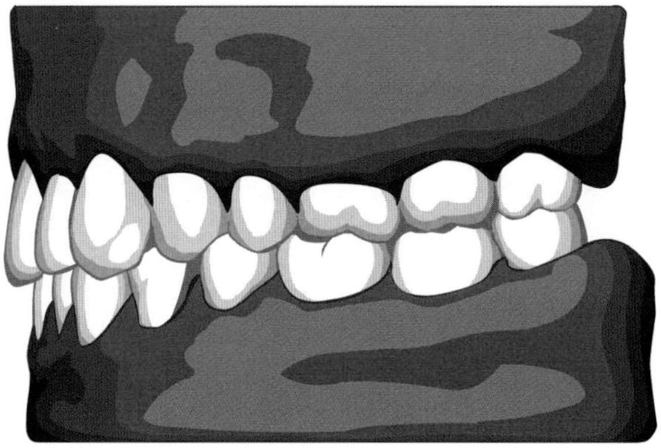

Brushing, flossing, rinsing and regular visits to the dentist are of course fundamental for good oral hygiene. Selecting oral care products free of toxic ingredients – sodium lauryl sulfate, fluoride and propylene glycol to name a few – also is important. The mouth can absorb toxins at a faster rate than if the toxins were digested. That is why many children's toothpastes contain warnings for ingestion.

But are there foods that can be beneficial or others that are harmful for the teeth? To answer this question we first have to know exactly what is the composition of our teeth.

Teeth are made up primarily of calcium. Nutrients essential for proper tooth development and maintenance include **vitamins A**, **C** and **D** and the minerals **calcium**, **phosphorus** and **fluorine**. Vitamin C is essential in forming the protein dentin called **collagen**. The tooth enamel contains keratin, a type of protein requiring vitamin A for its formation. Vitamin D is essential for the depositing of calcium and phosphorus that make up the matrix or structure of the jaw bones and teeth. The nutrient fluorine is incorporated into the tooth's structure before it erupts to combine with calcium and phosphorus to form a compound called fluorapatite, making the tooth more resistant to erosion. Many dentists believe the addition of topical fluoride in toothpastes, rinses and gels provides continued protection.

Fluorine vs. Fluoride

The mineral fluorine is extremely rare and is found naturally and in minute quantities in almonds, carrots, beet greens, turnip greens, dandelion, spinach and black tea. Refer to Appendix G: Mineral Chart for more flourine rich foods.

Trace amounts of fluorine may help with healthy teeth and bone formation. Today many health professionals recommend young children, even infants be given supplemental fluoride (sodium fluoride), a synthetic form of the natural mineral fluorine to support healthy teeth and guard against cavities.

Scientist Robert Carton, Ph.D., formerly with the U.S. Environmental Protection Agency stated, "Fluoride is somewhat less toxic than arsenic and more toxic than lead and you wouldn't want either in your mouth."

As early as 1961, as recorded in the Congressional Record, fluoride was exposed as a lethal toxin even though it is still used in many of our cities municipal water supplies. Decades later communities across America began to add fluoride to the water supply.

Recent studies in the Journal of Dental Research conclude that tooth decay rates in Western Europe, which is 98 percent unfluoridated, have declined as much as they have in the United States in recent decades. However, while fluoridation is encouraged by the U.S. government; most European nations – including Germany, France, Sweden and Holland -- prohibit fluoride on public health grounds.

According to Phyllis Balch, certified nutrition counselor, "Although many ailments and disorders – including Down syndrome, mottled teeth, and cancer – have been linked to fluoridated water, fluoridation has become the standard rather than the exception.[3]"

The American Dental Association has been an advocate of fluoride over the decades, but issued a directive that stated "Infants less than one year old may be getting more than the optimal amount of fluoride if their primary source of nutrition is powdered or liquid infant formula mixed with water containing fluoride." The ADA went on to advise: "If using a product that needs to be reconstituted, parents and caregivers should consider using water that has no or low levels of fluoride."

Canada's former top pro-fluoride authority, Dr. Hardy Limeback, a biochemist and professor of dentistry at the University of Toronto, told the Toronto Sunday Star in 1999 that parents should keep fluoride away from children under three, and that water fluoridation is unnecessary and may be risky.

"There is no point in swallowing fluoridated water," he said. "The only benefit comes with direct contact with the teeth."

Good Foods for Teeth

Whole grains, including oats, eggs and limes

Bad Foods for Teeth

Sugar, sodas (contains high fructose corn syrup and phosphoric acid), sticky candies and processed foods in general

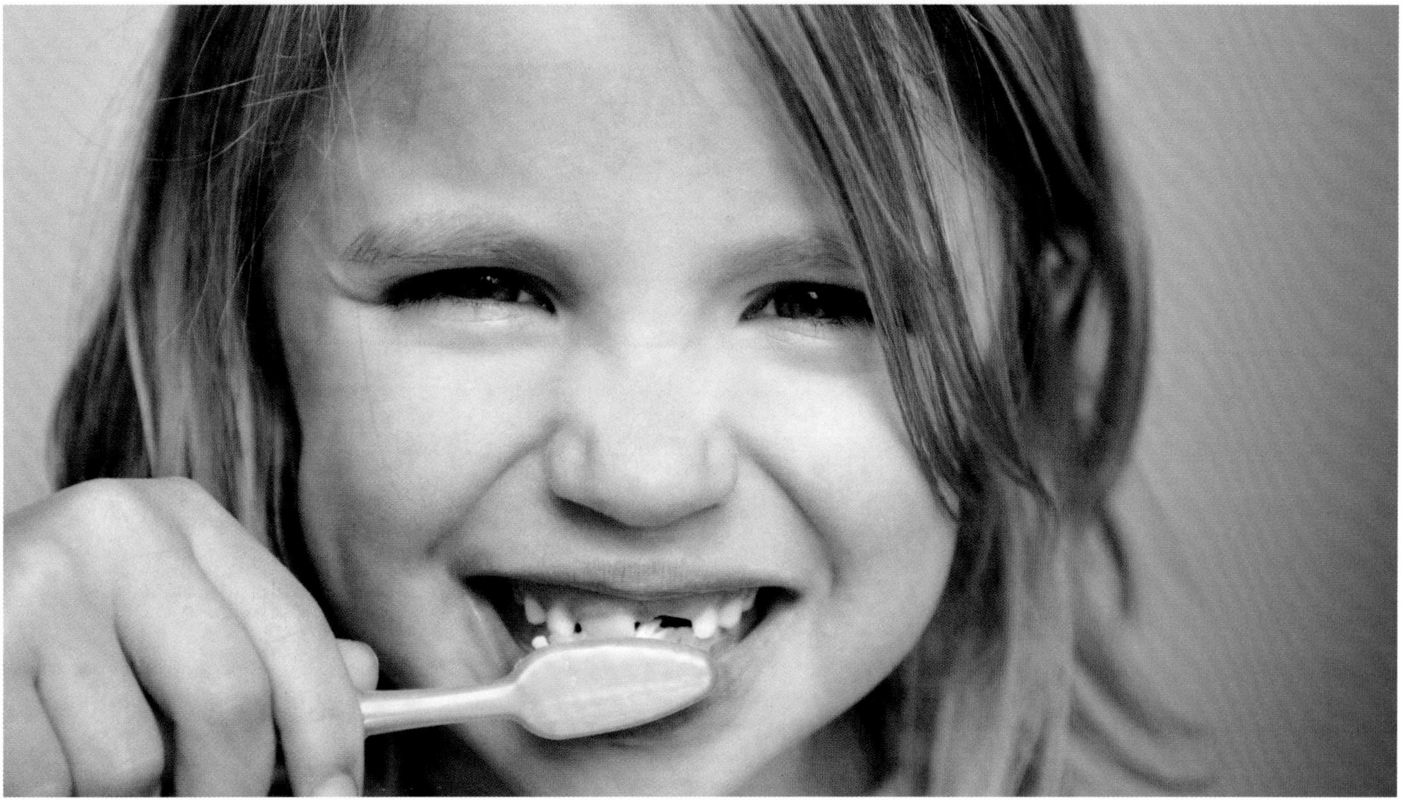

3 "Prescription for Nutritional Healing," fourth edition, by Phyllis A. Balch. Avery. 2006.

Unit 4 Chapter 1
Discussion Questions

1. What are your favorite Scriptures about bones?
2. Which bones do you use to run? Sit in a chair? Drink from a glass?
3. Have you ever broken a bone? How did the doctor treat it?
4. What are some ways we protect our bones?
5. Look over the calcium chart in Appendix N. Does it surprise you to see so many different foods that contain calcium?

Activities - plus the Nut Balls "Power" Recipe and activities.

Elementary

1. Read Exodus 13 with your family. As the Israelites left Egypt, Moses carried the bones of a special person? Which person was it and why did Moses do this?
2. Roll up a sheet of paper (8 1/2 x 11) about 1 inch wide into a cylinder. Repeat this three times to make three paper bones. Stand the bones up on their ends, placing a paper plate on top of the bones. Do the hollow bones support the plate? Slowly add weight (wooden blocks) to the plate. Count how many blocks the plate can hold before it collapses the bones. Roll three more sheets of paper as tightly possible so that there is no hollow section. Stand these bones up as before placing the same plate on top of them. Place weights on top of the plate until they collapse. Which bones were more supportive? Why?
3. Look around where you live for a home that is under construction. After a foundation is prepared, What is the next step? What happens if this step is skipped? How is your skeleton like the framework of a house?
4. Ask a dentist for a teeth chart or find one in a book or online. Look in a mirror and identify your incisors, canines, premolars, and molars. Are you missing any teeth? Do you still have some baby teeth?
5. Try two new foods from the calcium chart during a meal.
6. Based on the calcium recommendations in Appendix N, how much calcium should you consume each day?
7. Keep a daily record of the foods you eat for two days. Research to find out how much calcium is in those foods and calculate your daily intake of calcium for those two days. Did you reach the recommended calcium for your age?

Secondary

Choose any from above plus

1. What kinds of doctors specialize in bone and spine health?
2. Focus on one of the fields of study identified above and learn more about that specialty.
3. Collect the following materials: a large piece of cardboard; two large, two medium, and two small empty thread spools; a pencil; scissors, ruler, hole puncher, string, tape and a balloon. Draw five circles on the cardboard by tracing the base of the two large, two medium, and one small spools of thread. Cut the circles out and will punch holes through the center of them. Cut an 18 inch (45cm) length of string. Then thread the spools of thread together beginning with the largest spools, taping the string to the bottom of the largest spool (cardboard circles of corresponding sides will be threaded between each pair of spools). Blow up a balloon and will place it on top of the model. Identify the cervical, thoracic and lumbar vertebrae. How does an imbalance in one portion of the vertebrae affect the others?
4. Using chicken bones, preferably from the leg (drumsticks), clean the bones and place half in containers with vinegar. Place the other half in water. Compare and contrast the similarities and differences of the sets of bones. Were the bones placed in vinegar weaker and more flexible? Why?
5. Find out the RDA of calcium for each member of your family based on the chart in Appendix N. Have everyone in the family keep track of what they eat for two days. Find out the average calcium each member consumed each day. Did everyone get their recommended calcium for those days?
6. Plan a menu that includes all three meals and two snacks for a day that meets the average recommended calcium intake for everyone in your family. It has to include a variety of calcium rich foods and must be tasty.
7. Figure out how much spinach, collard greens, blackstrap molasses and sesame seeds each would equal the same amount of calcium as one eight ounce glass of milk. With your findings, make a chart to show the family. Be as creative with the chart as you would like.

Skeletal System Power

Seeds and Nuts

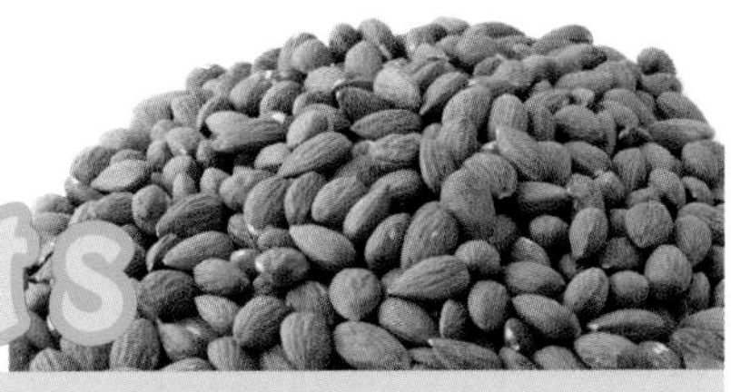

Seeds and nuts are amazing sources of calcium and other bone building minerals.
One quarter (¼) cup of sesame seeds has MORE calcium than an 8 ounce glass of milk!

Nut Balls

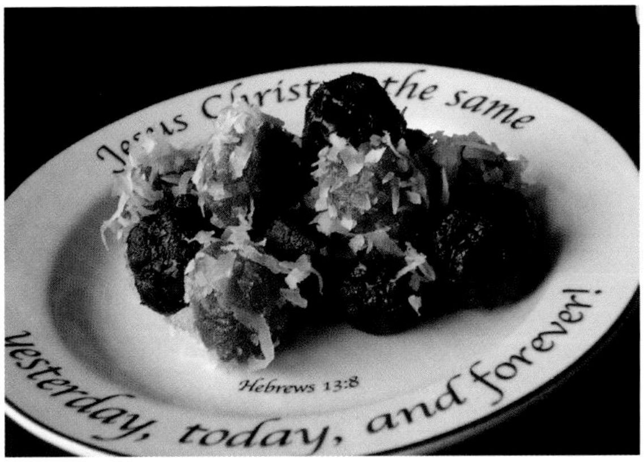

½ cup sesame seeds
1 cup almonds, chopped
½ cup pecans or walnuts, chopped
1 ½ cup pitted dates
Dash of salt

Coconut, shredded
Cocoa or Carob powder

Pulse all ingredients in food processor until a ball forms. Press into balls and roll in freshly shredded coconut or cocoa/carob powder.

Activities

Elementary

1. What is a drupe?
2. Identify which ingredients are nuts, which are seeds and which are drupes.
3. What does it mean to "pulse" something?
4. Dates are a staple in the Middle East and Mediterranean regions. In what type of climate are they typically grown? Are they grown in the U.S. or imported?
5. Make this tasty treat and share it with your friends. Wait to tell them about the healthy ingredients after they've tried it.

Secondary

Choose any from above plus

1. Look up "pulse" in the dictionary. What are other meanings of the word?
2. For those who do not like coconut, what are other ingredients that can be used?
3. Learn more about coconut. Study where and how it is grow and how the parts of the coconut are used.
4. Peanut allergies are very common these days. This recipe does not use peanuts, but does use almonds, pecans and walnuts. Are there allergies associated with these? Why or why not? How are these different from peanuts? Research this topic (including text from previous chapters of this curriculum) and prepare an oral or written report on the subject.
5. Calculate how many grams of protein are in this entire recipe by researching the protein content of each ingredient. Then, after making the nut balls, find out how much protein is in just one. Do the same for the calcium content. Are you surprised by your findings?

Chapter 2

Joints and The Muscular System

"For the word of God [is] quick, and powerful, and sharper than any two edged sword, piercing even to the dividing asunder of soul and spirit, and of the joints and marrow, and [is] a discerner of the thoughts and intents of the heart." Hebrews 4:12

"And not holding the Head, from which all the body by joints and bands having nourishment ministered, and knit together, increaseth with the increase of God." Colossians 2:19

"Then the king's countenance was changed, and his thoughts troubled him, so that the joints of his loins were loosed, and his knees smote one against another." Daniel 5:6

The Joints

Besides just bones, the joints allow us to bend and move the neck, shoulder, elbow, knee, hip, wrists, fingers, thumb, ankles, and toes. Without joints we would be stiff and unable to move about freely or do any of the tasks we may take for granted. The muscles that connect these joints together work in unison to allow us the freedom of movement we enjoy.

What are joints?

The place where two bones meet is called a **joint**. Some joints move and others do not. The skull is made up of joints called sutures, that while flexible at birth, they fuse together as a person grows and do not move. Along the side of the skull is the **parietal-temporal joint**, which also does not move.

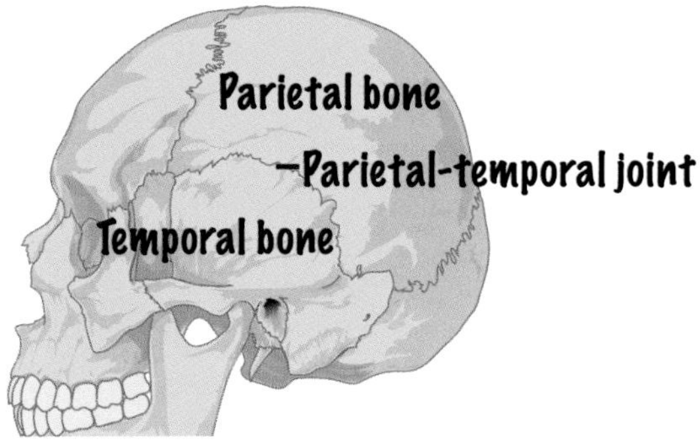

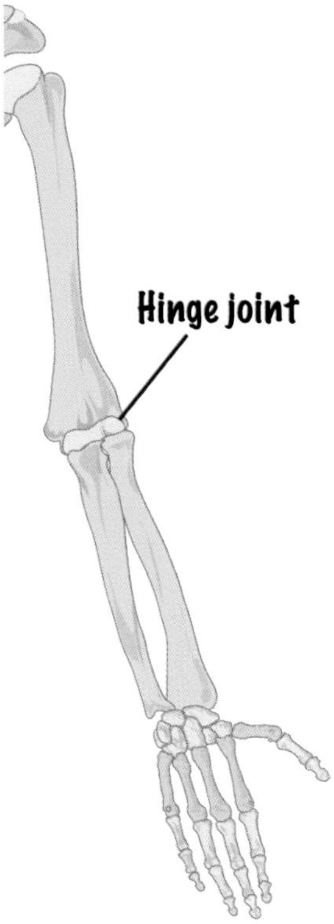

The vertebrae of the spine are actually individual joints that allow us to move, bend and twist. They only move just a little in comparison to the hip, knee and elbow, which have a wide range of motion. But even the arm and leg joints only move in one direction, much like a door hinge. Small **hinge joints** are in the fingers and hands.

The **ball and socket joints** are in the shoulders and hips. One end of the bone is rounded and fits into a socket or cup-like area of the other bone. They allow for more freedom of movement. You only have to watch a gymnast to see all the possibilities of movement the human body is capable of.

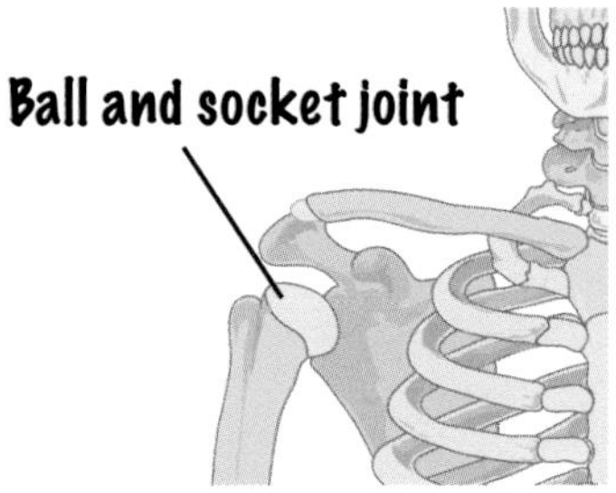

At the knee, there's a triangular-shaped bone called the kneecap - also known as the **patella** - that protects the knee joint.

Joints are cushioned with a special fluid called **synovial fluid** to help them move freely and not squeak and creak like a door hinge that needs oil. A diet rich in the **Omega-3 oils** is just one way to ensure this fluid is plentiful.

Joint Health Issues

Most of the diseases that occur within the skeletal system involve the joints. While osteoarthritis is a disease that causes the bones to become brittle and prone to fractures, most arthritic conditions involve the joints inability to move. Doctors often say that osteoarthritis is a pediatric disease with geriatric consequences. It is the healthy nutrition habits we learn now that can make or break our bones as we age.

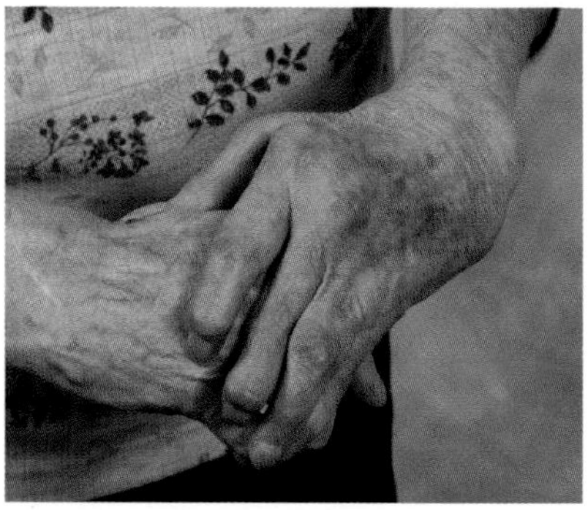

Rheumatoid arthritis (RA) is a disease of the joints generally regarded to be an autoimmune condition where the body attacks itself. (Autoimmune conditions will be explained further in Unit 5). Even though infectious agents such as viruses, bacteria, and fungi have long been suspected, none has been proven as the cause. Rheumatoid arthritis causes chronic inflammation of the joints. It can also cause inflammation of the tissue around the joints, as well as in other organs in the body. This chronic inflammation leads to the destruction of the cartilage, bone and ligaments, causing deformity of the joints.

Supporting the body with **Omega-3 fatty acids** is important to joint health and is also considered part of a natural approach to managing RA. Other herbs and nutritional support include turmeric[1], probiotics and essential oils topically for pain and inflammation relief.[2]

Psoriatic arthritis is closely tied to the condition psoriasis which affects the skin. People who have inflammatory arthritis and psoriasis are diagnosed as having psoriatic arthritis.

Bursitis occurs when the fluid filled sacs called bursa located within joints, muscles, tendons and bones become inflamed. It is most common in the elbows, feet, shoulders and hips. When in the shoulder, this is often called frozen shoulder and occurs in many women just after menopause. When it occurs in the feet, usually the big toe, it is called a bunion often caused by ill fitting shoes or the wearing of high heeled shoes for too many years. Injury, calcium deposits, infections or diseases such as arthritis and gout also contribute to bursitis. Since bursitis can be very painful and tender to the touch it may restrict movement. Nutrients to support joint health, including the bursa sacs include **protein** and **vitamin A**. Warm compresses over the area with alternating cold compresses may help to sooth the area. With the right nutritional support many cases of bursitis will resolve on their own. Stretching exercises and the topical use of therapeutic-grade essential oils have been used by many to hasten recovery and healing.[2]

Free Radical/Inflammatory Producing Food

Beef - antibiotic and corn fed
Dairy products
Fried foods
Hydrogenated fats
Processed sugar
Soft drinks
Trans fats

How does nutrition affect the joints?

Glucosamine

Found naturally in the body, glucosamine is made from glucose and the amino acid glutamine. Glucosamine is needed to produce glycosaminoglycan, a molecule used in the formation and repair of cartilage and other body tissues. The production of glucosamine slows with age.

Glucosamine is available as a nutritional supplement, with most manufactured in a laboratory from chitin, a substance found in the shells of shrimp, crab, lobster and other sea creatures. Over five million people take glucosamine, often in combination with chondroitin, for joint health. In additional to nutritional supplements, glucosamine also is used in sports drinks and in cosmetics.

---

1 "Turmeric Prevents Experimental Rheumatoid Arthritis, Bone Loss" Science Daily. Oct. 30, 2006.

2 See Appendix DD for authors' recommendations.

Since glucosamine supplements may be made from shellfish, people with allergies to shellfish should avoid glucosamine unless it has been confirmed that it is from a non-shellfish source. The source of glucosamine is not required to be printed on the label, so it may require a phone call to the manufacturer. The less commonly and more expensive form of glucosamine is made by the fermentation of a grain such as corn or wheat.

Glucosamine is often combined with chondroitin sulfate, a molecule naturally present in cartilage. Chondroitin gives cartilage elasticity and is believed to prevent the destruction of cartilage by enzymes. Sometimes glucosamine also is combined with methylsulfonylmethane or MSM.

Glucosamine may be labeled as: glucosamine sulfate, glucosamine sulphate, glucosamine hydrochloride, N-acetyl glucosamine, chitosamine

Bad Foods for Joints

alcohol, sugar, red meat, wheat (for some), milk (for some) – both wheat and milk contain proteins that are hard to break down for some people

Chondroitin

Chondroitin, also known as chondroitin sulfate, is a naturally occurring vital compound in connective tissue that is partly responsible for building and supporting the basic substance of cartilage. When present in the body, it is purported to promote healthy joints by warding off the effects of damaging enzymes, increasing water retention and enhancing the elastic properties of cartilage. This enhanced fluidity in the joints may have a rejuvenating effect on cells and tissues and assist in joint mobility and range of motion. Joint tissue contains chondroitin, but its natural production declines with age.

Though there have been no conclusive studies with people who take chondroitin to relieve osteoarthritis in their knees and hips, many still report that pain is abated and they are able to move about more freely after using it.

Scientists who have studied chondroitin report that the body is able to absorb as much as 15 percent when taken as a dietary supplement. The recommended daily dosage for those who take chondroitin sulfate as a supplement is 400 to 600 miligrams three times per day. Chondroitin is generally in a combination bone-joint health supplement.

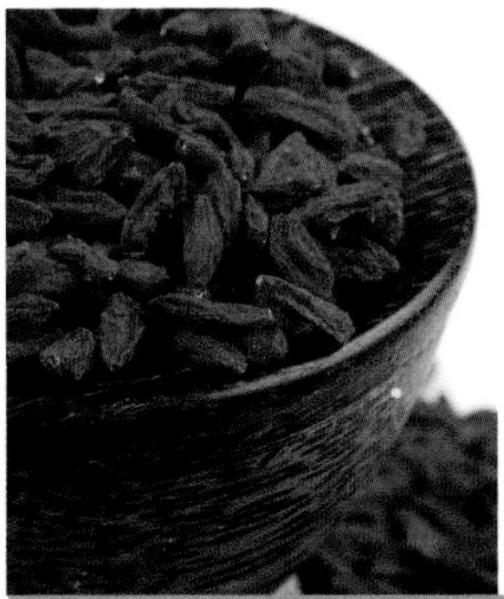

Antioxidants

Antioxidants help fight free radicals, which may be damaging to the joints. **Vitamins A**, **C** and **E** and the mineral **selenium** are known as the antioxidant vitamin and mineral powerhouses.

The highest know antioxidant substance is actually a spice – **clove**, with clove essential oil boasting the highest ORAC score of all at 1,078,700. The highest known food is the **NingXia Wolfberry** coming in at an ORAC rating of 33,000.

Aim for a diet high in antioxidant rich nutrients such as carrots, apricots, cantaloupe, peaches, and dark leafy greens. For extra vitamin A, eat grapefruit, oranges, papaya, mangoes, raspberries, pineapples, asparagus, red peppers, and broccoli. Vitamin C foods include avocados, whole-grain breads and cereals, sunflower seeds and nut butters. Vitamin E foods include whole grains. Selenium rich foods are brazil nuts, oatmeal, and brown rice.

As **manganese** is good for the bones, it is good for the joints as well. See Chapter 1 for a list of foods high in manganese.

Omega-3 fatty acids are considered the lubricants between joints. They are anti-inflammatory by nature and can reduce swelling and discomfort in joints. The correct balance of Omega-3 and Omega-6 fatty acids for joint health is 1000 mg of DHA and 400 mg of EPA from the Omega-3 family and 900 mg of GLA from the Omega-6 family. Borage oil is a good source of Omega-6 fatty acids. For a list of Omega-3 and Omega-6 rich foods, see Unit 1 and Appendix J.

The Muscular System

Smiling uses 17 facial muscles. Frowning takes 42 facial muscles. Reading for an hour causes the muscles around the eye to contract more than 10,000 times. Walking across the room puts more than 200 muscles to work.

The human body contains between 600 and 800 muscles. Why such a difference? There are a couple of muscle counting systems used in medical terminology. Depending on frame size, body type and body mass, the number of muscles in a body can vary.

What are muscles?

Muscles are made up of special tissue called **contractile tissue** that allows the muscles to expand and contract to create force and motion. There are three kinds of muscles: skeletal, smooth and cardiac.

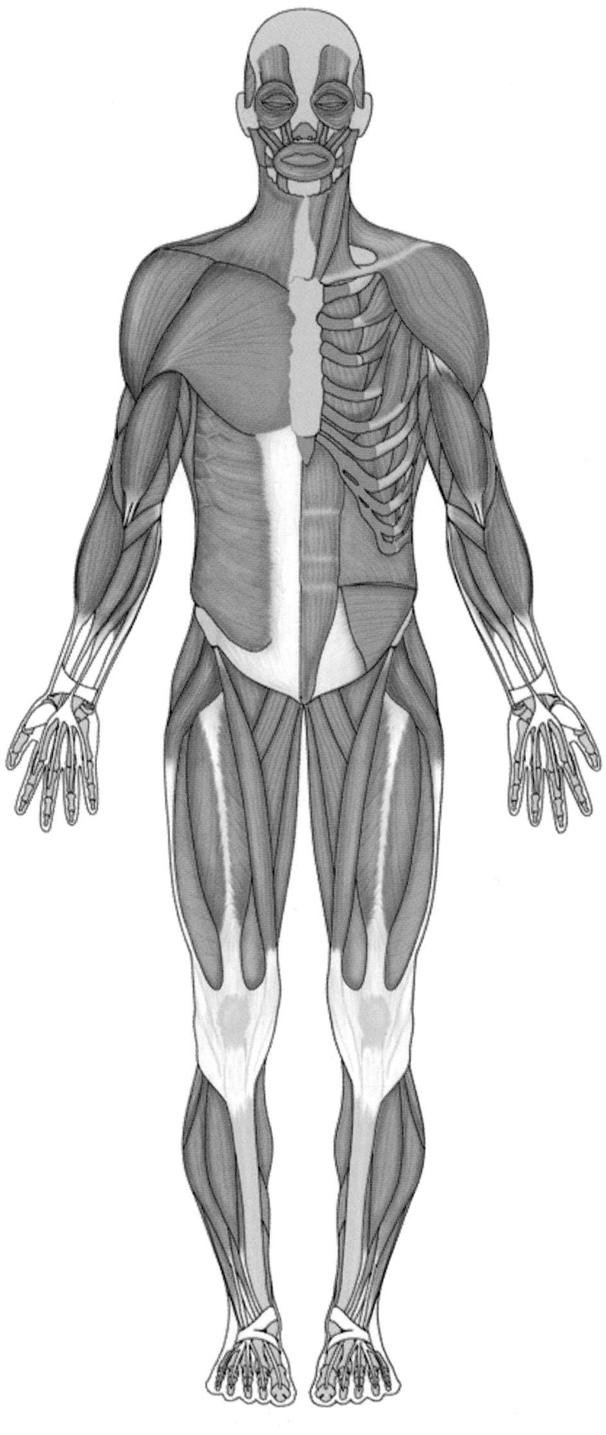

1. **Skeletal muscles** primarily joint bones together and are mostly controlled by conscious thought. When a child reaches for a book – his brain tells the muscles in the arm to extend and reach. These muscles combined with the bones are called the **musculoskeletal system**.

2. **Smooth muscles** are found inside our internal organs, in the walls of the veins and arteries and are controlled by involuntary processes. We do not have to think about them to have them work.

3. **Cardiac muscles** are found only in the heart. Further discussion of the cardiac muscles is in the Cardiovascular unit.

Muscles generally work in groups. This allows the exertion of force to swing a hammer or play a musical instrument. In order to function, the muscles have many blood vessels supplying oxygen and nutrients.

What are some of the muscles called?

There are many muscles and muscle groups in the body. Some of the main muscle groups are:

The **deltoid** muscles are in the shoulders and help with performing such tasks as swinging a softball bat and climbing a rope.

The **pectoralis major** muscles – or pecs for short - are in the upper part of the chest and help with upper body strength.

The **rectus abdominis** muscles – or abdominals or abs for short– are below the pectorals.

When asked to show their muscles, most people contract their **biceps brachii** - or biceps for short - which are the muscles in the inside of the upper arm.

Fun Fact
The tongue is operated by a group of 16 muscles.

The **quadriceps femoris** – or quads for short – are in the front of the upper leg, or thigh. Most athletes like runners and bikers have large quads.

When sitting in a chair, you are actually sitting on your **gluteus maximus** muscle.

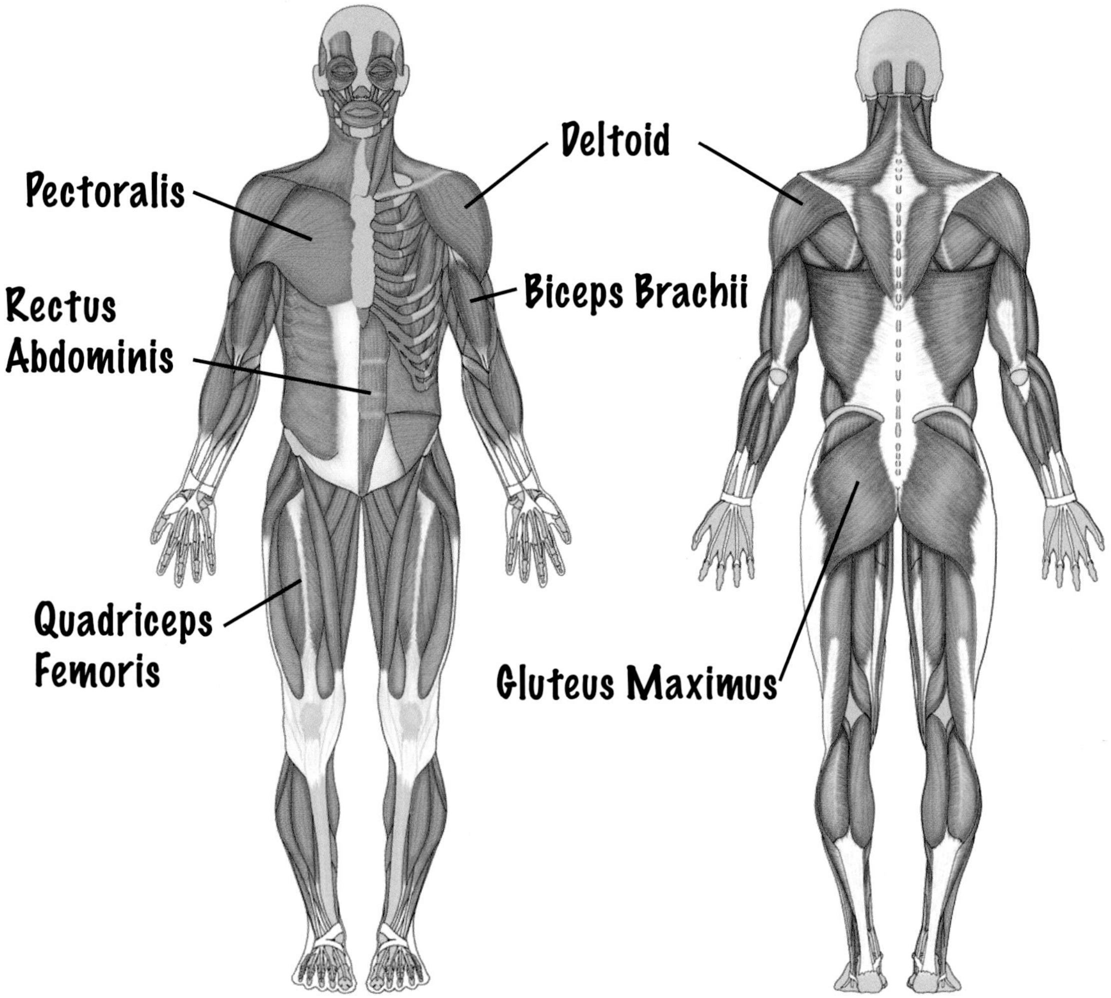

What do muscles do?

Our muscles are always at work. The heart, eyes and mouth muscles are the busiest. The eyes blink, the heart beats, the lungs expand and contract, we swallow and more. But they do more than just move us, they also help our bodies maintain our internal temperature. In fact, only about one-fourth of the energy generated by our muscles goes to movement. The rest is radiated as heat and is recycled back through all our tissues. When our temperature is too low, the brain tells the muscles to shiver in an attempt to generate heat.

Tendons and Ligaments

Tendons connect muscles to bones and are made of inelastic, cord-like tissue, meaning they do not stretch. Unlike muscles, which can be stretched and lengthened, tendons stay the same length. Since the length of a tendon always stays the same, it is interesting to note that successful bodybuilders have shorter tendons, while successful track athletes have longer tendons, specifically the Achilles tendon.

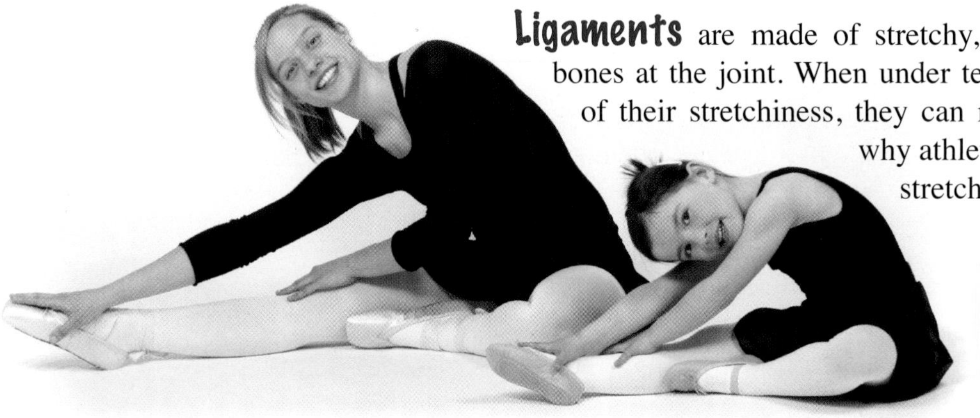

Ligaments are made of stretchy, elastic collagen connecting two bones at the joint. When under tension, ligaments stretch. Because of their stretchiness, they can make joints more supple. That is why athletes, dancers and gymnasts perform stretching exercises.

Fun Fact

Double-jointed people actually have more elastic ligaments.

Muscular System Health Issues

Health concerns affecting our muscles include; fibromyalgia, tendonitis, muscle cramps and muscular dystrophies.

Fibromyalgia (FM) is an autoimmune disorder of the soft tissues. The actual cause of FM is unknown, but it is believed that certain events may trigger its onset. Viral or bacterial infections (Epstein Barr, Chronic Fatigue, Lyme's), automobile accidents, rheumatoid arthritis and lupus have all been associated with the onset of fibromyalgia. The pain associated with fibromyalgia can cause a loss of sleep, which is when the body rejuvenates and repairs itself. Extreme fibromyalgia pain can be so intense that a person's mobility and quality of life are impaired. Many natural health professionals see an association between fibromyalgia and a toxic liver. UCLA researcher Ronald Lawrence, M.D., Ph. D. believes **MSM** (methylsulfonylmethane) offers a breakthrough in treatment for fibromyalgia.[3] The three M's have always been considered by nutritionists to aid in fibromyalgia symptoms: **magnesium**, **manganese** and **malic acid**. Avoiding caffeine, sugar, fried foods, refined foods and those with preservatives like MSG (monosodium glutamate) is often beneficial.

Muscle Cramps generally occur in the legs and toes and can be extremely painful. Some cramps are also known as Charlie horses, which are involuntary spasms or contractions of a muscle in the leg or foot. There are several causes for cramping of the muscles; poor circulation, arteriosclerosis, overexertion of a muscle and the nutritional deficiency of calcium and/or magnesium. Cramping may last a few seconds or several seconds. It can cause an athlete to stumble, or wake a person from a sound sleep. Sometimes the muscle contracts or a toe bends in weird way during a cramp. Rubbing, stretching or walking often can bring relief, but may leave a sore muscle for days afterwards. Essential oils rubbed topically can help a cramp subside quickly.[4] Prevent cramping prior to exercise with gentle warm-up stretching of the muscles. People prone to muscle cramping would do well to increase their intake of **magnesium**- and **calcium**-rich foods and avoid magnesium and calcium robbers like highly acidic food and soda.

---

3 "The Miracle of MSM: The Natural Solution For Pain" Stanley W. Jacob, M.D., Ronald Lawrence, M.D. Ph.D., Martin Zucker. New York: Penguin Putnam Books, 1999.

4 See Appendix DD for authors' recommendations.

Muscular Dystrophies (MD) are a class of muscle wasting diseases. In early stages some forms may be arrested and remission prolonged. As the muscle wastes away, mobility is impaired when the muscle is now replaced with scar tissue. Foods known to be beneficial to persons with MD include those rich in **vitamin E**, **choline**, **Omega-3 fatty acids**, **protein** and **enzymes**.

Tendinitis occurs when tendons become inflamed for a variety of reasons. When normal muscle movement becomes irritating and the smooth gliding motion of the tendon is impaired, the tendon will become inflamed and movement will become painful. The word tendonitis means inflammation of the tendon. The most common cause of tendonitis is overuse. A person just beginning an exercise program whose tendons are not accustomed to this new level of use may experience tendonitis. Athletes such as long time golfers, tennis players, etc. may begin to experience symptoms of tendonitis after some time. This overuse will cause inflammation of the tendon. The wrist, heels, elbow and shoulder are the most affected areas with tendonitis.

How does nutrition affect the muscular system?

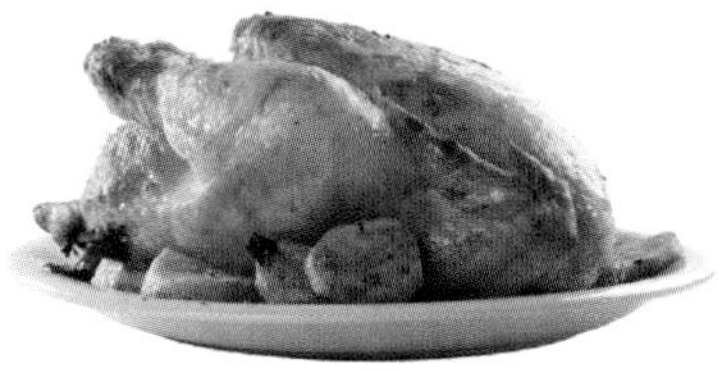

Selenium – this mineral has been studied for its requirement in producing unbiquinone (CoEnzyme Q) known to be beneficial as an anti-aging nutrient and for heart health. According to researcher Dr. Gerhard Schrauzer, selenium plays a significant role in preventing killer diseases.[5]

Some of the best food sources of selenium are Brazil nuts, crimini mushrooms, cod, salmon, tuna, turkey, sunflower seeds, brown rice and whole grains.

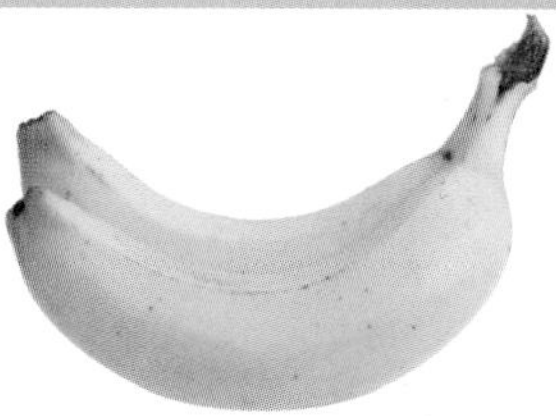

Magnesium – a macro mineral (meaning we need a significant amount of it daily) has many roles in the body. See Unit 2 about magnesium and its role to buffer the blood. For muscle health, magnesium is a muscle relaxer. Proper magnesium levels may prevent or reduce muscle spasms, muscle tremors and muscle weakness.

Some of the best food sources of magnesium are almonds, bananas, dark green vegetables, dried fruit, legumes, potatoes and whole grains.

Calcium - Low levels of calcium can cause tetany – excessive nerve activity, which includes spasms, muscle pain, tingling and/or numbness in the feet and hands. See Unit 4 Chapter 1 and Appendix G and N for a list of calcium-rich foods.

What is Protein?

Proteins are compounds made up of amino acids and are the building blocks for muscles. They are essential to life and are a part of every process within cells. Protein helps cells maintain their shape and is needed to rebuild body tissues such as our muscles. When carbohydrates and fats are not available for energy, the body will use protein as an energy source. Enzymes and hormones are also made from protein.

The typical American diet provides plenty of protein, more than the RDA in most instances. Fat cells store fat, muscles and the liver stores glucose, but did you know there is no place in the body to store protein? Excess protein is eliminated in urine and feces. We need to consume enough protein daily to allow our muscles to be healthy and perform everyday work and tasks for us.

---

5 "Miracle Food Cures from the Bible" Dr. Gerhard Schrauzer, Reese Dubin Prentice Hall Press, 1999.

How much protein do we need?

The RDA for **protein** in adults is equal to 0.8 g of protein per kilogram of body weight per day which translates to about 60 grams, and for children it is 0.5 grams per kilogram of body weight daily or about 35 grams. The average American diet provides from one to two times the RDA for protein. This may lead you to think that a protein deficiency is unlikely in the U.S. However, the RDA for protein has been derived from research studies performed on healthy individuals. Growing children, pregnant and lactating women, the elderly, and anyone undergoing severe stress (trauma, hospitalization, surgery), disease, disability or someone recovering from an injury, needs more protein. For a list of protein rich foods, see Appendix M.

When people consume too much protein, over 2.0 grams per kilogram of body weight daily, the extra protein can put undo stress on the kidneys. This is even more of a concern as we get older and our organs are less efficient and effective.

Very high levels of dietary protein have also been associated with increased urinary calcium excretion and the arthritic condition known as gout. The loss of calcium through urine could potentially be harmful for bone health adding to the risk of osteoporosis. Finally, protein requires **vitamin B6** in order to be metabolized and ultimately utilized in the body. Very high levels of dietary protein increase the requirement for this B vitamin.

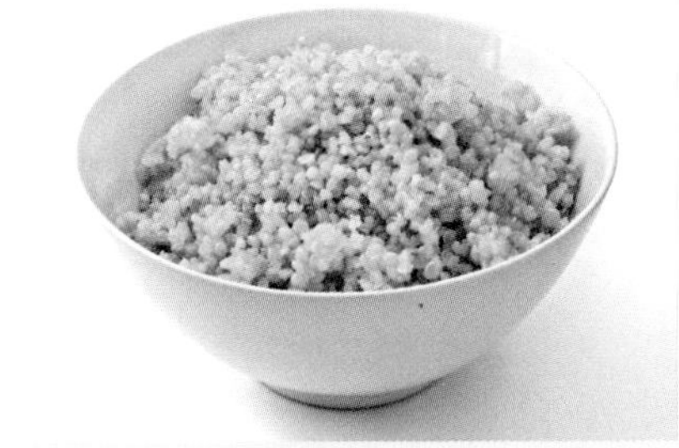

Fun Fact
Quinoa is a grain and a great protein source as it is actually a complete protein containing all nine essential amino acids and is also gluten free. Use it as a nutritious alternative to white rice and couscous.

Where do we get protein?

Animal and plant or vegetable foods are the two major protein sources. Animal protein foods include meat, poultry, fish, dairy products and eggs and contain all nine essential amino acids that cannot be synthesized in the body. A complete list of the amino acids and the foods they are contained in can be found in Unit 1 Chapter 4.

Plant protein sources, although good for certain essential amino acids, do not always offer all nine essential amino acids in a single given food. For example, legumes lack methionine, while grains lack lysine. What is needed to form a complete protein is to combine two or more plant protein sources. If vegans and vegetarians (people who only eat plant foods – fruits, vegetables, nuts, grains and seeds – nothing that comes from an animal) eat a variety of plant foods, they should be able to get adequate protein.

Quality Protein

While protein quantity is important, quality is equally vital. Animal protein sources, whether beef, poultry or fish, are best when they have been raised in their most natural habitat with no added hormones or antibiotics and in an organic environment void of harmful toxins such as pesticides, herbicides and other toxins. When purchasing beef, consider how the meat is raised, butchered and processed. Many retail grocery chains often use preservatives to keep their meat looking fresh longer. It is important to purchase locally raised animal protein that is fresh and from reputable sources.

Be a Label Reader!

Beware of **nitrates, such as sodium nitrate and sodium nitrite,** added to lunch meats and hot dogs. These nitrates are possible carcinogens. Try to avoid all processed meats and choose only uncured, organic meats that contain no nitrates, antibiotics or hormones.

Choose quality plant protein sources that are organic and, preferably, grown locally. As organic certification is costly, many local farmers do grow their produce without herbicides or pesticides. The key is to visit local farms or local farmers markets to visit with the farmers about their farming practices. This also may be a less expensive way to get quality, organic food. Visit www.localharvest.org or www.pickyourown.org to find local growers. If organic produce is not readily available, non-organic plant foods should be washed and peeled to lower the amount of pesticide residue. More information about selecting fresh produce is in Appendix D.

Below is a list of plant based protein foods. For a more detailed list of plant and animal protein foods, see Appendix M.

Rice Milk

Health food stores sell rice milk, which may be added to baked goods, soups, stews and beverages.

Wheat Germ

This is a natural source of good plant protein. Use it as a breakfast cereal or sprinkle it on salads. Use it in soups, casseroles or when making main dish foods. It also may be mixed in yogurt.

Nuts

Nuts may be eaten out of the shell or in the form of nut butters. Nuts are a good source of top-notch plant protein. They are a good source of essential unsaturated fatty acids, as well as many vitamins and minerals that work with protein for body cellular rebuilding.

Seeds

These are prime sources of good protein and other needed nutrients. Try sunflower seeds, sesame seeds or pumpkin seeds for snacks or mix in salads, in baking or with breakfast cereals.

Brewer's Yeast

This is a great source of high quality protein. Its amino acid pattern makes Brewer's yeast almost comparable to that of meat in protein structure. Sprinkle over salads, in stews and soups or mix in baked goods. Sprinkle over breakfast cereals or mix in most beverages.

Grains

All grains, like other seeds, are good sources of high quality protein. These sources are wheat germ, brown rice, wheat gluten, whole nuts, barley, whole rye, buckwheat flour and millet. Millet is almost perfect in its amino acid balance. It lacks tyrosine, but if wheat germ is added, millet will then have a complete protein with all essential amino acids. This grain has a substance known as nitriloside, which is taken up by protein and used to build or rebuild cells and tissues.

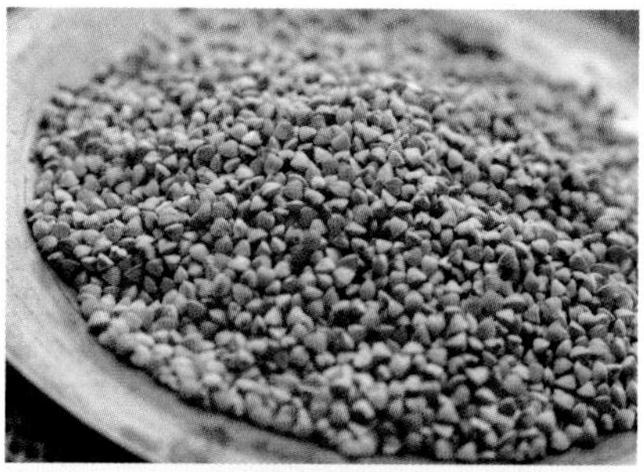
Buckwheat

Those who need more protein and plan to eat less meat and more plant foods should consider **Buckwheat**. It is a prime source of manganese. It reportedly has all the food values of animal protein. Buckwheat is immune to disease, requires little fertilizer and rarely is sprayed because it can smother weeds in swift growing. It is considered to be the **master plant protein source**. Buckwheat is available in about every food market and also is known as groats or kasha. Buckwheat honey also is considered to be a master protein.

Unit 4 Chapter 2
Discussion Questions

1. Read Hebrews 4:12 out loud with your family. What does this scripture mean to you?
2. What can you do because of your joints? What could you not do if you did not have joints?
3. What can you do because of your muscles? What could you not do if you did not have muscles?

Activities - plus the Traditional Hummus Dip with Basil "Power" Recipe and activities.

Elementary

1. Take a jar with a screw on lid. Tighten the lid securely. Now with a completely stiff hand, try to open the jar. Without the ability to bend the fingers around the lid, we cannot open an ordinary jar lid. Think about other daily activities with your hands you could not do if you did not have joints.
2. How many ways does your elbow and knee bend? Name one thing you could not do if we did not have an elbow joint.
3. You will need an adult, at least two participants, plactic wrap, a bowl and grapes. With an adults help, wrap the plastic wrap around both of your arms so that you cannot bend your elbows. Then, try to eat the bowl of grapes. Next, with the help of a partner, have the adult time how fast you both can eat the bowl of grapes.
4. Name three professions that must know the names of all the muscles in the body.
5. Calculate your body weight from pounds to kilograms and further calculate your protein needs. Track your protein consumption from all sources for one week to determine if your body's needs are being met. To figure out your protein needs, divide your weight in pounds by two.
6. Name one of the strongest animals on Earth that only consumes plant proteins. What does this animal eat?

Secondary

Choose any from above plus

1. Talk to someone who has arthritis and see what activities they are restricted from doing? Ask if they use prescription drugs to manage pain and if so what are their side effects. Ask if they have ever considered nutrition as a way to help their health condition.
2. Plan a meal for healthy joints and muscles.
3. Begin a daily plan of stretching before and after talking a walk, bike ride or other sport/exercise activity.
4. Plan your daily meal to ensure adequate protein intake from only plant sources. It may not exceed the standard caloric intake or be focused on one food group over another.
5. Using the protein chart in Appendix M, what do you see interesting in the plant sources of protein?

Additional Resources

Web sites:

1. For a great animation showing a knee joint with muscles in action, go to http://kidshealth.org/misc/movie/bodybasics/bodybasics_knee.html
2. http://kidshealth.org/kid/htbw/muscles.html
3. http://kidshealth.org/parent/general/body_basics/bones_muscles_joints.html
4. http://www.webmd.com/parenting/news/20060609/bone-joint-woes-hit-overweight-kids
5. http://www.myfamilyexercise.com/
6. http://www.fatfreekitchen.com/nutrition/high-protein-foods.html

Muscular System Power
Garbanzo Beans

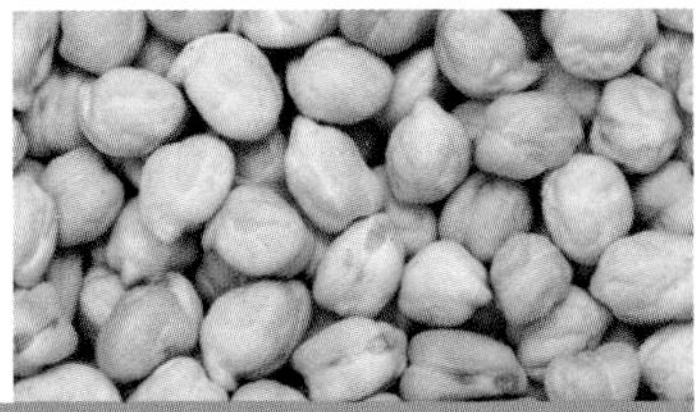

Garbanzo beans, or chickpeas, are a great source of muscle building protein!

Traditional Hummus Dip with Basil

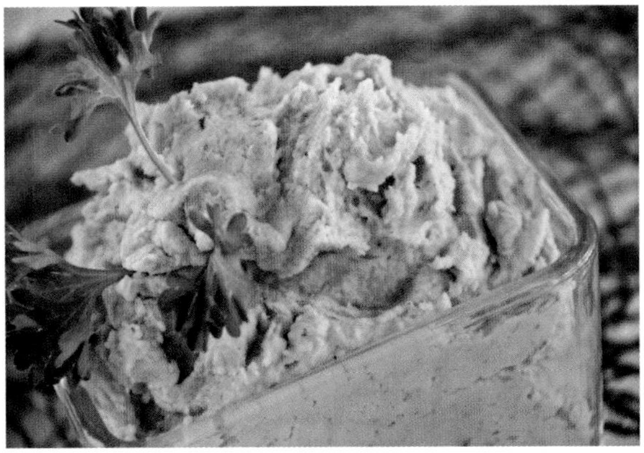

1-15 oz. can garbonzo beans, drained
4 Tbs. tahini (sesame seed butter)
4 Tbs. lemon juice
2 Tbs. hot water
2 cloves garlic, minced
½ tsp. sea salt
1 Tbs. fresh basil, minced
1/8 tsp. cumin
1/8 tsp. cayenne pepper
1Tbs. olive oil
1/8 tsp. paprika
1 Tbs. chopped parsley

Combine first eight ingredients in food processor or blender and blend on high for two minutes until smooth. Place in bowl and drizzle olive oil on it and sprinkle with paprika and parsley. Serve with fresh vegetables and/or whole grain flatbread.

Activities

Elementary

1. Before making this recipe, gather the ingredients. Based on the colors of the ingredients, what color will the end product be?
2. Garbanzo beans also are known as chickpeas. Research and find out why this is and in what countries are they called chickpeas.
3. What is the difference between roasting and baking?

Secondary

Choose any from above plus

1. Research to find out where hummus originated. Write or give an oral report about your findings.
2. What does gluten-free mean? Research this and prepare a written or oral report.
3. On your next trip to the grocery store, check labels for gluten. Does your store offer gluten-free alternatives?

Chapter 3

Skin, Hair and Nails

"But the very hairs of your head are all numbered." Matthew 10:30

Keeping skin healthy can't be overemphasized. It is not a matter of looking great; it is the body's first defense against disease and infection, and it protects the internal organs from injuries. As the largest organ in the body, the skin helps regulate body temperature and prevents excess fluid loss, and it also helps remove excess water and salt through perspiration. The skin gives us protection from fluids and chemicals, yet at the same time our skin acts like a giant sponge soaking in what we put on it. This ability is one reason many pharmaceutical companies use transdermal medications – a patch adhered to the skin for a slow release of medication. Learning to nourish the skin is only part of what makes healthy skin. Using only pure natural, chemical-free products on the skin will not only benefit the skins appearance, texture and over all heath, but directly impacts the rest of the body's health as well.

Skin conditions can affect anyone – young and old, men and women. Acne, dry skin, cracked skin, psoriasis, eczema and skin cancer, are just a few examples of common skin disorders. The good news is that there are a number of simple ways to keep skin healthy, and many natural options available to repair damaged skin.

Understanding a little about the structure of the skin, helps us know how best to care for this vital organ.

Fun Fact

The skin is part of the integumentary system which is the largest organ system in the body. It includes the skin, hair and nails and protects the deeper tissues, regulates body temperature, excretes waste and contains millions of sensory receptors for pain, pressure and temperature.

What makes up the skin?

Skin is composed of three layers: the epidermis, the dermis and the subcutaneous layer. The thickness of the dermis is variable depending on the location. For example, eyelid dermis is quite thin, but back dermis is about 1/2 inch thick.

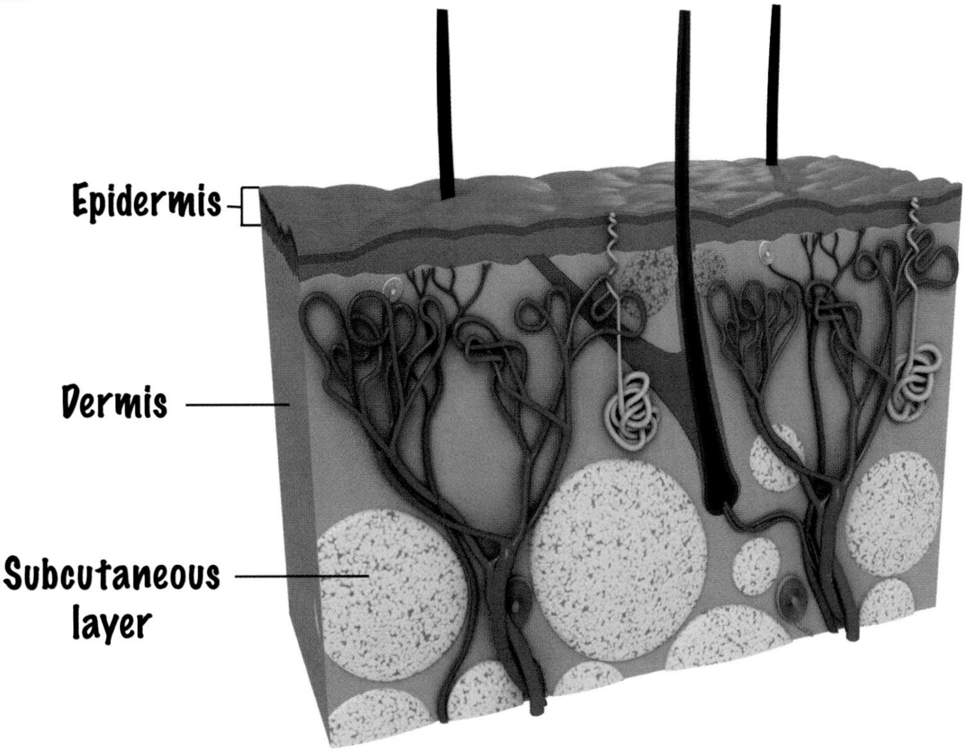

The **epidermis** is the outermost layer of skin and is about the thickness of a piece of paper. It has four layers: the stratum corneum, the granular layer, the squamous cell layer and the basal cell layer.

1. The **stratum corneum** or outer layer of the epidermis is the layer of skin that can be seen and felt. Proteins known as keratin, a fatty, waterproof envelope, and flat corneocyte cells make up the stratum corneum. This layer is the barrier between your body and the outside world.

2. The **granular layer** produces protein and lipids (fat) for the stratum corneum.

3. The **squamous cell layer** produces keratin for the stratum corneum and also transports water. Friction blisters occur in the squamous cell layer.

4. The **basal cell layer** is the lowest layer of the epidermis. This is where the skin cells are reproduced and give rise to the more superficial layers of the epidermis. The most common form of skin cancer, basal cell carcinoma, arises from this cell layer. Melanocytes, which produce melanin, or skin pigment, sit along this layer among these cells. Melanoma, one of the two main groups of skin cancer, originates from these pigment-producing cells.

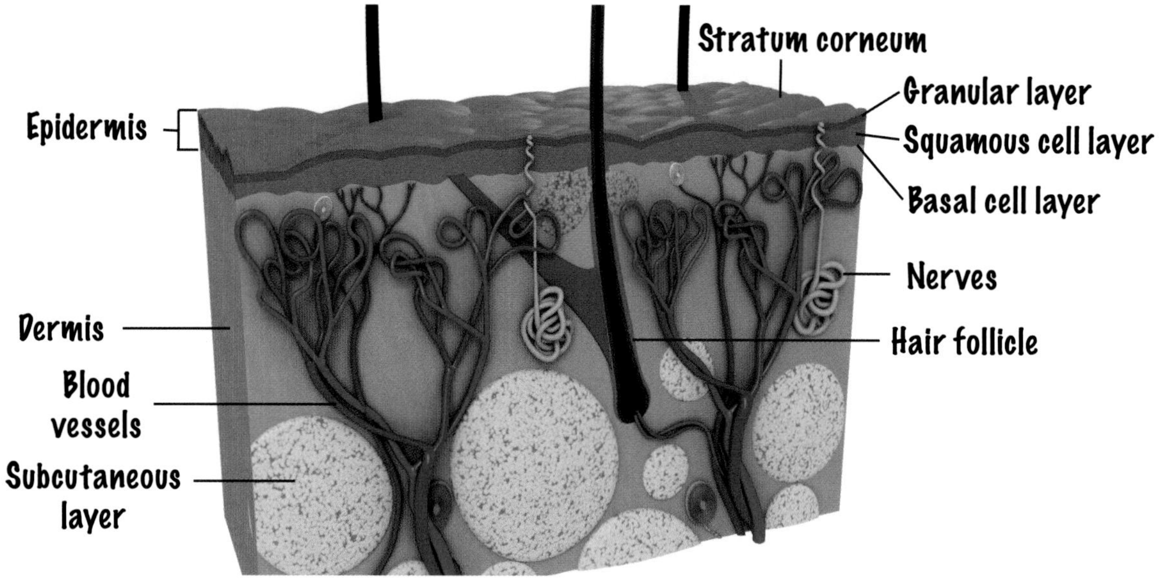

It takes about one month for skin cells to move from the basal cell layer to the top of the stratum corneum and slough off. One to two layers of these skin cells are sloughed off every day. Using scrubs on the arms and legs assists in the removal and production of new healthy skin cells.

The **dermis** is the deeper layer of skin. It is a diverse combination of blood vessels, nerves, hair follicles and sebaceous (or oil) glands. The proteins **collagen** and **elastin** are found in the dermis. They provide support and elasticity to the skin. The sun's rays can break down these proteins and, eventually, the skin begins to wrinkle and sag.

Only a slight prick from a pin or cut from glass or rock can result in the skin's tiny **blood vessels** to begin washing the area clean and sending millions of white blood cells to the area to begin the healing process. Washing the area and applying a first aid ointment and a bandage generally will allow the cut to heal on its own. However, there are various health concerns that slow or impair wound healing, such as diabetes. Some cuts will require stitches to heal.

The **nerves** in the dermis transmit sensory information to the brain such as pressure, temperature and pain.

There are millions of these sensory receptors in the skin.

Hair follicles produce and grow hair from dead cells.

The **subcutaneous layer**, or subcutis, is a layer of fatty tissue that provides nourishment to the dermis and upper layers of skin. It also conserves body heat and cushions internal organs against trauma.

Fun Facts

The largest human organ is the skin, with a surface area of about 25 square feet.
Humans shed about 600,000 particles of skin every hour – about 1.5 pounds a year. By 70 years of age, an average person will have lost 105 pounds of skin.
Humans shed and regrow outer skin cells about every 27 days – almost 1,000 new skins in a lifetime.

Sense of Touch

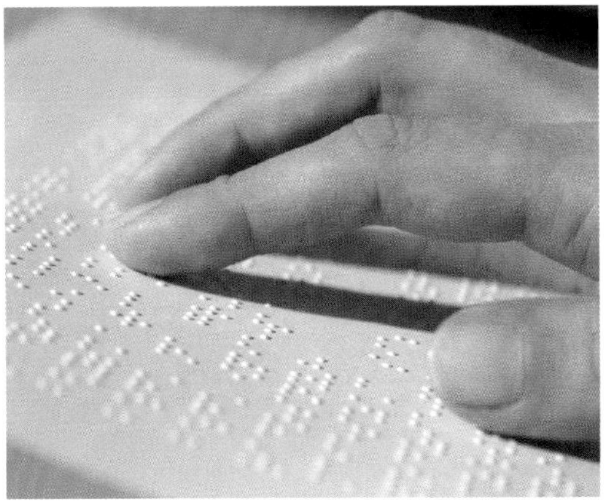

Is the brick on a house rough or smooth? Is the skin on a baby's face soft, oily or dry? While all of our skin can feel things, it is mainly the hands and fingers we use to touch or feel an object. Even with our eyes closed we can touch something and know what it is. The sense of touch can also keep us out of danger, especially in the case of a hot stove, oven or hot water.

The sense of touch originates in the bottom layer of the skin called the dermis. The dermis is filled with many tiny nerve endings which give us information about the things with which our body comes in contact. They do this by carrying the information to the spinal cord, which sends messages to the brain where the feeling is registered.

Why are some areas of the body more sensitive than others? This is due to the number of nerve endings. The fingertips are very sensitive. Blind people can use their fingertips to read bumps on a piece of paper. This is called Braille.

Nutrition and the Skin

Antioxidants

Antioxidant rich foods help to protect the skin from sun damage. We do not have to be sunbathers to get too much sun exposure. Just 10 minutes of unprotected sun can cause UVA and UVB damage to the skin. Antioxidants are also essential for the proper growth and function of the skin, helping to prevent dry, rough, cracked and premature aging of the skin.

Food sources: Fish oils, fruits high in antioxidants, winter squashes, dark greens, broccoli, watermelon, tomatoes, beet greens, cantaloupe, green algae.

"Growing up in Florida, well before the knowledge of the dangers of too much sun, as an adult I have had to deal with skin concerns related to the sun, even basal and squamous cell carcinomas on my face and arms. I now make sure my diet includes foods and supplements[1] that support skin health." - Debra Raybern

1 See Appendix DD for author's recommendations.

Vitamins

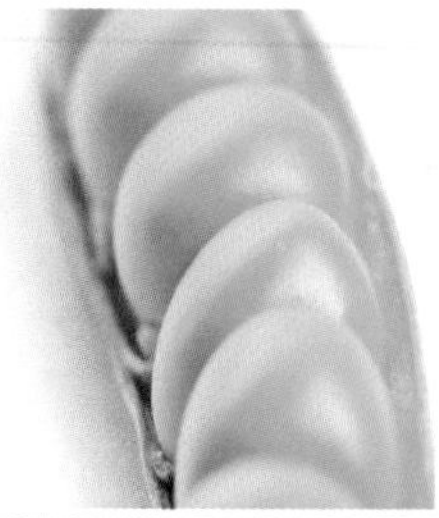

B-Complex Vitamins are for more than heart health and energy. B vitamins always are found as a group in foods, never isolates. These are your skins anti-stress vitamins, helping with acne and premature aging. Essential for wound healing, sunburns and aiding in new cell growth.

Food Sources: Egg yolks, whole grains, almonds, sunflower seeds, green leafy vegetables, peas, beans, wheat germ.

Vitamin C rich foods help produce collagen in connective tissue (the loss of which gives us premature wrinkles), strengthen capillary walls, help speed healing and battle environmental stresses.

Food sources: citrus fruits, rose hips, pineapple, bell peppers, green vegetables, apples, broccoli, acerola fruit, and berries.

Vitamin D and E are fat soluble antioxidants that oxygenate skin tissue helping to regenerate skin cells and prevent premature aging.

Food sources: Fish oils, tuna, alfalfa, sunshine (early morning light sun is best), whole grains, sprouts, green vegetables and eggs.

Minerals

Minerals important to the skin include iodine, sulfur, zinc and silicon.

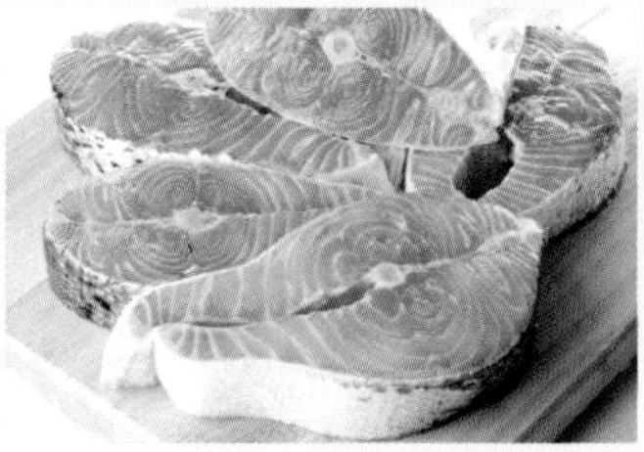

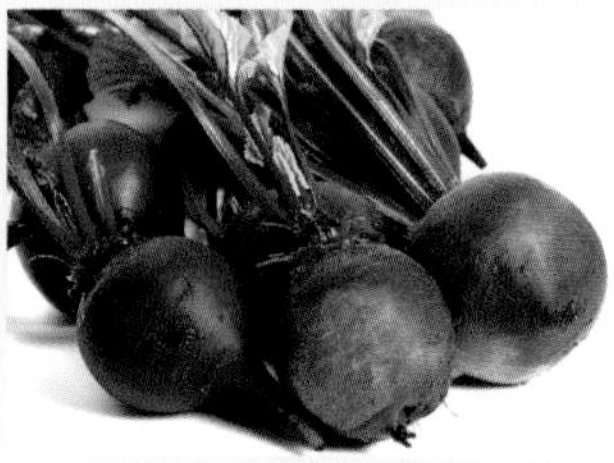

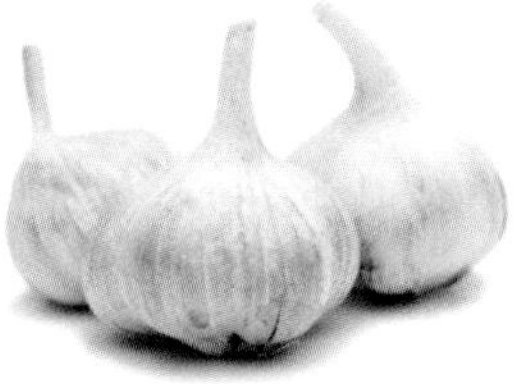

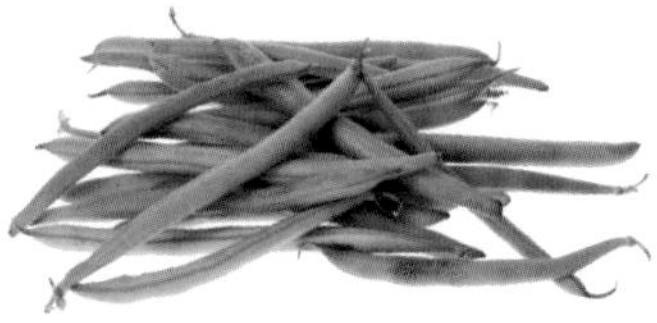

Iodine helps with acne, prevents roughness and wrinkles. Good sources are sunflower seeds, walnuts, fish and algae.

Silicon aids in collagen formation and strengthens bones and skin tissues. Good sources are the herb horsetail, flax seeds, wheat grass, sunflower seeds, berries, apples, grapes, onions, beets and nettle.

Sulfur is nicknamed the beauty mineral to keep skin clear. It also helps with nails and hair health. Good sources are turnips, dandelion greens, radishes, horseradish, garlic, cabbage and string beans.

Zinc promotes cell growth and helps with acne. Good sources are pumpkin seeds, onions, nuts, beets, fish, alfalfa, blue green algae and green leafy vegetables.

Herbs and Essential Oils

See Appendix T to learn about the many chemicals found in personal care products and how to make better, healthier skin care choices.

Hair

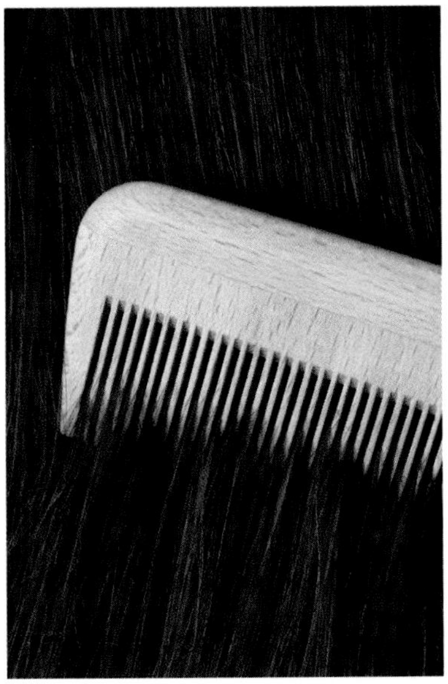

God says He knows how many hairs are on our heads. In Matthew 10:30 Jesus declared that even "the very hairs of your head are all numbered." So how many is that? The human head has approximately 100,000 hairs. To think about how many people exist and how each person and has different amounts of hair, simply boggles the mind!

Fun Fact

People with blond hair have more hair on their heads than do people with red or brown hair.

While hair is mentioned over 100 times in the Bible, it is usually in the context of God's love and protection for His people. For example, in Daniel 3:27, when God delivered Shadrach, Meshach and Abednego from the fiery furnace, "the hair of their head was not singed." In Luke 21:18, Jesus warned His disciples of persecution but told them not to fear because "not a hair of your head shall be lost." It is amazing how our Savior knows and loves us!

While comprised of water, lipids, traces of mineral elements and melanin, **keratin** is the main ingredient of the **hair shaft** and is made of fibrous proteins. Each hair is grown in the hair follicle. Once the hair has grown out of the follicle, it is dead. Surrounding each hair follicle are **sebaceous glands** which produce an oily matter called **sebum**. Sebum lubricates skin and hair.

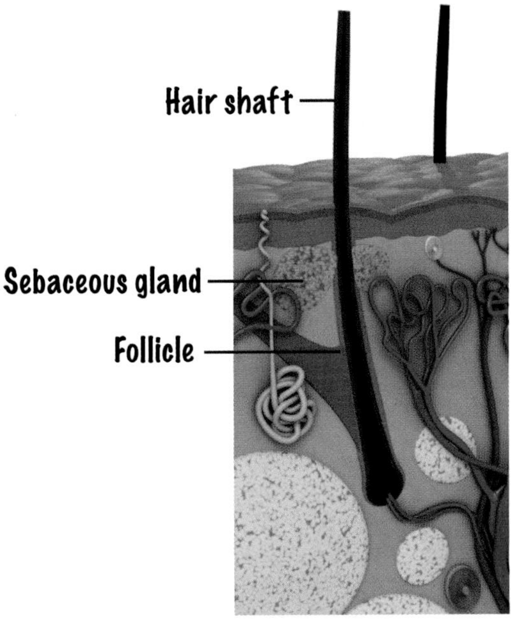

The hair, or shaft, has three layers.

1. The **cuticle** is the outer layer, and when the cuticle lies flat, the hair takes on a nice shine. This should not be confused with oily hair shine. The cuticle is actually scales that lie flat and slightly overlap each other, protecting the inner shaft from damage from chlorine, chemicals and sun. When the hair looks dull and damaged and breaks, the cuticle scales have separated.
2. Underneath the cuticle is the **cortex**. It is composed of fiber that is 90 percent of the hair's weight and contains keratin and melanin, which gives the hair its color.
3. At the core of the hair is the **medulla**. The cells composing the medulla quickly degenerate leaving air bubbles. The purpose of the medulla in hair is still unknown.

Depending on how long and how fast a person's hair grows, she might have hair that is several years old. On average human hair grows at about one-quarter inch per month with a life span of three to seven years.

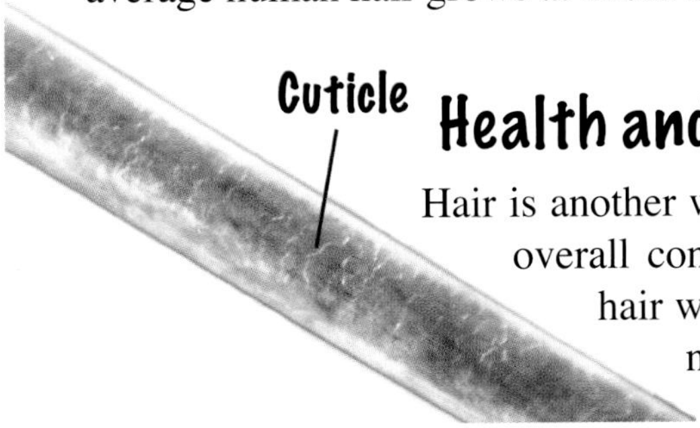

Health and Hair - Surviving or Thriving?

Hair is another way we can tell if our health is optimal.Our hair ultimately reflects the overall condition of our bodies. If the body is healthy and well nourished, the hair will be its shining glory. If a person has health problems or suffers from nutritional deficiencies, the hair may stop growing or show damage and become brittle.

Fun Facts

Wet hair is heavier than dry hair. Most healthy hair can hold 30 percent of its body weight in water. While a single hair can withstand the weight of 100 grams, a full head of hair in theory could withstand the weight of 12 tons, given that the scalp could withstand the weight.

A single follicle on the scalp produces approximately 0.35 millimeters of hair shaft daily. Certain vitamins and minerals must be present in adequate proportions, or there will be faulty or nonexistent hair growth. Research has shown that in our hurry-up world of fast food, and extreme work schedules we have developed extraordinarily poor eating habits. This extremely poor diet affects our general health and energy levels and makes our fingernails weaker and our hair thinner and far less healthy.

Stress, toxins in the environment, exposure to the sun, cigarette smoke (including second hand smoke), excess alcohol consumption and lack of sleep sometimes makes our bodies work overtime to maintain a standard of marginal health - not optimal. These factors may lead to our hair being compromised and weakened. Because we consider our hair to be expendable and not needed to maintain health, at least our physical health, it tends to be the last part of us to receive attention. The quality of our hair can indeed affect our emotional health, which we will soon learn can also play a significant role in our physical heath.

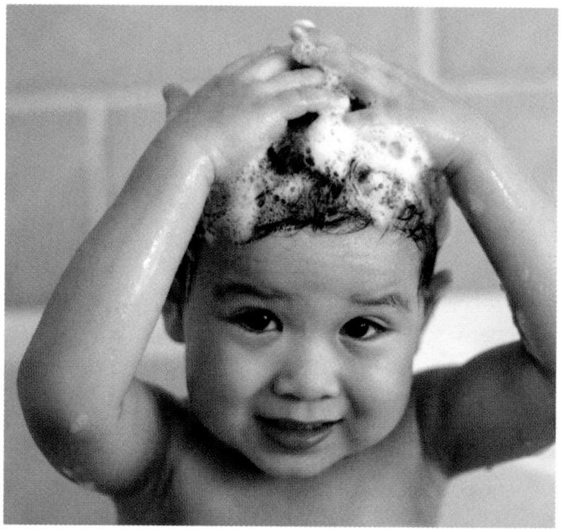

Another often overlooked factor in scalp and hair health is the shampoo, condition and other hair products we use. Many are filled with potentially toxic ingredients and many more are loaded with waxes that build up on the scalp and clog the follicle. Every hole in the scalp should have hair growing out of it. One of the most common potentially hazardous chemicals found in hair products is sodium laureth sulfate and its derivatives. See Appendix T for a list of chemicals to avoid in your personal care products.

Nutrition and Hair

Taking proper, whole food daily vitamins and minerals plays a huge role in keeping hair healthy. Any nutritional deficiencies can lead to thinning hair or even total baldness. It is a well-known fact that an under-active thyroid can result in frizzy or brittle hair while an overactive thyroid turns hair greasy and limp. The goal is healthy, nutrient dense foods and supplementation.

In an older person the total number of the capillaries supplying the hair follicles (which carries nutrition to the hair) with blood is considerably diminished. Increasing the amount of nutrients of various types such as vitamins, minerals, proteins and amino acids is the best way to keep the hair healthy.

If the body is in good health, a person can maximize her hair growth cycle through taking the proper blend of **amino acids** and **B-vitamins**.

It also is important to include foods rich in **vitamin B6**, **biotin** (vitamin B7), **inositol** and **folate** (vitamin B9), and it may be advisable to be sure these nutrients are included in your supplemental program. Certain minerals including **magnesium**, **sulfur**, **silicon** and **zinc** also are very important in maintaining healthy hair. **Beta-carotene** is important to hair growth because it is converted to vitamin A as the body needs it, also helping maintain normal growth and bone development, protective sheathing around nerve fibers, as well as promoting healthy skin, hair and nails.

For more specific nutrient information for the hair, refer to the "Nutrition and the Skin" section in this chapter.

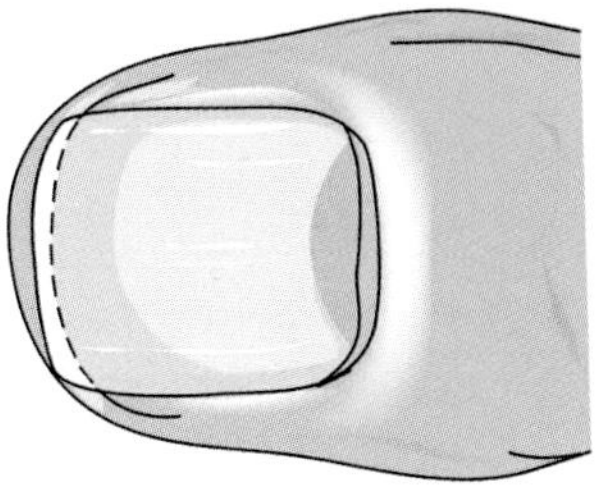

Nails

Nails are made of **keratin**, a type of protein, and **sulfur**. It takes approximately seven months to fully grow a fingernail, at a rate of about .05 to 1.2 millimeters a week.

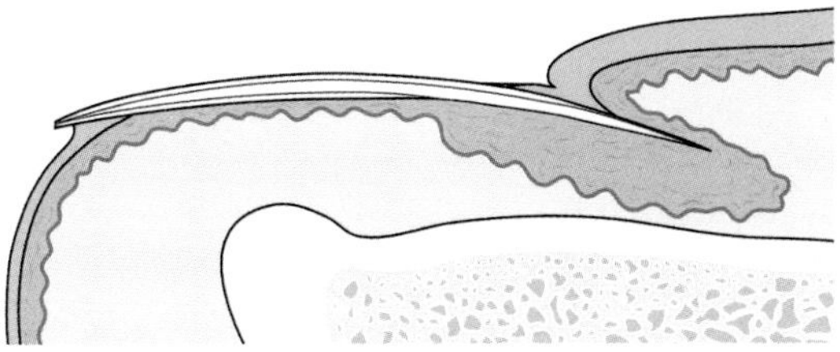

Healthy nails are pink on the nail bed indicating a rich blood supply. Changes in the look, shape, or color of our finger nails may indicate a nutritional deficiency or disease somewhere in our body long before other symptoms manifest. Nails should not be ignored; they can serve as an early warning signal for poor health.

Many women with not-so lovely nails often have acrylic nails glued on top of their natural nails. This is an extremely bad practice. The glues and acrylics are toxic and can penetrate into the bloodstream; the fake nails cut off oxygen to the nail making it weak and thin. Many a nail fungus had its beginning with a manicure or pedicure. The area where the acrylic nail attaches to the natural nail bed is a breeding ground for bacteria.

For the sake of the body's health, natural nails should be allowed to grow out, and we should take steps to make them strong and healthy by getting the whole body in balance. Although nails may be soft at first, they will strengthen and grow quickly if they are kept short and cared for properly.

Excessive exposure to water and detergents or soaps can cause the nails to swell. When they dry, they shrink, which results in loose brittle nails. Rubber gloves should be used when washing the dishes or getting your hands in lots of water.

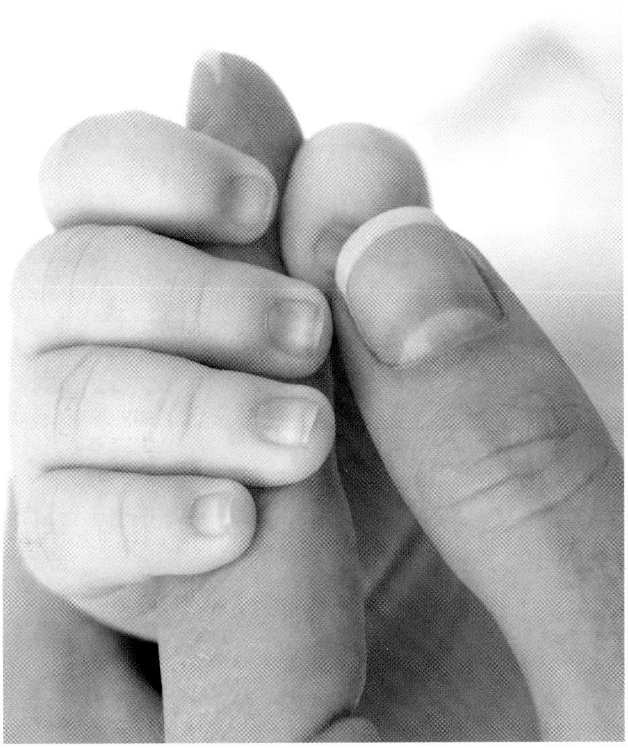

Awhile back, doctors used to look into eyes and at nails during regular check-ups. Why? Because fingernails are a window into the body's health. Changes in the look, shape or color of fingernails can indicate a nutritional deficiency or imbalance somewhere in the body long before other symptoms manifest. Though doctors may not look intensely at nails anymore, the fingernail guide in Appendix U may be of help in evaluating overall health and lists authors' supplement recommendations.

Unit 4 Chapter 3
Discussion Questions

1. Who do we think had the longest hair in the Bible? Name one man and one woman and tell their bible account regarding their hair. ANSWER – Sampson, Mary – washing Jesus feet with her hair
2. In this age of strange hairdos and bright hair color dyes, what are your family views on the length of hair for boys and girls? Are these views based on scripture, if so what ones?
3. Tattoos are quite popular in our culture. Does God's word have anything to say about marking the skin? Lev. 19:28

Activities - plus the Cabbage Slaw "Power" Recipe and activities.

Elementary

1. Have a family member collect five different items from around the house. Put on a blindfold. Have the family member help you touch each one first with your elbow and then your knee. Can you identify them? Lastly, touch each one with your fingers. Was it easier to identify the objects? Why?
2. Mystery Veggies: Have a family member or your mother collect five different vegetables from the refrigerator or from the grocery store and put each one in a separate bag. Reach into each bag and try to identify the veggies. Try the same activity with five different pieces of fruit.
3. Find out who invented Braille and write a report about it.
4. Measure your hair from the crown of the head to the end. If each inch represents one month, how old is your hair?
5. Look at the list of vitamin rich foods good for the skin and pick out a food that you have never tasted. Find that food in your kitchen or go to the grocery store to get it and taste it. What did you think of the taste? If you did not like it very much, try it again for the next three days prepared in three different ways whether raw, cooked, in a recipe, etc.
6. Read Appendix S and T. Locate and collect all the products in your home that include ingredients from any of the chemical lists in the Appendices. Make a list of all the found chemicals and list their known harmful effects. Prepare a written or oral report to share with your family and discuss a possible plan to remove as many of the toxins as you can.

Secondary

Choose any of the above plus

1. Write a paper on tattoos. Cover biblical references, our culture and the health and wellness aspects and state your desire to have or not have a permanent tattoo on God's temple.
2. Collect all the shampoo bottles in the home and read the ingredients. Then look up each on the Internet to see if they are potentially hazardous.
3. Prepare a snack for your family that contains a food rich in zinc. Look in recipe books, online or create your own recipe.

Additional Resources

Web sites:

1. http://library.thinkquest.org/3750/touch/touch.html
2. http://www.answersingenesis.org/articles/am/v2/n3/amazing-human-hair
3. http://christianteens.about.com/od/advice/f/tattoo.htm

Skin, Hair and Nail Power

Cabbage

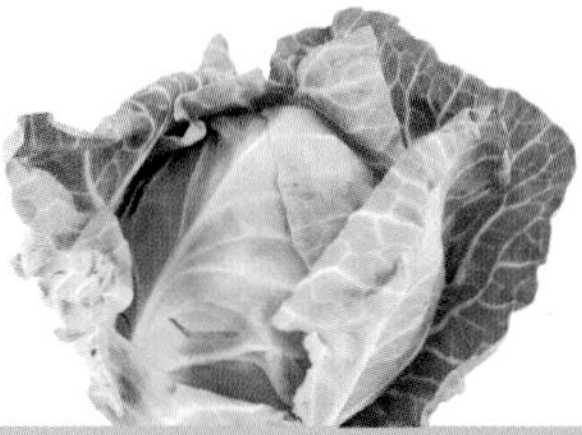

Cabbage is a wonderful source of sulfur.
Sulfur promotes skin, hair and nail health and is nicknamed the beauty mineral.

Cabbage Slaw

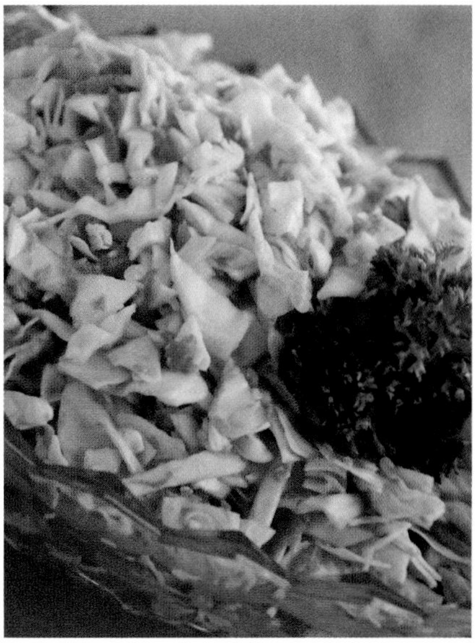

1 small head of green or red cabbage, or use ½ head of each for great color, chopped
1 carrot, peeled and shredded
2 Tbs. sesame seeds
2 Tbs. Blue Agave Nectar
1 tsp. apple cider vinegar
¼ tsp. lemon juice or 1 drop Young Living lemon essential oil
¼ cup olive oil mayonnaise

Add all ingredients in a large bowl and stir until well combined.

Activities

Elementary

1. Gather all ingredients and make sure to get both green and red cabbage. Taste each kind of cabbage. Do they taste the same? Different?
2. Where is cabbage grown? How is cabbage grown? Share your findings in an oral and written report.
3. What is sauerkraut? Find out if it tastes the same or different than raw or cooked cabbage.
4. If you have mayonnaise in your refrigerator, read its ingredients. Does it contain olive oil? What kind of oil does it have? If it is not olive oil, which do you think is healthier? You may refer back to Unit 1 about Fats or you can research on the Internet.
5. What is apple cider vinegar? How is it different from regular white vinegar? How is it made? Share your findings in an oral or written report.

Secondary

Choose any from above plus

1. Research to find out the main nutrients in cabbage. How many minerals are found in cabbage? How much of each mineral is in one cup of cabbage? Are the nutrients the same in raw versus cooked cabbage?
2. What other common dishes have cabbage in them? If you do not know of any, research on the Internet to find two different recipes containing cabbage and prepare one of them as a side dish to a meal this week.
3. What are the origins of sauerkraut? How is it made? Is it as healthy as raw or cooked cabbage? Is it healthier? Give an oral or written report with your findings.
4. Research to find a homemade olive oil mayonnaise recipe. Make sure the ingredients are healthy and make it for the recipe above.

Chapter 4

Exercise

"I have taught thee in the way of wisdom; I have led thee in right paths. When thou goest, thy steps shall not be straitened; and when thou runnest, thou shalt not stumble" Proverbs 4:11 and 12

It's easy to see that Americans, young and old, are out of shape. A trip to the mall or supermarket is not without seeing someone on oxygen, having difficulty getting around due to weight issues. A look in the grocery cart reflects Americans' obsession with self-indulgence. So many lack discipline. Why? Modern conveniences have made it too easy to become inactive. The men and women of the Bible walked everywhere, worked the land and made their food from scratch.

Fun Fact

The average Amish man takes 18,245 steps a day, and the average Amish woman takes 14,196 steps. Other Americans, by contrast, take about 5,000. - Your Body, A Users Guide, Time Inc. 2008

Society has changed a lot over the past 100 years. Most people are no longer working the land for their food. Instead, they drive to the store and buy it, and many times it comes already prepared - no work, no labor. Machines have taken over many of the physical tasks of food preparation. Neglecting the body by leaning on the Bible verse, "Bodily exercise profits little," is only valuable for those who are living as they did in the Old and New Testament. No matter a person's lifestyle, all Christians should heed Romans 12:1, "I beseech you therefore, brethren, by the mercies of God, that ye present your bodies a living sacrifice, holy, acceptable unto God, which is your reasonable service." Without caring for our bodies, how will we fulfill His will?

Engaging in physical activity or exercise is beneficial in weight control, but above and beyond those benefits, heart disease, diabetes, arthritis, high blood pressure, certain cancers and other health conditions can benefit from exercise. As a person ages, exercise also aids in keeping flexible, and studies show that women can help maintain bone density with weight bearing exercise.

Stepping on the bathroom scale is not always an indicator of health. By calculating age, weight and height and taking into account a person's gender, the Body Mass Index or BMI was created to help people to determine if they were in an ideal weight range for their height. The higher the BMI number, the greater the risk of developing certain health problems - such as coronary artery disease or adult-onset diabetes. While BMI is one of the quickest and easiest ways to determine body fat composition, it is not perfect because of our unique body compositions. It is not ideal for kids, competitive athletes, weight lifters, pregnant or nursing women, or frail or inactive elderly persons.

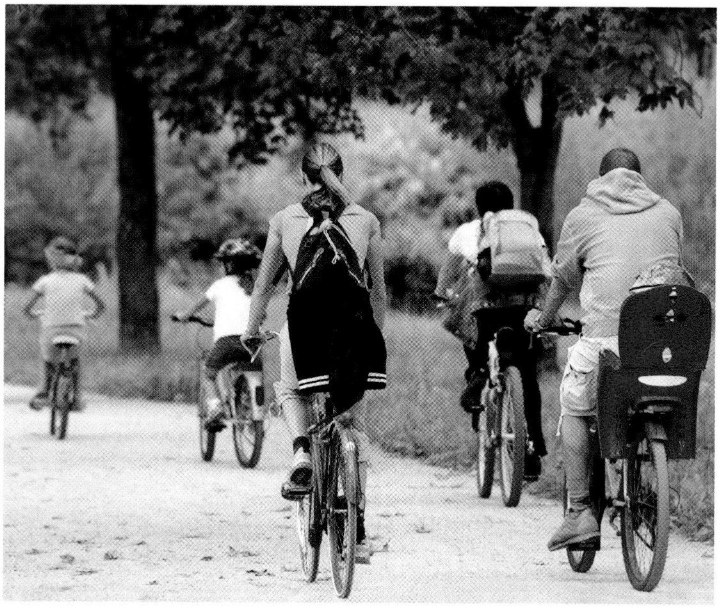

In Proverbs 19:15-16, it says, "Slothfulness casteth into a deep sleep; and an idle soul shall suffer hunger. He that keepeth the commandment keepeth his own soul; but he that despiseth his ways shall die." We must be good stewards of the bodies we have been given and maintain it as we age.

What happens to our bones, muscles and joints when we exercise?

One of the most important benefits of exercise is to strengthen the bones, muscles and joints. When we exercise, muscles become stronger, bones become more dense and stronger and joints become more flexible. Along with good nutrition, weight bearing exercise is a great way to build strong, healthy bones. Our heart is a muscle and even benefits from exercise creating greater heart or cardiovascular health. When bones, muscles and joints are cared for, they will give a lifetime of good service.

What are the different types of exercise?

Exercise involves three types:

1. Aerobic exercise
2. Strength training
3. Flexibility exercises

Aerobic Exercise

Aerobic exercise increases heart rate, works muscles and raises the rate of respiration as well as builds endurance. During aerobic exercise, the heart beats faster and a person breathes harder. When done regularly and for continuous periods of time, aerobic activity strengthens the heart and improves the body's ability to deliver oxygen to all its cells. For most people, 30 minutes a day, five days a week is enough to maintain proper health. Someone just beginning an exercise program should start slow with five or 10 minutes per day and work up to more time each week. Start by taking a brisk 10-minute walk after each meal. Here are some additional examples of aerobic exercise:

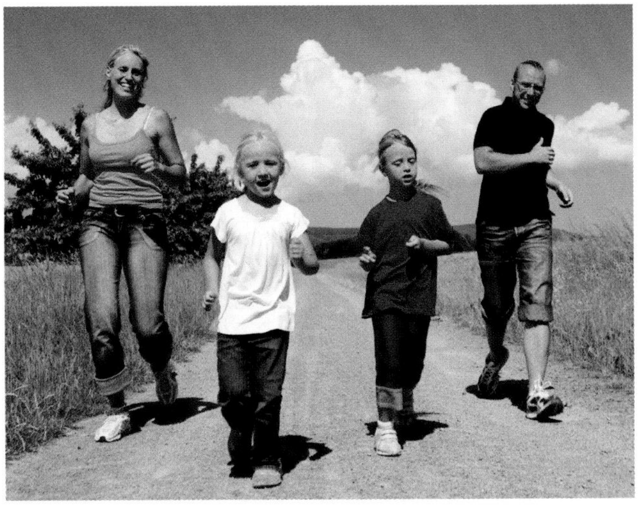

- Brisk walking outside or inside on a treadmill
- Running
- Dancing – jazz, ballroom, tap
- Low-impact aerobics classes
- Swimming or water aerobic exercises
- Ice or roller-skating
- Sports that require physical exertion – basketball, baseball, football, tennis, etc.
- Outdoor biking or indoor stationary bicycling
- Aerobic exercising with a recorded program

Strength Training

Strength training helps build strong bones and muscles and makes everyday chores easier. With more muscle, more calories are burned, even at rest. Strength training should be done three to five times per week. Strength training exercises involves training with weights, elastic bands or other resistance equipment. Push-ups, stomach crunches and pull-ups are examples of strength training exercises that young children can perform. They also incorporate strength activities in their play when they climb, do a handstand, do flips, slide into a split or wrestle.

Flexibility Exercises

Flexibility refers to the range of motion of a joint. Differences in flexibility vary from person to person; one person can do the splits with ease, while others never seem to bend and stretch. Maintaining flexibly as we age may mean the difference in bending to tie our shoes or reaching an item from a shelf. Even simple tasks can become impossible without flexibility. An inactive and unhealthy lifestyle can bring about decreased muscular flexibility and weaker joints as parts of the bone must bare more weight than they should. Back pain can be caused by tight hamstring muscles causing the hips and pelvis to rotate back, flattening the lower back and causing back problems.

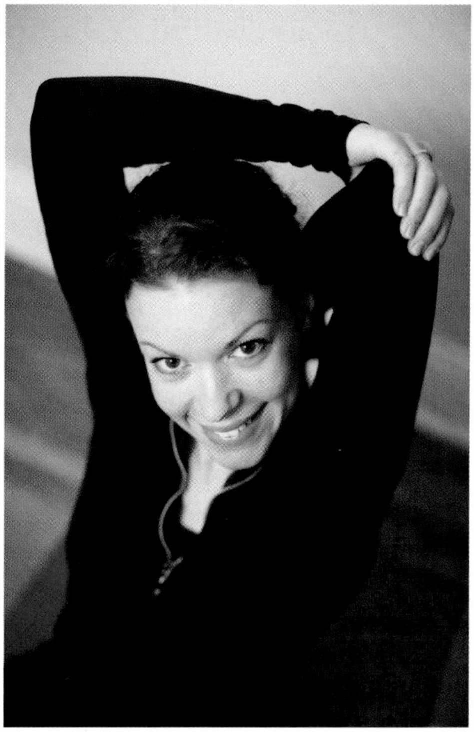

Various forms of flexibility or stretching exercises increase flexibility. Many people use ballet, pilates, yoga and callanetics for stretching exercises. A search on the Internet provides daily stretching exercise options. See the Additional Resources section of this chapter for web addresses.

"My favorite stretching and deep muscle toning exercise is Callanetics. The Callanetics Exercise Method is a very personalized and unique form of exercise that utilizes precise positioning to isolate specific muscle groups. Then it uses tiny, yet powerful movements that cause the muscles to work even deeper, requiring more muscle fibers to be recruited. More muscle fibers recruited means quicker toning and results I can feel in one hour and see in as little as two. Each muscle group is warmed, worked and then stretched to ensure total body health increasing strength, flexibility and endurance.[1]" - Debra Raybern

Harmless as Doves and Wise as Serpents

In his book, "Yoga and the Body of Christ," author Dave Hunt studies the history of yoga and reveals its origins in India through pagan worship prior to the birth of Jesus and was adopted by other religions to achieve higher spirituality. Hunt warns that no form of yoga, including Hatha Yoga (also known as physical or non-spiritual yoga), has Biblical endorsement. He also outlines in the words of Hindu organizations how yoga is used by missionaries to propagate the religion around the world. Healing and health come only through the one true God. In all areas of life, we should allow the Word of God and the Holy Spirit to give us wisdom.

Stand up and sit up straight!

Posture often deviates from good to poor as we age. Slumping, rolling the shoulders forward and other forms of bad posture can sometimes cause muscles on one side of the body to become weaker than the other side. This can cause the spine to be pulled to one side, which may then lead to the shifting of vertebrae, pinching of nerves and back pain. The effects of poor posture can be rehabilitated through exercise.

Stretches to eliminate lower back pain

These exercises can be done as often as needed to loosen the quad and lower back muscles.

1. The person with back pain should lie on the floor with plenty of room to extend the legs straight.
2. With the back flat on the ground, pull the right leg toward the chest and hold for 10 seconds.
3. Then extend the leg straight and slowly raise it so the toes are pointing up.
4. Place the hands behind the thigh or knee and slowly stretch the leg toward the chest, keeping it straight.
5. Slowly lower the right leg and repeat steps one to four with the left leg.
6. Once finished, bring both legs to the chest and rock the legs only from side to side. The hips will come off the floor, but the shoulders should stay flat against the floor.

If the person is not strong enough to perform the exercises alone, another person can assist providing gentle pressure to stretch the leg toward the chest. The helper should not push or pull, but allow the muscles to do as much of the work as possible.

1 http://www.callanetics.com/method.php

How often should we exercise and for how long?

For healthy adults younger than age 65, the American Heart Association and the American College of Sports Medicine recommend at least 30 minutes of moderate-intensity aerobic activity (brisk walking or swimming) five days a week or at least 20 minutes of vigorous aerobic activity (such as running, dancing, step aerobics, etc) three days a week, plus strength training exercises twice a week.

A new study from the University of Pittsburgh published in Archives of Internal Medicine in July 2008 noted that moderate exercise profits little and more vigorous exercise produces real health benefits.

NOTE: Before you begin any exercise program, you should consult your health professional to be sure you are physically fit enough for vigorous exercise.

Fun Fact

A 2005 Time Inc. survey determined that Americans are notorious for lying about the amount of exercise they engage in weekly. Thirty-three percent of survey participants said they exercise at the 30 minute standard, but government surveys suggest the number is more like 26 percent or less.

What can we do to get moving and make it count?

Walking is still considered to be the best of all exercises. Moderate exercise is walking at about 3.5 miles per hour while maintaining conversation with the heart rate not above the acceptable limits for exercise.

When at rest, the average human heart beats at 70 beats per minute (bpm) in males and 75 bpm for females. The infant neonatal heart beat typically ranges between 130 and 150 bpm. These rates vary, but can be significantly lower for athletes.

Maximum heart rate is the number of times the heart can constrict in a minute based on age. The maximum heart rate is about 220 minus a person's age. For moderate intensity activity, a person's target heart rate should be 50 to 70 percent of his or her maximum heart rate. For vigorous intensity activity, a person's target heart rate should be 70 to 85 percent of his or her maximum heart rate.

Age	Target Heart Rate 50% - 85%
15-25	102-165 bpm
26-35	97-157 bpm
36-45	92-148 bpm
46-55	87-140 bpm
56-65	82-131 bpm
66-75	77-123 bpm
76 - 85	72-114 bpm

Measuring Heart Rate

The heart rate can be taken on the surface of the skin near an artery where a pulse can be felt. The most common places to measure the pulse or palpations are the radial artery at the wrist and the carotid artery at the neck.

1. Place the index and middle finders together on the opposite wrist so that they line up with the index finger. On the neck, place the same fingers on the front of the neck to either side of the center of the throat. Do not use the thumb, especially when taking another person's pulse, because the thumb may pulse, giving a false reading.
2. Count the number of beats in one minute. The per minute rate can be estimated by counting for 10 seconds and multiplying by six or counting for 15 seconds and multiplying by four or counting for 30 seconds and multiplying for two.

Children and Exercise

Healthy adults often have an exercise program either at home or a gym, but for children, exercise means playing and being physically active. Parents should take time daily to be sure their children are actively engaged in some form of exercise. This may include a gym class, soccer or other sport practice or dance class. Playing tag, running around the yard and riding a bike also are good forms of exercise for children.

In addition to the health benefits of regular exercise, children who are physically fit sleep better and are better able to handle the physical and emotional challenges that a typical day presents, including school work.

Start early to help your children build healthy exercise habits now. They will reap a life time of rewards and will hopefully pass the good habits on to their children.

How much exercise is enough for children?

Parents need to ensure that their kids get enough exercise. One of the best ways to get children of all ages – that might include mom and dad's participation – to be more active is to limit the amount of time spent watching television or playing video games.

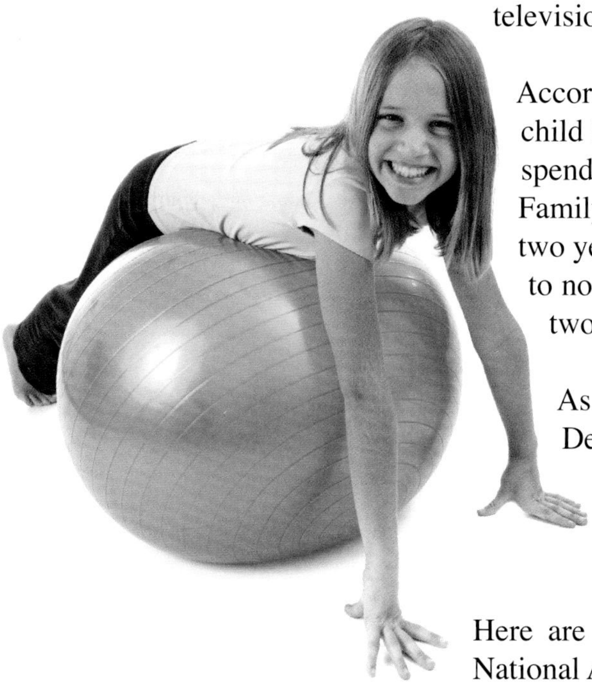

According to the American Academy of Pediatrics (AAP), the average child is watching about three hours of television a day. The average child spends five and a half hours on all media combined, according to the Kaiser Family Foundation. The AAP recommends that children under the age of two years watch no television at all and that screen time should be limited to no more than one to two hours of quality programming a day for kids two years and older.

As far as exercise goes, the 2005 dietary guidelines from the U.S. Department of Agriculture (USDA) and the Department of Health and Human Services (HHS) say that all children two years and older should get at least 60 minutes of moderate to vigorous exercise on most, preferably all, days of the week.

Here are the current activity recommendations for kids, according to the National Association for Sport and Physical Education (NASPE):

Infants – No specific requirements; physical activity should encourage motor development.
Toddlers – 1 ½ hours, 30 minutes planned physical activity and one hour unstructured play time.
Preschooler – Two hours, 60 minutes planned physical activity and one hour unstructured play time.
School age – One hour planned physical activity, broken into 15 minute intervals.

Fun Fact

The President's Challenge, formerly known as the President's Sports Award, is a program for both children ages six and up and adults who engage in regular and active exercise. Not based on performance, this is open to everyone and can be incorporated into physical education class. Go to www.presidentschallenge.org

Benefits of Regular Exercise

Exercise …

- Reduces the risk of heart disease, high blood pressure, cholesterol concerns, diabetes, obesity, osteoporosis and some cancers which in turn reduces the risk of premature death.
- Keeps muscles, joints, tendons and ligaments flexible to make bending, walking and in general moving around easier.
- Has been shown to be helpful for mild depression and anxiety.
- Makes people feel and look healthy.
- Promotes better sleep patterns.
- Increases cognitive function.
- Reverses dementia.[2]

Successful exercising is not about breaking records on the first day. It is about gradual, consistent improvement. Even people who were once active and have done less physical activity over the years should ease into exercise. Pushing the body past its ability can do more harm than good.

Exercise Safety Tips

- **Protect the skull and brain by wearing a helmet for bike riding and other sports where the head is at risk.**
- When skateboarding, skating or riding a scooter, be sure to add wrist guards and elbow and knee pads for added protection.
- **Sports, such as football, soccer and baseball require special protective equipment and players should wear them correctly.**
- While a trampoline might be a lot of fun, children and even adults should not play on a trampoline. Many kids end up with broken bones from jumping on them. Leave the trampoline to a supervised gymnastics class.

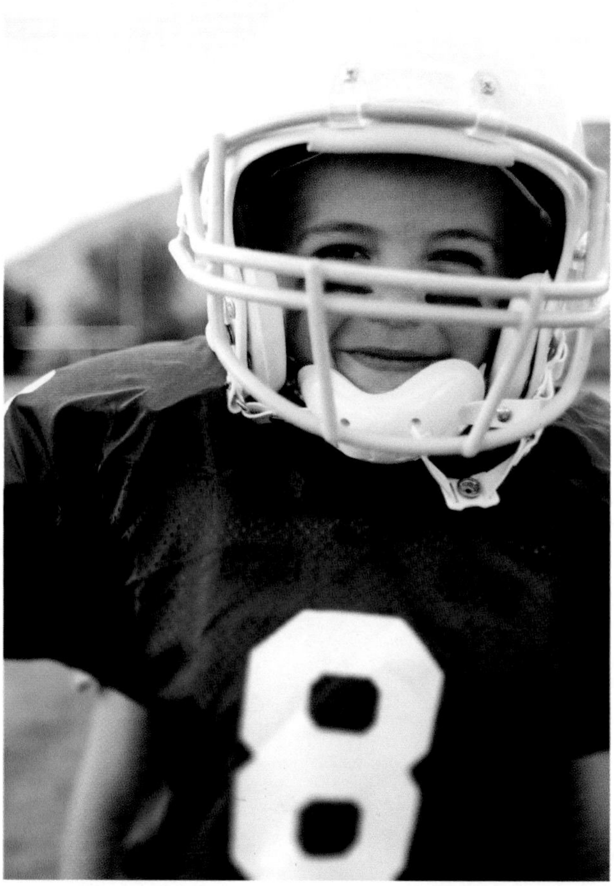

Exercise Disguised

1. Take the stairs and not the elevator.
2. Take brisk walks during breaks at work or school.
3. Vacuum with vigor and a really clean home is another side effect.
4. Rake leaves and work in the garden; these can work up a sweat and increase heart rate.
5. When shopping, park a further distance from the store and walk quickly to and from the car.

2 http://www.wvdhhr.org/bph/oehp/hsc/dementia/prevent.htm

Fuel for Exercising

In Luke 12:22-23, Jesus told his disciples "Take no thought for your life, what ye shall eat; neither for the body, what ye shall put on. The life is more than meat, and the body is more than raiment." This does not mean that we should not care for our bodies, but just not worry or be anxious about caring for it.

Food provides the body with necessary energy. **Carbohydrates** are the body's chief source of fuel. Athletes feel better and perform optimally when they exercise after eating foods high in carbohydrates and low in fat. The body stores excess carbohydrates as **glycogen**, primarily in the muscles and liver. Then, the muscles use stored glycogen when needed for energy.

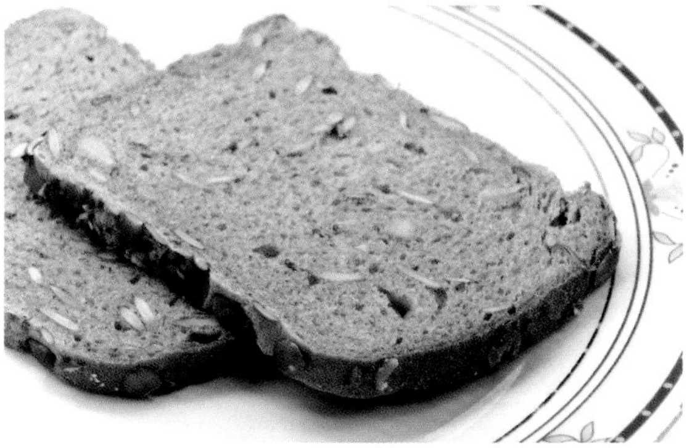

Whole grain cereals, breads, pasta, rice, starchy vegetables (potatoes) and fruit are good sources of carbohydrates. Avoid high fiber carbohydrates right before exercise as they may give you gas or cause cramping. Fructose, a simple sugar found in fruit, can increase the tendency for diarrhea with high-intensity exercise.

For the regular exerciser, a diet containing at least 40 percent to 50 percent of calories from carbohydrates allows the body to store glycogen.

Protein and fats are important for muscle repair and growth, however it is not the body's top fuel choice. Most people can easily get the protein they need from their regular diet. Fats, as well as carbohydrates, can provide fuel for muscles during exercise. The primary supply of fat should come from unsaturated sources such as nuts, fatty fish or vegetable oils. Fatty foods should be avoided just before exercising, as fats remain in the stomach longer, causing bloating and heaviness. Fried foods should be avoided all together.

Exercise and Eating

Refraining from eating before exercising can be just as bad as eating too much. Low blood sugar levels that result from not eating can make a person feel weak or tired, and affect his or her mental abilities as well, causing a person to react slower and increasing the chance of injury. To get the most from a workout, follow these guidelines:

- Wake up early enough to eat a full breakfast. Don't rely on last night's dinner. Those nutrients and calories are already used up; the blood sugar is generally at its lowest point. If exercising within an hour after breakfast, eat a smaller breakfast or have a balanced breakfast meal-in-a-glass with protein, carbohydrates and healthy sugars.[3]

- Eat large meals at least three to four hours before exercising giving the food time to leave the stomach. If having a small meal, eat two to three hours before exercising.

- Skipping meals may cause low blood sugar, which can make a person feel fatigued and light-headed. Even if there is not much time to eat before a workout, it is best not to skip food; select quick and health choices, such as a balanced snack bar or fruit and yogurt.

- Following exercise, help the muscles recover and replace their glycogen stores by eating a snack or meal that contains both protein and carbohydrates within two hours if possible.

---

3 See Appendix DD for authors' recommendations.

Hydration

Hydration is very important before, during and after exercise. While many people drink water for hydration, athletes often drink sports drinks to replenish the minerals called **electrolytes** lost during perspiration. So which is the better choice?

What are electrolytes?

Electrolyte drinks are waters infused with sodium, calcium, potassium and sometimes flavor. Electrolytes serve three general function in the body:

1. They are mostly minerals the body needs.
2. They control osmosis of water between body compartments.
3. They help maintain the acid-base balance required for normal cellular activities.

As the body perspires or sweats, many of the electrolytes in the body are lost to evaporation. The electrolyte composition of sweat may vary, but it is comprised of mainly the following components:

- Sodium
- Potassium
- Calcium
- Magnesium
- Chloride
- Bicarbonate
- Phosphate
- Sulfate

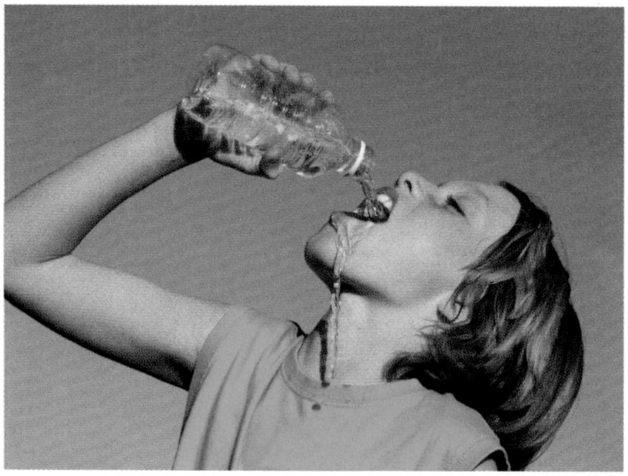

The ideal sports drink will contain the correct ratio of electrolytes, B-complex, chromium, amino acids and contain very low salt. Americans already consume more salt than the body requires. New research suggests there even are benefits from having protein in sports drinks. See the home made electrolyte recipes in the Additional Recipes section of this unit.

Are electrolyte drinks necessary or even safe?

Well, that depends. If a person is training for a triathlon, playing professional high-intensity sports or losing lots of water to sweating, then yes. These people should be drinking electrolyte-infused water. But if not, if a person engages in 30 to 60 minutes of aerobic exercise daily, the answer is no.

Elizabeth Quinn, trainer and health professional, says that athletes who consume electrolytes under normal exercise conditions risk over-hydration. "It is unnecessary to replace losses of sodium, potassium and other electrolytes during exercise since it is unlikely that a significant depletion of the body's stores of these minerals will occur during normal training. However, in extreme exercising conditions over five or six hours, the consumption of a complex sports drink with electrolytes is recommended."

Most sport drinks typically contain very high levels of sugar and are not recommended for regular use by children. Water is considered the only essential beverage for children during exercise. Electrolyte and sports drinks can be made at home and supply all the necessary nutrients without harmful sugars (see Unit 5 Additional Recipes).

Determining an athlete from a person who regularly exercises is important; there is a difference. Water is generally the best way to replace lost fluid, unless as previously stated, a person is exercising for more than 60 minutes.

What about water?

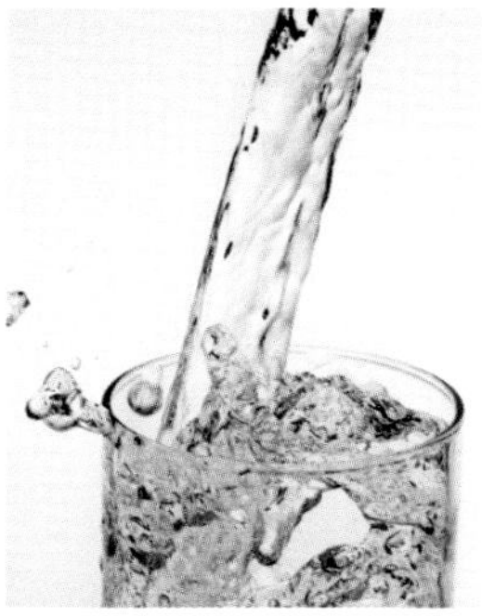

The American College of Sports Medicine recommends that people drink eight glasses of water every day and more on days when the temperature and humidity are high.

Those who exercise should drink at least one glass of water before and after a workout and every 10 to 15 minutes during the workout to replace fluid lost in perspiration. Avoid substituting coffee, tea or soda for water, because they often contain caffeine, which acts as a diuretic that causes the body to lose even more water.

The body uses the water in its blood to carry nutrients such as sugar (glucose) to cells and to remove waste products from the cells. The presence of water in the body ensures that a person can safely sustain physical activity. During exercise, the body produces heat, which leaves the body as perspiration taking with it the electrolytes. If the fluid and its nutrients lost during exercise are not replaced the heart rate increases and the body's temperature rises, putting a person at risk of dehydration.

Signs of dehydration

Thirst, headaches, fatigue, loss of coordination, mental confusion, irritability, dry skin, elevated body temperature, diminished urine output

Exercise Tips

1. Exercise with a partner.
2. Schedule time to exercise time on the calendar so as not to forget and to be accountable.
3. Start with warm-ups and stretching exercises to prepare the muscles.
4. Pick enjoyable exercises or exercise equipment to avoid boredom and burnout.
5. Make it fun by listening to music or watching a video.
6. Do not become discouraged. Transforming the body takes time.
7. Keep hydrated! Have a bottle of water handy to remember to drink 16 ounces of water before exercising and to sip on during and after exercising.
8. Do not do aerobic exercise on an empty stomach, but also do not get up from a meal and immediately go for a five-mile run.
9. Stop if there are feelings of dizziness, inability to catch one's breath, faintness or pain.

Isaiah 35:3-10 has an incredible encouragement for the children of Israel and hope for restoration. Staying on the Holy Highway, following His way, not our own will lead us to life rather than destruction. Be encouraged by this inspirational passage:

"Strengthen ye the weak hands, and confirm the feeble knees. Say to them that are of a fearful heart, Be strong, fear not: behold, your God will come with vengeance, even God with a recompense; He will come and save you. Then the eyes of the blind shall be opened, and the ears of the deaf shall be unstopped. Then shall the lame man leap as an hart, and the tongue of the dumb sing: for in the wilderness shall waters break out, and streams in the desert. And the parched ground shall become a pool, and the thirsty land springs of water: in the habitation of dragons, where each lay, shall be grass with reeds and rushes. And an highway shall be there, and a way, and it shall be called The way of holiness; the unclean shall not pass over it; but it shall be for those: the wayfaring men, though fools, shall not err therein. No lion shall be there, nor any ravenous beast shall go up thereon, it shall not be found there; but the redeemed shall walk there: And the ransomed of the Lord shall return, and come to Zion with songs and everlasting joy upon their heads: they shall obtain joy and gladness, and sorrow and sighing shall flee away."

Unit 4 Chapter 4
Discussion Questions

1. What are your favorite ways to exercise?
2. How do your parents like to exercise?
3. Do you have the right protective equipment for the kind of exercising you enjoy?
4. What are some examples of physical strength in the Bible?
5. What are your favorite Scriptures about exercise?

Activities - plus the Chicken Nuggets "Power" Recipe and activities.

Elementary

1. Choose three regular household chores and think of ways to incorporate exercises that strengthens and tones muscles and burns calories.
2. Find a widow or elderly person at church or in your community who needs help with yard work. After receiving permission, organize your family to get the yard clean. Make sure that everyone is safe by stretching first and then encourage them to work quickly, increasing their heart rates and getting good exercise. Schedule the time to work following an appropriate meal and be sure to have enough water on hand for your family to drink before, during and after exercise.
3. Learn more about the Presidential Fitness Program and determine if you or other members of your family would like to participate. Have an adult help you find the Web site: www.presidentschallenge.org
4. Keep an exercise and food journal for 30 days to track your healthy choices and record your thoughts.

Secondary

Choose any from above plus

1. Learn to measure your heart rate.
2. Once you can take your heart rate, use the scale in this chapter to determine your heart rate intensity.
3. Go to http://www.presidentschallenge.org/tools_to_help/bmi.aspx to calculate your BMI. Then calculate the BMI for your family members. Keep in mind that BMI doesn't always work well for kids, competitive athletes, weight lifters, pregnant or nursing women, or frail or inactive elderly persons.
4. Arrange an exercise schedule for your family. Help them keep track of their progress and encourage them to continue.
5. Teach your family members how to determine their heart rate and then how to determine their heart rate intensity.
6. Find a local fun run or other activity that interests you and that is three to six months away. Train for the event and record your progress.

Additional Resources

Authors' favorite exercises:

Pilates
Callanetics
T-Tapp - www.t-tapp.com

Web sites:

1. http://www.ehow.com/how_2049140_increase-flexibility.html?ref=fuel&utm_source=yahoo&utm_medium=ssp&utm_campaign=yssp_art
2. http://www.womenfitness.net/flexibility_increase.htm

Exercise Power Chicken

Exercised muscles need protein for repair and strengthening. Chicken is a great source of protein, Make sure your chicken is organic, cage free and free from antibotics and growth hormones.

Chicken Nuggets

"Because my children used to be addicted to fast food chicken nuggets, I came up with this healthier version using coconut oil and sweet potato puree that makes really crunchy, yummy chicken nuggets. Now my children don't feel like they are missing out on one of their old favorites!" – Sera Johnson

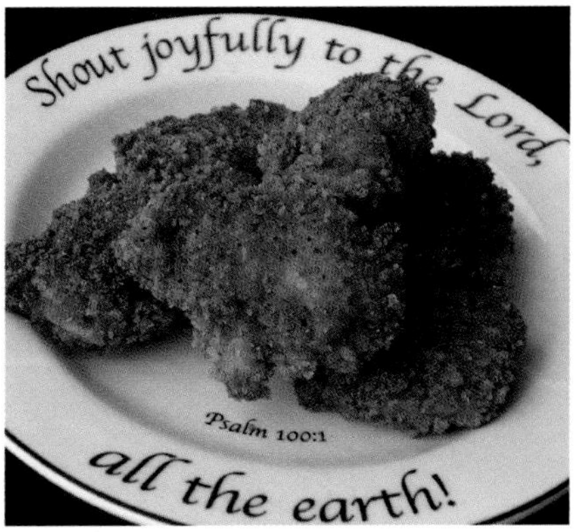

1 pound organic chicken breast, cut up into nugget sized pieces
1 egg
2 oz. sweet potato puree
2 cups organic Italian bread crumbs
Celtic sea salt to taste
Pepper to taste
¼ cup organic raw coconut oil

In a medium bowl, add egg and sweet potato puree and beat well together. Add the nugget sized chicken breast to completely coat. In a shallow dish, combine the bread crumbs, salt and pepper. Add the coconut oil to the heated skillet. Evenly coat each chicken nugget in the bread crumb mixture and place in the skillet. Cook thoroughly 2-3 minutes on each side until brown.

For a low fat option, place the breaded chicken in a baking dish in a 375° oven for 30-35 minutes or until brown and thoroughly cooked.

Activities

Elementary

1. When selecting chicken for this recipe, see what other labels are on the packaging. What do these mean? If your chicken does not come with labels, interview the farmer who provided the chicken to understand more about the terms free range, organic and cage free.
2. Proper care should be taken when cooking with raw meat and eggs. Have an adult help you go to this link on the United States Department of Agriculture (USDA) Web site: http://www.fsis.usda.gov/Factsheets/Basics_for_Handling_Food_Safely/index.asp to learn more about working with such foods.
3. What is salmonella?
4. How can people get and avoid salmonella?

Secondary

Choose any from above plus

1. Go to http://nutrition.mcdonalds.com/bagamcmeal/itemDetailInfo.do to get the nutrition facts for their Chicken McNuggets. Scroll down to see the list of ingredients and compare it to the recipe above.
2. Do the same experiment for French fries. Before looking at the ingredients, write down the ingredients you would need to make fries at home. Now check McDonald's Web site. How many ingredients are in an order of small fries?
3. Locate the nutritional facts for the top three restaurants where your family eats.
4. Based on what you learned in Unit 1 about trans fats and fried foods, do you believe that the nutritional value, as identified by the USDA is accurate? Prepare an oral or written report on your beliefs.

Unit 4 Additional Recipes

Use organic ingredients when possible.

Sun Dried Tomato Chickpea Dip

1 can (16 ounce) garbano beans (chickpea), drained and rinsed
3 Tbs. sun dried tomatoes in oil
1-2 tsp. roasted garlic
2 tsp. parsley
2 Tbs. olive oil
2 Tbs. lemon juice

Combine the garbanzo beans, tomatoes, parsley, and garlic in a food processor; pulse several times. Use a spatula to push mixture from sides of processor bowl. Pulse the mixture again while drizzling in the olive oil and lemon. Pulse until combined. Season with salt and pepper. Serve with fresh vegetable sticks or whole grain flatbread.

Millet Salad

Though not widely consumed in the U.S., millet is an ancient grain with a history as an important food in many countries as a good source of manganese and phosphorus.

1 cup cooked millet
1 medium tomato, diced
1 small onion, finely diced
½ cucumber, seeded and diced
3 Tbs. olive oil
1 tsp. apple cider vinegar
1 drop Young Living tarragon essential oil OR 1Tbs. fresh tarragon, diced and allowed to marinate in the vinegar for one hour, then strain out tarragon

Mix in a bowl and serve as a side dish. Top with Feta cheese crumbles.

Quinoa with Grilled Vegetables & Cashews

Not only is quinoa high in protein, but the protein is a complete protein, meaning it includes all nine essential amino acids, Quinoa, while high in protein is gluten free, high in iron and manganese.

1 cup quinoa
2 cups water
Pinch of salt
Cook according to package directions.

Vegetables
¼ cup each: yellow squash, zucchini, red bell pepper, mushrooms (crimini are the most nutritious) and fresh green beans.

Rinse quinoa under running water, place in saucepan with salt and water and bring to a boil. Turn heat to low, cover and simmer for 15 minutes. Once cooked, the grain will be somewhat transparent and the germ will partially detach making it look like it has a tail.

While the quinoa is cooking, sauté a variety of vegetables in coconut or olive oil. Combine cooked quinoa and sautéed vegetables. Serve on a bed of shredded Romaine lettuce. Top with diced tomatoes and onions.

Noodle, Egg and Onion Casserole

1 ½ cup macaroni (this can be whole wheat, gluten free, etc.)
2 Tbs. butter or coconut oil
1 egg for each person

Topping sauce:
1 large tomato, diced
1 small onion, finely diced
1/4 cup olive oil
1 tsp. apple cider vinegar
1 drop YL Tarragon essential oil
Salt and pepper to taste

Combine ingredients of topping sauce in a bowl, mix well and set aside for one hour before serving.

Cook macaroni product per package directions and drain. Melt two tablespoons coconut oil in hot skillet, add macaroni and stir to coat. Stir in scramble eggs and stir until egg is fully cooked. Spoon onto plates and top with the tomato and onion sauce.

Protein Power Shake

1 serving of high quality protein shake mix – authors' choice is Young Living's Pure Protein Complete (whey based) or Power Meal (vegetarian)
1 banana
4 strawberries
2 oz. rice milk or water
1 cup of ice

Place ingredients in a high power blender and blend until smooth. Makes one to two servings. For more protein boost, substitute the strawberries with 2 Tbs. organic peanut butter or any nut butter and 1 Tbs. carob powder.

Electrolyte Recipe 1

14 ounces filtered water
2 oz. NingXia Red Infusion Juice
15 drops liquid IONIC mineral (Mineral Essence or Concentrace Drops)

Electrolyte Recipe 2

14 ounces filtered water
1 tsp. un-sulfured molasses
one drop Young Living lemon oil

Grilled Salmon

Wild Alaskan Salmon is preferred for this recipe. Select about 1/3 pound of salmon per serving. This recipe uses three pounds.

Combine the following to make a rub:
2 Tbs. celery seed
1 Tbs. paprika
1 Tbs. ground nutmeg or one drop of Young Living nutmeg essential oil
1 Tbs. chili powder
1 Tbs. finely diced garlic
1 Tbs. finely diced onion
1 Tbs. Celtic Sea salt
½Tbs. Blue Agave Nectar
1 Tbs. fresh ground black pepper

Rub the mixture on the salmon and drizzle it lightly with olive oil. Place the salmon on the grill, flesh side first. Let cook for about seven to ten minutes each side. To bake the salmon, preheat the oven to 375° F. Cook the salmon for seven to ten minutes without flipping. It is finished when it easily flakes with a fork.

Whole Chicken and Homemade Chicken Stock

This is a simple, inexpensive and delicious way to get multiple healthy meals from the same pot. It does take some planning, so be sure to start in plenty of time.

1 whole organic chicken
5 medium carrots
1 full head of celery
5 cloves of garlic
2 medium white or yellow onions
Celtic Sea salt and pepper

Wash the vegetables and peel the carrots if not organic. Chop the carrots and celery into three to four inch sticks. Quarter the onion and peel the garlic. Do not discard the leafy parts of the celery and carrot tops, but place them in a container or plastic bag and refrigerate. Separate about ¼ of the carrots, celery, onion and garlic; refrigerate the rest of the vegetables for use in the stoup recipe below.

Rinse the chicken, including the cavity, with cold water. Pat it dry with a paper towel. Insert the carrots, celery, onion and garlic into the cavity. Place the chicken in a slow cooker or crock pot. Wash hands thoroughly with soap and warm water. Sprinkle the chicken with salt and pepper. Place the lid on the cooker and set it on low for

12 hours or high for about six hours. Do not add water.

After the cooking time is completed, turn off the cooker and let it stand for 20 to 30 minutes. The chicken will be tender when removed from the cooker and is not likely to stay in one piece. Discard the vegetables. Remove the meat from the bones and place on a platter. Put the bones back in the slow cooker with the juices. Serve the chicken immediately as a main course with your favorite sides. Or refrigerate a pound of the chicken for use in the Chicken Noodle Stoup recipe below.

Take the leafy parts of the celery, carrot tops and one quarter of the onion and two whole cloves of garlic and place them in the juice. Add three to five cups of water, depending on the size of the slow cooker. This typically makes about ½ quart; add more water for more stock. Set it on low for eight hours or on high for four. When time elapses, turn it off and let it stand for 20 to 30 minutes. Place a pitcher on the counter next to the slow cooker. Put a strainer on top of the pitcher and ladle the contents of the cooker into the strainer. Discard all of the things in the strainer. The chicken stock in the pitcher should be used immediately in the stoup recipe below or poured into ice cube trays and frozen. To measure the amount of stock, use measuring cups to pour into the ice cube trays. These cubes can be stored for use in future recipes.

Chicken Noodle Stoup

This recipe is thicker than soup, but thinner than stew, making it a stoup. Personalize it by adding homemade noodles or other ingredients for a family favorite.

1 cup of quinoa or rice noodles (or favorite healthy homemade version)
2 medium carrots, peeled and chopped
2 cloves garlic, minced
2 Tbs. extra-virgin olive oil or coconut oil
1 medium zucchini
1 medium yellow skinned onion, peeled and halved
Celtic Sea salt and pepper
1 tsp. each dried sage, rosemary and thyme or a drop each of the essential oil
1 quart of homemade chicken stock
1 (14-ounce) can diced organic tomatoes or coarsely ground tomatoes
1 pound cooked chicken, diced
2 Tbs. chopped flat-leaf parsley
4 Tbs. of arrowroot powder (for thickening)

In medium soup pot preheated over medium-high heat, add oil, garlic and two quarters of the onion, finely chopped, and stir to coat in the oil. Add ½ cup of stock and reduce by letting it cook a minute or so. Add the tomatoes, noodles, remaining stock and arrowroot powder to the pot, cover the pot and raise heat to high. Bring the stoup to a boil, then add cut chicken and simmer eight to 10 minutes until noodles are just tender and chicken is warmed through. Finely chop the remaining vegetables and add to the stoup for about five minutes. These will be crunchy. Serve stoup in shallow bowls. Top stoup with chopped parsley and pass crusty homemade bread at the table for dipping and mopping.

Unit 5

The Cardiovascular and Immune Systems

People with healthy hearts often take for granted the rhythmic beating of this essential organ and the intricate silent workings of the immune system. However, without them it is impossible to live beyond a few seconds. Think of the heart as the engine that keeps the body running and the immune system as the filter for everything eaten, touched and smelled. Without the protection of the heart and blood, which God calls the "life of the flesh" in Leviticus 17:11, we would cease to exist.

Thus far, **Nutrition 101: Choose Life!** has covered many of the body systems, and we have learned the importance of nutrition, supplements and exercise in keeping them functioning and disease free. Now is a crucial time to learn what we can do to keep our hearts and immune systems healthy and serving our body, so we have the health to serve others.

It has been said "it is no measure of health to be well adjusted to a profoundly sick society." In the United Sates deaths from heart disease continue to climb despite modern medicine and pharmaceutical drugs. An estimated 1,500 people die from cancer every day, and this number is projected to double in the next 20 years. Let's implement healthy changes and reverse this prognosis.

Restoring the body's health may take time, especially if it has been in poor health for a long period of time. But what does the Word of God say about disciplining the flesh? Hebrews 12:11 reads "Now no chastening (discipline) for the present seemeth to be joyous, but grievous; nevertheless afterward it yieldeth the peaceable fruit of righteousness unto them who are exercised thereby." Disciplining the body, although uncomfortable for a season, is well worth it.

Forming new habits and breaking old ones is never easy. However, we have assurance that when we make changes in our health for the better, we will reap a pleasant reward – great health!

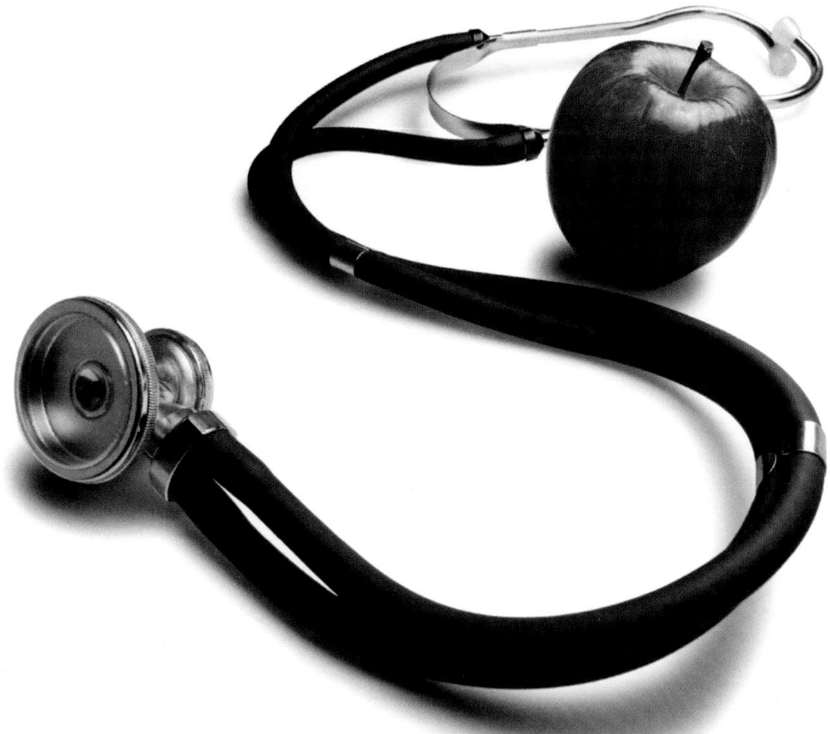

Chapter 1

The Cardiovascular System

"My heart is fixed, O God, my heart is fixed: I will sing and give praise." Psalm 57:7

If a child places his hand lightly on the side of his neck, closes his eyes and is very still, he will feel more than just his heart beat. The pulsating movement is the blood rushing through the blood vessels with every beat of the heart. The heart beats an average of 70 times per minute or 100,000 times per day and pumps an amazing 2,000 gallons of blood each day. By the end of a long life, a person's heart may have beaten – or expanded and contracted – more than 3.5 billion times.

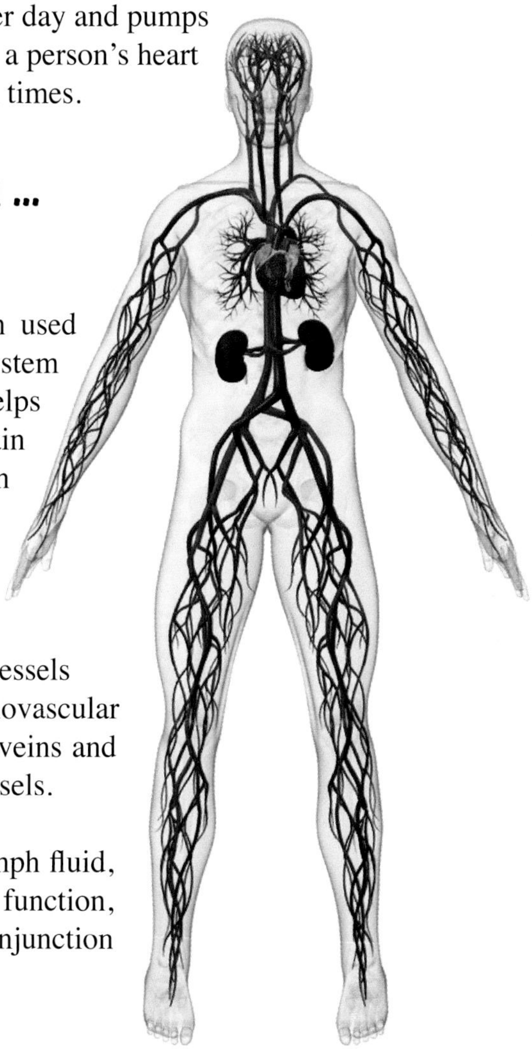

Circulatory System and Cardiovascular System ...

Is there a difference?

The names circulatory system and cardiovascular system are often used synonymously. The **circulatory system** is known as the organ system that moves nutrients, gases and waste to and from cells. It also helps fight diseases and helps stabilize body temperature and pH to maintain homeostasis. This system may be seen strictly as a blood distribution network, but some consider the circulatory system as composed of two systems together - the cardiovascular system, which distributes blood, and the lymphatic system, which distributes lymph fluid.

The **cardiovascular system** is comprised of the heart, blood vessels (arteries, veins and capillaries) and blood. Humans have a closed cardiovascular system, meaning that the blood never leaves the network of arteries, veins and capillaries, unless by injury or the cutting of one of the component vessels.

The **lymphatic system**, on the other hand, is made up of the lymph fluid, lymph nodes and lymph vessels and is an open system. Because of its function, the lymphatic system will be discussed in Chapter 3 of this unit in conjunction with the immune system.

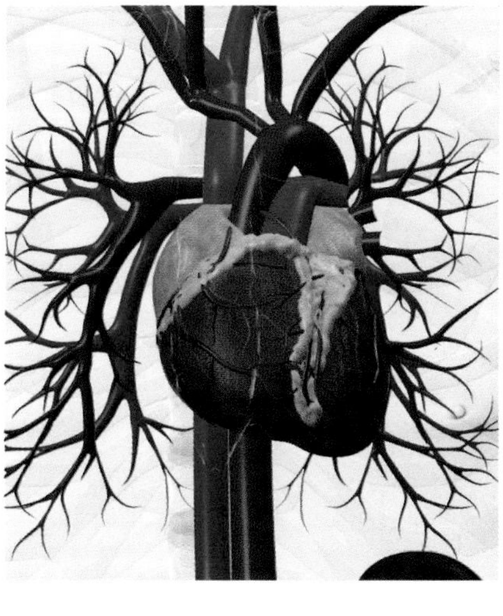

The Heart

"And I will give them an heart to know me, that I am the Lord: and they shall be my people, and I will be their God: for they shall return unto me with their whole heart." Jeremiah 24:7

Weighing in between seven and 15 ounces, the human heart is about the size of the average person's fist and sits under the rib cage and just slightly left of the sternum – the bone connecting the ribs. When Americans say the Pledge of Allegiance to the U.S. or Christian flags, they place their hands on the left side of the chest over the heart. This symbolizes love and loyalty – virtues associated with the heart by various cultures. World literature is filled with references to the heart in regard to emotion. In the New King James version of the Bible the heart is mentioned 830 times.

Although most children may believe the heart is shaped like a valentine, it is a more complex and unromantic shape. It is a muscle that works as a pump, pushing blood to the organs, tissues and cells of the body, in order for the blood to deliver oxygen and nutrients to the cells and remove carbon dioxide and other waste products made by the cells. When the heart contracts or squeezes, it pushes blood out of the heart and to the body. When it expands or relaxes, blood rushes back to the heart, and it fills with blood again.

The heart is surrounded by a double-layer membrane, or sac, called the **pericardium**. The outer layer surrounds the heart's major blood vessels and is attached to the spinal column and diaphragm by ligaments that hold it in place. The inner layer is attached to the heart muscle, also known as the **myocardium**. Between the two layers is a coating of fluid that lets the heart move as it beats while reducing friction.

Parts of the Heart

"A wise man's heart is at his right hand; but a fool's heart at his left." Ecclesiastes 10:2

Chambers

The heart has four **chambers.** The upper chambers are called the **left** and **right atria**, and the lower chambers are called the **left** and **right ventricles**. A wall of muscle called the **septum** separates the left and right atria and the left and right ventricles. The left ventricle is the largest and strongest chamber in your heart. The left ventricle's chamber walls are only about a half-inch thick, but they have enough force to push blood through the aortic valve and into your entire body.

Valves

There are four types of **valves** that regulate the flow of blood through the heart. The **tricuspid valve** regulates blood flow between the right atrium and right ventricle. The **pulmonary valve** controls blood flow from the right ventricle into the pulmonary arteries, which carry blood to the lungs to pick up oxygen. The **mitral valve** lets oxygen-rich blood from the lungs pass from the left atrium into the left ventricle. The **aortic valve** opens the way for oxygen-rich blood to pass from the left ventricle into the aorta, the body's largest artery.

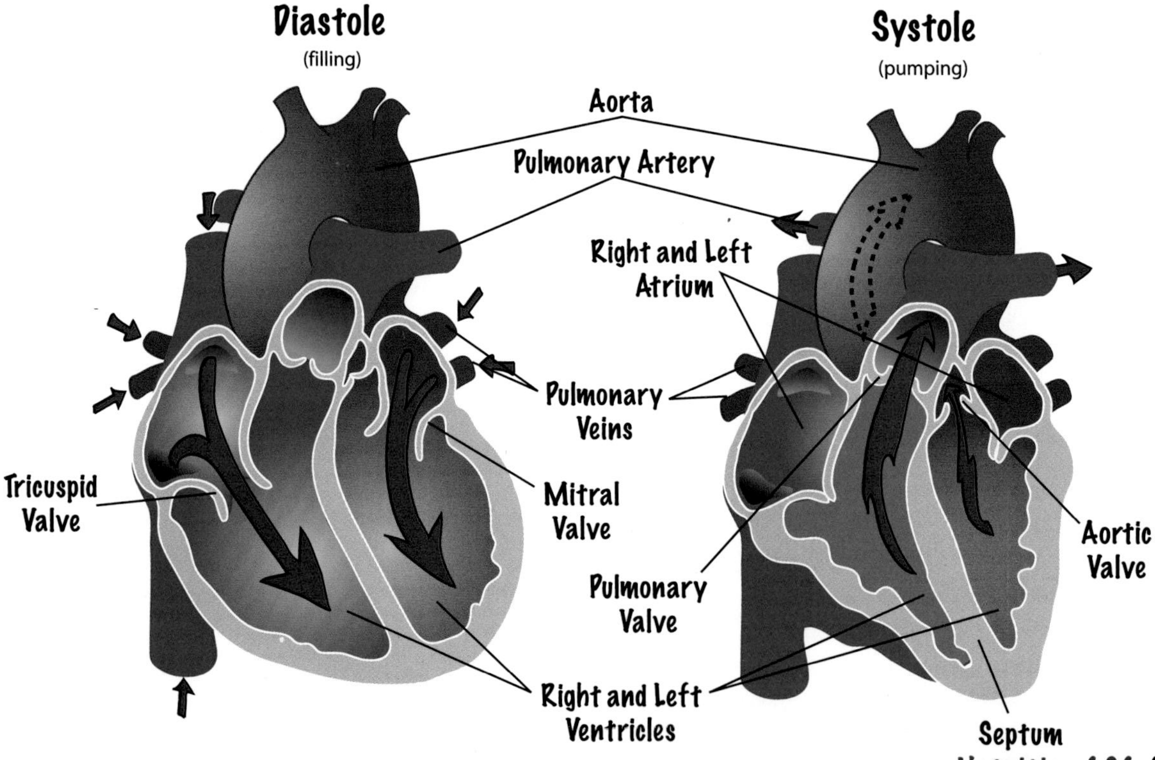

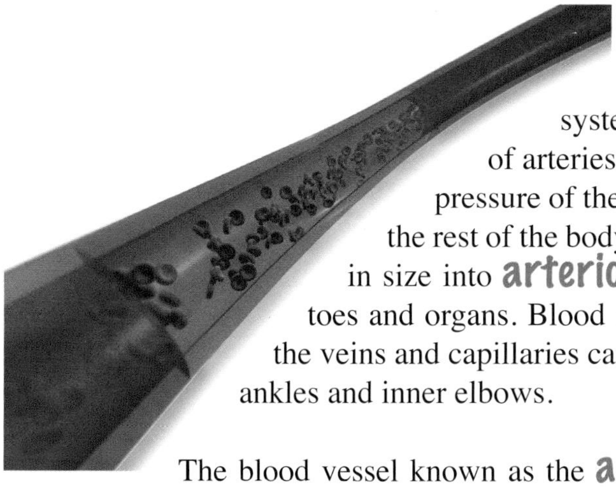

Blood Vessels

Several types of **blood vessels** make up the circulating system of the blood. This system is a lengthy and complex network of arteries, veins and capillaries, which are elastic to allow for the constant pressure of the blood flowing through them. They carry blood from the heart to the rest of the body. Beginning at the heart as large **arteries**, the vessels decrease in size into **arterioles** and then into tiny **capillaries** as they reach the fingers, toes and organs. Blood is returned to the heart through **venules** and **veins**. Some of the veins and capillaries can be seen through thin skin layers of the body such as the wrists, ankles and inner elbows.

The blood vessel known as the **aorta** is the main blood supplier to the body and branches off into two main coronary blood vessels also called arteries. These two coronary arteries branch off into smaller arteries, which supply oxygen-rich blood to the entire heart muscle. The right coronary artery supplies blood mainly to the right side of the heart, while the left coronary artery supplies blood to the left side of the heart. The right side of the heart is smaller than the left because it pumps blood only to the lungs. The left side of the heart is larger and more muscular because it pumps blood to the rest of the body.

Fun Fact

If a person's blood vessels were connected as a single vessel, they would circle the earth two and a half times!

How does the heart work?

Ever wondered why doctors and paramedics use electric shock to revive a person whose heart has stopped beating? It is electrical impulses from the myocardium that cause the heart to contract. This electrical signal begins in the sinoatrial (SA) node, located at the top of the right atrium. The SA node is sometimes called the heart's natural pacemaker. An electrical impulse travels through the muscle fibers of the atria and ventricles, causing them to contract. Although the SA node sends electrical impulses at a certain rate, the heart rate may still change depending on physical demands, stress or hormonal factors.

Word Power

Defibrillator

Pronunciation:
\dē-fi-brə-lā-tər\
Function: noun
Date: 1952
: an electronic device that applies an electric shock to restore the rhythm of a fibrillating heart

Blood

Made of blood cells and a liquid called plasma, blood is mostly made of water and is a particular type of body fluid that transports nutrients and oxygen to cells and carries waste away from cells.

Plasma is 90 percent water and makes up 55 percent of the total blood fluid. In addition to water, plasma also contains dissolved proteins, glucose, mineral ions, hormones, carbon dioxide, platelets and blood cells.

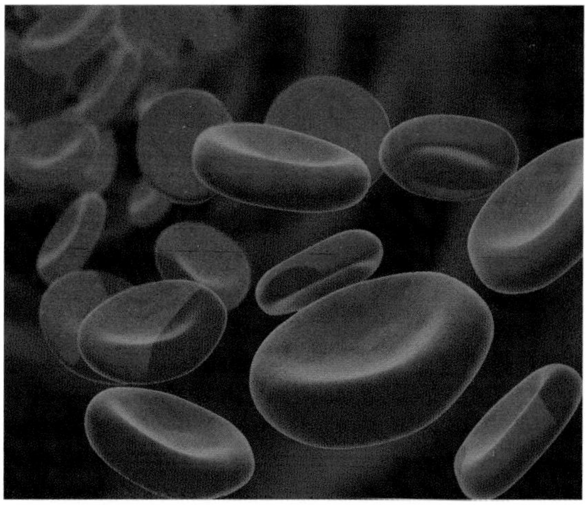

The most abundant blood cells are **red blood cells** or erythrocytes. The red blood cells are shaped like indented disks and contain hemoglobin, which is an iron-containing protein that facilitates the transportation of oxygen. The hemoglobin is bright red when it is oxygenated. While red blood cells live for about four months, every day new red blood cells are made in the bone marrow to replace the dead cells or those that are lost from the body.

White blood cells, also known as leukocytes, defend the body against foreign material such as bacteria and viruses and are found throughout the body both in the blood and in the lymphatic system. There are fewer white blood cells than red blood cells. Because white blood cells can live from a few days to a few months, the bone marrow is constantly making more. Someone fighting off an infection or disease typically has a higher than usual white blood count. See more about white blood cells in Chapter 3 of this unit.

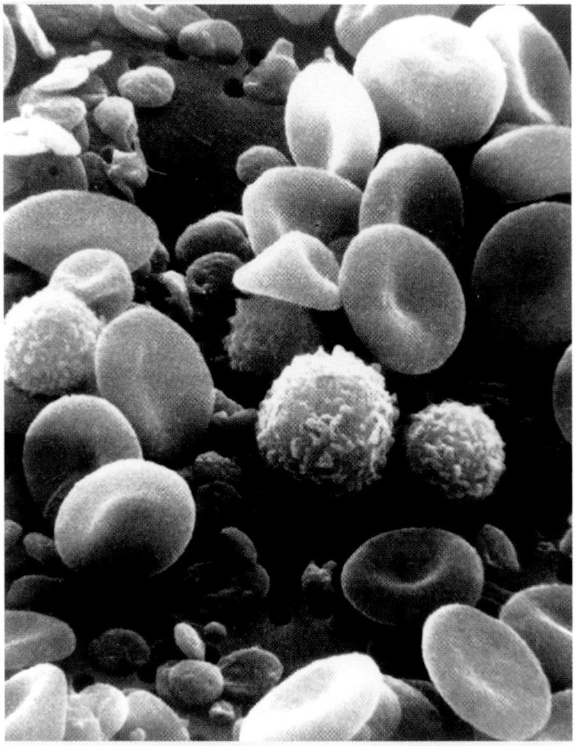

Actual scanning electron microscope image of red blood cells, a few white blood cells and several tiny platelets.

Platelets are tiny oval shaped cells that help the blood clot. Blood clotting is a natural process in which platelets and a sticky substance called fibrin rapidly form a clump to stop bleeding after a blood vessel has been cut or injured. Eventually the clot will form a protective scab over a wounded blood vessel, allowing it to heal. If the body did not have the ability to form blood clots, people would bleed to death after even a minor cut. In some individuals this clotting mechanism does not work properly making even the smallest of cuts dangerous. Vitamin K is known as the blood clotting vitamin and is abundant in dark green leafy vegetables.

Sometimes, blood clots form even when a person has not been injured. Although most blood clots tend to dissolve on their own with no long-term problems, there are situations in which blood clots can cause medical problems. Blood clots become dangerous when they block blood flow through an artery or vein which may result in a stroke or heart attack. Other blood clotting concerns range from mild spider/varicose veins to a life-threatening pulmonary embolism.

Just a small cut on the finger can bleed due to the tiny capillaries that provide a constant flow of blood. Without this constant blood flow the tissues would die, which is a condition known as gangrene.

Blood Tests

Blood tests, using blood drawn from a vein or artery usually in the wrist, finger or forearm, are analyzed at a laboratory and can reveal biological and physiological information about an individual. For instance, the results may help determine if the body is low in iron, which is usually termed anemic.

Physicians also can check kidney and liver function or look for deficiencies of major minerals such as magnesium, calcium, potassium and sodium. Blood sugar levels of diabetics are monitored with daily finger prick testing. Physicians specializing in diseases of the heart and cardiovascular system, known as cardiologists check the blood for cholesterol levels. While a cardiologist concentrates on the heart and venous structure, a hematologist specializes in the blood itself, checking for specific blood diseases.

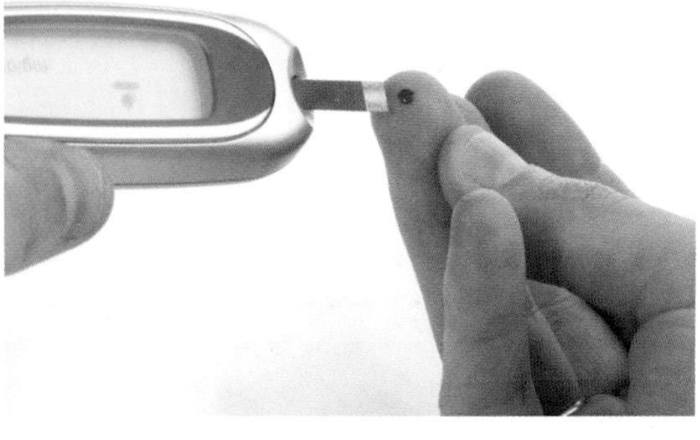

Blood Types

During 1900 and 1901, Karl Landsteiner was in the process of learning why blood transfusions sometimes caused death and at other times saved lives. It was during this time at the University of Vienna that he discovered the four blood groups or types. In 1930, he was awarded the Nobel Prize for this discovery.

There are four principal types: A, B, AB and O. Each type is also classified by an Rh factor – either positive (+) or negative (-). There are two antigens and two antibodies that are mostly responsible for the ABO types. The specific combination of these four components determines an individual's type in most cases and is inherited from his or her parents. See the blood types possibilities chart in the Activity Guide for this chapter.

When a blood transfusion is necessary, both the donor and the recipient patient's blood must be compatible. If not, the patient's body will react to the incompatible donor cells, leading to complications, maybe even death.

Other Important Organs to the Circulatory System

Lungs

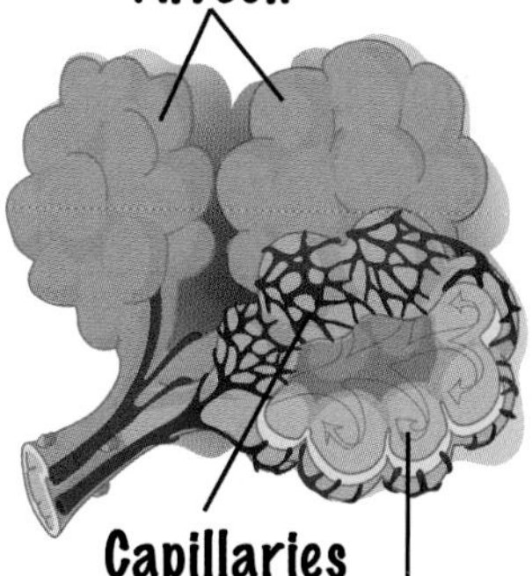

The lungs typically are associated with just the respiratory system. However, the lungs also are an important part of the circulatory system as they help transport oxygen into the bloodstream and remove carbon dioxide from the bloodstream. As discussed in Unit 3, the exchange of oxygen and carbon dioxide happens between the capillaries and alveoli deep within the lungs. Without the lungs, the blood would not have oxygen to carry to the cells and the body would die.

Kidneys and Urinary Tract

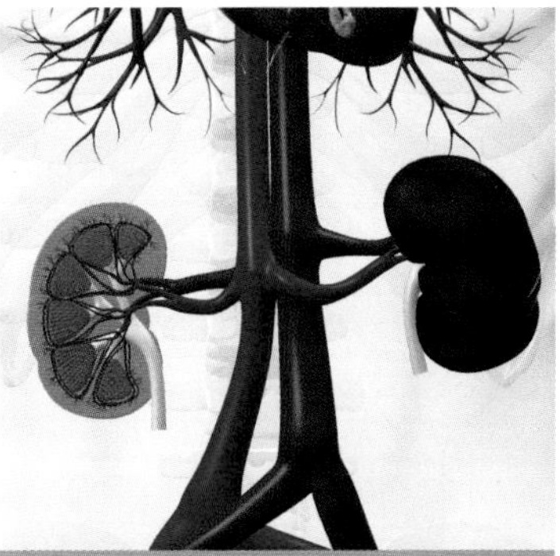

Fun Fact
Every minute, nearly one quart of blood goes through the kidneys.

The kidneys and urinary tract, which includes the kidneys, ureters, bladder and urethra, aid the circulatory system by extracting excess salts, toxins and water that end up in the blood in a fluid called urine. They also help maintain a balance of water in the body. The cells need a certain amount of water inside and out, and the kidneys help to make sure all the cells have the proper amounts.

Most everyone is born with two bean-shaped kidneys. Few people are born with just one kidney, which really isn't a problem since a person can actually live with just one. If one kidney has to be removed, the remaining kidney will take over the job of filtering all the blood.

The kidneys also help regulate blood pressure and the levels of vital salts in the blood. The hormone erythropoietin is created in the kidneys, which stimulates and controls red blood cell production. Additionally, the blood and body pH balance is regulated by the kidneys. The kidneys will be covered in greater detail in Unit 6.

Liver

The liver is a very complex organ. In fact, it also is a gland. As the liver helps the digestive system by producing bile, which helps break down fats, it also helps filter nutrients and by-products of digestion out of the blood. The hepatic portal vein brings blood from the spleen, pancreas, stomach, small intestines and large intestines into the liver, so the liver can filter out the nutrients. Other functions of the liver involving the circulatory system include the decomposition of red blood cells and plasma protein synthesis. The liver will be covered in greater detail in Unit 6.

Digestive System

The digestive system plays an important role with the circulatory system in that through digestion of food, nutrients are extracted and sent into the bloodstream to be filtered in the liver or kidneys and then sent back through the blood to all the cells in the body. Without the digestive system, the circulatory system would not have a supply of nutrients to carry to the rest of the body.

Unit 5 Chapter 1
Discussion Questions

1. What does Ecclesiastes 10:2 mean to you?
2. Have you ever observed your blood following a scrape? What did you notice?
3. Has anyone you know ever donated blood? If so, ask them why they chose to donate blood. How did it make them feel to give their blood?
4. Why do you think God gave us two kidneys if we can function with just one?

Activities - plus the Heart Healthy Oatmeal with Fruit "Power" Recipe and activities.

Elementary

1. Use a stethoscope to listen to your own or a family member's heart and listen to hear similarities or differences. Count the number of beats per minute. Is the beat loud or soft? Who has faster heart beats? Males or females? Older or younger? Or does it vary?
2. After completing the previous question, repeat the rhythm of your heart beat aloud. Make up a song about your heart that goes to the beat of your heart.
3. See if your family knows anyone with a pacemaker and ask that person specific questions, such as why he or she had to have one inserted, does that person feel it working and what benefits have been experienced from the pacemaker.
4. What is a sphygmomanometer? How is it used and by whom?
5. What is CPR? What jobs require a person to know CPR?
6. To visually display a heart beat, use some modeling clay and a toothpick. Take a small piece of the clay and roll it into a ball about the size of a dime. Stick the toothpick vertically into the ball and place the clay on the wrist, palm up. The side of the clay touching the skin may need to be flattened slightly to maintain contact. Move the clay around until you find the spot with the strongest beat. Describe and explain what you see.
7. Make a model of your heart with modeling clay by referring to the heart illustration. Start by using a clump of clay the size of your fist. Once you are finished, hold the clay up to your chest to get an idea of how large your heart is inside your chest.
8. Create valentines for your family and loved ones using the paper and embellishments of your choice. In each one include a Bible scripture about the heart and a fun fact you learned from this chapter or other study on the circulatory system.

Secondary

Choose any from above plus

1. Research the origin of the shape known as the heart and why it is so different from the actual shape of the human heart.
2. Find out what your blood type is. What are the blood types of your parents and siblings? What conclusions can you draw from your findings?
3. How do you measure blood pressure? What is a normal blood pressure reading? What is too high or too low? What are health risks associated with low or high blood pressure?
4. Blood drives are routinely held in communities across the country in order for hospitals to store blood for emergency transfusions. Plasma donation also is accepted by some of these agencies. What is the difference between donating blood and plasma?
5. What are the requirements for donating blood and or plasma?
6. The practice of retrieving umbilical cord blood is widely advertised to expectant moms. Research this topic and determine whether you are in favor of or oppose it. Prepare an oral or written report expressing your views.

Circulatory System Power Oats

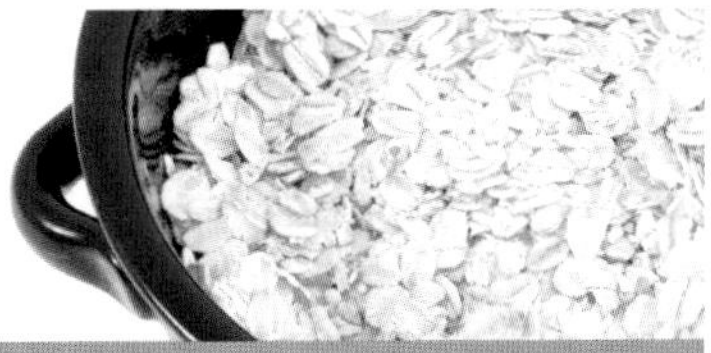

Oats are high in antioxidant and a unique fiber called beta glucans that help lower cholesterol and promote heart health.

Heart Healthy Oatmeal with Fruit

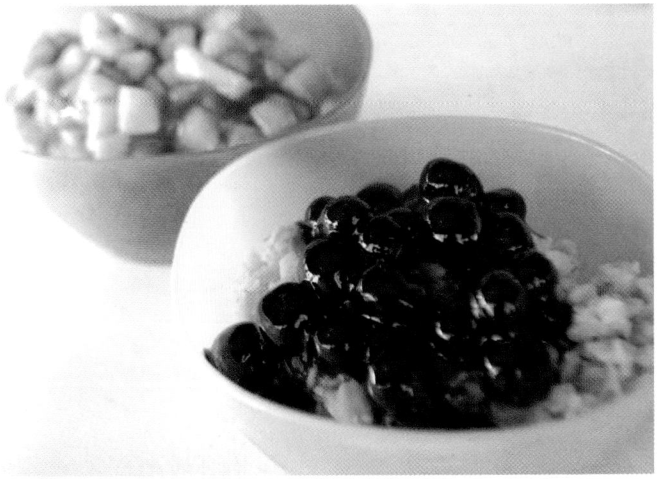

The fruit toppings in this recipe will make great healthy pie fillings and dessert toppings.

1 cup steel-cut or old fashioned rolled oats (not instant)
2 cups water, rice milk or almond milk

Blueberry Topping:
1 cup blueberries
1/3 cup Blue Agave Nectar
½ Tbs. arrowroot powder
½ Tbs. water
1 tsp. vanilla extract
1/8 tsp. almond extract

Cinnamon Apple Topping:
1 cup apples – cubed
1/3 cup Blue Agave Nectar
½ Tbs. arrowroot powder
½ Tbs. water
½ Tbs. vanilla extract
1 tsp. cinnamon or to taste

Cook oatmeal according to package directions, or bring water, rice milk or almond milk to a boil and then add oats. Add less water for thicker oatmeal or more for thinner oatmeal. For toppings, place fruit, blue agave, vanilla and/ or almond extract and/or cinnamon in medium saucepan and bring to simmer while stirring. In a separate small bowl, combine arrowroot powder and water and stir to a thick consistency. Slowly add arrowroot mixture while stirring so the arrowroot doesn't stick to the bottom. Stir until thoroughly combined and thickened. Top a bowl of cooked oatmeal with one of the fruit toppings. Double or triple the fruit topping recipe to make a healthy pie filling.

Activities

Elementary

1. What is arrowroot powder?
2. From what part of the plant is the arrowroot powder extracted?
3. What does the phrase "staple foods" mean?
4. Draw a line down the middle of a piece of paper. On one side list common staples, and on the other side list healthy alternatives.
5. Acquire real vanilla bean. Observe how it looks, feels, tastes and contrast it with liquid vanilla.

Secondary

Choose any from above plus

1. Arrowroot powder contains calcium ash. Why is this important and what does it do in the human body?
2. Find a favorite family recipe that contains cornstarch and use arrowroot powder instead. Replace any other ingredients that you deem unhealthy. Prior to whipping up the recipe, be sure to determine the appropriate conversions for each item your substitute. For example, two teaspoons of arrowroot powder are equal to one tablespoon of cornstarch and 1 ½ teaspoons of arrowroot powder are equal to one tablespoon of flour.
3. What is the difference between pure vanilla extract and imitation vanilla? Compare the two in your pantry or at the store.
4. Prepare an oral or written report on the history of vanilla and include information about the introduction of imitation vanilla.

Chapter 2

Heart Health and Nutrition

"Nevertheless he left not himself without witness, in that he did good, and gave us rain from heaven, and fruitful seasons, filling our hearts with food and gladness." Acts 14:17

According to the Center for Disease Control (CDC), heart disease is currently the leading cause of death and a major cause of disability among Americans. While cancer briefly took the top spot, it ranked second in the latest compilation of statistics, and stroke remained the third leading cause of death overall.

Over 80 million Americans suffer with some form of cardiovascular disease, including high blood pressure, angina and raised lipid levels. Statistics report that 40 percent of women with heart disease will eventually die of it and that every 33 seconds, heart disease or stroke kills someone. However, the CDC states that most of these conditions can be prevented.

Are you at risk for heart disease?

Most men are stricken with heart disease in their middle years, whereas women tend to get heart disease 10 to 20 years later, often after menopause. Some of the factors that may increase the risk for heart disease are: a family history of heart disease, exercising less than three times per week, eating non-heart healthy foods, taking nutritional supplements that do not contain heart healthy ingredients, unfavorable blood tests, shortness of breath, low thyroid function, gum disease, a root canal or tooth extraction, pneumonia, staph infection, herpes, chronic fatigue syndrome, Epstein Barr, mononucleosis or Lyme's Disease.

Heart Disease

Heart disease is actually an umbrella term used for several specific heart ailments. The following is a listing of the most common types of heart and artery diseases.

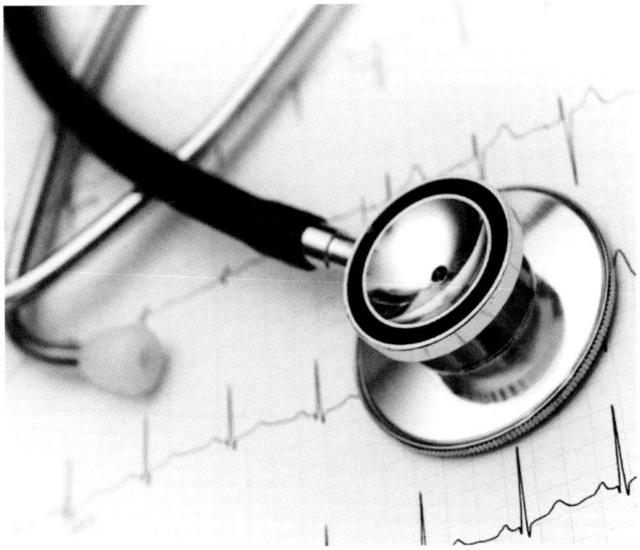

Angina is chest pain or discomfort experienced when the heart muscle does not receive enough blood due to coronary heart disease.

An **aneurysm** is an abnormal bulge in the wall of an artery, especially the aorta, which carries blood from the heart to the rest of body.

Arteriosclerosis is the hardening of medium or large arteries.

Coronary artery disease occurs when the arteries that supply blood to the heart muscle lose their flexibility and narrow as plaque, a buildup of cholesterol and other material, grows within artery walls. This is the most common type of heart disease according to the CDC.

Congestive heart failure is when the heart pumps very weak causing fluid retention in the lungs.

A **heart attack**, also referred to myocardial infarction, most often occurs when a clot in the coronary artery blocks the supply of blood and oxygen to the heart, causing an irregular heartbeat, or arrhythmia, and a severe decrease in the heart's pumping power.

Heart failure is a blanket term for any weakening of the heart's ability to pump enough blood, which is usually caused by coronary artery disease, high blood pressure and diabetes.

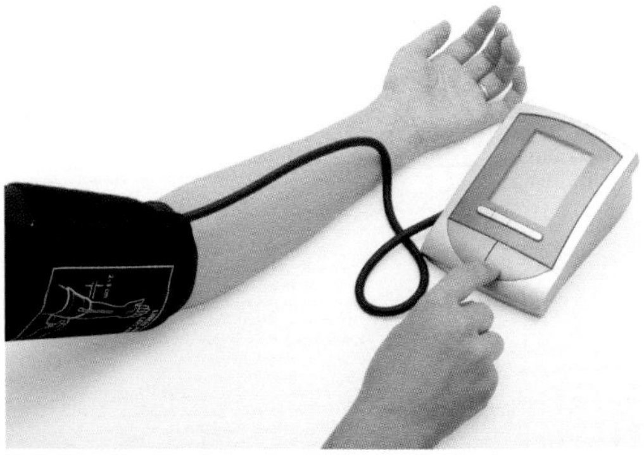

High blood pressure is when blood exerts excess force against vessels.

A **stroke** is when blood vessels supplying blood to the brain have been disturbed causing rapid, decreased brain function.

Cholesterol

The traditional method of early heart disease detection has been through laboratory blood work, with a prime focus on cholesterol levels. Cholesterol actually has a bad reputation as the culprit in all heart disease, when in fact, cholesterol is critical. It is vital in the digestion of fats, manufacturing of hormones, as an essential component in cell membranes, to the health of the immune system and in the absorption of fat soluble vitamins (A, D, E and K). Cholesterol is not only obtained from a person's diet, but according to renowned cardiologist Lee Cowden M.D., the human liver synthesizes about 3,000 mg of cholesterol in a 24-hour period, a quantity equivalent to 24 eggs. In fact, in most people less than five percent of the cholesterol in the bloodstream gets there through diet. Dr. Cowden adds, "when cholesterol levels are too low, depression, lung disease and even cancer can be the result.[1]"

There are two different types of vehicles for cholesterol transportation in the blood, LDL and HDL. **LDL** stands for **low density lipoprotein** – a fat with a protein coating – and **HDL** stands for **high density lipoprotein**. Both transport cholesterol to and from the liver. When a cell is damaged, LDL transfers the cholesterol from the liver to the cell for repair. HDL brings excess cholesterol in the blood back to the liver for storage. The real culprit is oxidized or damaged cholesterol which can stick to blood vessel walls and cause plaque formation. Oxidation of cholesterol is caused by processed foods, poor quality foods, environmental toxins, stress and negative emotions. This oxidation can cause problems for those with low or high cholesterol levels.

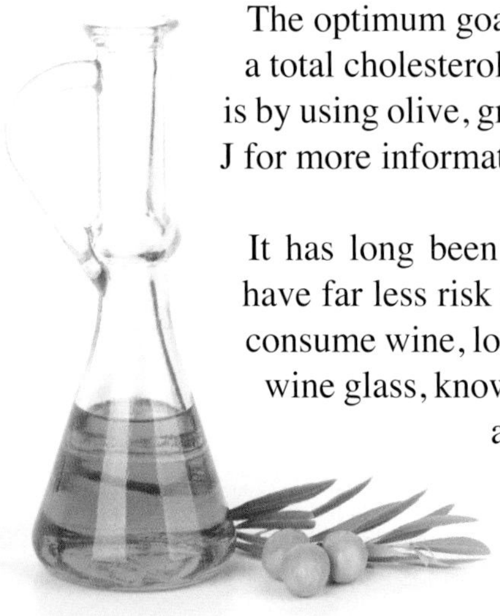

The optimum goal for most adults according to many cardiologists and laboratories, is to have a total cholesterol of less than 200. One of the easiest ways to decrease LDL and increase HDL is by using olive, grapeseed, flaxseed, sesame and coconut oils in food preparation. See Appendix J for more information on healthy fats.

It has long been known that the French and Mediterranean cultures eat high fat foods but have far less risk for heart disease. This is due in part to their use of olive oil. The French also consume wine, long believed to promote heart health by raising HDL levels. But before filling a wine glass, know that researchers at the University of Wisconsin compared wine to red, purple and white grape juice and found that purple grape juice was just as effective but without the potentially damaging effects of the alcohol. Some vineyards also offer non-alcoholic wine-grape juices that are harvested with the same quality of grapes, but fermenting is not allowed to occur.

1 "Heart Disease, Stroke and High Blood Pressure" Burton, Goldberg, Future Medicine Publishing, 1998.

Triglycerides

But wait, there's more. It's not just the cholesterol levels that indicate a possible risk factor, **triglycerides** are another form of blood-borne fat that contributes to heart disease. They also come from both diet and liver synthesis. Most fat in food and in the body exist in the form of triglycerides. Any excess calories eaten that are not immediately used by the body are converted to triglycerides and stored in fat cells.

The following chart is used by many health professionals in assessing risk factor by the numbers.

	Ideal	Normal	Borderline	High	Very High
Total cholesterol	<170	170-200	201-239	240-280	>280
LDL cholesterol mg/dL	<100	100-129	130-159	160-189	>190
HDL cholesterol mg/dL	>65	45-64	35-44	20-34	<20
Triglycerides mg/dL	<100	100-150	151-200	201-500	>500
Homocysteine mmmol/L	<8	8-12	13-30	31-100	>100
CRP mg/L	<1	1-3	3-5	5-7	>7

Homocysteine

One of the major indicators for heart and cardiovascular disease is **homocysteine**. Researchers believe that elevated homocysteine levels pose as much a threat as cholesterol, plus it has been linked to such diseases as diabetes, some types of cancer and Alzheimer's.

Homocysteine is an amino acid, a normal by-product of protein metabolism that in elevated amounts causes damage to the inner lining of the blood vessels and oxidizes cholesterol. This damage is then covered by cholesterol to facilitate healing, which in turn promotes atherosclerosis (hardening of the arteries) and increases blood clotting tendencies. As much as 10 to 20 percent of heart disease is linked to elevated homocysteine, regardless of cholesterol level. A German study in 1991 studied the arteries of 163 males and concluded that the arterial narrowing was due more to blood levels of homocysteine than of cholesterol.[2] Checking for homocysteine levels in the blood is not routine, but it may be requested by a patient, especially when he or she has a history of heart disease, has any of the risk factors previously listed or is over 40 years of age.

To reduce homocysteine levels, the body must convert homocysteine to cystathionine. This conversion requires sufficient levels of **vitamin B6**, **folate** and **B12**. If the conversion is not able to happen, oxysterols are produced. Antioxidant foods rich in **vitamins C** and **E** are among the nutrients the body can use to neutralize oxysterols.

2 "Heart Disease, Stroke and High Blood Pressure" Burton, Goldberg, Future Medicine Publishing, 1998.

Inflammation

Recent research demonstrates that inflammation of the blood vessels is an underlying cause of heart attacks, strokes, certain cancers, Alzheimer's, Parkinson's, diabetes and leukemia. Some inflammation can be traced to bacteria and viruses that take up residence in the walls of blood vessels, especially those nearest the heart itself. Other inflammation is considered "silent inflammation" caused by stressors to the body such as environmental toxins, processed food toxins and emotional discord.

Inflammation can be measured through blood tests by determining the level of C-Reactive Protein (CRP). The Nov. 14, 2002, issue of the New England Journal of Medicine confirmed that an elevated CRP in women is a strong predictor of future cardiovascular events regardless of cholesterol level. Since this also is a non-routine test, the doctor must request this to be added to blood work.

Gum Disease

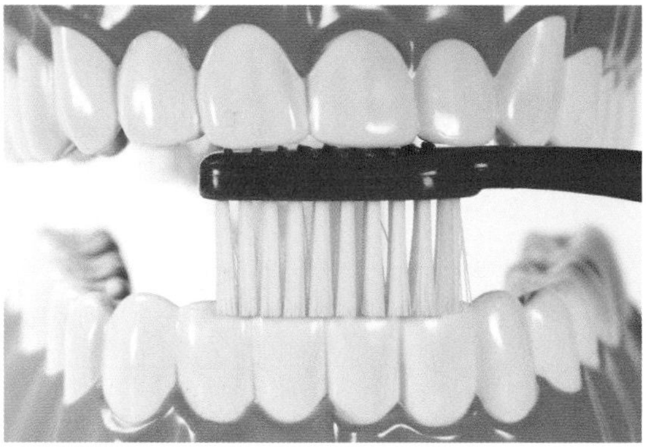

Research suggests that gum disease presents a far more serious threat to the health of millions of American's than previously thought. The September 2003 issue of "Stroke: Journal of the American Heart Association" published a study linking atherosclerosis, the build up of artery-clogging plaque that can lead to heart attack and stroke, to tooth loss as related to gum disease.

Researchers at the University of Minnesota recently reported their findings linking "bacteria in the mouth to the formation of potentially fatal blood clots. Chronic inflammation of the gums due to plaque can lead to inflammation of the arteries."

Additionally, studies presented showed that the bacteria in plaque also are linked to a potentially fatal disease called infective endocarditis, where the sac around the heart becomes inflamed. This is why dentists ask their patients if they have a history of heart disease. Certain heart conditions like valve problems and murmurs are at high risk for heart attack during many dental procedures. Doctors and dentists alike have known for years that at-risk individuals must take an antibiotic prior to having their teeth cleaned, drilled or other procedures. Other related diseases worsened due to dental plaque and bacteria include chronic pulmonary disease, diabetes, bronchitis, pneumonia, emphysema, weakened immune system, poor wound healing, low birth weight in infants and possibly influenza and hepatitis B.

Toothbrushes

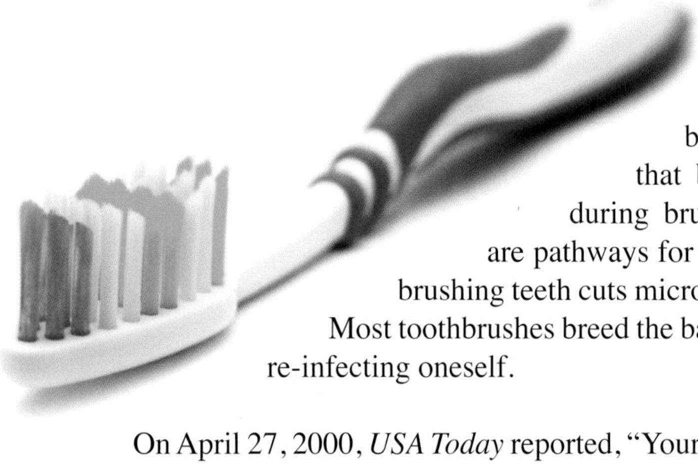

Dental bacteria reside along the gum line and in pockets caused from tooth extraction, bone loss, cavities and root canals. Researchers are unsure what causes the bacteria to become mobile, but it has been suggested that bacteria can be dislodged and enter the bloodstream during brushing, flossing or chewing. Infected, bleeding gums are pathways for dislodged bacteria to enter the bloodstream. The act of brushing teeth cuts microscopic slits in the gums with plastic toothbrush bristles. Most toothbrushes breed the bacteria from previous brushings, resulting in perpetually re-infecting oneself.

On April 27, 2000, *USA Today* reported, "Your toothbrush may be a biohazard. The most serious threat to your everyday health may be hanging in plain sight in your bathroom." In 1996, a research study in the United

Kingdom analyzed 28 toothbrushes. The results of the study found up to 100,000,000 colony-forming germ units on the tested toothbrushes. While many of these germs can be easily fought by the immune system, there are some bacteria that could very well cause health issues once entered into the body, especially those with compromised immune systems. Because of the short distance between the heart and mouth as many blood vessels from the mouth funnel directly into larger veins that go to the heart, the heart may become vulnerable to some bacteria.

Protect the Heart with Good Dental Habits:

1. **Daily oral hygiene** - Brush the teeth at least twice per day and floss regularly. Visit the dentist regularly for cleaning and check for gum disease. Be sure to use a toothpaste or herbal tooth powder that does not contain chemicals, such as propylene glycol and sodium lauryl sulfate,[3] that are hazardous to the health

2. **Sanitize toothbrushes** - Use three percent hydrogen peroxide to rinse your toothbrush after each brushing, or place the brushes in boiling water for three to five minutes after every brushing.

Those who do **not** have a history of gum disease, and have incredibly healthy, brush and floss regularly, visit the dentist and stay away from sugar-laden foods, still must take another step. Anyone who has frequently bleeding gums when brushing or flossing, has ever had a tooth pulled, a root canal or is contemplating mercury removal, then step three is mandatory because these are germs, not degenerative conditions.

3. **Daily Supplementation** - The American Medical Journal reports that most doctors now recommend taking a multi-vitamin and mineral supplement.

Smoking and Heart Health

According to the American Heart Association, cigarette smoking is the most important preventable cause of premature death in the United States and accounts for nearly 440,000 of the more than 2.4 million annual deaths.[4] Cigarette smokers have a higher risk of developing several chronic disorders, which include fatty buildups in arteries (artherosclerosis), several types of cancer and chronic lung problems. Studies show that cigarette smoking decreases HDL – good cholesterol – and is a major cause of coronary heart disease, which leads to heart attack.

Salt

Salt has taken its share of criticism concerning heart disease, especially elevated blood pressure. The recommend daily allowance of salt or sodium is 2,300 mg. This amount equals one teaspoon. When salt is refined, the other naturally balancing minerals are removed. If the diet is lacking these minerals from other food sources and contains excessive sodium, it could be hard on the kidneys. The kidneys play a very important role in removing excessive salt in the body. So make sure the kidneys are functioning properly and salt intake is moderate.

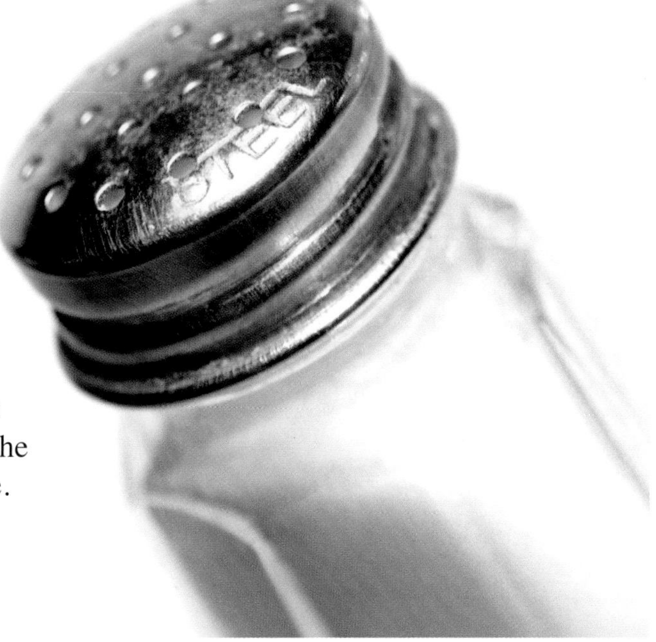

3 See Appendix DD for authors' recommendations.
4 http://www.americanheart.org/presenter.jhtml?identifier=4545

What can be done about heart disease?

Researchers at the Maine Medical Center found that 50 percent of all bypass operations in the U.S. are not necessary, and 80 percent of all heart diagnostic procedures were inappropriate. The U.S. government states that 90 percent of all bypass operations give no benefit to the patient and does not improve survival rates.[5] So what can be done for someone at risk or has heart disease?

Dangers of Pharmaceutical Drugs

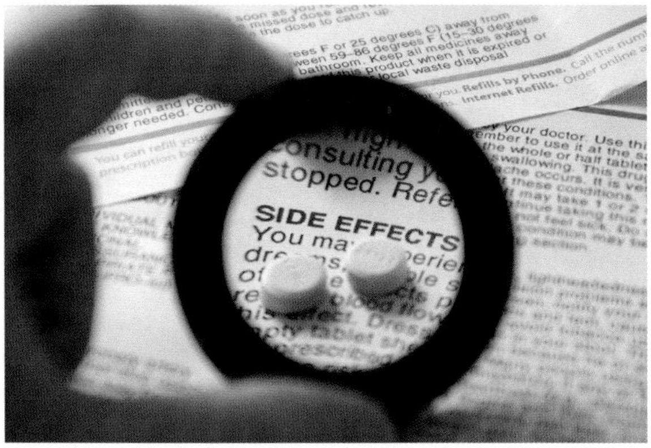

The use of pharmaceutical drugs may control symptoms, but with such use comes the added risk of sometimes debilitating or fatal side effects, assuming the drug taken is effective. Recently, the former senior vice president for genetics research and pharmacogenetics of drug manufacturer Glaxo-Smith-Klein reported that half of all drugs were ineffective.[6]

Death from pharmaceutical drugs affects over 250,000 people yearly. Researchers in Sweden found men with only slightly elevated blood pressure taking an anti-hypertensive drug had a four times greater risk of heart attacks as those not taking the drugs.[7] A study of 900 elderly people with hypertension showed that while taking popular calcium channel blockers the likelihood of dying from heart attack, heart failure and stroke doubled.[7]

These reports and studies show that pharmaceutical drugs only treat or mask the symptoms of the disease – the root cause still exists.

Chelation

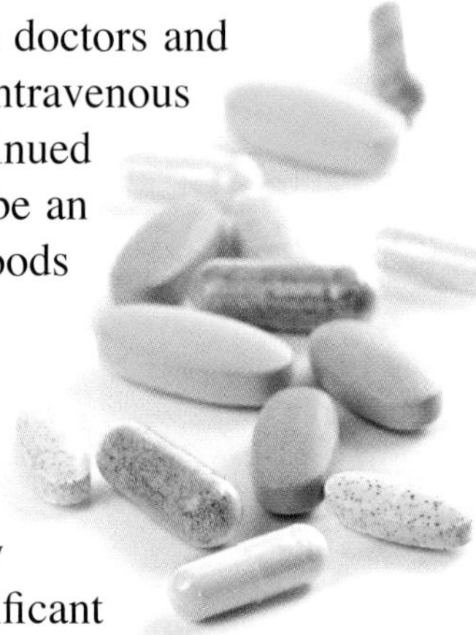

Various forms of chelation or plague-removing therapies are employed by alternative doctors and is gaining in popularity. While deemed effective in mild cases of arterial blockage, intravenous chelation is costly and takes many hours per week. Oral chelation must be continued indefinitely to achieve and maintain the desired results and is considered by most to be an insurance policy and not treatment. Natural chelators include garlic, vitamin C rich foods and vinegar.

Heart Healthy Diets

Without question, most Americans do not eat a heart-healthy diet, and even those few that do are not getting the vitamins and minerals necessary for the body to use in significant amounts to prevent heart disease. Even the Journal of the American Medical Association reports that taking a multivitamin supplement could significantly reduce your risk of cancer and heart disease.[8] Could this suggestion address the underlying causes of heart disease, as well as normal risk factors – eliminating viruses and bacteria, lowering cholesterol, homocysteine and CRP levels? Taking a dozen different supplements could help bring the numbers in line and a handful of natural supplements could even slowly but surely scrub those arteries clean as a whistle. However, if the underlying pathogens are not dealt with, then sooner or later the problem will reoccur.

---

5 "What Doctors Won't Tell You" Lynne McTaggart, Avon Books, 1998.

6 "Glaxo Chief: Our Drugs Do Not Work on Most Patients" Steve Connor http://www.ghchealth.com/glaxo-chief-our-drugs-do-not-work-on-most-patients.html

7 "Heart Disease, Stroke and High Blood Pressure" Burton, Goldberg, Future Medicine Publishing, 1998.

8 "JAMA Recommends a Multivitamin" The Journal of American Medical Association, 2002: 287;3127-3129.

As stated numerous times in **Nutrition 101: Choose Life!**, it is very important to eat a diet rich in whole grains, quality proteins, fresh vegetables, nuts, seeds and fresh fruit. It's also important to limit or eliminate the intake of over-processed, sugar-laden foods, which encourage plaque buildup and the growth of bacteria, elevate triglycerides and weaken the immune system response.

Saturated Fat

Saturated fat has long been regarded as a major factor of heart disease. However, several studies have indicated that other culprits are to blame. William P. Castelli, M.D., director of the renown, ongoing Framingham Study stated in 1992, "the more saturated fat one ate, the more cholesterol one ate, the more calories one ate, the lower people's serum cholesterol." It has become evident that something other than cholesterol and saturated fat are causing coronary disease.

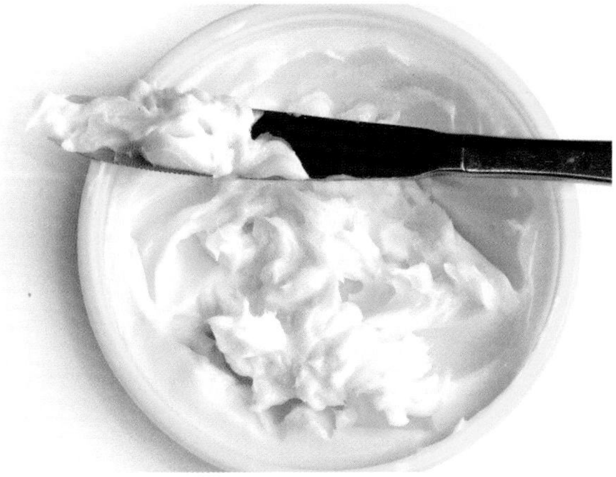

While margarine has often been touted as a heart-healthy alternative to butter, a Framingham Study of 832 men free of coronary heart disease (CHD) were fed a diet of margarine, and over an extended 21 year follow-up, the study concluded that margarine intake increases the risk of CHD.[9]

A study in "Preventative Medicine" stated that "very low total cholesterol, less than 160ml/dl, has been shown to increase the risk of mortality from lung cancer by 1.75 times for men and 3.29 times for women."[10]

For more information about dangerous fats and healthy fats, see Appendix J.

Nutrients - see the Vitamin and Mineral Charts for foods high in these nutrients

Iron is a trace mineral critical to life because of its role in helping transport oxygen from the lungs to body tissues and returning carbon dioxide from tissue to lungs. Iron makes up the central core of hemoglobin, a protein that gives blood its red color. Iron also enhances cardiac performance.

Vitamin K is one of the few vitamins found both in foods and made in the human body's intestinal tract in the presence of certain beneficial bacteria. It has been called the band-aid due to its major role in blood clotting.

Vitamin B12 works with folate or folic acid (vitamin B9) in the synthesis of DNA, aids in the formation of healthy red blood cells and assists the function of iron absorption and utilization. Vegetarians are at risk for depleted B12 as this vitamin is found in animal protein, eggs and dairy. Contrary to claims, the form of B12 found in a select few plant foods is biologically inactive in humans.[11] Therefore it is important for vegetarians to supplement B12.

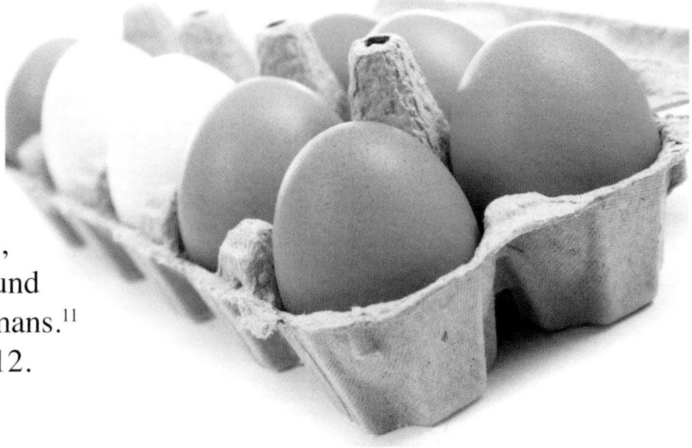

9 "Margarine Intake and Subsequent Coronary Heart Disease in Men".Matthew W. Gillman, L. Adrienne Cupples, David Gagnon, Barbara E. Millen, R. Curtis Ellison and William P. Castelli, Lippincott Williams & Wilkins, 1997.

10 Preventative Medicine, 1995; 24:557-62

11 "Nutrition Almanac" sixth edition, McGraw Hill, John D. Kirschmann and Nutrition Search, Inc. 2007.

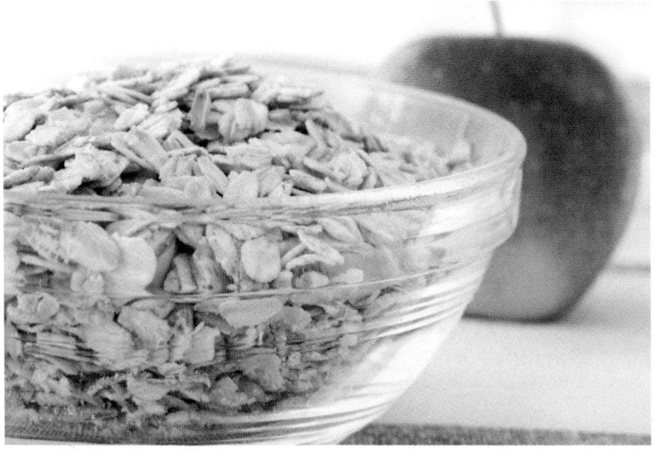

Folic acid, also known as folate, is essential to the formation of blood cells and works in conjunction with B12 and vitamin B6 to reduce homocystein levels.

Vitamin C helps to strengthen arteries, raises the good cholesterol (HDL), lowers the bad cholesterol (LDL), may reduce blood pressure and assists in preventing blood clots by inhibiting platelet aggregation.

Beta glucans are beneficial to the body's immune system and also have the ability to lower unhealthy cholesterol levels. Found abundantly in oats, this may be one of the mechanisms along with fiber to lower cholesterol levels.

Vitamin E is thought to prevent disease of the circulatory system. Many studies give high praises to vitamin E supplementation in regards to cardiovascular health. Vitamin E can act as a blood thinner and more is not always better. When supplementing, vitamin E can come in eight different forms. The one to select is *d*-alpha-tocopherol. Supplements designated with *l*-alpha-tocopherols are synthetic forms and should be avoided.

Fiber comes in two forms, soluble and insoluble. Both are dietary fibers and are the parts of plants (vegetables, grains, legumes, and fruits) that we do not digest. When regularly eaten as part of a diet low in saturated fat, trans fat and cholesterol, soluble fiber has been shown to help lower blood cholesterol. Foods high in soluble fiber include oat bran, oatmeal, beans, peas, rice bran, barley, citrus fruits, strawberries and apples. Insoluble fiber doesn't seem to help lower blood cholesterol, but is an aid in normal bowel function. Foods high in insoluble fiber include whole wheat breads, wheat cereals, wheat bran, cabbage, beets, carrots, Brussels sprouts, turnips, cauliflower and apple skin. See more about fiber in Appendix K.

Natural Heart Tonic Herbs

Hawthorne is one of the most significant heart herbs. Hawthorne (Crataegus) contains a combination of flavonoids that can protect the heart against oxygen deprivation and the development of abnormal rhythms. The berries and leaves have been used for centuries as cardio tonics for angina, hypertension, arrhythmia and congestive heart failure. No herb has a greater history of nourishing the heart. Hawthorne strengthens the heart, is free of side effects and has several major medical studies to back up its effectiveness. After one report, hawthorne gained recognition by the German Federal Ministry of Hearth as a cardio tonic.[12]

Hawthorne works by dilating the coronary arteries and improving circulation, which may reduce angina symptoms. While results do not occur rapidly, hawthorne use results in gentle, sustained positive effects on degenerative age-related heart issues.

Cayenne has been called the cure all of herbs. The late Dr. John Christopher, famous master herbalist and founder of The School of Natural Healing, said with confidence about someone having a heart attack, "If they are still breathing, I [give] them a cup of cayenne tea – a teaspoon of cayenne in a cup of hot water – and within minutes they are up and around."[13]

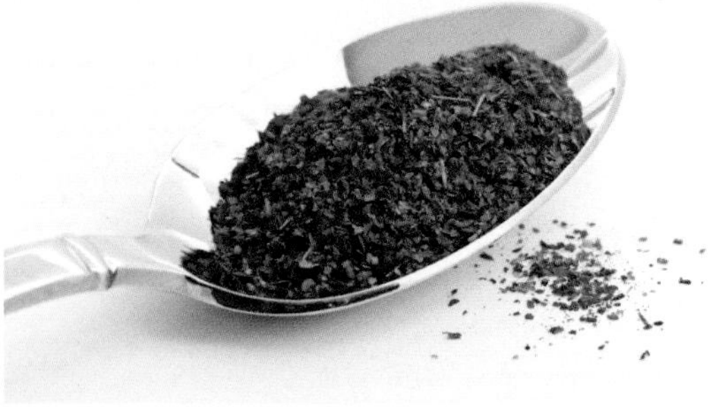

12 Ammon and Handel, Planta Medica, 1981; 43:209

13 If you feel you are experiencing a heart attack, please seek immediate medical attention.

Cayenne is a pepper with high amounts of the substance capsicum. It is one of the fastest-acting aids for the heart because it feeds the heart immediately.

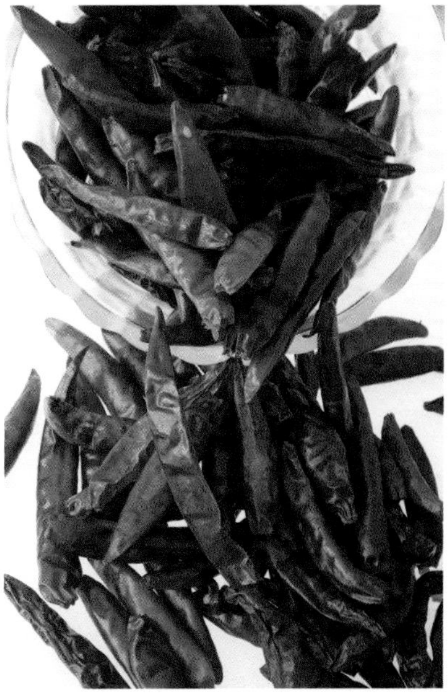

Cayenne helps maintain health in the bloodstream. When the blood becomes blocked -- which leads to oxygen starvation, organ dysfunction, disease and, in severe cases, heart attack – cayenne pepper works like a drain opener that blasts through the blockages, delivering oxygenated blood into sick or dying organs faster than any other medicine or herb.

There are numerous books touting the virtues of cayenne and over 3,000 scientific studies listed in the National Library of Medicine which support the use of cayenne in preventing and reversing many common health ailments. It is said by many herbalists that cayenne has more health benefits than any other single food or herb on earth.

Cayenne taken internally as a tea may quickly stop bleeding — even from a severe cut or wound. Cayenne has a natural, powerful, equalizing effect on blood-pressure. When it hits the bloodstream, which it does immediately, it adjusts the blood pressure from the top of the head to the bottom of the feet. Thus, the high pressure at the wound site is alleviated, and clotting can start at once. Powdered cayenne may be applied with light pressure to open wounds. Bleeding should slow to a stop, giving adequate time to asses the wound and decide if professional medical help is necessary.

Fun Facts

The hotness of a pepper is measured in Scoville Heat Units. The higher the number the hotter the pepper, and for heart health – the hotter the better! Cayenne peppers range from 0 to 300,000 heat units. The **spice-cabinet** variety averages 5,000 heat units. **Paprika** has no heat and is rated 0 heat units. **Jalapeño** peppers are between 50,000 and 80,000 heat units; **Serrano** peppers are approximately 100,000 heat units. **African Bird Peppers** average 200,000 heat units and **Mexican habañeros** are between 250,000 and 300,000 heat units.

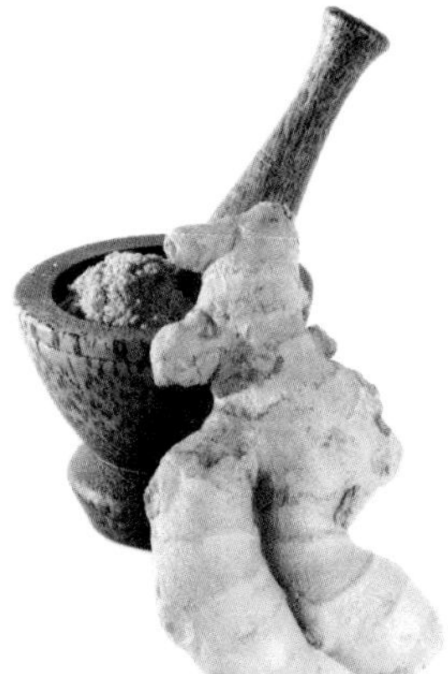

Ginger is another important herb for a healthy heart. It has been observed that by eating a little bit of ginger every day, it will help to prevent heart attack, reduce cholesterol, normalize blood pressure and even prevent blood clots.

Ginger's heart-helping attributes are similar to that of garlic. Ginger interferes with the long sequence of events necessary for blood clots to form. This helps to prevent clots that can lodge in narrowed coronary arteries and set off a heart attack.

Garlic, known scientifically as Allium sativum, contains more than 100 biologically useful chemicals. Garlic has been used medicinally for at least 3,000 years, but until recently its benefits were considered little more than folklore. According to a report in the Journal of the American Medical Association, the therapeutic roles of garlic have been described in more than 1,000 scientific studies.[14]

Garlic may prevent the oxidation of LDL cholesterol and the liver from producing excess fat and cholesterol. The American Dietetic Association suggests that in order to obtain the potential health benefits of garlic, one must take 600 - 900mg (about 1 fresh clove) per day.

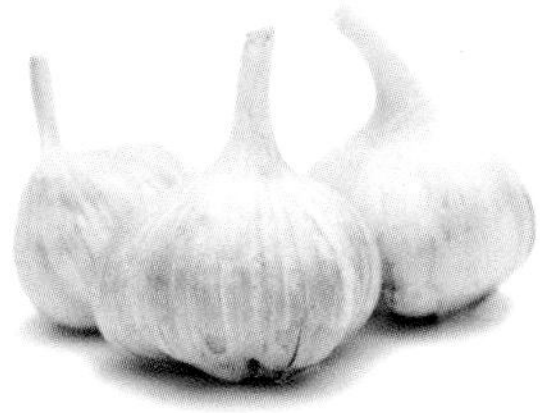

14 Journal of the American Medical Association Nov. 28, 1990;264:2614

Adesh K. Jain, M.D., of the Clinical Research Center at Tulane University School of Medicine, New Orleans, reported that garlic can lower blood levels of "total" cholesterol and the dangerous LDL from an average of six percent among those taking the garlic tablets (900 mg), compared with only a one percent drop among those taking a placebo.[15] The garlic takers also benefited from an 11 percent decrease in LDL, compared with a three percent reduction in the placebo group.

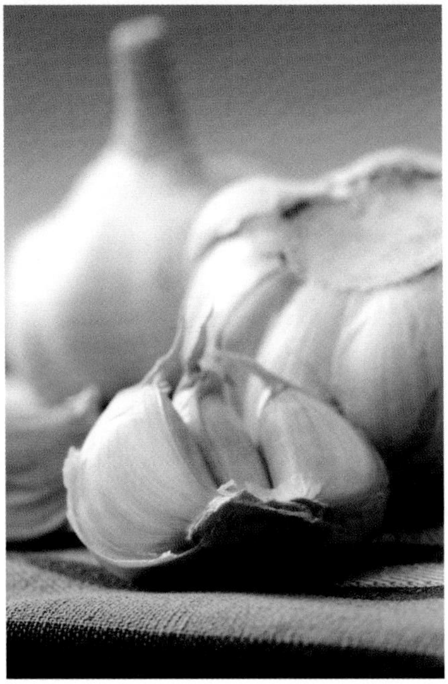

Garlic also is an anticoagulant or a natural blood thinner. H. Kieswetter, M.D., of the University of Saarlandes in Hamburg, Germany, recently found that garlic could help patients suffering from peripheral arterial occlusive disease, characterized by blood clots in the legs.[16] Typically, patients with the condition are asked to walk regularly because increased blood flow reduces the number of clots. However, patients are discouraged easily because peripheral arterial occlusive disease causes extreme pain after walking only a short distance. In his study, after a period of time, Kieswetter's patients taking the garlic powder tablets were able to walk further without any pain than those who did not take the garlic. They also had a decrease in blood pressure after taking just one garlic powder capsule.

The **NingXia wolfberry** is one of the greatest heart healthy fruits on earth. Not to be confused with other species of wolfberry, the NingXia wolfberry is one of the highest known sources of potassium and magnesium.

This is quite important as Dr. Stephen Coca of Yale University stated in a study that "Increases in dietary potassium benefit several disease states. These include the treatment of hypertension (high blood pressure), stroke prevention, arrhythmia prevention, and treatment of congestive heart failure." The study goes on to state that low magnesium concentration may contribute to the pathogenesis of coronary atherosclerosis or acute thrombosis.[17]

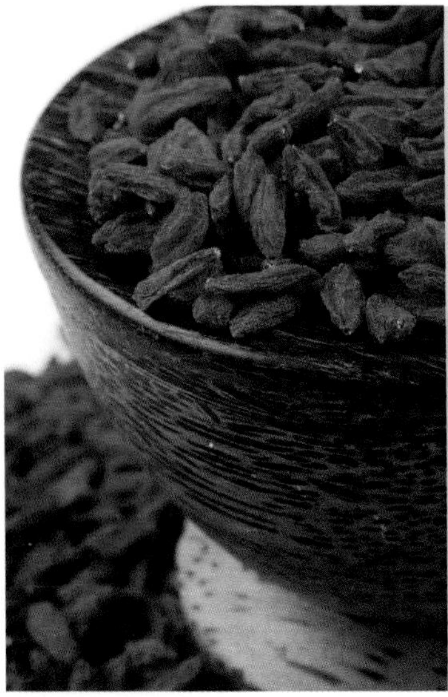

Bad Foods for Cardiovascular System

sugar
fried foods
hydrogenated oils
partially hydrogenated oils

Good Foods for Cardiovascular Health

almonds, apple, asparagus, beets, black beans, blueberries, broccoli, Brussels sprouts, cabbage, carrots, cauliflower, coconut oil, fish oils, flax seed, kidney beans, NingXia wolfberry, oats, oranges, red bell peppers, spinach, sweet potatoes, tomatoes, turnips, walnuts, whole-grains

15 "The Wonders of Garlic: This 'Miracle Food' Protects You Against Heart Disease, Cancer and Infections" Jack Challem, The Nutrition Reporter, 1995. http://www.thenutritionreporter.com/garlic.html

16 Clinical Investigator May 1993;71:383-6

17 "The cardiovascular implications of hypokalemia" Coca SG, Perazella MA, Buller GK. Am J Kidney Dis. 2005.

Unit 5 Chapter 2
Discussion Questions

1. Why do you believe so many people have diseases that the Center for Disease Control describes as preventable?
2. What are the heart healthy foods you have eaten this week?
3. What are some foods that are bad for the cardiovascular system that you have eaten this week?
4. Do you know anyone with any of the diseases listed in this chapter?

Activities - plus the Rice Stuffed Tomatoes "Power" Recipe and activities.

Elementary

1. Carefully measure the amount of salt you add to foods during a day and see how much this is. Then be sure to add up the amounts in pre-prepared foods that already contain salt and see where you stand. Next time at the grocery store or in the family pantry, look for the amount of sodium found in foods. Discuss ways you can reduce salt intake, without reducing flavor.
2. Tobacco use is very dangerous. Draw a picture that shows why you think it is good to be tobacco-free.
3. To understand how bacteria travels through the bloodstream, use the following experiment. The materials needed include a stalk of celery with leaves, a clear glass of water and food coloring. Drop one or two drops of food coloring in the glass. Stand the celery in the glass of water. Observe what happens. Try the experiment again with a new stalk of celery and detect any changes.
4. Using the recipe for the toothbrush cleaner in the chapter, create this mixture for your family and remind them to use it after each brushing.
5. If you do not already have healthy habits for taking care of your teeth, begin following these steps outlined in the chapter. At your next dentist appointment see what improvements he or she notices.
6. Look through the newspaper or magazines for pictures of foods that are good for your cardiovascular system and foods that are bad for it. Paste your selections on a piece of construction paper under the category "good" or "bad." Put the finished product in the kitchen for your family to learn about these foods.
7. Pick out two of the heart healthy foods listed and make up your own afternoon snack recipe for the family.

Secondary

1. Research the history of the famous Framingham Heart Study. When and why did it get its start? Why is this ongoing study so important? Present your findings in a written or oral report.
2. Create a crossword puzzle with the following terms from this chapter: cholesterol, low density lipoprotein, HDL, inflammation, Dr. Cowden, angina, vitamin B12, oral hygiene, drugs and cayenne. Arrange them in a down or across format and write clues for each term. Have your family complete it together and see how long it takes them.
3. Select one of the diseases listed in the chapter above and learn how it is diagnosed and the allopathic methods of treatment. Prepare your findings in a written or oral report.
4. Research the names of the top five pharmaceutical companies. Visit their Web sites or search the Internet for any drug recalls they have had in the past five years. How many and why?
5. Learn more about the damaging effects of smoking and tobacco from the Center for Disease Control (http://www.cdc.gov/tobacco/).
6. Pick out one of the heart healthy foods that you have never tasted and create or find a recipe to make as part of a family meal.

Additional Resources

Web sites:

1. www.eurekalert.org
2. www.germterminator.com
3. http://childrensheartinstitute.org/educate/heartwrk/hearthse.htm
4. www.framinghamheartstudy.org

Books: "Healthy Heart", David Hoffman, B.Sc., F.N.I.M.H., Storey Books, 2000.

Circulatory System Power

Tomatoes

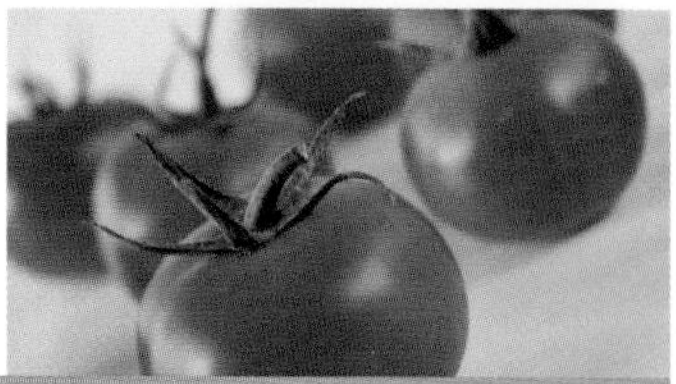

Tomatoes are high in lycopene which supports heart health and helps prevent cancer.
For the most lycopene content, choose organic tomatoes.

Rice Stuffed Tomatoes

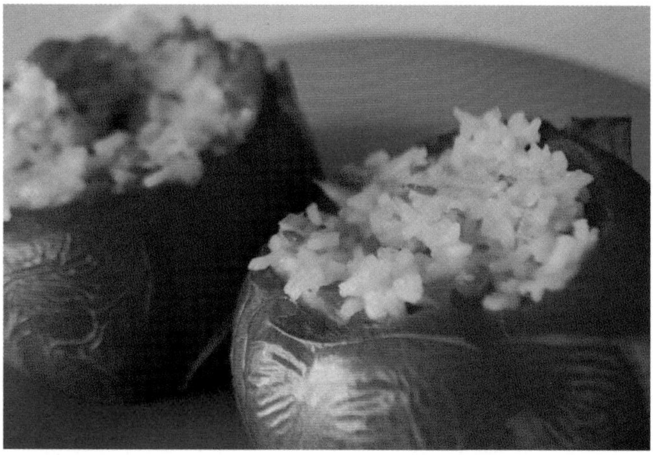

2 large tomatoes
Extra virgin olive oil or coconut oil
½ cup vegetable broth

Filling and sauce:
Diced tomato flesh
½ cup diced onions
½ cup diced carrots
½ cup diced celery
½ cup yellow bell pepper
1 cup cooked rice
2 cloves minced garlic

Cut the tops off of the tomatoes and scoop out the flesh to leave them empty for the filling and sauce. Saute the filling ingredients in olive or coconut oil. Then, add the vegetable broth. Spoon into empty tomatoes. Place in 375 degree oven for 15 minutes. Serve along baked chicken or fish or add diced, cooked chicken to the rice for a main dish.

Activities

Elementary

1. After removing the tops of the tomatoes, but before scooping out the flesh, compare the tomato to the heart.
2. Make some of the filling in olive oil and some in coconut oil. Which do you prefer? Why? How do they differ?
3. Do a taste test with your family after you make this recipe. Blindfold members and ask them to identify the ingredients. See who can guess the most.
4. Celery is one of the top 12 foods experts suggest to buy organic. Why do you think this is true? Research the answer to determine if you are correct.

Secondary

Choose any from above plus

1. How many varieties of tomatoes are there?
2. What are the top 12 foods to buy organic?
3. What do these have in common? What conclusions can you draw from this?
4. Experiment with this recipe by switching the roles of the yellow bell pepper and the tomato. (Be sure to discard the seeds from the pepper.) How is this different? If you do not like it, find a way to improve it.

Chapter 3

The Immune System

"And the Lord will take away from thee all sickness, and will put none of the evil diseases of Egypt, which thou knowest, upon thee; but will lay them upon all them that hate thee." Deuteronomy 7:15

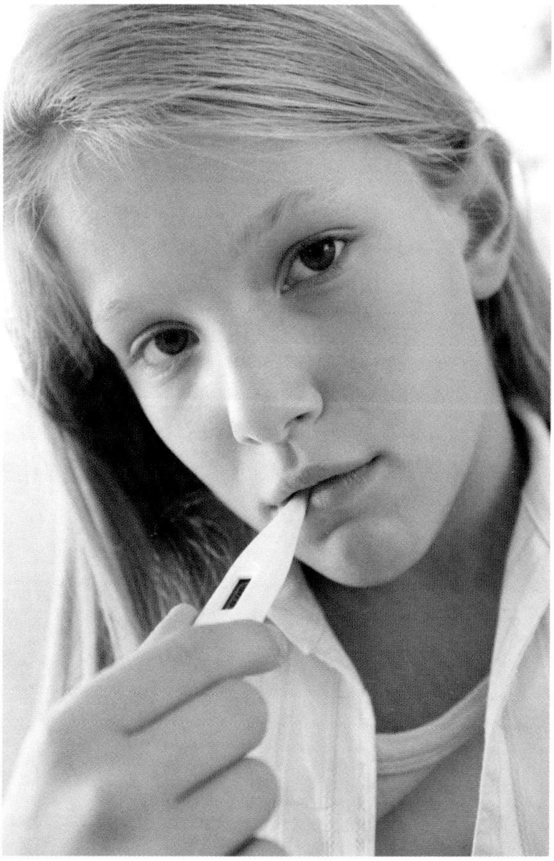

West Nile virus, influenza, the common cold, strep throat, viruses, bacterial infections, cancer, parasites, flesh eating bacteria... What do all these illnesses and diseases have in common? They all are wreaking havoc across America as they invade bodies with weakened immune systems. However, for bodies with strong immune systems, they have little or no power. The body has the God-given natural ability to protect itself from all invaders, provided it is operating at peak performance.

Race car drivers routinely check, monitor and upgrade components on a race car to be sure it operates at peak performance. Even the family car gets gasoline, water, oil and an occasional bath to keep it running and looking good. Without daily maintenance, soon the car would be in the junk yard. The body is much the same. Daily maintenance is required to keep it working efficiently.

What is the Immune System?

The body's immune system is a very complicated and intricate system, but its basic strategy is simple - to recognize the enemy, mobilize forces and attack. It can be likened to an army on a "seek and destroy mission." Its job is to protect the body from harmful foreign invaders, such as bacteria and viruses and self-mutated cells. Any cells the immune system does not recognize, including once good but worn out, dead cells, are targets for destruction and removal. These invaders commonly are referred to as **pathogens** (disease-creation) and include bacteria, viruses, fungi, pollen, toxic pollutants, cancer cells, old dead cells and waste products not previously eliminated. Many pathogens are breathed in through the nose, while others enter the body through the skin. Some pathogens result from mutated cells and waste material that the body was unable to eliminate.

The **innate immune system** is the body's first, generic way of getting rid of a pathogen, meaning that it triggers certain responses to defend against infection. However, it does not create lasting immunity, or defense, to the pathogens as the adaptive immune system does.

> **Inflammation** is one of the first responses to an infection or irritation by the body's innate immune system. The injured cells release chemicals that trigger inflammation to try to keep the pathogens from spreading and to promote healing of the damaged cells once the pathogens are removed.
>
> The chemicals released at the site of infection sensitize pain receptors, widen nearby blood vessels and attract white blood cells. An inflammatory response includes symptoms of redness, heat, swelling, pain and possible dysfunction of the organs or tissues involved.

White blood cells, also known as **leukocytes**, attack foreign invaders by either eating them or producing antibodies, which kill the pathogens. Leukocytes are very different than red blood cells and most body cells because they are not tied down to a particular organ or tissue and are able to move freely throughout the entire body. They are made in the thymus, spleen and bone marrow and are stored in clumps of tissue called lymph nodes.

There are many different types of leukocytes each with unique jobs. The two main categories of leukocytes are:

1. **Phagocytes** – The primary responders in the innate immune system that eat pathogens.

2. **Lymphocytes** – The primary responders in the adaptive immune system that help the immune system destroy pathogens and then remember and recognize the former invaders. They identify and mark pathogens so that the phagocytes can then ingest and destroy them.

Phagocytes, literally meaning "cells that eat," are the main defense of the innate immune system. Once the inflammatory response has been initiated due to an invading pathogen, chemicals are released that call for phagocytes to come and eat up the pathogens. The phagocytes engulf the pathogens and release chemicals that cause the pathogen to be digested – a process known as **phagocytosis**. There are several different types of phagocytes, including macrophages and neutrophils.

Macrophages are nicknamed "big eaters" because they are large cells that engulf microbes after they have been targeted for destruction by the immune system. They have a short life of only seven to 10 days. Macrophages contain granules consisting of chemicals and enzymes that allow them to digest the ingested microbe, usually destroying it. Macrophages are not found in the blood, but rather they reside strategically in tissues where the body organs interface with the bloodstream. For example, macrophages are found where lungs receive air and where the liver cells connect to blood vessels. Similar cells in the bloodstream are called monocytes. Go to www.wikipedia.org/wiki/macrophage to see video of macrophages ingesting pathogens.

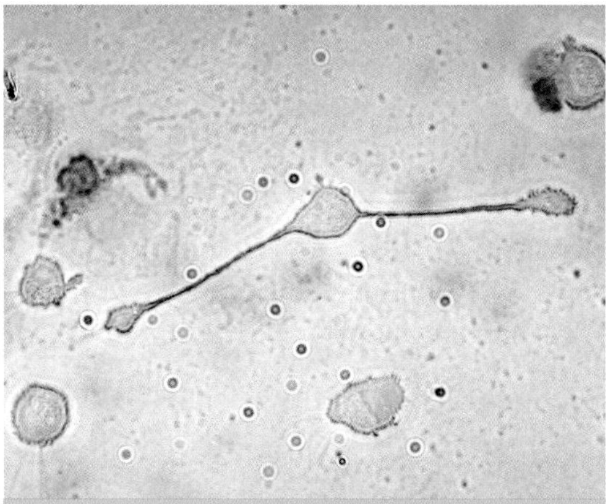

Macrophage from a mouse reaching out to ingest pathogens.

Neutrophils are cells that engulf cellular debris or foreign material in the bloodstream and can rapidly congregate at the site of injury as the first line of defense when cells are damaged. They also are increased with inflammatory conditions. Increased concentrations of neutrophils can indicate acute infections, adrenal dysfunction, gout or rheumatoid arthritis. Decreased concentrations can indicate chronic infections, bone marrow depression, anemia and lupus.

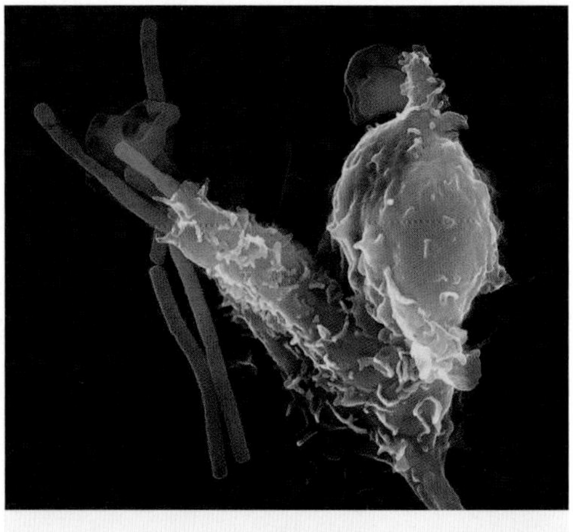

Neutrophil phagocytosing an anthrax bacteria.

The **adaptive immune system** is composed of specialized cells and processes that eliminate pathogens. These adaptive immune responses train the immune system to recognize and remember these pathogens so that the next time that particular pathogen enters the body, the immune system can fight it off faster and easier each time creating long-lasting immunity to that pathogen. The main responders in the adaptive immune system are white blood cells called **lymphocytes.**

Lymphocytes are small, round leukocytes that, instead of eating a pathogen, identify pathogens and create antibodies to destroy them. The antibodies help the immune system remember and recognize those pathogens if they invade again. There are two main types of lymphocytes – T cells and B cells.

T cells are the communicators. They identify pathogens and then produce proteins, or cytokines, that trigger the immune response. T cells identify pathogens by their antigen. Every cell, including a pathogen, contains antigens. **Antigens** are tiny cell markers on the surface of a cell that tell the T cells if that cell is friend or foe - part of the body or an invader. When a T cell recognizes an antigen as foe, it is activated and begins to divide and produce proteins that activate B cells and killer T cells.

B cells are called upon when a pathogen is located and then produce antibodies specific to the pathogen. **Antibodies** are like y-shaped keys that lock onto the antigens of pathogens and help destroy them by allowing phagocytes to eat them or allowing chemicals in the blood to destroy them. Some B cells become **memory B cells**, which have antibodies that remain in the system so that when the same pathogen strikes again, the antibodies immediately race to destroy them.

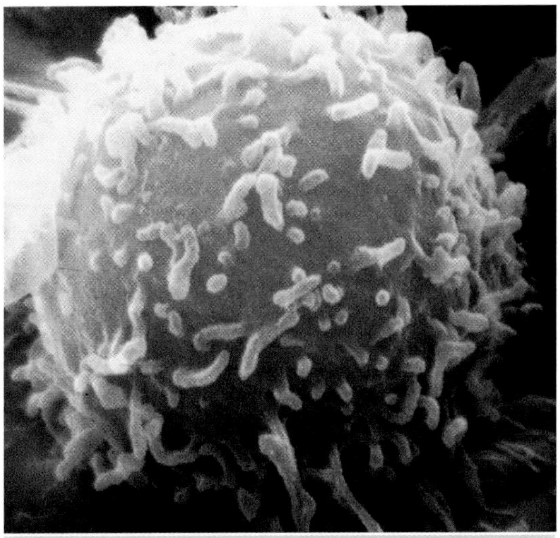

A scanning electron microscope (SEM) image of a single human lymphocyte.

The Lymphatic System

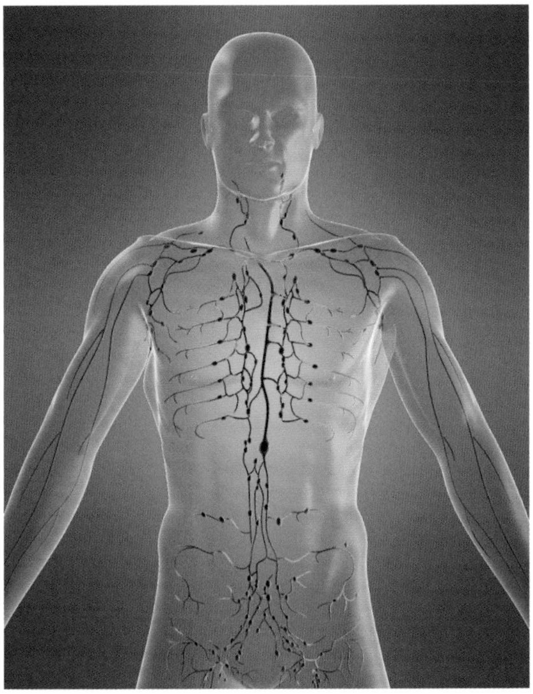

"He gives power to the weak, and to those who have no might He increases strength." Isaiah 40:29

The immune system has its own system of circulation called the **lymphatic system**, which is a network of lymph vessels, organs, ducts and nodes that run throughout the body and permeate every organ except the brain. Its job is to collect and return fluid surrounding cells called interstitial fluid, to absorb and transport fatty acids and fats to the circulatory system and to transport lymphocytes to lymph nodes where immune responses are initiated.

The **lymph vessels** carry a watery fluid called **lymph** that is formed when interstitial fluid enters the lymph vessels through filtration. **Interstitial fluid** is the means by which nutrients are transferred from the blood to the cells and waste is carried away from the cells. Once inside a lymph vessel, the interstitial fluid becomes lymph. As it flows through the lymph vessels, lymph nodes and other lymphoid tissue and organs, it picks up lymphocytes. The lymphatic

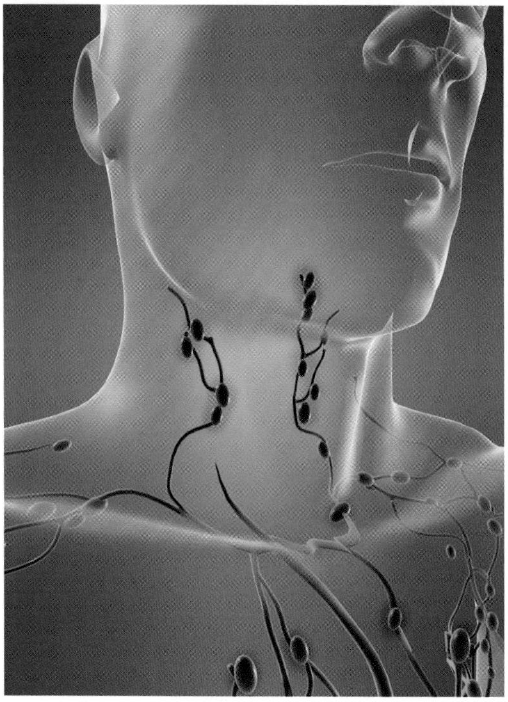

system does not have a main pump like the cardiovascular system has the heart. Lymph is not pumped through the lymphatic system like blood is pumped. It is pumped by the skeletal muscles.

Lymph nodes are organs made up of lymphoid tissue. They house lymphocytes and filter out destroyed pathogens and foreign particles from the lymph. Lymph nodes may expand and become swollen during infections as B cell numbers and activity increases. Infections can be caused by numerous things from viruses to cancer cells. When lymph nodes become swollen or clogged, the excess lymph has nowhere to go and backs up into the surrounding tissues and can cause a condition known as edema. One of the best ways to get the lymphatic system pumping is exercise. A particular exercise that helps the lymphatic system to pump is rebounding, which is jumping in place on a small trampoline.

The lymphatic system also includes certain structures that are dedicated to the production of lymphocytes such as the spleen, thymus gland, bone marrow and lymphoid tissue in the digestive system. Other important lymphoid tissue is the appendix, tonsils, adenoids and Peyer's patches.

The **thymus gland** is highly important as it orchestrates the workings of the immune system and is located in the neck, tucked behind the top of the collarbone. The thymus is big and robust in young people, but declines with age. When a child is born, the thymus is bigger than the heart. The shrinking starts at puberty and by the time a person is sixty, it may only be the size of a walnut. This correlates with the decline of the immune system and is one reason the elderly are more prone to illness. The reduction in the function of the immune system is one of the most visible signs of aging.

Stress

One culprit to the body's ability to defend itself properly is stress. In short, stress burns up nutrients. When the body is out of nutrients – its fuel – it can no longer run efficiently. One of the first systems affected by a lack of nutrients is the immune system. This is one reason why people under a great deal of stress are more susceptible to illness and feel tired most of the time. They are simply out of gas. For people in a stressful circumstance it is especially important to eat healthy foods and refrain from skipping meals,

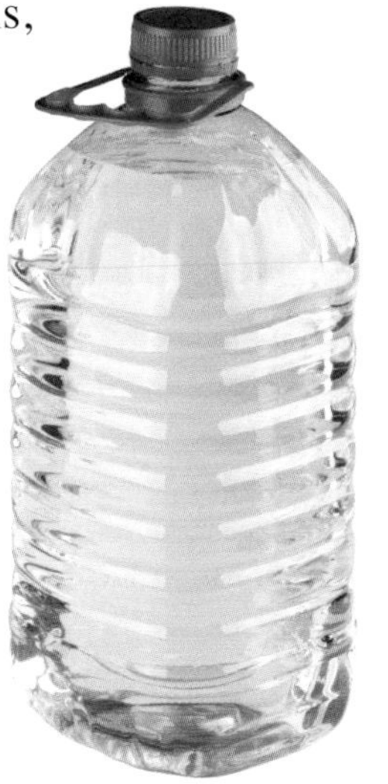

Air and Water

A lack of fresh air and pure clean water also contribute to poor immune system health. Breathing air filled with pollutants in an environment without fresh air from open windows contributes to the creation of free radicals. These free radicals must be neutralized with antioxidant-rich foods or supplements. Whenever possible, open up a door or window and let in the fresh air. Even on colder days, just an hour of fresh air will eliminate many household contaminants.

Drinking pure water quickly helps the body to eliminate cells the immune system destroys without clogging up the bloodstream or lymphatic system.

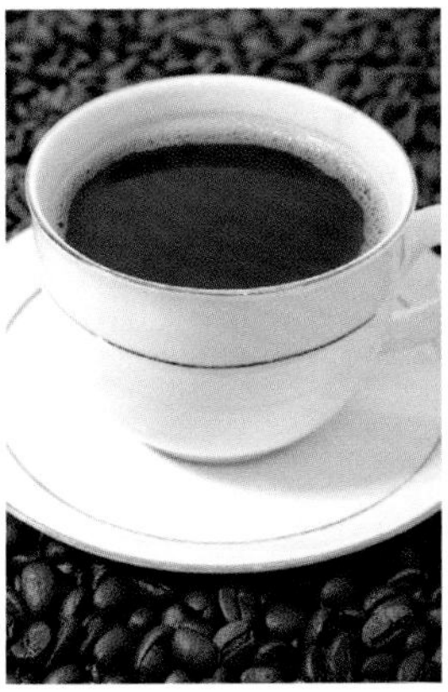

Immune-Suppressing Food

Foods that suppress the body's immune system include caffeine and sugar. Caffeine in excess raises the body's cortisol levels. Even a slight increase in sustained cortisol levels may compromise the immune system for up to 18 hours. Sugar, even amounts as little as one teaspoon per day, may suppress the immune system, too.

Antibiotics

While antibiotics may destroy harmful bacteria in the body, they also destroy the beneficial bacteria in the gut that is required for optimal health. A large percentage of the immune system resides in the intestines in the form of billions of healthy bacteria that feed on bad bacteria and excess fungus and yeast. When the good bacteria is destroyed, the ever fragile balance in the intestines is compromised, resulting in overgrowth of yeast and fungus and many health issues. See Unit 2 for more detailed information on the intestines, good bacteria and probiotics.

Another issue is the overuse of antibiotics, which has created super bugs. Super bugs are antibiotic resistant strains of bacteria, such as MRSA (methicillin-resistant Staphylococcus aureus), that have wreaked havoc among hospitals and nursing homes for years. In recent years, MRSA outbreaks have been reported in gyms and schools.

Vaccines

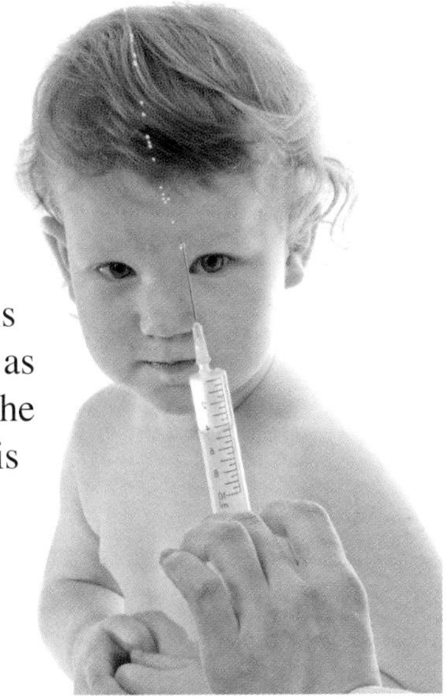

There is much controversy over whether or not one should be vaccinated. After extensive research to both sides of the issue, the authors have chosen not to vaccinate. We instead prefer the use of excellent nutrition and the use of therapeutic-grade essential oils to boost the immune system and protect ourselves from disease. This is a very personal family matter, and the best advice to be given on the subject is for each family to research and read as much as possible to become as informed as possible. Then, armed with the facts and with much prayer, families can make the decision that is right for them. See the Additional Resources section at the end of this chapter for links to informative Web sites about vaccination.

Disorders and Diseases of the Immune System

There are four main categories of immune system disorders.

1. **Immunodeficiency disorders** occur when a part of the immune system is not present or is not working properly. These can be primary, such as being born with the inability to produce a particular kind of antibody, or they can be acquired, such as HIV/AIDS and immunodeficiencies, specifically caused by medications like chemotherapy treatment for cancer.

2. **Autoimmune disorders** are when the immune system mistakenly attacks healthy organs and tissues while thinking they are pathogens. Common autoimmune disorders are lupus and juvenile rheumatoid arthritis.

3. **Allergic disorders** happen when the immune system overreacts to antigens in the environment called allergens. Responses with allergic disorders can cause swelling, watery eyes, sneezing and life threatening reactions such as anaphylaxis. Common allergic disorders include asthma, eczema and environmental, seasonal, drug, food and toxin allergies.

4. **Cancers of the immune system** occur when cells grow out of control. The most common types are lymphoma, which involves the lymphoid tissue, and leukemia, which involves abnormal overgrowth of leukocytes.

Boosting the Immune System

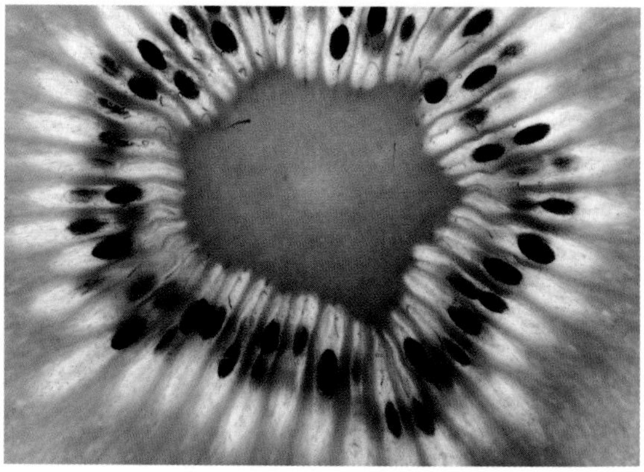

"And by the river upon the bank thereof, on this side and on that side, shall grow all trees for meat, whose leaf shall not fade, neither shall the fruit thereof be consumed: it shall bring forth new fruit according to his months, because their waters they issued out of the sanctuary: and the fruit thereof shall be for meat, and the leaf thereof for medicine." Ezekiel 47:12

Understanding how the immune system works is the first step. The next step is learning ways to make a sluggish immune system work better or an over active immune system calm down and work correctly.

Nutrients - see the Vitamin and Mineral Charts for foods high in these nutrients

There is no one nutrient that completely controls the working of the immune system, all are needed for a healthy body. But there are a few that have a greater impact on the immune system than others.

Vitamin C supplements can come in all shapes, sizes, colors and flavors. From fizzy drink mixes and fortified juices to chewable tablets, vitamin C tops the list of supplements marketed and sold. Look for whole food sourced vitamin C. It may be labeled as ascorbic acid, but as long as it is derived from whole food sources it is a good choice. It is quite difficult to take too much vitamin C, but in excess, it will cause loose stools. When taking vitamin C, spread it out over the course of the day.

Zinc is best taken in a combination multi-whole food vitamin. Zinc's role in immune system health can be seen in proper T cell function and proper lymphocyte activity. Zinc is directly involved in antibody production to help fight infection. It also plays a major role in keeping the thymus going.

Elenolic acid, found in olive leaf and the NingXia wolfberry, is largely known for its anti-viral capabilities. One study by Upjohn, a major American pharmaceutical company, investigated this compound in olive leaf for its ability to fight viruses. By the late 1960's they proved that it could stop every virus it tested against but found that while safe in even large doses, the elenolic acid when separated from the rest of the herb would attach itself to blood proteins, making it useless in humans. Olive leaf extract only became available in the US in 1995. While the mechanism as to how it works may not yet be explained, there is no doubt elenolic acid works against all known viruses.

Supplementation

A great supplementation program can be targeted to kill germs and support the immune system. For more details on supplementation recommendations, see Appendix DD.

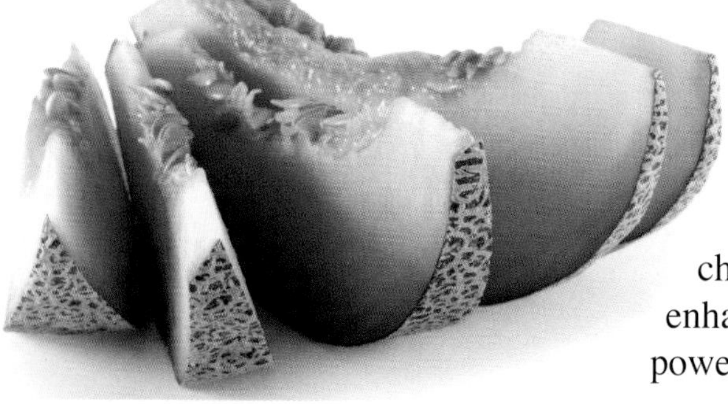

Beta glucans are a great nutraceutical to help build white cells and increase macrophage activity. Common in many foods including cantaloupe and oats, beta glucans have been researched for over 60 years. Evidence shows beta glucans' ability to lower cholesterol, drastically reduce septic morbidity from infections, enhance macrophage activity and accelerate wound healing. It is a powerful anti-viral and anti-bacterial agent safe in large doses.

Herbs

Certain herbs will stimulate the white blood cells of the immune system into action very quickly, like **Echinacea**. Often at the first onset of cold or flu like symptoms, a blast of super high quality Echinacea is enough to stop the illness dead in its tracts. But Echinacea should not be taken as a tonic herb on a daily basis as it will become ineffective as the body grows accustomed to its presence.

The herb **cat's claw** boosts macrophage activity and is reported to have many anti-cancer effects. It is reported to possess tremendous anti-inflammatory properties and has the ability to boost phagocytosis – the phagocytes' ability to "eat" pathogens. It is being researched for its effects against leukemia. A compound in cat's claw – rynchophylline is known to inhibit blood platelets from sticking together and lessens the formation of arterial plaque.

Astragalus is an herb well known for its immune calming properties which may make it beneficial for those suffering from autoimmune conditions.

Good Foods for the Immune System	Bad Foods for the Immune System
Whole grains – especially oats (not quick oats)	Alcohol
Vegetables	Artificial sweeteners
Fruit – especially cantaloupe	Caffeine in excess
Legumes	Candy
Nuts	High fructose corn syrup
Seeds	High sugar desserts and juices
High quality protein	Refined sugar
	Sodas

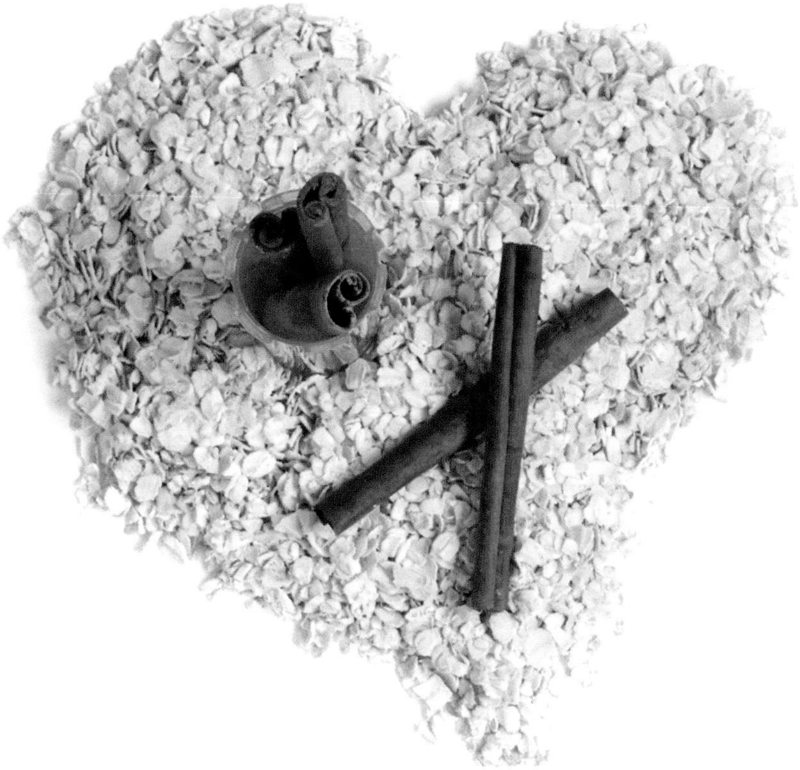

Unit 5 Chapter 3
Discussion Questions

1. How is our immune system like an army?
2. What are the differences between the innate and adaptive immune systems?
3. How can you tell a T cell from a B cell?

Activities - plus the Mixed Berry Salad "Power" Recipe and activities.

Elementary

1. Find "cyte" in the dictionary and learn its meaning. From what language is it derived?
2. Find out what Peyer's Patches are, what they do and where they are found in the body.
3. What is anaphylaxis? What does a person have to do when they are experiencing anaphylaxis?
4. What vaccines are recommended for a person your age? Research what they are for and list all the ingredients in each vaccine. Was it easy or hard to find out the ingredients? Are you surprised at any of the listed ingredients?
5. Draw a picture of a white blood cell phagocytosing a germ.
6. Write a fun story about what the immune system does when a germ invades the body. Be creative. As an optional activity, turn the story into a play and act it out for your family.
7. Look at Appendix I and find out how much vitamin C you need a day for your age.
8. Refer to the Vitamin Chart in Appendix F, find the foods high in vitamin C and list those that you like and eat regularly. Find those that you do not eat or have never tried and pick two to prepare with a family meal. Look through the additional recipes sections of the units for recipe ideas, find healthy recipes online or in a cookbook that contain these ingredients.

Secondary

Choose any from above plus

1. Research scientists Ilya Mechnikov and Paul Ehrlich. Prepare a written or oral report discussing what they discovered and why their discoveries were important.
2. Learn more about super bugs and research the outbreak closest to your home. What warnings were given to the public about the outbreak? How was it contained?
3. Are B cells the only cells in the body that have memory? Review previous chapters and conduct independent study in order to share your findings with your family.
4. Play the Immune System Defender game at http://nobelprize.org/educational_games/medicine/immunity/game/index.html.
5. Review your state laws about vaccinations. Are they mandatory? Find out what is required for someone who chooses not to vaccinate to attend a public school.
6. Look at Appendix I and figure out the RDA for zinc for everyone in your family and create a daily meal plan for one entire day in which each meal includes a different food containing zinc. Refer to the Mineral Chart in Appendix G for a list of foods high in zinc.

Additional Resources

Web sites:

1. Immune System video - http://videos.howstuffworks.com/hsw/6074-disease-defense-the-immune-system-video.htm
2. Vaccine Web site: http;//www.vaccineinfo.net
3. Article Titled "Private Study Links Vaccinations to Neurological Disorders" - http://www.naturalnews.com/022642.html
4. http://www.healthdangers.com/drugs/vaccinations/index.htm

Immune System Power

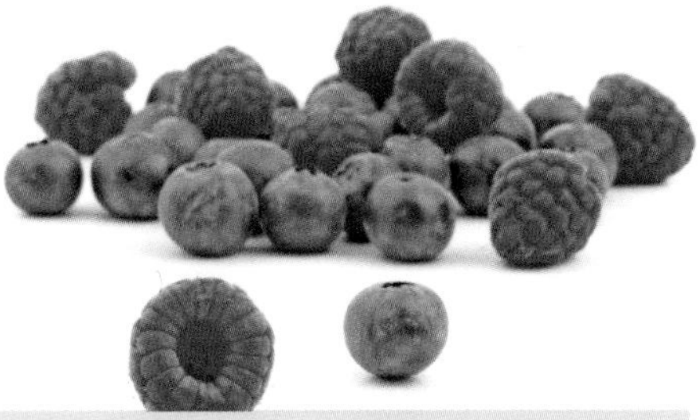

Berries

Berries are high in vitamin C and antioxidants and are great immune system supporters.

Mixed Berry Salad

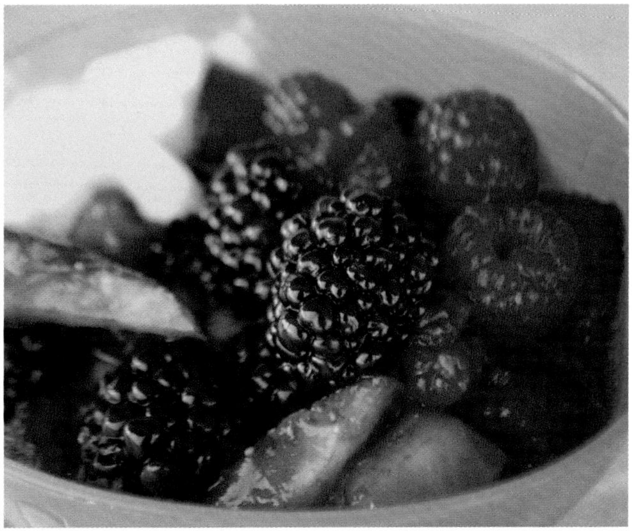

1 cup fresh blueberries
Chosen for their high ORAC rating and being rich in phenolic acid, anthocyanins and ellagic acid that may inhibit tumor growth
1 cup fresh blackberries
Chosen for their ability to capture free radicals and prevent damage to the liver and colon cells
1 cup fresh raspberries
Chosen for their fiber content, selenium and vitamin C all associated with fighting disease
1 cup fresh sliced strawberries
Chosen because they are rich in folate, vitamin C and potassium. Harvard researchers have found promising results on many cancers.

Combine in a bowl, drizzle two tablespoons blue agave nectar and let sit overnight. Spoon onto a bed of unpasteurized kiefer or yogurt.

Activities

Elementary

1. Three of the four fruits in this recipe are members of the Rosoideae family. Identify them and what this means?
2. What is kiefer?
3. Do more people in the world consume milk from cows or goats?
4. These ingredients contain seeds. What is the difference between hybrid and non-hybrid seeds?
5. What is an heirloom seed?

Secondary
Choose any from above plus

1. Locate a farm in your area that grows and allows people to pick their own berries. Arrange a field trip for your family during the appropriate season.
2. Blueberries are indigenous to North America. Prepare a written or oral report about the history and diverse uses for this fruit.
3. Based on Appendix H, is this recipe more acidic or alkaline? Which individual ingredients are more alkaline?
4. Find a poem that references any of the berries and memorize it.

Chapter 4

Carbohydrates and Sugar

"I will behave myself wisely in a perfect way. O when wilt thou come unto me? I will walk within my house with a perfect heart." Psalm 101:2

What are carbohydrates?

Carbohydrates, also known as carbs, are the body's primary energy source and are required for proper organ function. Carbohydrates come in a variety of forms, most commonly and abundantly as sugars, fibers and starches. Because of their versatility, they are found in a wide array of foods such as bread, beans, milk, popcorn, potatoes, cookies, spaghetti, soft drinks, corn and pie.

Though often vilified, carbohydrates are an important part of a healthy diet. The best sources of carbohydrates include whole grains, vegetables, fruits and legumes. They promote good health by delivering vitamins, minerals, fiber and a host of important phytonutrients to every organ and cell of the body. There are two kinds of carbohydrates – simple and complex. While both supply simple sugars, or glucose, to the cells of the body, it is the complex, unrefined carbohydrate that really "does the body good."

Word Power
Phytonutrients
Pronunciation: \fī-tō-nü-trē-ənt, -nyü-\
Function: *noun*
Date: 1994
: a bioactive plant-derived compound (as resveratrol) associated with positive health effects

What makes up carbohydrates?

Carbohydrate molecules are made of carbon, hydrogen and oxygen and are arranged into small units called sugars, or **monosaccharides**. Small monosaccharides, such as glucose, are quickly digested and immediately used for energy by the body's cells. These single unit sugars also are known as simple sugars or **simple carbohydrates**.

When 10 or more monosaccharides are linked together, they form **polysaccharides**, or **complex carbohydrates**. These larger carbohydrate molecules include fibers and starches. The digestive system must first break these polysaccharides down into monosaccharides, or glucose, providing a more sustained energy supply.

Simple Carbohydrates

Simple carbohydrates or simple sugars, are made of monosaccharides, which are single unit sugars, and disaccharides, which are two combined monosaccharide molecules. **Monosaccharides** include **glucose**, **fructose** and **galactose** and are easily digested and immediately used as fuel for the body.

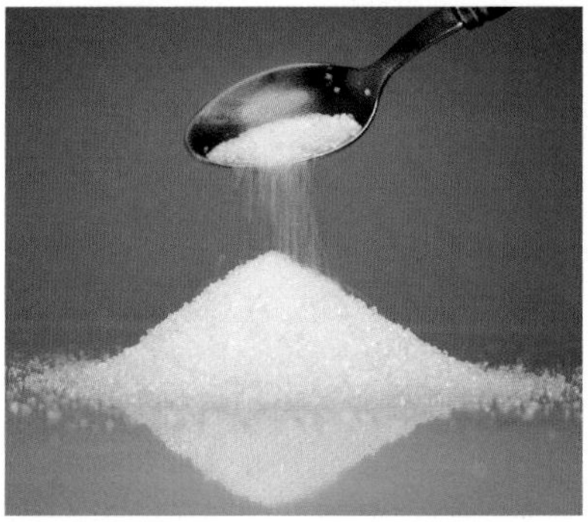

Disaccharides include **sucrose** (table sugar), which is made up of one glucose molecule and one fructose molecule, and **lactose** (milk sugar), which is made up of one glucose molecule and one galactose molecule. Sucrose and lactose also are easily broken down into glucose as energy, given that the appropriate enzymes exist to break them down. For instance, the enzyme lactase is needed to break down lactose into the simple sugars glucose and galactose. Lactase is produced in the villi of the small intestines. Those with a deficiency of the enzyme lactase cannot break down lactose properly, resulting in gastrointestinal problems.

Examples of simple carbohydrates are ripe fruit, milk, honey, table sugar and high fructose corn syrup.

Problems with Simple Carbohydrates

Simple carbohydrates provide quick energy, but they also raise blood sugar levels quickly. When too many simple carbohydrates are consumed at one time, blood sugar levels are raised too high and too fast. What follows is a dramatic drop in the blood sugar. This roller coaster in the blood sugar causes a jolt of energy followed by feelings of shakiness, being tired and run down. When blood sugar levels are raised abruptly and lowered frequently, it can lead to blood sugar dysregulation conditions, such as hypoglycemia and diabetes.

Fun Fact
Blood sugar levels, or glucose levels, refer to the amount of glucose in the blood that is being transported from the intestines and liver to the body's cells for energy. While blood sugar levels normally fluctuate throughout the day around meals, the normal blood glucose level is about 90 mg/100ml.

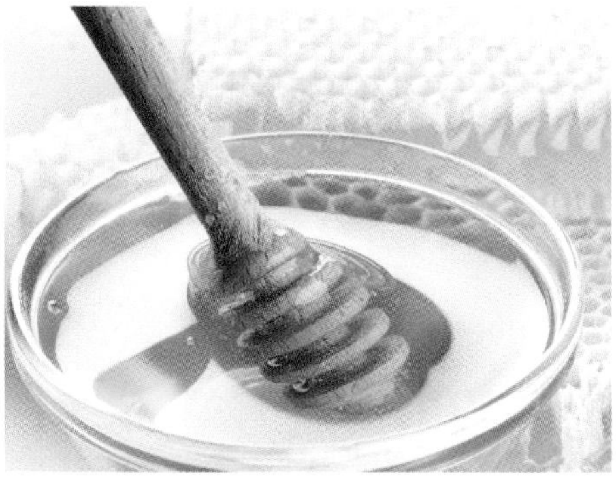

Not all simple carbohydrates are created equal. While fruit is a simple carbohydrate, it does contain many important nutrients, like vitamins and some fiber. Simple carbohydrates like table sugar and high fructose corn syrup are void of any nutrients and are easily over-eaten, causing the rapid fluctuation in blood sugar levels. These simple carbohydrates may contribute to weight gain, interfere with weight loss and promote diabetes and heart disease.

Simple carbohydrates, such as fruit and honey, should be eaten in moderation, while table sugar and high fructose corn syrup should be avoided all together. See Appendix P to find out about healthier sweet alternatives to table sugar and high fructose corn syrup.

Bad Simple Carbohydrates
table sugar, high fructose corn syrup, processed honey, candy, sugared sodas and other highly processed foods with added fructose and sucrose

Better Simple Carbohydrates
(eat in moderation and/or along with complex carbohydrates)
fruit, unprocessed raw honey, molasses, raw cow or goat milk

Complex Carbohydrates

Complex carbohydrates, or **polysaccharides**, do the body a world of good. They are comprised of starch and fiber in foods such as vegetables, legumes (dried beans) and whole grains. **Starch** is the photosynthesized glucose produced and stored in plants as their source of energy. Foods high in starch are rice, wheat, corn, potatoes, lentils and peas. **Fiber** is the indigestible part of a plant that surrounds the starch and aids in digestion and elimination by slowing down the digestion process for the absorption of nutrients and water, moving food along the digestive tract and easing elimination. Due to the high fiber content, complex carbohydrates digest much slower, therefore entering the bloodstream slowly. This helps the body avoid the blood sugar rush experienced with most simple carbohydrates. Complex carbohydrates contain plenty of minerals, vitamins and fiber, which also may satisfy hunger for longer periods of time.

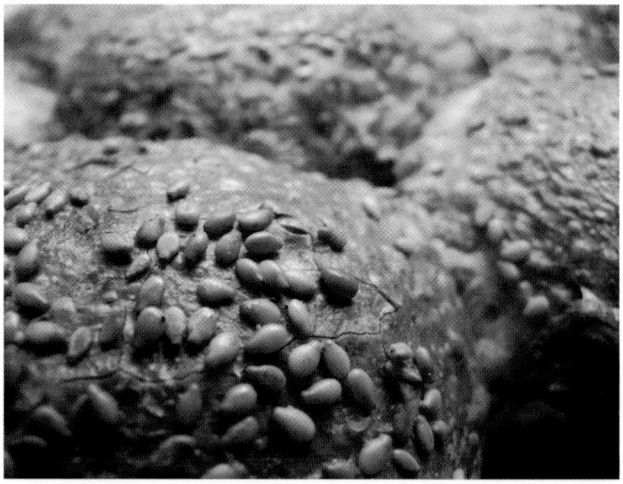

Problems with Complex Carbohydrates

Complex carbohydrates, such as grains, often are refined and added into baked goods to make them lighter colored and lighter textured resulting in a seemingly more desirable product. However, during refinement, the fiber from the grain is removed exposing the starch. This causes the complex carbohydrate to be digested much faster and act more like a disaccharide, or simple carbohydrate, while increasing blood sugar levels more rapidly. Even when processed foods have added fiber, the fiber is no longer surrounding the starch to make it digested more slowly. The result is the same as with a disaccharide, or simple carbohydrate.

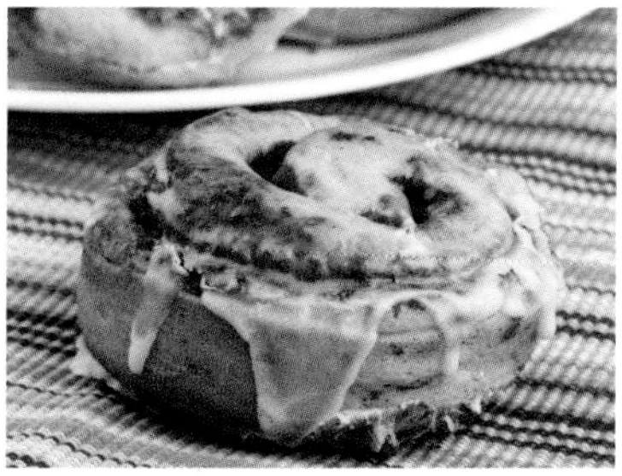

Be a Label Reader!

Watch out for the word "enriched" on labels of bread products. The fiber, wheat germ and bran of the grain had been stripped away along with all the vitamins and nutrients during the processing of the flour. Companies add back, or "enrich", the flour with vitamins and minerals creating a false sense of nutrition as those nutrients are not as readily absorbed and used without the help of the original fiber, wheat germ and bran of the grain.

Fun Fact

Carbohydrates, especially starches, if eaten in excess, cause cancer. In a study reported in internationally recognized medical journal, "The Lancet," women who ate large amounts of pasta, rice, white bread and other starches had a 39 percent increased risk of breast cancer. Lancet, 1996, VOL. 347

Bad Complex Carbohydrates

processed and bleached flours, rice and other grains, white bread, donuts, cakes, rolls, cookies, muffins, pastries and tortillas made from processed flours

Good Complex Carbohydrates

potatoes, sweet potatoes, peas, lentils, wheat, rice, millet, barley, quinoa, oats (not "quick" oats), whole grain breads (not "enriched")

How does glucose get to the cells to be used as energy?

Polysaccharides and disaccharides are broken down into monosaccharides, or glucose, by digestive enzymes all along the digestive tract. In the intestines, the glucose is absorbed into the bloodstream and taken to the liver to be stored as glycogen or distributed back into the bloodstream to be sent throughout the body to the cells and used as energy.

As the sugar levels, or glucose levels, rise in the bloodstream, the pancreas is stimulated to produce a hormone called insulin which functions to get the sugar out of the blood and into the cells to be used as energy. Insulin also helps the liver store excess glucose as glycogen to be used later, and it stops the use of fat as an energy source.

Simple and complex carbohydrates affect the production of insulin differently. When digesting simple carbohydrates, blood sugar levels spike and cause insulin levels to spike, resulting in a rapid increase of energy. After such a rapid increase in blood sugar levels comes a rapid decrease in blood sugar levels and energy. These roller coaster glucose levels explain why many people who turn to a candy bar for a quick supply of energy feel so sluggish when the sugar high comes to an end. However, complex carbohydrates take longer to digest and help to keep insulin levels low and, in the process, aid the body in burning fat for energy.

What happens when too much glucose is produced?

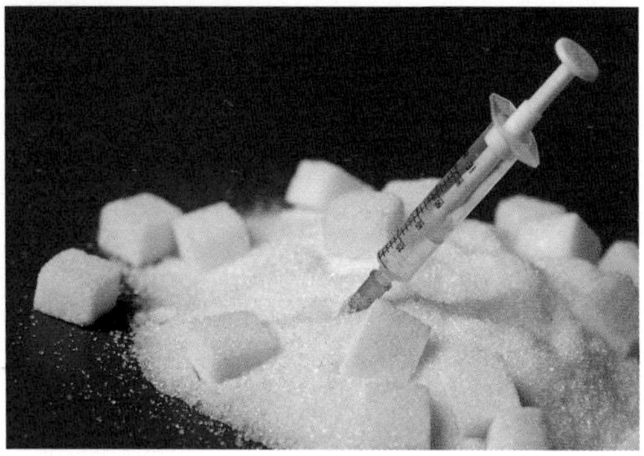

If the body produces too much glucose, it will be stored in the liver and muscle cells as glycogen, to be used when the body needs an extra burst of energy. The body uses the immediate store of glycogen for short bursts of exercise. For extended periods of exercise, such as long distance running and more strenuous workouts, the body will turn to its fat reserve to draw extra energy.

Too much glucose also stimulates the production of too much insulin, which may lead to dysregulation conditions of blood sugar levels, such as diabetes and hypoglycemia.

How much of the diet should include carbohydrates?

The recommendation of the Institute of Medicine suggests that 40 to 65 percent of an adult's dietary energy should come from carbohydrates, while the World Health Organization (WHO) recommends 55 to 75percent. The WHO also recommends that no more than 10 percent of carbohydrate consumption come from simple carbohydrates. When in the form of healthy vegetables, fruit and whole grains, the benefits of carbohydrates are good for overall health.

How to eat more complex carbohydrates

- Choose fresh, whole fruits instead of candy or cookies for snacks and desserts.
- Buy 100 percent whole grain bread and pasta instead of regular white bread and pasta.
- Eat lots of green and brightly colored vegetables every day.
- Substitute raw crunchy vegetables for French fries or chips.
- Stay away from sugar-sweetened beverages. Drink water, herbal teas, and freshly squeezed 100 percent fruit or vegetable juice (not from concentrate and always organic).
- Start meals with a salad or broth-based soup. This helps to create a feeling of being full and makes it easier to skip the sugary desserts.

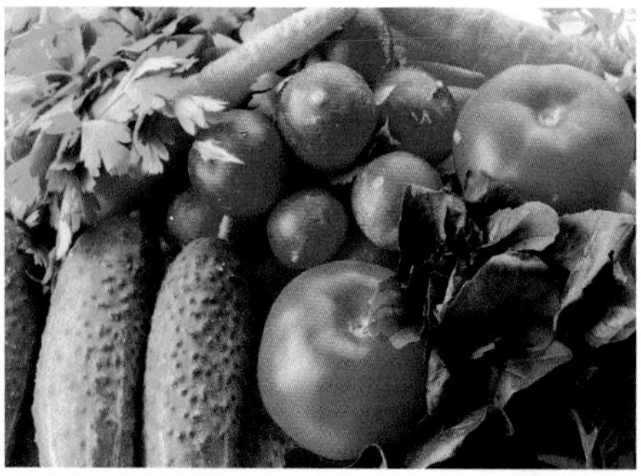

Should anyone completely avoid carbohydrates?

Except in rare occasions, no one should avoid all carbohydrates. The advent of popular diet plans, Atkin's, the Zone, South Beach and others may lead one to believe that all carbohydrates are bad. Nothing could be further from the truth. None of the authors of even these highly successful weight loss programs advocate zero carbs. As discussed in this unit, carbs are the body's fuel. But as they can be digested rapidly – especially when void of balanced fiber as seen in simple and processed carbs – they can spike blood sugar readings, which are not beneficial for most diabetics. The key to carbohydrate consumptions again lies in the kind of carbohydrates you choose – simple or complex, whole or refined - and the quantity.

What has really happened is that many people are eating more carbohydrates then they are using up in a day and are usually eating carbs void of good nutrients in over-processed, quick meals and fast foods. A low carbohydrate diet usually incorporates more protein, which study after study concludes is not harmful to the heart, liver, bones or kidneys.

When should someone eat zero carbohydrates?

Many diabetics may go on a very low to no-carbohydrate diet for generally not longer than two week intervals.[1] Although, it may be necessary for severe diabetics to avoid carbohydrates for a longer period of time.[2] People with various health concerns, such as candida (yeast or fungal overgrowth), Irritable Bowel Syndrome, Chron's Disease and Polycystic Ovarian Syndrome, would all benefit from short-term zero carb intake. This generally is regarded for adults and should not be followed by teens or young children without supervision of a qualified health professional.

As detailed in Unit 2, fiber is vital to the digestive and elimination systems and to maintaining normal blood sugar levels. Completely avoiding complex carbohydrates would eliminate the much needed fiber from the diet and could worsen blood sugar levels, causing wild fluctuations.

For mild to moderate diabetics, at least half of the grains eaten should be whole grains, such as whole wheat, whole oats, brown or wild rice, buckwheat, quinoa, bulgur, whole grain rye and whole grain barley. In addition, people with diabetes should consume other healthy carbohydrate foods like high fiber vegetables and harder flesh fruits, such as apples and pears rather than peaches and banana with lower fiber. The ideal meals are a tasty balance of healthy carbs, lean proteins and heart-healthy fats. See Unit 6 for more information on diabetes.

The **Nutrition 101: Choose Life! Food Pyramid** in Appendix B shows the carbohydrate intake meets the recommendations without excess as in traditional food pyramids.

Sugar

When looking at the huge increase in sugar in Americans' diets this past century — particularly in processed foods — it appears to march in step with the epidemic increase in many diseases. According to the US Department of Agriculture, in 2000, the average American consumed 148.9 pounds of caloric sweeteners.[3] That's 40 teaspoons for every man, woman and child every day or nearly three pounds per week! The biggest sources are corn sugar and corn syrup found in beverages like juice drinks and soda.

Refined sugar has no nutritional value and no fiber. It has just 99.7 percent pure calories ... no vitamins, no minerals, no proteins. To metabolize processed sugar, the body actually must give up minerals, specifically magnesium. So rather than needing 400 milligrams of magnesium per day, the average adult would need much more magnesium if consuming sugar. One of the effects of magnesium deprivation is muscle cramps such as toe cramps and Charlie horses.

Sugar and Cow Bones?

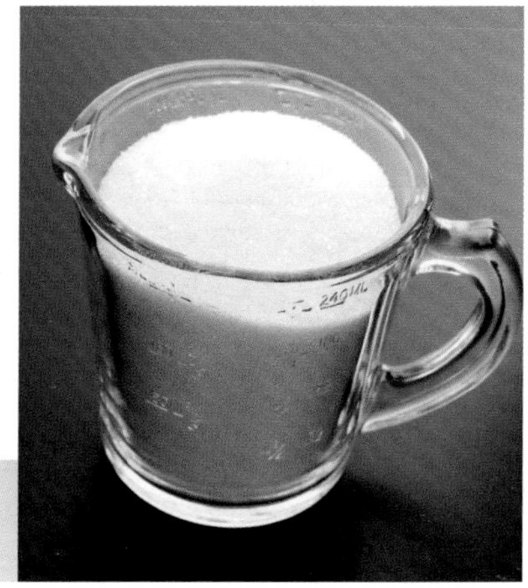

In the past, charred cow bones, known as bone char, were used extensively to remove color from raw cane sugar in the refining process. Modern technology, such as filters using granular carbon or an ion exchange system, has largely replaced the bone char process but it is still used in a few refineries. Therefore, refined sugar cannot be categorized as vegetarian. Bone char is not used in making white beet sugar and it is not used in making raw cane sugar.

Fun Fact - Juice "cocktails" such as cranberry cocktail usually have 10 teaspoons of sugar.

1 Please consult the health care practitioner of your choice before beginning any diet.
2 See Unit 6 for more diabetes information.
3 "U.S. Per Capita Food Supply Trends: More Calories, Refined Carbohydrates, and Fats" Judy Putnam, Jane Allshouse, and Linda Scott Kantar, Economic Research Service, USDA, Dec 2002.

Sugar and the Immune System

Sugar suppresses the immune system in several ways. First, it causes the pancreas to secrete abnormally large quantities of insulin, which is the key that allows cells to use glucose as energy. Excess insulin remains in circulation in the bloodstream long after sugar has been metabolized. One of the main side effects of excess insulin is the suppression of the release of growth hormone in the pituitary gland. Growth hormone is a primary regulator of the immune system, so a person who eats a lot of sugar every day is going to experience critical growth hormone deficiency and consequent immune deficiency caused by the constant presence of insulin in the bloodstream.

Fun Fact

How many times have you reached for a Gatorade® or a Sprite® when you were sick or an ice cream when your throat hurt? While these things seem to bring temporary relief, they are actually prolonging the healing process and making you susceptible to more germs.

Those who have high metabolisms and think they can eat all the sugar they want are greatly mislead. Sugar still suppresses the immune system and makes way for sickness and disease to strike the body.

Secondly, white blood cells need vitamin C to be able to engulf and digest pathogens. This process is known as phagocytosis. When vitamin C is present, it is transported into the white blood cell through its outer membrane.[4] However, sugar has a similar molecular structure to vitamin C. If too much sugar is in the blood, the white blood cells will take in the sugar instead of the vitamin C, which greatly decreases phagocytosis. Instead of actively moving around to search and destroy invading germs, the white blood cells are left in a frozen state while the germs wreak havoc on the body. The immune system becomes suppressed and unable to fight off pathogens.

Fun Fact

It is estimated that one can of soda containing 9 to 11 teaspoons of sugar can suppress the immune system for up to 6 hours.

"A few years ago, I had been feeling very fatigued, so I had a live blood cell analysis done. It revealed the presence of sugar crystals in my blood, and my white blood cells were not moving at all. At that time, I was still eating a lot of sugar and, in fact, had just eaten two of my son's birthday cupcakes the previous day. It was amazing that my white blood cells were STILL effected by the sugar the following day." – Sera Johnson

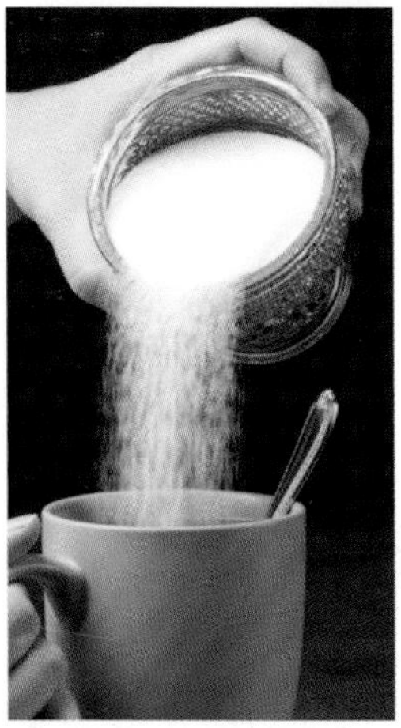

How can sugar make a person fat?

Most people consume far more sugar than their bodies can possibly use for energy. When this happens, the extra sugar is turned into triglycerides and stored as fat.

Refined white sugar is treated as a toxin by the immune system. This is due to its unnatural chemical structure and the industrial contaminants it retains from the refining process. Excess toxins in the body are stored in fat cells as the body's effort to protect itself. Sugar is a major factor in obesity and also has a major role in cardiovascular disease as well.

Sugar and the Heart

In the 1960's, Dr. John Yudlin, a British physician, researched the link between sugar consumption and heart disease. In 1964 one of the world's leading medical journals "The Lancet" published his research demonstrating how a person who consumes 120 grams sugar, or eight tablespoons (half a soda pop) each day, is five times more likely to develop heart disease than a person consuming less than 60 grams daily. Elevated sugar levels contribute to elevated thromboxane, one of the body's blood clot triggering compounds.

4 "The membrane transport of ascorbic acid" Mann GV. Ann NY Acad Sci, 1975; 258: 243-252.

Glycemic Index

The glycemic index, or GI, ranks carbohydrates according to their effects on blood glucose levels. Foods with a low GI raise blood glucose levels slowly, while foods with a high GI raises blood glucose levels very quickly. The standard value of 100 is based on the rise of blood sugar after ingesting glucose. The index ranges from 20 for fructose and barley to about 98 for a baked potato. Sucrose, or table sugar, ranks at 60.

Foods with a high glycemic value should be avoided by people with diabetes and hypoglycemia. Foods high in bad fat such as ice cream and sausage also should be avoided because they interfere with insulin production in the pancreas and impair glucose tolerance.

Glycemic Index Values For Some Common Foods

Sugars

Fructose	20
Glucose	100
Honey	75
Maltose	105
Sucrose	60
High Fructose Corn Syrup	62
Maple Syrup	55
Agave Nectar (from the agave salmiana plant[5])	32
Raw Blue Agave Nectar (from the agave tequilana plant[6])	11

Fruits

Apples	39
Bananas	62
Orange juice	46
Oranges	40
Raisins	64

Vegetables

Beets	64
Carrot, cooked	36
Carrot, raw	31
Potato, baked	98
Potato, boiled	70

Grains

Bran Cereal	51
Bread, white	71
Bread, whole grain	50
Corn	59
Cornflakes	80
Oatmeal	49
Pasta	45
Rice	70
Rice, puffed	95
Wheat Cereal	67

Legumes

Beans	31
Lentils	29
Peas	39

Other Foods

Ice Cream	36
Milk	34
Nuts	13
Sausages	28

Be a Label Reader!

Sugar by any other name still has the harmful effects of sugar. When examining labels for sugar, an easy rule is to look for words ending in -ose or –ol in the ingredients. The following are a few of the sugar homonyms commonly used on labels: sucrose, dextrose, corn syrup, malt, fructose, glucose, carbitol, mannitol, lactose, evaporated cane juice or concentrated fruit juice.

5 Madhava brand
6 Young Living brand

High Fructose Corn Syrup

High fructose corn syrup (HFCS) is chemically derived from corn, is as sweet as sugar, but is much cheaper to use than sugar and has a longer shelf life. It has replaced processed sugar in nearly 50 percent of processed foods, and that percentage is ever increasing. In 1997, The Journal of Nutrition stated, "High fructose corn syrup has no fiber or nutrients. While fructose doesn't raise blood sugar as fast as sugar, fructose raises triglycerides and actually increases insulin resistance, the root cause of Type II Diabetes".[7]

Excess table sugar and HFCS are both bad, but recent evidence show that HFCS is the worst. While table sugar is made of glucose and fructose that is bound and needs to be digested before it is separated and used as energy, HFCS is chemically made of unbound glucose and unbound fructose that immediately increases blood sugar levels upon consumption.

Medical doctor Dana Flavin says that HFCS also may lead to a fatty liver that is not functioning properly and encourages weight gain.[8] As HFCS inhibits leptin, which is the body's natural appetite suppressant, it promotes overeating that leads to weight gain.

New evidence shows that manufacturing is adding mercury to HFCS from the chemicals used in the process. Half of the products made with HFCS may contain trace amounts of toxic mercury.[4]

Dangers of Artificial Sweeteners

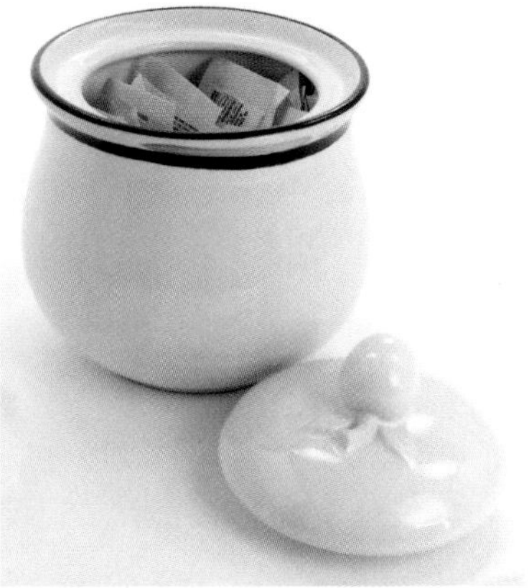

In an effort to shrink the bulging American waistline and allow diabetics the opportunity to enjoy something sweet, the artificial sweetener market is ever expanding. And with adolescent diabetes on the rise and parents being more cautious of sugar content, the artificial sweetener industry has infiltrated an even broader market – children.

While artificial sweeteners once were commonly seen only in diet sodas and sugarless gum, they now are showing up in cereals, juice, flavored milk, ketchup, snack foods, bread, cookies, pasta sauce and more. In 2004, 11 percent of the new food products introduced contained artificial sweeteners, which was double that of the two years pervious.[9] Sales in granulated sugar have dropped due to the public perception that natural is somehow not as good as artificial. With such an infiltration into so many food sources, there is great concern with the safety of artificial sweeteners.

Word Power

Mutagen

Pronunciation: \'myü-tə-jən\

Function: noun

Date: 1933

: an agent (as a chemical or various radiations) that tends to increase the frequency or extent of mutation

The fastest growing artificial sweetener is sucralose, also known as Splenda®. Sucralose is made chemically by combining chlorine molecules with sugar molecules. Dr. Susan Schiffman, a sweetener specialist and a professor of medical psychology at Duke University Medical Center, is among the many doctors and nutritionists that have safety concerns about sucralose. In a "New York Times" article, she noted that in the Food and Drug administration's 1998 report giving approval for sucralose they said it is "weakly mutagenic in a mouse lymphoma mutation assay." which means that it caused minor genetic damages in mouse cells, and further tests said sucralose is a possible carcinogen.[9]

---

7 The Journal of Nutrition, 1997, Vol. 127

8 "Mercury from chlor-alkali plants: measured concentrations in food product sugar" Dufault *et. al.*, Environmental Health 2009. http://www.ehjournal.net/content/8/1/2

9 "Sugar is Latest Super Market Demon" Melanie Warner, The New York Times, May 15, 2005.

Dr. Schiffman said, "The sucralose people keep saying, 'It's just a little bit of a mutagen.' Well, I don't want a little bit of a mutagen in my food supply. How do you know what happens in a long-life span or to the next generation or to your eggs and sperm? I don't feel like the issues have been answered.[8]"

There are many forms of artificial sweeteners, which include Splenda (sucralose), Sweet'N Low® (saccharin), Equal® and NutraSweet® (aspartame), acesulfame K and neotame. Artificial sweeteners are considered non nutritive sweeteners because they provide no calories when consumed. They have no calories because they do not nourish the body in any way, and because they are chemically made, the body identifies them as toxins and has to remove or store them to deal with later.

Artificial sweeteners are chemicals, not food! They are never a good idea to consume for anyone, but especially pregnant and lactating women, children and teenagers. Despite the reduced sugar content, the possible link to irreversible cell damage is not worth the risk. See Appendix P for more information about the specific artificial sweeteners.

Natural Sugar Substitutes

Not reserved just for special occasions anymore, sugary desserts and drinks abound. Many doctors recommend a reduced intake of sugar for prevention and treatment of diabetes, infections, and heart disease, and for ailments such as flu, cold, bronchitis, and urinary tract infections. They also suggest eliminating sugar from the diet to keep the immune system strong and guard against calcium loss. When a family starts making more healthy choices, naturally healthy sugar substitutes are a must.

Natural sweeteners tend to be less refined than white table sugar and contain small to generous amounts of vitamins and minerals. White sugar is refined to 100 percent sucrose. It is a refined carbohydrate that the body has a hard time using without the associated vitamins and minerals that were present in the plant, beet or sugar cane before refining.

Examples of natural sugar substitutes include **raw blue agave nectar**, **honey**, **maple syrup** and **molasses**. For a more complete list of natural sugar substitutes, how and when to use them and where to get them, see Appendix P.

Be a Label Reader!

While agave is becoming an ever popular sugar substitute, beware that not all agave is created equal. Much agave on the market has been highly processed (which is cheaper for companies to make), acts like high fructose corn syrup in the body and does not have a low glycemic index value. Beware of the word "agave syrup" or "light agave." Look for organic, raw blue agave nectar.

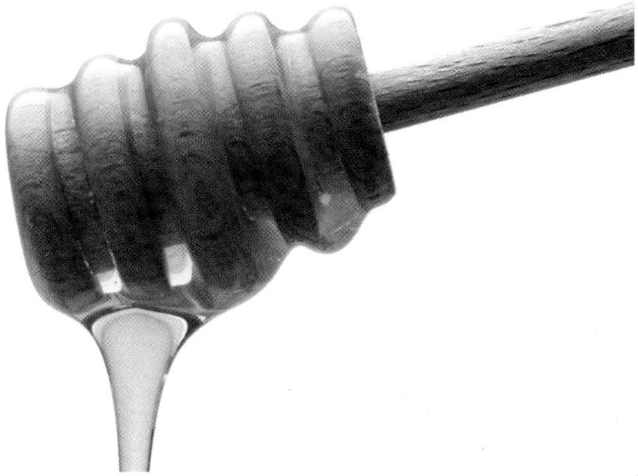

Unit 5 Chapter 4
Discussion Questions

1. Have you ever felt an afternoon crash and had a hard time keeping your eyes open while working, reading or even driving? Think about what you had for lunch. What kind of carbohydrates did you consume? How much of them did you eat?
2. Have you ever had a Charlie horse or muscle cramp? Why did this happen?
3. Did you learn something in this chapter that surprised you?
4. How many of the natural sweeteners have you tried?
5. What Bible stories include sweet foods?

Activities - plus the Almond Butter Chip Bars "Power" Recipe and activities.

Elementary

1. At the beginning of the chapter, it said that carbohydrates are often vilified. What does "vilify" mean? Write or give an oral report explaining why this term has been associated with carbohydrates.
2. Grow a sweet potato without soil to demonstrate how stored carbohydrates and photosynthesis work. Gather several wooden toothpicks, an organic sweet potato and a large glass container. First insert three toothpicks around the sweet potato near the large end so they stick out to the sides in different directions. Then, fill the glass container with water at least ½ full. Put the sweet potato into the container small-end first. The rest the toothpicks will rest on the rim and hold up the sweet potato. Fill the container with enough water so that about 3/4 of the sweet potato is submerged. Put the jar in a sunny spot for several days. Add water as needed. A vine will begin growing from the top of the potato. Explain what happened.
3. At the grocery store compare regular white sugar to organic unrefined sugar. What do you see?
4. While at the grocery store, find products that are labeled "all natural" and then check the ingredient list for artificial sweeteners.
5. "Carb Art" - Make carbohydrate artwork. Using dried lentils, beans and craft glue, create a mosaic with the carbs on cardboard, heavyweight poster board or canvas. Give it as a gift or display it in your home.

Secondary

Choose any from above plus

1. Repeat exercise #3 above. Did you find any? If so, research and then prepare a written or oral report on how an artificial sweetener can be labeled and approved as natural.
2. Using a chemistry text as a resource, draw a picture of what makes up a single glucose molecule and a sucrose molecule. Show in the drawing how the oxygen, hydrogen and carbon atoms are combined for each type of molecule.
3. Research to find out how refined sugar is made. Does sugar sound appetizing after what you have learned? Give you findings in an oral or written report.
4. The Corn Refiners Association (CRA), a trade organization of seven corn-refining companies, began a massive multimedia campaign in the United States to defend high fructose corn syrup (HFCS) against its critics. Review the CRA's Web site on HFCS. Find five inconsistencies on the site with what you've learned about HFCS and natural sweeteners either from this study or through independent research.
5. Using one of your family's favorite recipes that contains sugar, substitute a healthy sweetener for sugar. Use the conversion suggestions in Appendix P and experiment with the recipe until you get the right balance. Serve it during one of your family meals.
6. Take your Carb Art to the next level by embellishing other mediums such as pottery, picture frames, plywood or making jewelry.

Additional Resources

Web sites: Institute for Agricultural and Trade Policy: www.iatp.org

Books:

1. "21 Days to a Healthy Heart" Alan L. Watson, Bronze Bow Publishing, Inc. 2002.
2. "Sweet Deception: Why Splenda, NutraSweet and the FDA May Be Hazardous to Your Health" Joseph Mercola M.D., Nelson Books, 2006.

Immune System Power

Blue Agave Nectar

Organic, raw blue agave nectar is a great, low-glycemic alternative to using refined white sugar in recipes. Try to avoid refined white sugar as it is an immune system depressor.

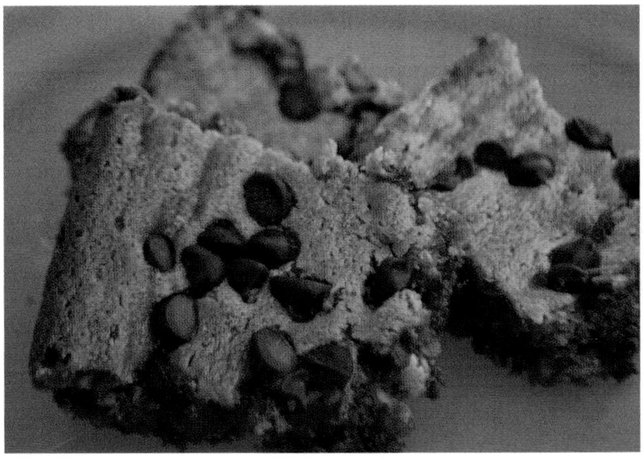

Almond Butter Chip Bars

1 – 16 ounce organic creamy almond butter (not "No Stir")
1 cup Blue Agave Nectar
2 eggs
1 tsp. vanilla extract
1 tsp. baking soda
½ tsp. sea salt
1 cup organic carob chips or organic dark chocolate chips

Mix almond butter with a hand blender until creamy. Add blue agave, eggs, vanilla, baking soda and sea salt. Mix well until all ingredients are thoroughly combined. Mix half of the carob chips or dark chocolate chips into the batter. Pour batter into a well greases 9x13 inch baking dish. Top with the rest of the carob or chocolate chips. Bake at 325° F for 25 to 30 minutes. Once out of the oven, it will look like a puffed up soufflé. Let it sit for five minutes before cutting and serving. Substitute other organic nut butters for unique flavors.

Activities

Elementary

1. Where are almonds most commonly grown in the U.S.?
2. Chapter 4 reported that in 2000 the average American consumed 148.9 pounds of caloric sweeteners, equal to 40 teaspoons for every man, woman and child every day or nearly three pounds per week. Find out how many teaspoons are in a pound. If you have a pound of a dry ingredient in the pantry, see if the answer to this question matches what the nutritional label says.
3. If you purchase eggs at the store, how many eggs come in a carton? What are the various sizes available?
4. What are the various grades of eggs sold in the grocery store and what do they mean?
5. Some eggs are white and others are brown. What is the difference in the coloring of eggs?

Secondary

Choose any from above plus

1. Besides almond, find other available butters in your market or online.
2. Experiment with this recipe by using almond butter or other alternatives to see what you like best.
3. The wording on egg cartons can be confusing. Visit a store and write down the terms used on the cartons and research to understand what these truly mean. Even research those that you think you know. (Examples: Omega-3, Cage-free, Free-range, organic, pasteurized)
4. Help plan a field trip to a farm with hens that produce eggs. Have a list of at least three questions ready for the person who provides the tour.

Unit 5 Additional Recipes

Use organic ingredients when possible.

Heart Healthy No Bake Chocolate Bars

Enjoy these bars as a breakfast or snack.

1 cup shredded coconut, unsweetened
1 cup ground hazel nuts, flax seeds, or Chia seeds
2 cups rolled oats
½ cup Blue Agave Nectar
¼ cup butter
Pinch of salt
1 tsp. vanilla
2 Tbs. cocoa powder

Combine coconut, ground nuts, oats, cocoa powder, salt and set aside. Combine butter, Agave and vanilla in a saucepan and heat until it begins to bubble. Pour over dry ingredients, stir and press into a 9 x 13 inch pan. Let cool until solid. Cut into squares and enjoy.

Classic Fresh Tomato Salsa

4 medium tomatoes, ripe
1 small onion
2 large jalapeno peppers
4 cloves garlic
½ cup fresh cilantro
2 Tbs. lime juice
1 tsp. cumin powder
dash salt
dash pepper

Dice all vegetables and combine with other ingredients, or place all ingredients in a food processor. Makes about seven cups and can be refrigerated for up to three days. Serve with non-GMO (genetically modified) organic corn chips, whole grain pita chips or fresh vegetables.

Sunshine Salad

2 ½ cups sweet potatoes, grated
2 ½ cups apples, grated
¾ cup shredded unsweetened coconut
¾ cup almonds, julienned
1 – 20 ounce can crushed pineapple, drain and reserve juice
2/3 cup raisins
juice of one lime

Mix ingredients together and drizzle ¼ cup of reserved pineapple juice into the mixture. Best when chilled for 8 hours before serving.

Tex Mex Soup

2 to 3 cups of hot beef stock or chicken stock
1 zucchini cut in one-inch slices
1 cabbage wedge cut in one-inch pieces
1 stalk green onion
3 cloves garlic
1 celery stalk with top
1 sliver green or red pepper
1 jalapeno slice
1 Roma tomato
2 sprigs cilantro
1 small carrot sliced
1 one-inch slice of cheddar cheese (optional)
Salt and pepper (optional)
¼ cup cooked rice, three or four non-GMO corn tortilla chips or ¼ cup of pinto beans (optional)

Combine ingredients into blender and run on low speed until all ingredients are chopped. Then switch to high and blend for one to one-and-a-half minutes. Turn blender to lowest speed and open top center and add rice, chips or beans. Blend only a few seconds, turn off machine and serve. Mixture will be warm because of the hot broth used. If it is not desired warmth, heat on medium in a saucepan for a few minutes.

Italian Pasta Sauce

This pasta sauce is a great base for many different types of Italian dishes from spaghetti to lasagna.

1 medium yellow onion
3-4 cloves freshly minced garlic
Organic extra virgin olive oil
2 – 28 ounce cans organic crushed tomatoes or 6-8 ripe tomatoes, chopped
3 fresh basil leaves, finely chopped (may use more to taste)
Sea salt and pepper to taste

Coat the bottom of a large stock pot with olive oil. Add the onions and garlic and sauté. Add the canned or fresh tomatoes, basil, sea salt and pepper. If adding fresh tomatoes, add a cup of water or more if it is still too thick. Simmer for up to five hours stirring occasionally. If desired, add cooked, ground organic beef, chicken or turkey while the sauce simmers. Serve over pasta or use in a baked pasta dish. Any leftover sauce can easily be kept in the freezer.

Carrot Cake

2 ½ cups carrots sliced
1 ¾ cup Blue Agave Nectar
4 eggs

cup olive oil
½ tsp. salt
3 tsp. cinnamon
2 tsp. baking soda
2 ¾ cup whole wheat flour

Cook carrots in small amount of water until tender. Drain and slow to cool. Puree carrots. In a large bowl, beat together agave and eggs. Add oil and carrots, blend well. Add remaining ingredients and blend. Pour into 9" by 13" greased and floured cake pan. Bake at 350° F for 35 to 40 minutes. Cool and then frost.

Honey or Blue Agave Cream Cheese Frosting

For a lower glycemic index value, substitute blue agave for honey

½ cup butter
8 oz. soft cream cheese
½ cup unprocessed honey
2 tsp. vanilla

Blend all ingredients until smooth and creamy. Use as icing for cakes and muffins.

Unit 6

The Endocrine System and Emotions

"Finally, brethren, whatsoever things are true, whatsoever things are honest, whatsoever things are just, whatsoever things are pure, whatsoever things are lovely, whatsoever things are of good report; if there be any virtue, and if there be any praise, think on these things. Those things, which ye have both learned, and received, and heard, and seen in me, do: and the God of peace shall be with you." Philippians 4:8-9

The function of the endocrine system, along with its hormone production and regulatory tasks of nearly every component of the human body, comprise the final unit in this study; in reality, it may be the most important unit of all. As we discuss the many functions of the endocrine system glands and how even minor imbalances can lead to dysfunction, it will bring together everything covered thus far as a complete program for health and wellness.

The way a person thinks and feels along with his or her attitudes and habits are determining factors in wellness or ill health. Emotions of anxiety, stress, worry and fear can lead to chronic digestive complaints and poor nutrient assimilation. Feelings of hopelessness, despair and laziness can lead to a sluggish, constipated digestive system.

When we fret or fuss, stew or simmer, worry, lie, are fearful, hold any negative emotion too long or choose not to forgive, we must stop and take a moment to think of the impact on our health. Although the food we eat and the chemicals we are exposed to are important factors in our health, many of the health conditions we face have roots in emotional and spiritual strongholds.

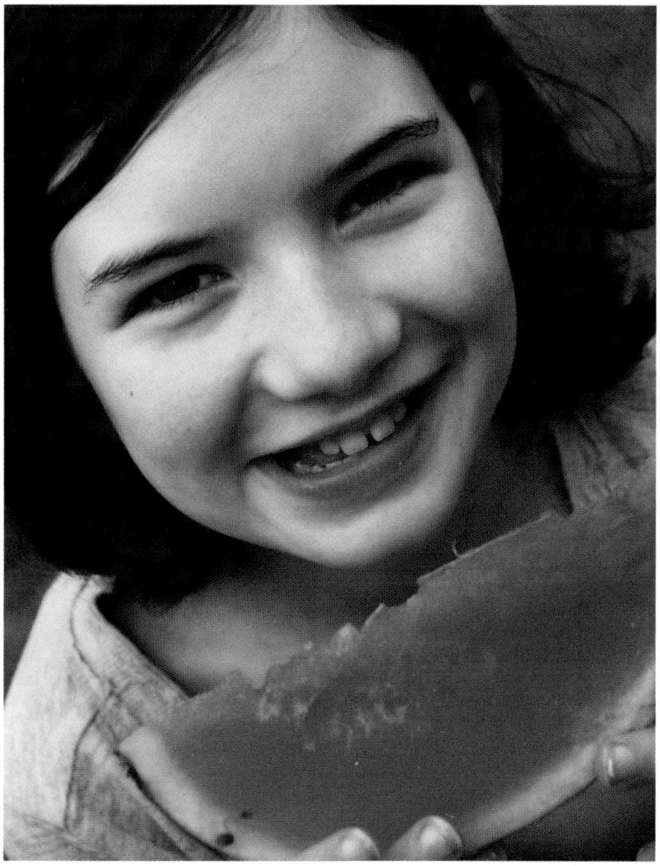

Chapter 1

The Endocrine System

"But the fruit of the Spirit is love, joy, peace, longsuffering, gentleness, goodness, faith, meekness, temperance: against such there is no law." Galatians 5:22-23

There are chemicals running throughout our bodies that are essential to life! They are good chemicals that the body needs to function in many ways – to regulate mood and emotions, for cell growth and development and to regulate metabolism and reproductive functions. These chemicals are called hormones and are produced and regulated by the endocrine system in a very intricate and delicate way. Too much or too little of these hormones will cause an imbalance that can have serious consequences to optimal health.

When the endocrine system is working at peak performance, a person feels great, looks great and his or her body is more able to defend itself against almost all infection and chronic disease. Today's lifestyle is a major culprit that undermines the endocrine system. Lack of exercise, poor or insufficient sleep, poor nutrition intake, prescription medication use and environmental toxin exposure all impact the endocrine system.

What is the endocrine system?

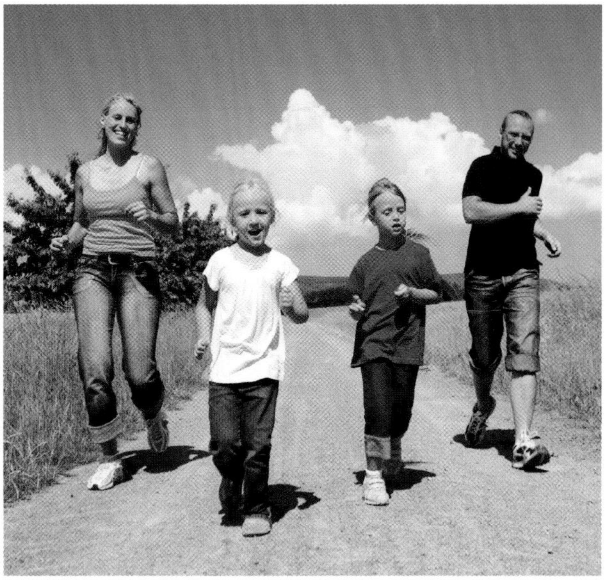

The **endocrine system** includes the hormones and the glands, such as the adrenal, pituitary, pancreas and thyroid glands to name a few, and is the master manipulator of the body. While the endocrine system regulates most slow processes of the body, it often works with the brain and nervous system to help with faster processes during certain situations, such as getting a rush of adrenaline when being startled or under stress. The gland called the hypothalamus located in the brain helps link the two systems together.

Besides the nervous system, the endocrine system also works with the reproductive system, kidneys, digestive system, liver, pancreas and fat cells. This collaboration helps maintain and control body energy levels, reproduction, growth and development, internal balance of body systems – or homeostasis – and responses to surroundings, stress and injury.

What are hormones?

Hormones are chemical messengers that are created in glands and travel throughout the body to specific areas with specific jobs. They carry special instructions and information from one set of cells called target cells to other cells. Some hormones travel through the bloodstream while others are released from a gland into the tissue immediately surrounding the gland such as salivary glands, or exocrine glands, releasing secretions directly into the mouth.

What are glands?

Glands are groups of cells that produce and give off, or secrete, hormones. They make hormones by gathering material from the blood, processing it and then secreting the finished chemical, or hormone, into certain areas of the body.

Some glands secrete hormones directly into the tissue surrounding them, such as sweat glands. Other glands, such as endocrine glands, secrete hormones directly into the bloodstream to be sent to other parts of the body. The major glands of the endocrine system include the hypothalamus, pituitary gland, pineal body, thyroid gland, parathyroid glands, adrenal glands and reproductive glands.

Major Endocrine Glands

The **hypothalamus** is the main connection of the nervous system to the endocrine system via the pituitary gland. It is located in the lower central part of the brain beneath the thalamus and right above the brain stem and controls the pituitary gland by stimulating how much or how little hormones are secreted by the pituitary gland. Widely regarded as the center of management for the immune system, the hypothalamus also is the center of emotions and memory.

The **pituitary gland** is the master of the endocrine system as it produces hormones that control many other glands. No bigger than a green pea, the pituitary gland sits beneath the hypothalamus at the base of the brain. The hypothalamus regulates the amount of hormones released by the pituitary depending on factors such as emotions and changes in seasons. It is divided into two parts: the anterior lobe and the posterior lobe.

> The **anterior lobe** regulates the activity of the thyroid, adrenals and reproductive glands and produces hormones. These hormones include growth hormone which stimulates the growth of bone and other body tissues and plays a role in the body's handling of nutrients and minerals. This includes prolactin which activates milk production in women who are breast feeding; thyrotropin, which stimulates the thyroid gland to produce thyroid hormones; and corticotrophin, which stimulates the adrenal gland to produce certain hormones. The pituitary also secretes endorphins, which are chemicals that act on the nervous system and reduce feelings of pain.
>
> The **posterior lobe** helps to regulate the balance of water in the body by producing antidiuretic hormone. It also triggers the contractions in a woman about to have a baby by producing oxytocin.

The **pineal body**, or **pineal gland**, is located in the middle of the brain and secretes melatonin, which is a hormone that helps regulate sleep and wake patterns, also known as the circadian rhythm. The pineal gland is stimulated to produce melatonin by nerves from the eyes. When it gets dark, more melatonin is released and promotes sleep. In the winter months when nights are longer, more melatonin is released.

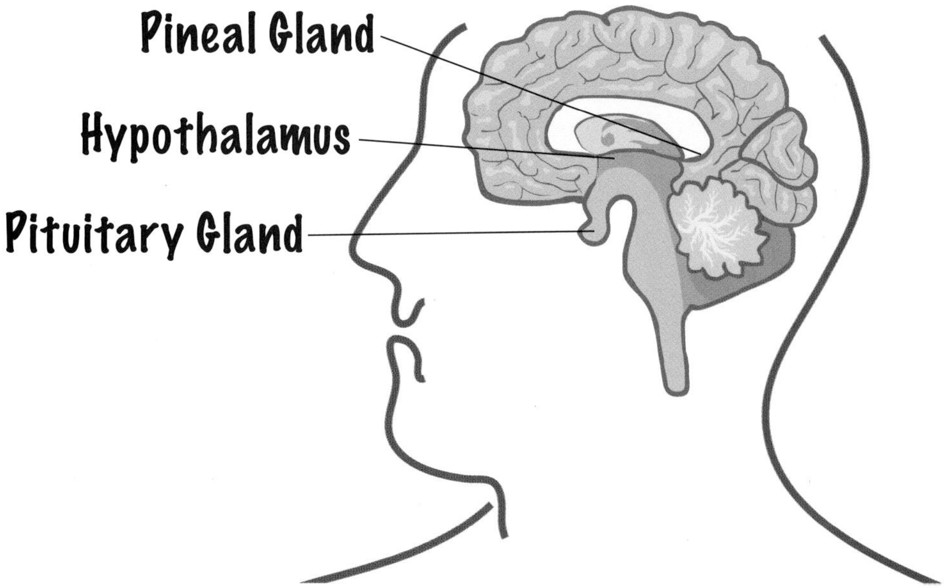

The **thyroid gland** is located in the front part of the lower neck and is shaped like a bow tie or butterfly. It produces two hormones that help kids' and teens' bones grow and develop, and they also play a role in the development of the brain and nervous system in young children and teens. The two hormones thyroxine and triiodothyronine are produced by the thyroid and control metabolism, which is the rate at which cells burn fuels from food to produce energy. The pituitary gland controls the production and release of thyroid hormones by secreting a hormone called thyrotropin. The more thyroid hormone there is in a person's bloodstream, the faster chemical reactions occur in the body.

Surrounding and attached to the thyroid are four tiny glands that function together called the **parathyroid glands**. They release parathyroid hormone, which along with the hormone called calcitonin made by the thyroid, regulates the level of calcium in the blood.

The **adrenal glands** are considered a major player in the endocrine system and are vitally important to health in general. The two triangular shaped adrenal glands each sit one on top of each kidney. They have two parts, each of which produces a set of hormones and has a different function. The **adrenal cortex** is the outer part and produces hormones called corticosteroids that regulate salt (sodium) and water balance in the body, the body's response to stress, metabolism, the immune system, and sexual development and function. The inner part of the adrenal glands is called the **adrenal medulla**, which produces epinephrine, also called adrenaline. Adrenaline increases blood pressure and heart rate when the body experiences stress.

The **reproductive glands** are a very important part of human growth, development, reproduction and overall health. As this subject may be a sensitive issue for younger audiences, a deeper discussion on the reproductive system and related health issues can be found in Appendix V.

As a quick overview, the male **testes** secrete hormones called androgens, the most important of which is testosterone. These hormones tell a boy's body when it's time to make the changes associated with puberty.

A female's **ovaries** produce eggs and secrete the female hormones estrogen and progesterone. Estrogen is involved when a girl begins to go through puberty. These hormones also play a role for women in pregnancy.

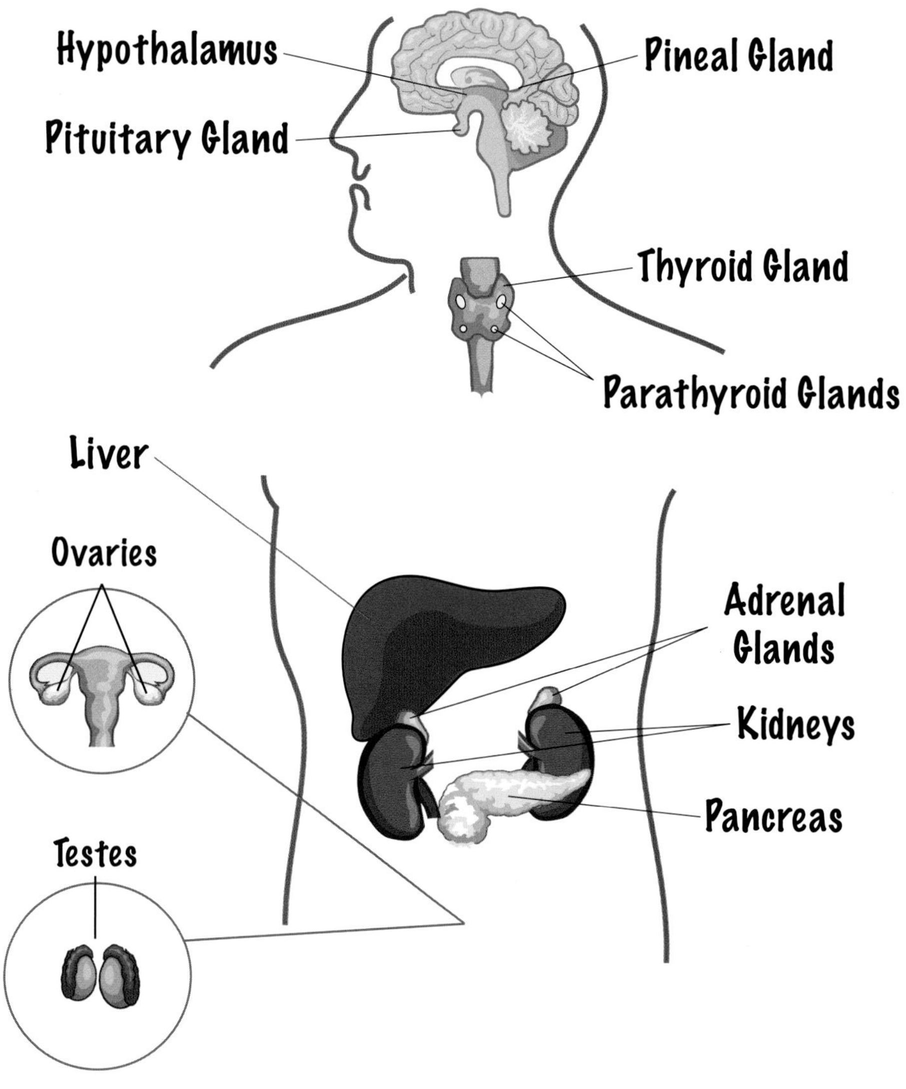

Organs, Glands or Both?

While the endocrine glands are the main hormone producers, there are several organs in the body that also produce and release hormones, such as the pancreas, liver and kidneys, which makes them glands as well.

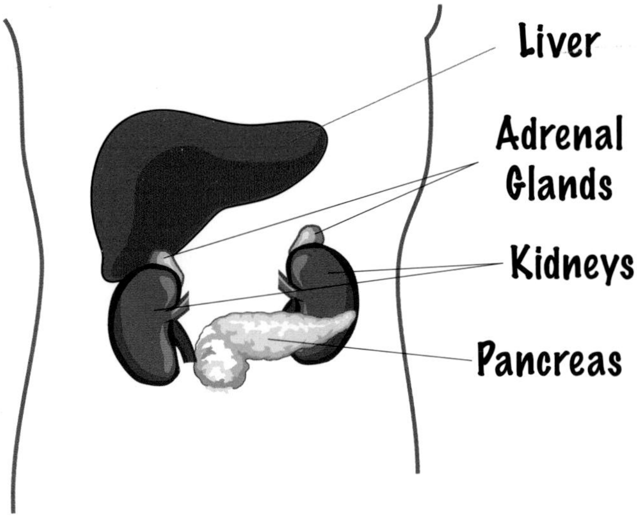

Pancreas

Even though it plays a role in the digestive system by producing and secreting digestive enzymes, the **pancreas** is part of the body's hormone-secretion system as well. The pancreas produces two important hormones, **insulin** and **glucagon**. They work together to maintain a steady level of glucose, or sugar, in the blood and to keep the body supplied with fuel to produce and maintain stores of energy.

The pancreas is a long spongy grayish-pink organ about six inches long that stretches across the back of the abdomen behind the stomach. The top of the pancreas is on the right side of the abdomen and is connected to the duodenum, which is the first section of the small intestine. The narrow end of the pancreas, called the tail, extends to the left side of the body.

The pancreas is a compound gland. It is compound in the sense that it is composed of both exocrine and endocrine tissues. The exocrine function of the pancreas involves the creation and secretion of pancreatic juices and enzymes for digestion. These powerful enzymes digest fats, proteins and carbohydrates. As pancreatic juices are made, they flow into the main pancreatic duct. This duct joins with the common bile duct, which connects the pancreas to the liver and the gallbladder. Exocrine tissue also makes bicarbonates that work to neutralize stomach acids.

The Pancreas and Hormones

The endocrine portion of the pancreas resides in the million or so cellular islands called the **islets of Langerhans**, which are embedded between the exocrine tissues of the pancreas. When glucose levels are too low in the bloodstream, alpha cells in the islets secrete glucagon signaling the liver to convert stored glucogen into glucose. Beta cells in the islets secrete insulin, which tells the body's cells to take in glucose from the bloodstream.

Liver

Located just below the diaphragm to the right of the stomach, the **liver** is the body's largest internal organ. It also is the largest gland in the body. The liver filters one quarter of the body's blood volume every minute and blocks harmful substances from getting into the blood, These substances include environmental toxins, worn out blood cells, toxins from medications, pesticides and herbicides obtained in food, and other chemicals, and many other harmful pathogens.

> **Fun Fact**
> Heavier than the brain, the liver weighs a whopping three and a half pounds!

Once a red blood cell is old and is no longer useful, big white blood cells residing in the liver called macrophages eat the old red blood cells. The hemoglobin from the old red blood cells contains iron that carried oxygen from the lungs to all the cells of the body. The liver recycles this iron, stores it for later use or turns it into bile, which it excretes as a digestive juice. Bile contains bilirubin, which is a yellow-orange pigment from the iron. When a liver is sick or sluggish, the bile backs up and the liver is not able to filter the blood. This causes the skin, eyes and urine to take on a yellow-orange color known as jaundice and is a good sign that the liver is very constipated.

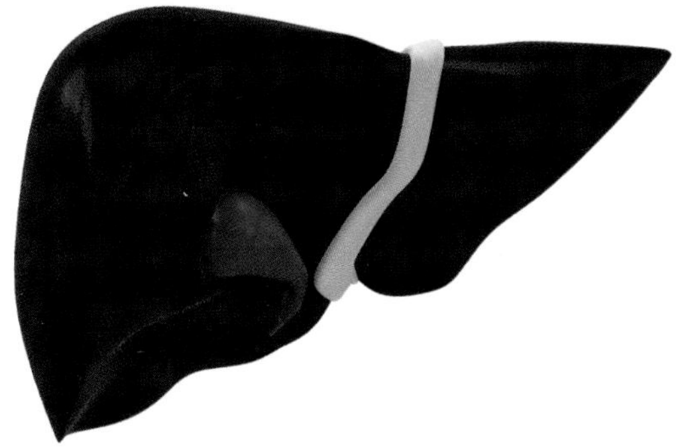

The Liver and Hormones

While the liver's connection to hormones is often overlooked, it plays a large role in the body's hormonal balance. The liver is responsible for breaking down many hormones, including cholesterol, testosterone and estrogen. Once the hormones have done their job in the body, the liver breaks them down so as to keep a healthy hormonal balance. The liver even produces and secretes a few hormones which include a hormone called Insulin-like Growth Factor 1 (IGF-1) that plays an important role in childhood growth. Another hormone secreted is a hormone called thrombopoietin which regulates the production of platelets by the bone marrow.

Kidneys

Kidneys are bean-shaped organs each the size of a fist that surround the spine. The right kidney sits below the diaphragm and behind the liver while the left kidney sits below the diaphragm and behind the spleen. Because of the liver, the right kidney is a little lower than the left.

The kidneys clean and filter the body's entire blood volume each hour while monitoring the quality of blood so that the body is not poisoned by the end-products of its own metabolism. They also help regulate blood pressure and the assimilation of vitamins into the bloodstream. Vitamins not used are excreted through the urine. Sometimes when urine is quite yellow it indicates the kidneys need a little more support or cleansing.

The kidneys also help to maintain proper acid/alkaline pH levels, which is important for disease prevention, weight balance and emotional health. Solely responsible for regulating the body's fluid balance, the kidneys help keep enough water on hand to prevent dehydration while at the same time prevent the holding of water – a condition often referred to as edema.

Fun Fact

Some people are born with only one kidney. The body is well able to function with only one kidney, which makes it possible for people to donate a kidney to a person who has lost the function of both.

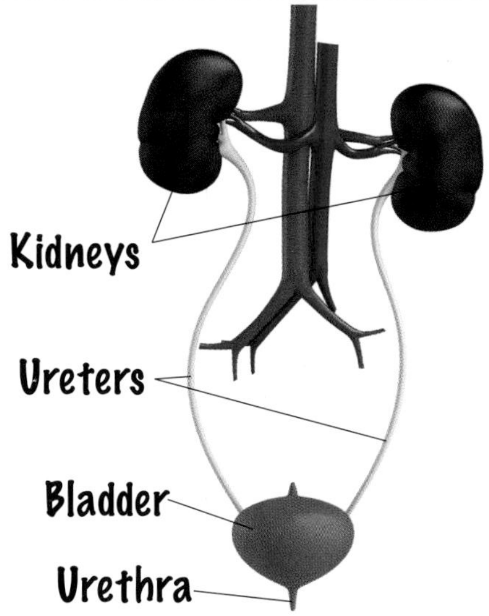

The Urinary Tract

The **urinary tract** includes the **kidneys**, **ureters**, **bladder** and **urethra**. Altogether, they filter and eliminate waste from the body. Once the kidneys have filtered waste from the blood, such as nitrogen waste products, excess sodium, urea, uric acid and excess water. It combines this waste into a liquid called **urine** which travels through the ureter and accumulates in the bladder and can be eliminated from the body through the urethra.

Kidneys and Hormones

Besides removing waste as an organ, the kidneys are also a gland and produce and secrete three important hormones:

- erythropoietin, which stimulates the bone marrow to make red blood cells
- rennin, which regulates blood pressure
- calcitriol, the active form of vitamin D, which helps maintain calcium for bones and for normal chemical balance in the body.

Fun Fact

Some cases of anemia may be linked to lowered kidney function, not just poor iron assimilation.

How does the endocrine system work?

Once an endocrine gland secretes a hormone, the hormone travels from the gland through the bloodstream to the target cells that were designed to receive its message. As it travels to the target cells, special proteins bind to some of the hormones and act as carriers that control the amount of hormone available for the cells to use.

The target cells and hormones each have receptors so that specific target cells will receive and communicate with only the correct hormones. When the hormone reaches its target cell, it locks onto the cell's receptors, and these hormone-receptor combinations transmit chemical instructions to the inner workings of the cell.

When hormone levels reach a specific normal amount, the endocrine system helps the body to keep that level of hormone in the blood. For example, once the thyroid gland has secreted the right amount of thyroid hormones into the blood, the pituitary gland makes sure that level remains normal. If it senses the levels too low, the pituitary gland adjusts its release of thyrotropin, the hormone that stimulates the thyroid gland to produce more thyroid hormones.

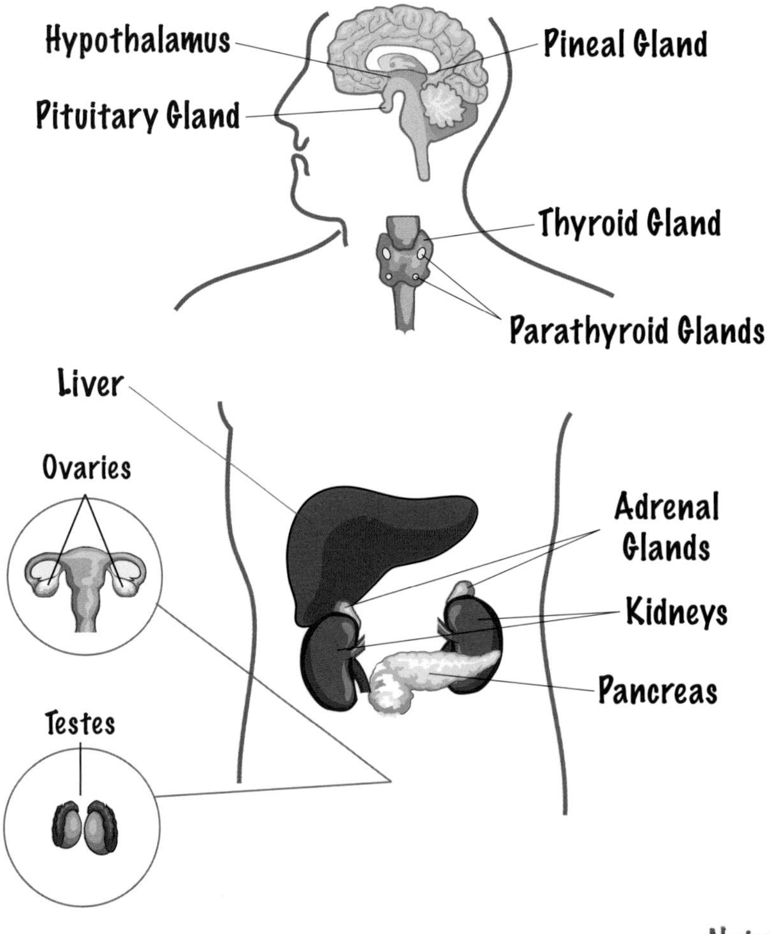

Unit 6 Chapter 1
Discussion Questions

1. Why is the endocrine system so important?
2. Could you function without an endocrine system?
3. Could you function without hormones?
4. Can you locate the various endocrine glands on your body?

Activities - plus the Ultimate Pizza "Power" Recipe and activities.

Elementary

1. Get a frozen pea and hold it up to your head to get an idea of how big the pituitary gland is inside of your brain. Write a poem expressing how amazing it is that God made such a tiny thing to do so many important things in the body.
2. With modeling clay, create a model of the thyroid and parathyroid glands.
3. What is the body's largest organ? Review this chapter and make a list of the ways glands support this organ.
4. Using a scale, find an item nearby that weighs the same as your liver.

Secondary

Choose any from above plus

1. Research the circadian rhythm in humans and the history of its discovery. What is it? What factors affect it? What biological processes does it regulate? Do other living things have a circadian rhythm? Give your findings in an oral or written report.
2. Research to find out when and on who the first successful kidney transplant was performed. Give your findings in an oral or written report.
3. What are the types of jaundice typically affecting adults? Which ones are predominantly found in newborn babies?
4. What hormones, organs and glands are necessary for proper digestion?

Endocrine System Power
Tomatoes

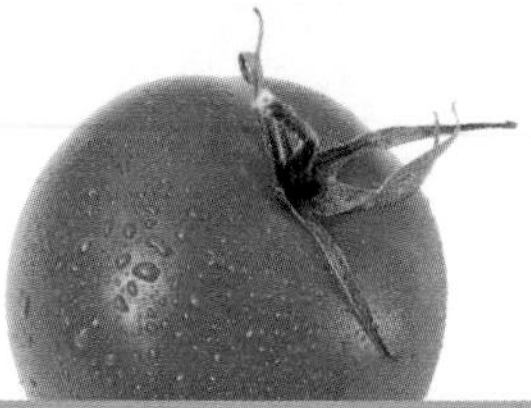

Tomatoes are high in lycopene which helps support normal blood sugar levels.

Ultimate Pizza

This is a family favorite! Each time you make this pizza, try adding a new healthy ingredient.

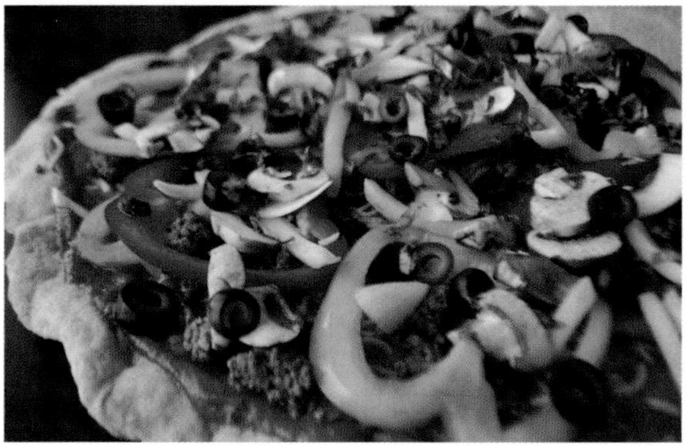

Honey wheat pizza crust

(makes 2 pizza crusts)
1 ½ cups organic whole wheat flour
1 ½ cups organic unbleached all-purpose flour
1 Tbs. active dry yeast
¼ tsp. sea salt
2 Tbs. olive oil
1 Tbs. honey
1 cup warm water

Pizza Sauce

½ cup onion, diced
2 cloves garlic, minced
3 Tbs. plus ¼ cup extra virgin olive oil
2 Tbs. fresh basil, minced
1 tsp. ground oregano
½ tsp. to 1 tsp. ground black pepper or to taste
1 can organic diced tomatoes, drained
1 can organic tomato puree
3 Tbs. organic tomato paste
2 tsp. Blue Agave Nectar

Toppings

Lean ground meat – beef, turkey or chicken
Shredded chicken
Onions (white, yellow or red)
Bell peppers
Mushrooms
Black olives
Tomatoes
Artichoke
Asparagus
Spinach
Squash
Zucchini
Organic mozzarella
Organic feta

For the crust - In a separate bowl, combine the whole wheat and all-purpose flour. In a large mixing bowl, combine 1 ¼ cups of the flour, yeast and sea salt; add warm water, oil and honey. Beat with an electric mixer on low speed for 30 seconds and then scrape bowl. Beat on high speed for three minutes. Using a wooden spoon, stir in as much of the remaining flour as possible. Turn dough out onto a lightly floured surface and knead in remaining flour for six to eight minutes to make a moderately stiff, smooth and elastic dough. Divide dough in half, cover with a damp cloth and let rest for 15 minutes. Sprinkle pizza pan or pizza stone with olive oil. Press dough out with olive oil sprinkled on top. Bake in 400 degree oven for 10 minutes or until lightly brown on the edges.

For the sauce - In small sauté pan, add olive oil. Once hot, add onions and garlic and sauté until onions are translucent. Add basil, oregano and pepper. In blender, add diced tomatoes, tomato puree, remaining olive oil, sautéed onions, garlic and spices and raw blue agave (the secret ingredient) and blend until smooth.

Top baked pizza dough with sauce and then with favorite toppings, especially the vegetables. Get creative! Bake another 10 minutes or until crust is lightly brown and cheese, if any, is melted. Enjoy!

Activities - continued on the following page.

Ultimate Pizza - continued

Activities

Elementary

1. Why are fresh herbs superior to dried herbs? If you do not grow herbs, check the produce section of your market to select herbs needed for this recipe. (If fresh herbs are not available, select organic dried herbs.) After using the fresh herbs, find out how to store any leftovers and how long they will last.
2. Help prepare the ingredients for the dough. Why must the water be warm?
3. When topping your pizza, see how many different colors you can add.
4. For many among the Italian-American population, the first American pizzas were known as tomato pie. Present-day tomato pie commonly is found in the Northeastern United States. Research the difference between tomato pie and pizza.
5. Research the differences between the various types of onions. Examine and taste the various kinds and observe any differences you find.

Secondary

Choose any from above plus

1. Complete activity #5 above. Then, research the varieties of onions and their nutritional or medicinal value. On an index card, write the names and characteristics of the onions kept in your pantry and attach it to the bin or shelf where the onions are stored.
2. Although historically attributed to the Italians, pizza dates back to the 6th century B.C. Find out more about the first documented culture to enjoy pizza and share this information with your family as you enjoy eating the Ultimate Pizza.
3. What is the difference between active yeast and inactive yeast? Why is it good to limit your intake of active yeast?
4. Check out the menu offerings of various pizza restaurants where you live or online. Use these as inspiration to create healthier versions of pizza varieties.

Chapter 2

Endocrine Health and Vitamins

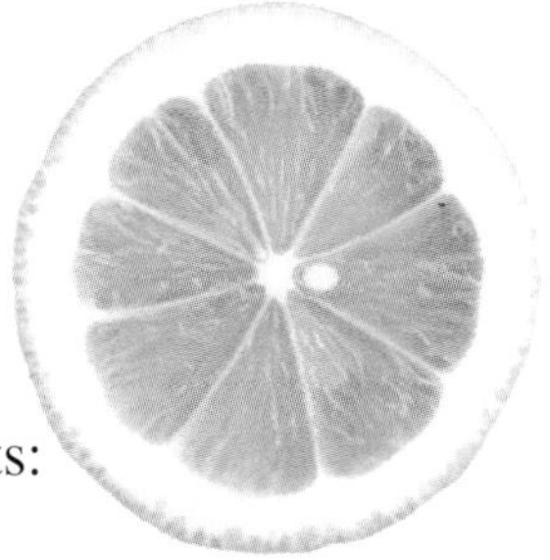

"My son, forget not my law; but let thine heart keep my commandments:
For length of days, and long life, and peace, shall they add to thee.
Let not mercy and truth forsake thee: bind them about thy neck;
write them upon the table of thine heart:
So shalt thou find favour and good understanding in the sight of God and man.
Trust in the Lord with all thine heart; and lean not unto thine own understanding.
In all thy ways acknowledge him, and he shall direct thy paths.
Be not wise in thine own eyes: fear the Lord, and depart from evil.
It shall be health to thy navel, and marrow to thy bones."
Proverbs 3:1-8

The endocrine system is very intricate and affects every body system through its chemical messengers – hormones. However, it is very delicate and can easily become imbalanced by toxins, nutrient deficiencies, poor eating habits, physical and emotional stress and even lack of sleep. Too much or too little of any hormone can be harmful to the body. For example, if the pituitary gland produces too much growth hormone, a teen may grow excessively tall. If it produces too little, she may be unusually short. When in balance, the endocrine system helps to create a solid foundation of optimal health.

Hypothalamus

The hypothalamus is the main connection of the endocrine system to the brain. **Vitamin C** is the number one nutrient needed by the hypothalamus for optimal performance. See Appendix F for a list of foods high in vitamin C.

Pituitary Gland

Health issues with a poor functioning pituitary gland include too little growth-hormone production causing stunted growth. Too much growth-hormone production may result in gigantism in adolescents. Hypoglycemia also may occur in infants and young children with growth-hormone deficiency.

Tumors in the pituitary can cause excessive production of corticotropin and can over stimulate production of corticosteroids in the adrenals, causing Cushing syndrome. Large doses of corticosteroids taken by children to treat autoimmune diseases, such as lupus, also may cause Cushing syndrome. Symptoms of Cushing syndrome may take years to develop and include obesity, growth failure, muscle weakness, acne, easy bruising of the skin, high blood pressure and psychological changes.

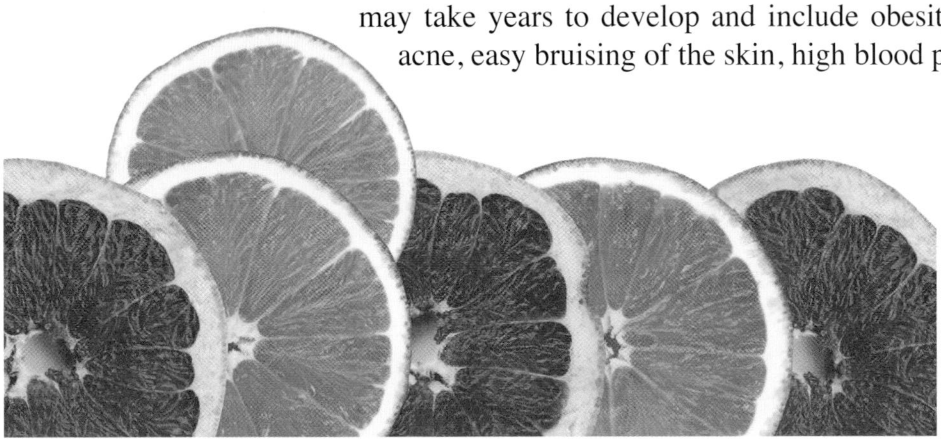

Vitamins C and **E** concentrate in the pituitary and aid in its function. The pituitary gland is one of the largest tissue stores of vitamin C. See Appendix F for a list of foods high in vitamins C and E.

Thyroid Gland

Hyperthyroidism is a condition in which the levels of thyroid hormones in the blood are very high. In children and teens, hyperthyroidism is usually caused by Graves' disease, which is an immune system problem that causes the thyroid gland to become very active. Excessive amounts of aluminum in the body may accumulate in the thyroid and may cause over activity. Symptoms of an overactive thyroid include weight loss, nervousness, tremors, excessive sweating, increased heart rate and blood pressure, protruding eyes and a swelling in the neck due to an enlarged thyroid gland, or goiter.

Hypothyroidism is a condition in which the levels of thyroid hormones in the blood are very low. Hashimoto's thyroiditis is an immune system problem that often causes damage to the thyroid and blocks the production of thyroid hormones. Thyroid hormone deficiency slows body processes and may lead to fatigue, a slow heart rate, dry skin, weight gain and constipation. Children and teens with this condition may also grow more slowly and reach puberty at a later age.

Studies show that excessive consumption of monosodium glutamate (MSG) may cause atrophy of the thyroid.

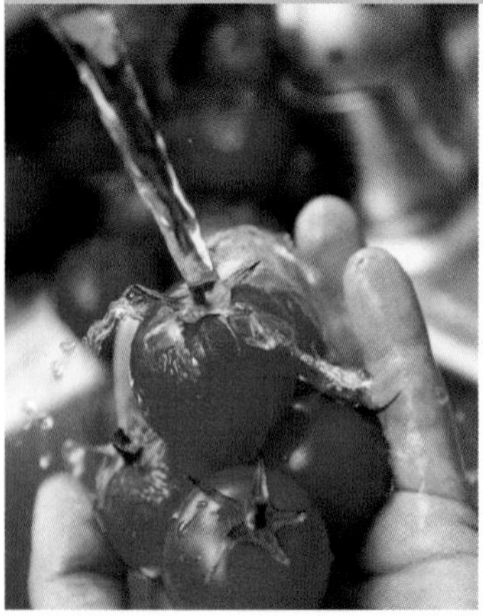

Nutrients for thyroid support include **beta-carotene** and **lycopene** which both concentrate in the thyroid and presumably enhance its function. Beta-carotene is a precursor to vitamin A and is found in yellow and orange fruits, orange vegetables and in green leafy vegetables. Lycopene is found in tomatoes and may help prevent cancer.

The minerals **boron**, **iodine** and **zinc** also may improve thyroid function. Nearly 20 percent of the body's iodine is used by the thyroid gland. See Appendix G for a list of foods high in iodine and zinc.

Vitamin A is required for optimal function of the thyroid as it contains higher concentrations of vitamin A than any other gland. Thyroid malfunction may occur as a result of vitamin A deficiency and also of **vitamin B2** deficiency. See Appendix F for a list of foods high in vitamins A and B2.

Essiac, which is a mixture of herbs that primarily contains Sheep Sorrel, is claimed to enhance the function of the thyroid gland. **Therapeutic-grade essential oils** such as lemongrass, myrrh, spearmint and wintergreen may help support the thyroid.[12]

Parathyroid Glands

Health issues of the parathyroid include hyperparathyroidism caused by a tumor on one of the parathyroid glands. The benign tumor called an adenoma causes the release of too much parathyroid hormone which pulls calcium out of the bones then causing excessive amounts of calcium in the blood. Hyperparathyroidism may lead to osteoporosis.

Nutrients to support the parathyroid glands include **boron**, which is found in plants, with highest concentrations in plants grown in arid climates. Supplementation is generally not needed as long as plenty of fresh vegetables and fruit are consumed. A few exceptions are in cases of compromised bone health and post-menopausal women who are magnesium deficient. Studies have shown that three milligrams of boron a day resulted in improvements in calcium and magnesium retention, and elevated levels of estrogen and testosterone.[3]

---

1 Use only therapeutic-grade essential oils that are of the highest quality and may be ingested. Beware of most essential oils that are for external use only and/or have expiration dates. See Appendix DD for the authors' recommendations.

2 "Essential Oils Desk Reference" Fourth Edition, Essential Science Publishing, 2007.

3 Alexander G. Schauss, Ph.D, AIBR Life Sciences Division, Tacoma, WA http://www.traceminerals.com/products/boron.html

Pineal Gland

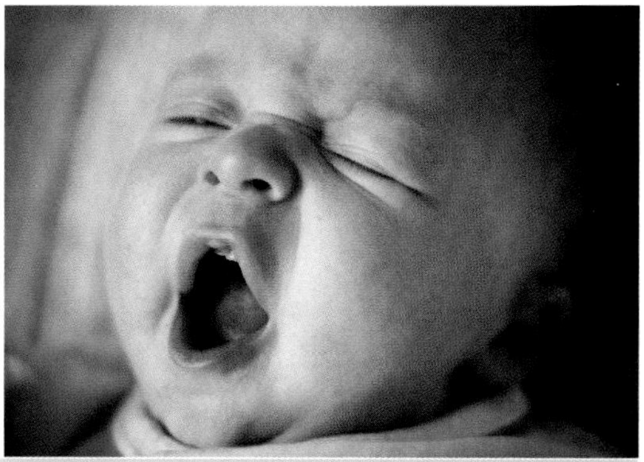

As the pineal gland helps regulate sleep patterns and the amount of melatonin production in the body, too much melatonin can cause health problems. In northern-most regions of the world where there is little to no sunlight during winter days, too much melatonin is an issue for many resulting in **seasonal affective disorder** (SAD). Those affected with SAD often oversleep and experience depression, tiredness, weight gain and sadness. Treatments include being exposed to bright lights for several hours a day to reduce the amount of melatonin in the body.

Fun Fact - Early morning sunshine is a great way to wake up the pineal gland and get ready for the day.

Adrenal Glands

Adrenal insufficiency is a health issue of the adrenal glands. This condition occurs when the adrenal glands do not produce enough corticosteroid hormones. The symptoms of adrenal insufficiency may include weakness, fatigue, abdominal pain, nausea, dehydration and skin changes.

Pantothenic acid, also known as **vitamin B5**, and **vitamin C** are two of the primary nutrients needed by the adrenals. Physical and mental stress and the presence of mercury increase adrenal activity and deplete vitamin B5 and C from the glands. **Vitamin B5** has been observed to activate the adrenal glands and may revive exhausted adrenal glands,[4] while a vitamin B5 deficiency may lead to the destruction of the adrenals. The adrenals are one of the largest tissue stores of **vitamin C**. If vitamin C stores are low, the adrenals will pull the vitamin C from other locations in the body leading to inadequate immune function. As learned in the previous unit, white blood cells need vitamin C to be able to kill and digest pathogens. If vitamin C is not readily available, pathogens are free to damage the body and the immune system suffers.

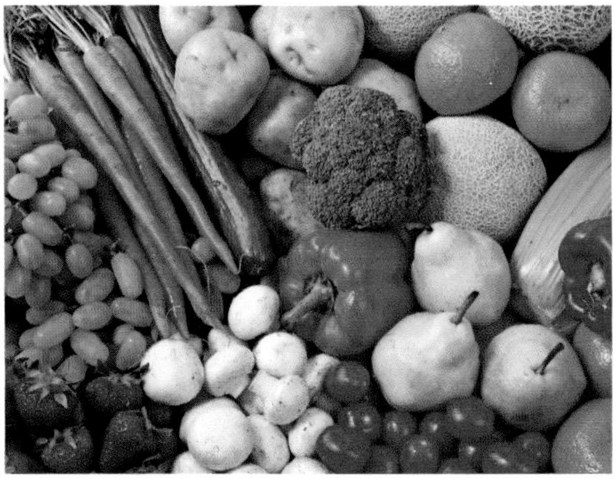

Vitamin A and **choline** concentrate in the adrenal glands and also may improve their function. For a list of food high in vitamin A, C, B5 and choline, see Appendix F.

Calcium, **chromium**, **zinc** and **magnesium** may be required for healthy function of the adrenal glands. See Appendix G for a list of foods high in these minerals.

Another aid to adrenal gland support is good **sleep**. See Appendix X about good sleep for good health.

Fun Fact

To see if the adrenal glands may need some support, look in the eyes up close in a mirror. Look at one eye, paying attention to the pupil. Does it slowly expand and contract as the eye focuses, or does it appear to have its own heartbeat? Is it about one-third the size of the iris or larger? If it seems to have its own heartbeat or is larger than half the circumference of the iris, the adrenals may need supplementation with vitamin C and pantethenic acid, or vitamin B5, as well as better sleep.

---

4 "Nutritional and botanical interventions to assist with the adaptation to stress" Kelly, G. S. Alternative Medicine Review. 4(4):249-265, 1999.

Reproductive Glands

See Appendix V for health-related issues of the reproductive glands and the nutrients that best support them.

Pancreas

Diseases of the pancreas include pancreatitis and cancer of the pancreas. The most common health issue involving the pancreas is diabetes which, according to the American Diabetes Association, affects 23.6 million Americans and 57 million Americans with pre-diabetes.

Pancreatitis is inflammation of the pancreas, which is caused when the digestive enzymes become activated inside of the pancreas instead of in the duodenum and start digesting the pancreas itself. Causes of pancreatitis are gallstones, gallbladder disease, alcoholism, cystic fybrosis, some drugs and autoimmune conditions, which can lead to destruction of the pancreas, bacterial infections and Type 2 diabetes.

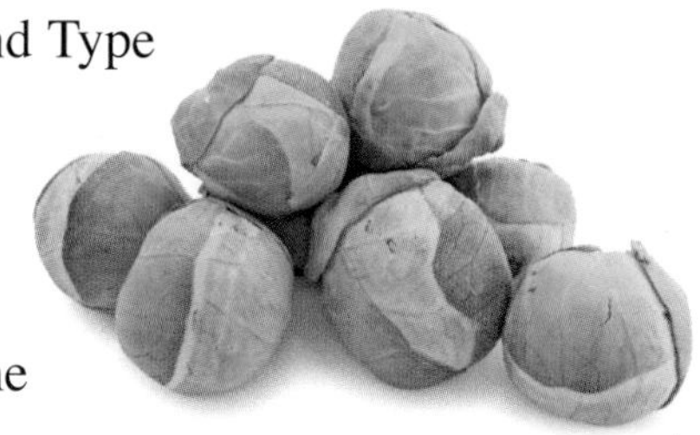

Cancer of the pancreas is the fourth leading cause of cancer death in the United States, killing about 34,000 people a year.[5] Risks are based on smoking, age, gender (more common in men), chronic pancreatitis and exposure to some industrial chemicals. See Appendix W for more information about cancer.

Fun Fact

While not a food many kids or adults willing included in their diet, Brussels sprouts are an amazingly powerful food everyone should eat more often. According to several studies, Brussels sprouts detoxify aflatoxin, a fungus linked to cancer, particularly liver cancer.[1] Aflatoxin has been found in peanuts, corn and rice. A diet rich in Brussels sprouts has been shown to reduce DNA damage, which also may decrease cancer risk. They contain vitamin A and beta-carotene which play important roles in supporting the immune system and are rich sources of iron, lutein and zeaxanthin.

1 "IARC Handbooks of Cancer Prevention Volume 9: Cruciferous Vegetables, Isothiocyanates and Indoles" International Agency for Research on Cancer, World Health Organization, IARC Press, Lyon, 2004.

There are two main types of diabetes – Type 1 and Type 2. **Type 1 diabetes**, previously known as juvenile diabetes, occurs in young children and teens when the pancreas fails to produce enough insulin. It is usually an autoimmune disorder, which means that some parts of the body's immune system attack and destroy the beta cells of the pancreas that produce insulin. To control their blood sugar levels and reduce the risk of developing diabetic problems, Type 1 diabetics generally require regular injections of insulin.

With **Type 2 diabetes** the body does not respond normally to insulin and becomes resistant to it so that glucose is not received by the cells. The condition is often combined with reduced insulin secretion. Children, teens and adults with this condition tend to be overweight. Complications with Type 2 diabetes include heart disease and stroke. Some Type 2 diabetics can control their blood sugar level with dietary changes, exercise and nutritional supplements. However, some may require medications and even insulin injections. See Appendix DD for more information on overcoming diabetes naturally.

Chromium is an important mineral in helping to regulate blood sugar. Chromium is found in foods such as onions, tomatoes and romaine lettuce.

5 "SEER Cancer Statistics Review, 1975-2005" Ries LAG, Melbert D, Krapcho M, Stinchcomb DG, Howlader N, Horner MJ, Mariotto A, Miller BA, Feuer EJ, Altekruse SF, Lewis DR, Clegg L, Eisner MP, Reichman M, Edwards BK (eds). National Cancer Institute. Bethesda, MD, http://seer.cancer.gov/csr/1975_2005/, based on November 2007 SEER data submission, posted to the SEER web site, 2008.

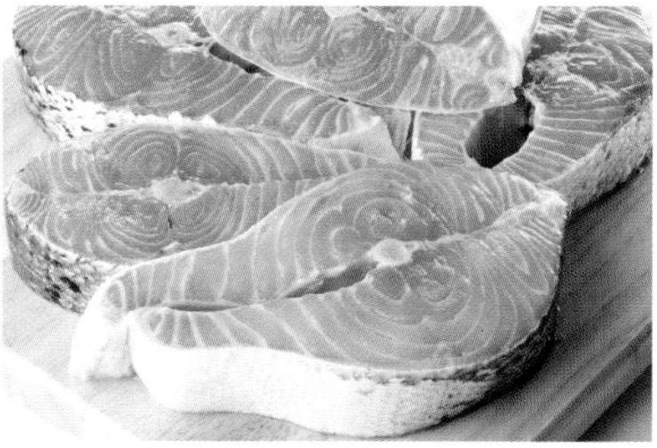

The antioxidant nutrients **vitamin C** and **E** aid the body in blood sugar balance. Diabetics often deal with bacterial infections, and vitamin C helps to boost the immune system to aid in fighting off the infections. See Appendix F for a list of foods high in vitamin C and E.

Omega-3 fatty acids are helpful to cardiovascular health and studies have shown that populations that eat fish regularly have low incidences of Type 2 diabetes.

Foods high in **fiber** and **protein**, such as legumes, have a beneficial effect on blood sugar regulation.

Cinnamon stimulates insulin receptors and significantly increases cells' ability to use glucose. Cinnamon bark essential oil is the most potent form of cinnamon.[6]

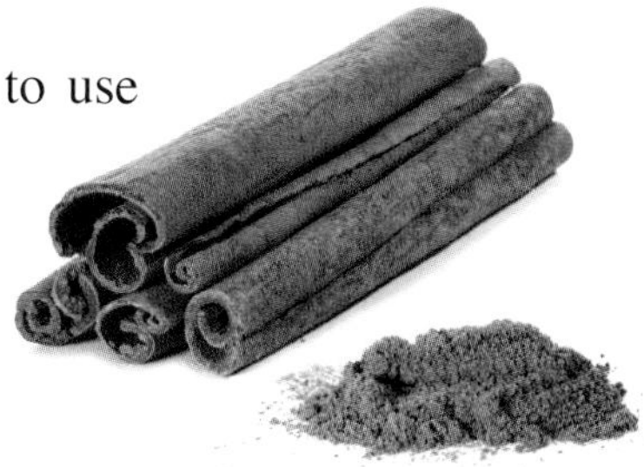

See Unit 6 Chapter 3 for more detailed information about diabetes.

Liver

Because the liver breaks down and even produces hormones, it is crucial to the health of the endocrine system and to all the systems in the body. If the liver gets sick or sluggish, it is unable to do its job of cleaning out the bloodstream, and thus the whole body, of harmful waste and toxins. Numerous health conditions can be a direct result of a clogged up, poorly functioning liver - bad breath, constipation, allergies, food cravings, fatigue, digestion problems, cancer, IBS, slow metabolism, weight gain, hormonal imbalances, and the list goes on. If the liver could not do its job at all and completely failed, a person would be dead in a matter of hours.

How do you protect the liver?

Stop doing the things that make it sluggish – eating fatty foods, too many sugary foods and excessive red meat, drinking alcohol, using harmful household chemicals, taking prescription and over the counter medications – and start doing things that promote a healthy liver.

Cleansing

Now for the fun part, getting the liver clean and restoring optimal health.

Note: When doing any type of liver cleanse, be sure the colon is working well first, otherwise the toxins flushed from the liver can cause constipation and ill feelings common with improper cleansing.

Fun Fact - One of the best liver cleanses to start with is eating all raw vegetables and fruits for five days.

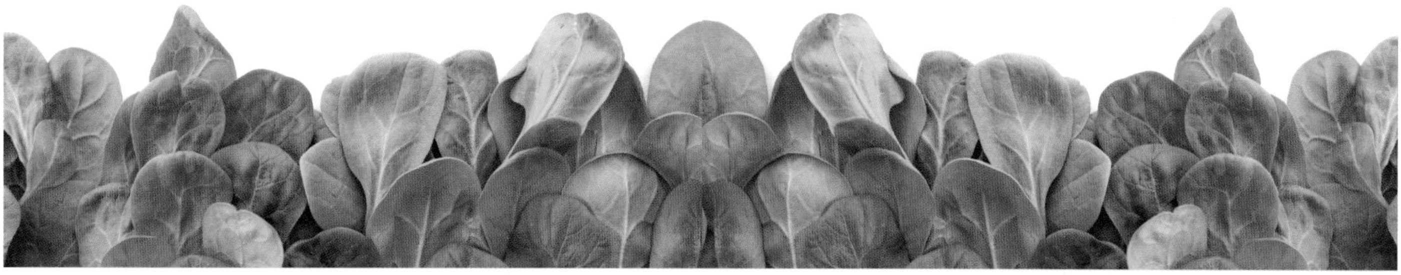

6 See Appendix DD for authors' recommendations.

Nutrients for the Liver

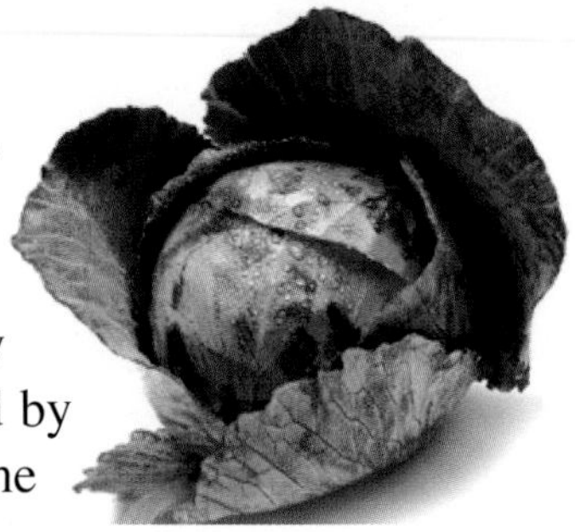

Biotin, also known as vitamin B7, is a B-complex vitamin and may improve the function of the liver.

Choline may be essential for the normal function of the liver and may prevent dietary fats from accumulating in the liver. **Fatty degeneration of the liver**, caused by a fatty liver and a leading cause of liver transplants, may occur as a symptom of choline deficiency.

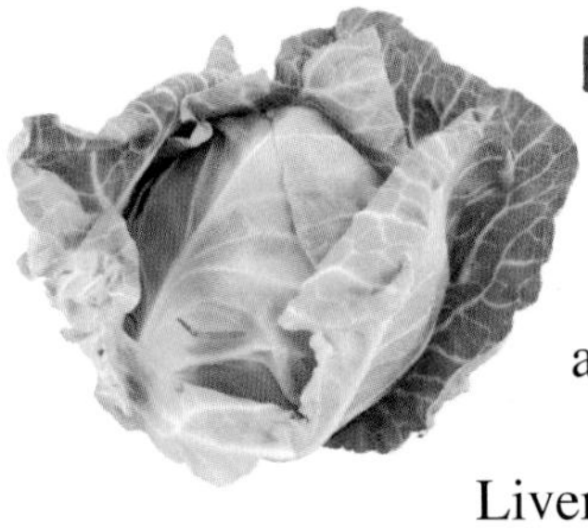

Folic acid may enhance the function of the liver by inhibiting the ability of homocysteine to damage the liver. **Inositol** may facilitate the removal of fats from the liver.

Lipoic acid may protect the liver from the toxic effects of many pharmaceutical drugs and toxins, such as toxic mushrooms, alcohol, carbon tetrachloride and toxic minerals.

Liver malfunction may reduce the body's absorption of vitamin A, therefore, supplementation with whole food **vitamin A** may improve the function of the liver. The niacinamide form of **vitamin B3** may inhibit the ability of alcohol to damage the liver. **Vitamin B5**, especially the pantethine form of vitamin B5, may protect the liver from the toxic effects of alcohol and carbon tetrachloride and may inhibit the ability of ibuprofen to destroy liver cells.

Ailments of the liver may increase the body's **vitamin B6** requirements and under-functioning of the liver may occur as a result of vitamin B6 deficiency. **Vitamin C** may prevent oxidative damage, the damage caused by free radicals, in the liver caused by tobacco smoking and alcohol.

See Appendix F for a list of foods high in these vitamins.

Kidneys

The most common causes of kidney disease are diabetes and high blood pressure. **Diabetes** keeps the body from utilizing glucose in the bloodstream. The excess glucose in the blood can act as a poison to the kidneys and damage them. **High blood pressure** damages the small blood vessels of the kidneys hindering them from being able to filter waste from the blood. Other causes of kidney disease are excessive toxins in the body, some prescription drugs, overused over-the-counter drugs and physical trauma. People with permanent kidney failure must undergo dialysis or kidney transplantation to stay alive.

Symptoms of poorly functioning kidneys include:

bladder infections
kidney infections
incontinence and urinary urgency
kidney stones
kidney failure
skin rashes
fatigue
cancer
elevated blood sugar
brain fog

Fun Fact
Some cases of anemia may be linked to lowered kidney function, not just poor iron assimilation.

All of which can be prevented, even healed, if a person is willing to adopt a healthy food program, exercise, establish a periodic cleanse routine, nourish the kidneys and have a healthy attitude.

So how do we keep these two fist-size organs healthy?

1. Drink plenty of good clean water. Drinking half your body weight in ounces is a good rule to follow. Adding a squeeze of fresh lemon can help alkalize the water for better health.
2. Eat about 75 percent of your food raw. This includes vegetables, fruits, nuts and seeds as they will still retain not only their enzymes and nutrients but their higher water content as well.
3. Avoid all sodas and coffee, as both are highly acidic.

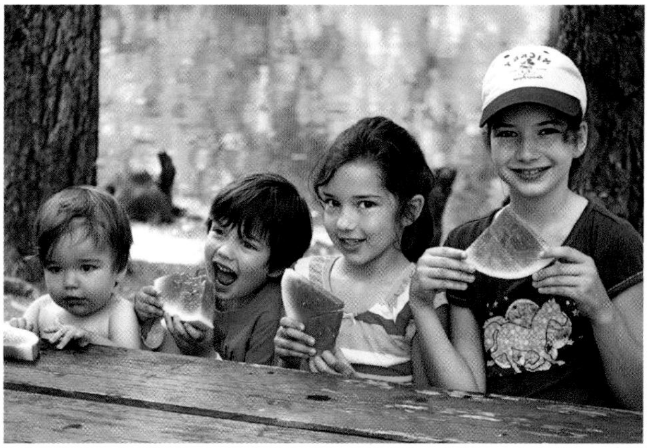

Treat your kidneys with love and care. So along with joining the LLC (Liver Lovers Club), consider enrolling in the KLC (Kidney Lovers Club) as well. Both are free and will pay you back with a lifetime of great health.

Foods good for the kidneys are those that are packed with high water content such as melons, canteloupe, cucumber, cranberries, summer and zucchini squash, parsley, fennel and beets.

Bad items for the kidneys include heavily salted and smoked foods.

Vitamins for the Kidneys

Biotin may enhance the function of the kidneys. **Choline** deficiency may cause kidney dysfunction. **Vitamin B1** concentrates in the kidneys. **Lipoic acid** may prevent the kidney damage, a common side effect of diabetes known as diabetic nephropathy, that may inhibit damage to the kidneys.

Environmental Toxins

Carbon tetrachloride was once widely used as a solvent, pesticide and in fire extinguishers, but once it was discovered that it caused severe damage to the liver and kidneys, manufacturers stopped using it. However, in 2008, a study of common cleaning products found carbon tetrachloride in very high concentrations due to the manufacturers' mixing of soap with **sodium hypochlorite**.[7]

Good Foods for the Endocrine System

Whole grains, legumes, nuts, all vegetables - celery, moderate use of sea salt, hard fleshed fruits – apples, pears, citrus fruits (not juices), fish, eggs, chicken, flax, chia seeds, sesame seeds, sunflower seeds

Bad Foods for the Endocrine System

Refined sugar, sodas, caffeine, chocolate, bananas and dried fruits (contain too much fruit sugar for diabetics), alcohol, fried foods

7 "Halogenated Volatile Organic Compounds from the Use of Chlorine-Bleach-Containing Household Products" Odabasi M Environmental Science & Technology, 2008, **42** (5): 1445–1451.

What are vitamins?

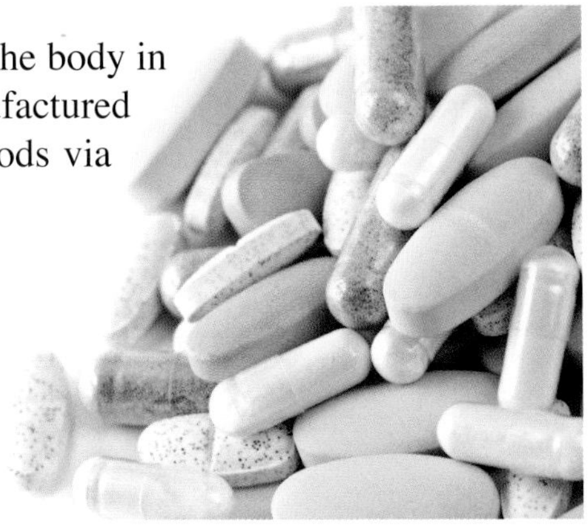

Vitamins are organic micronutrients that are required in small amounts by the body in order to sustain human life. Vitamins, with few exceptions, cannot be manufactured by the body and must therefore be obtained from supplements or from foods via the diet.

What do vitamins do?

Vitamins have several different functions in the body. A few include functioning as:

- Hormones – vitamin D
- Antioxidants – vitamin E
- Precursors to coenzymes that assist enzymes in metabolic functions of the body – B complex vitamins. For example, vitamin B7 or biotin, are part of enzymes involved in breaking down fats and making fatty acids.

Vitamins come in two classes – fat-soluble vitamins and water-soluble vitamins.

Fat-soluble vitamins are absorbed through the intestines with the help of lipids, or fats, and are more likely to accumulate in the body. They include **vitamins A, D, E** and **K**. Things that interfere with fat-soluble vitamin absorption are the artificial fat Olestra, which binds to fat-soluble vitamins, and a carbohydrate called chitosan, which is derived from the shells from crustaceans and is strongly speculated to impair the absorption of fat-soluble vitamins. Refer to appendix F for food rich in fat-soluble vitamins and the effects of deficiency.

Water is an essential transport mechanism within the body for **water-soluble vitamins**, which means a person must drink plenty of water to utilize these vitamins. Water-soluble vitamins include **vitamin C** and the **B vitamins** - **B1** (thiamine), **B2** (riboflavin), **B3** (niacin), **B5** (pantothenic acid), **B6** (pyridoxine), **B7** (biotin), **B9** (folic acid) and **B12** (cobalamin). The best utilization of water-soluble vitamins occurs when the required or therapeutic daily dosage is consumed in four evenly spaced divided dosages. When the entire daily dosage is consumed all at once, the levels of these vitamins in the blood end in a very high, but largely wasted peak. Following such a spike in blood levels is rapid excretion through urination and low levels for the remainder of the day. Peak absorption of water-soluble vitamins occurs one hour, or less, after ingestion. The half-life of water-soluble vitamins is four hours. Refer to appendix F for food rich in water-soluble vitamins and the effects of deficiency.

Word Power

Soluble

Pronunciation: \säl-yə-bəl\
Function: *adjective*
Etymology: Middle English, from Anglo-French, digestible, laxative, from Late Latin *solubilis,* from Latin *solvere* to loosen, dissolve
Date: 15th century
1 : susceptible of being dissolved in or as if in a liquid and especially water
2 : subject to being solved or explained <*soluble* questions>

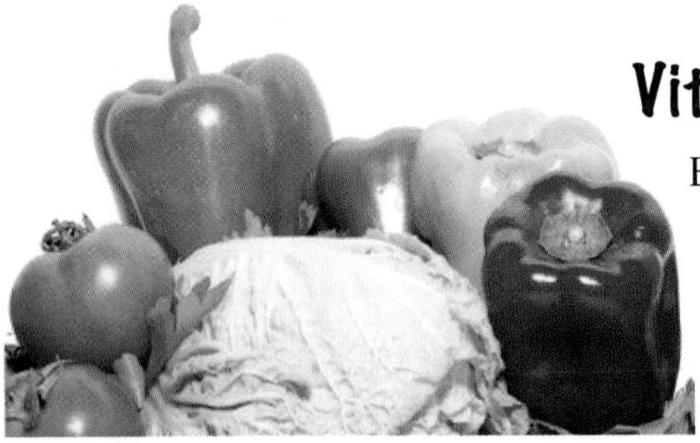

Vitamins in Food

Excessive heat during cooking destroys many of the vitamins in food. Besides retaining important enzymes, fresh, raw vegetables and fruits are some of the highest sources of vitamins. Therefore it is very important to include a variety and large quantity of fresh, raw vegetables, fruit, nuts and seeds to the daily diet.

Vitamin Supplementation

While vitamin supplementation may be needed in individuals with specific vitamin deficiencies, vitamins are best utilized and absorbed from the whole food in which God placed them. Many studies have found that certain vitamins extracted and consumed alone are not as readily absorbed in the body as when there are other nutrients present.

For example, when derived from natural sources, 80 to 95 percent of vitamin C is absorbed.[8] However, when it is isolated in a laboratory by a manufacturer, it often does not have the components that allow it to be metabolized by the body, rendering it ineffective. Synthetic and so-called natural forms of vitamin C vary little in bioactivity.[9] A quality vitamin C supplement will allow the body to absorb a vitamin by coupling it with the components needed for proper absorption: rutin, citrus bioflavonoids, calcium, zinc, magnesium and potassium.

Many people experience great health benefits by including more nutrient-rich foods and juicing in their diet. However, there are times when additional supplementation is needed. If vitamin supplementation is needed, a whole food multi-nutrient supplement is highly recommended.[10] For those who have been determined by a health care professional to need specific B vitamin supplementation, unless prescribed by a health professional, the B vitamins are best taken as a complex, which includes all of the following in proper ratio:

Biotin
Choline
Folic acid
Inositol
Lipoic acid
Para aminobenzoic acid
Vitamin B1
Vitamin B2 or riboflavin*
Vitamin B3
Vitamin B5
Vitamin B6
Vitamin B12

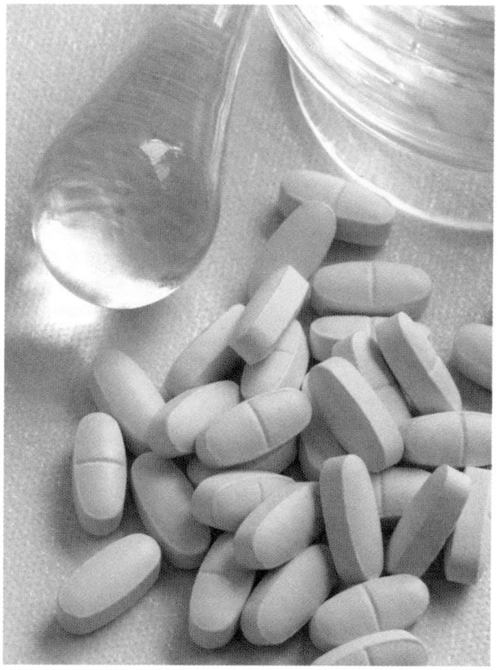

***Note:** Excessively large dosages of supplemental vitamin B2 may cause the excretion of other B vitamins via the urine, so proper ratios are very important.

With or without food?

Vitamin supplements that are consumed on an empty stomach are absorbed more rapidly than those consumed in conjunction with food, but their absorption levels peak far more quickly. Any vitamins not absorbed are eliminated. Supplemental vitamins that are consumed with food take longer to reach the bloodstream, but their peak bloodstream levels are sustained for longer periods of time allowing for greater absorption. With any given vitamin supplement, it is best to follow the recommendations of a nutritionist or to follow the directions listed on the supplement.

---

8 "The Water Soluble Vitamins. In: Advanced Nutrition and Human Metabolism" Groff, J.L., Gropper S.S., and Hunt S.M. Minneapolis: West Publishing Company, 1995, p. 222-237.

9 "Vitamin C. In: Modern Nutrition in Health and Disease" Ninth Edition. Jacob, R.A., Edited by Maurice Shils, James Olson, Moshe Shike, and A. Catharine Ross. Baltimore: Williams & Wilkins, 1999, p. 467-482.

10 See Appendix DD for authors' supplement recommendations.

Unit 6 Chapter 2
Discussion Questions

1. What are some bad habits in your lifestyle that might undermine your endocrine system?
2. What steps can you take to support your endocrine system?
3. What are the things we typically perform maintenance on? How often do we do these in comparison to doing maintenance/cleansing on our bodies?
4. Do you know anyone with diabetes? Is it Type 1 or 2?
5. What does bioactivity mean?

Activities - plus the Brussels Sprouts with Lemon Pepper Dressing "Power" Recipe and activities.

Elementary

1. Draw and color pictures of three foods important to the endocrine system.
2. The endocrine system is very small, but yet very powerful and important. Name as many fruits, vegetables, nuts and seeds that you can think of that are small, but yet powerful and important. Use Appendix D for support.
3. What food closely resembles the kidneys? Can you think of any other food that resembles an organ?
4. Choose your favorite vegetable or fruit. Refer to the Web site www.whfoods.com to find out what vitamins that vegetable or fruit has. Then, refer to Appendix F. Does it have more fat soluble or water soluble vitamins?
5. Research scientist Elmer Verner and his various discoveries. Prepare a written or oral report about the one discovery you believe is the most significant.

Secondary
Choose any from above plus

1. What is a synthetic growth hormone? How are they used in commercial food production? Prepare a written or oral report about the dangers of consuming such foods.
2. Check your household cleaners for carbon tetrachloride or sodium hypochlorite. If you find any, find out how to dispose of them properly.
3. Read Appendix X. Then, go to the National Sleep Foundation's Web site (www.sleepfoundation.org) and search the Sleep Topics. Select a topic that affects someone you know. Ask permission to observe the activities or tendencies of the person who is affected for a week. Make some sleep recommendations to the person and help him or her implement them. See how this helps the person.
4. Research the leading cause of liver failure. Find a person on a cholesterol lowering drug and ask if they have experienced any side effects. You will want to research the drugs, so you can ask them about the side affects associated with each.
5. March is national and worldwide kidney month. Create some activities for your family during every week of the month to support or improve the health of you kidneys. Mark the activities on the calendar even if it is a long time away.
6. Brussels sprouts have many health benefits including cancer prevention. Search the Internet or look in a favorite recipe book to find another fun, interesting recipe that incorporates Brussels sprouts as a side dish at a family dinner.

Additional Resources

Web sites:

1. http://www.helpguide.org/life/healthy_diet_cancer_prevention.htm
2. www.juicing-for-health.com

Books:
"The Super Antioxidant Diet" Robin Jeep & Richard Couey, PhD, Hampton Roads Publishing Co., 2008.

Endocrine System Power

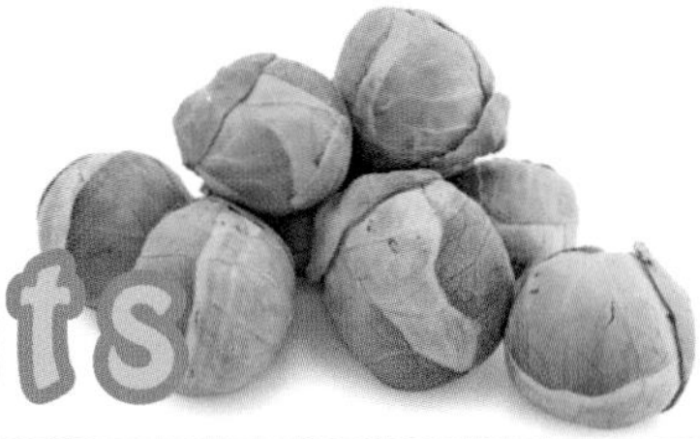

Brussels Sprouts

Brussels sprouts may decrease cancer risk. They contain vitamin A and beta-carotene which play important roles in supporting the immune system and are rich sources of iron, lutein and zeaxanthin.

Brussels Sprouts with Lemon Pepper Dressing

Cut four Brussels sprouts for each person into quarters and steam for five minutes. While steaming, prepare the dressing:

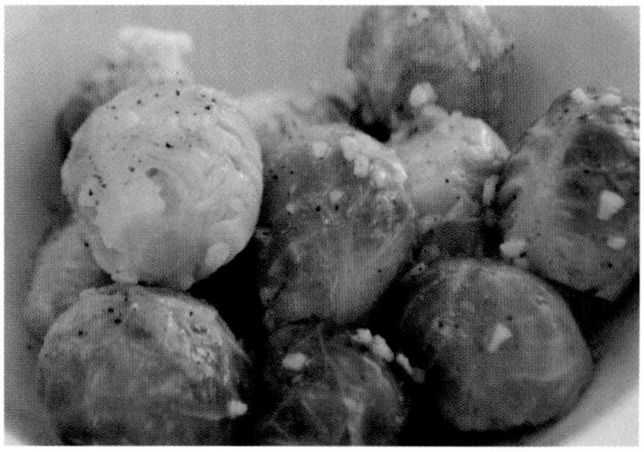

3 Tbs. extra virgin olive oil
2 tsp. fresh squeezed lemon juice OR one drop Young Living lemon oil
2 cloves garlic, minced
Salt and pepper to taste

Whisk dressing ingredients together in a small bowl. Place the steamed Brussels sprouts in a larger bowl, add the dressing and toss.

Activities

Elementary

1. Brussels sprouts are from the cruciferous family. What does this mean?
2. What other vegetables are considered cruciferous?
3. How did Brussels sprouts get their name?
4. What are goitrogens? How do they affect people with thyroid conditions?

Secondary

Choose any from above plus

1. Prior to the making this recipe, put the following six nutritional facts on separate index cards or pieces of paper. Before the meal, help set the table and place the pieces of paper under various plates. After saying the prayer and before passing the food, tell everyone to look under their plates for a fact on Brussels Sprouts. Take turns reading them aloud as you pass the food and enjoy the tasty dish. Brussels Sprouts are low in fat and sodium, high in dietary fiber and are cholesterol-free. Brussels Sprouts also contain high levels of naturally occurring vitamin C and specific health-promoting compounds called glucosinolates with antioxidant properties, and proven health benefits in the area of cancer prevention. Brussels Sprouts have three times the level of vitamin C of an orange. Unlike most vegetables, Brussels Sprouts are rather high in protein, accounting for more than a quarter of their calories. Four-to-six sprouts contain the adult daily requirements for vitamin C. Brussels sprouts also an excellent source of vitamin D and folate during pregnancy.
2. Which phytonutrient in Brussels sprouts has anti-bacterial compound that reduce the risk of stomach ulcers and stomach cancers?
3. Which phytonutrients in Brussels sprouts are proven to reduce the incidence of cancer, reverse cancer by killing cancer cells and inhibit cancer development?
4. What is the link between cruciferous vegetables and cancer?

Chapter 3

Diabetes

"Who forgiveth all thine iniquities; who healeth all thy diseases." Psalm 103:3-4

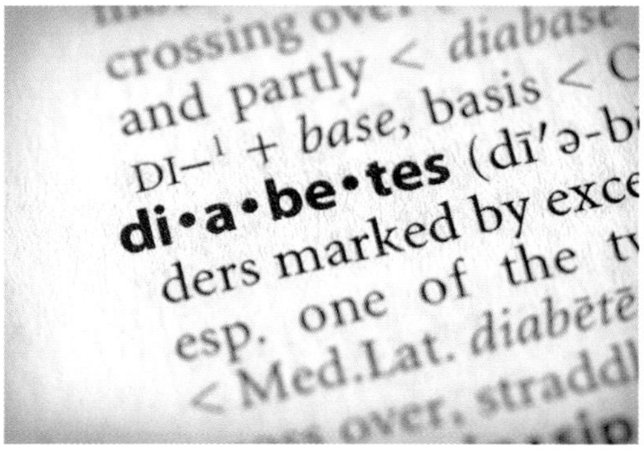

As mentioned in Chapter 2, diabetes is a group of diseases known as Type 1 immune-mediated, Type 2 insulin-resistant diabetes mellitus and gestational diabetes mellitus, which occurs during some pregnancies. It is defined as high levels of blood glucose resulting from defects in insulin production, insulin action, or both. Basically, it is too much sugar, or glucose, in the blood. The disease can lead to serious health complications and premature death. Adults, children and pregnant women share many similar symptoms: an unusual thirst, a frequent desire to urinate, blurred vision, and a feeling of being tired most of the time without any apparent reason.

From the American Diabetes Association (ADA), 2007 statistics revealed that a staggering 23.6 million Americans have diabetes and 57 million are pre-diabetic. Diabetes statistics are climbing at an alarming rate. Around 200,000 people younger than 20 years of age have diabetes Type 1 or 2. Diabetic researchers are suggesting massive screenings to stave off "the beginnings of an epidemic." The ADA is predicting by 2020, 65 percent of all people in the U.S. will be diabetic or pre-diabetic.

Diabetes History

The earliest recognition of diabetes was in the *Ebers Papyrus,* a medical text written around 1500 B.C., describing a condition of "passing too much urine." After an observation that the urine from people with diabetes was sweet, the Latin term *mellitus* was added by physicians in the 18th century. In 1776, scientists discovered that sugar glucose was in the blood, which led to the reasoning that diabetic people passed sugar from the blood to the urine. It wasn't until 1889 that two German physiologists discovered by accident that the pancreas was involved in diabetes. At this time in history medical science used bloodletting, opium and special diets, but most patients died without help. In 1921, Dr. Fredrick Banting, discovered isolated groups of cells from the islets of Langerhans in the pancreas and created an extract that led to the diabetic treatment in use today.

Although many theories exist about the causes of diabetes, no one is exactly sure what causes the disease. Researchers have found many factors that appear to be linked to the cause: genetics, auto-antibodies, viruses, fungi, cow's milk, chemicals, man-made drugs and oxygen-free radicals.

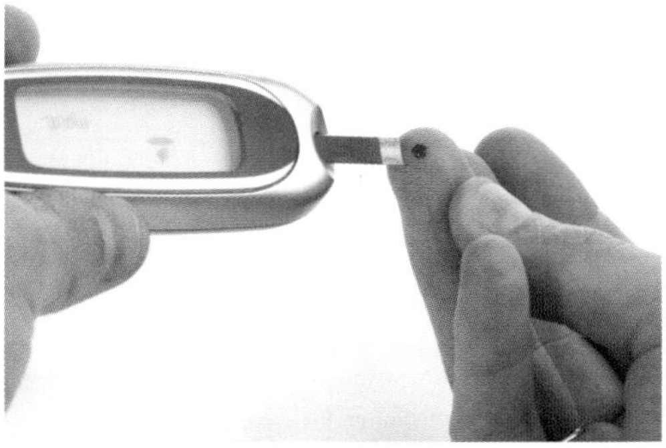

Type 1

Type 1 diabetes is a condition where the immune system mistakenly destroys the insulin-producing beta cells of the pancreas. This is called an **autoimmune response**. Beta cells are the only cells in the body that make the hormone insulin which regulates blood glucose. The heredity factor generally is believed to be the main cause of Type 1 because it appears to run in families. Also, Type 1 is more common in certain racial groups. According to scientists, doctors and researchers, there is no way to prevent or cure Type 1 diabetes.

Genes

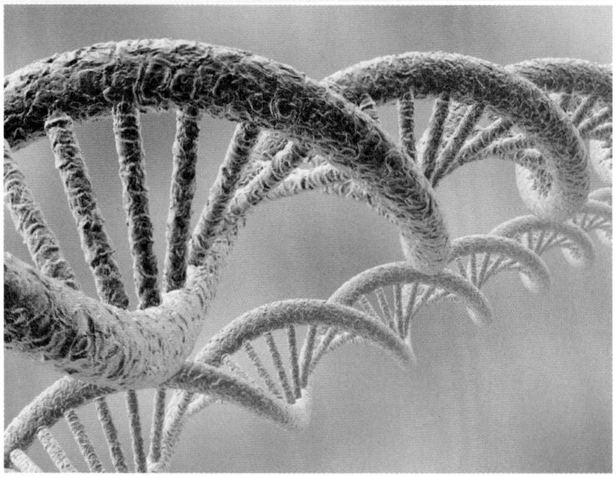

The genetic factor can be explained by understanding the role of DNA in the cells. Within every human is a blue print of instructions for the body on how to grow, live and function. Each cell of the body contains 46 chromosomes, which are made up of DNA and proteins. DNA, deoxyribonucleic acid, is a chemical sequence of units with genetic information within millions of bases in a long string. Along the strand lie the genes which are unique segments of DNA that tell your cells what kind of protein to make. Researchers have identified several genes known as diabetes susceptibility genes, but they have not found a single gene responsible for all people that seem to inherit diabetes.

A set of genes that may be responsible for a person to more likely become diabetic is the human leukocyte antigens, or HLAs.[1] These genes assemble in the body to identify a person's own cells as "self" and are called antigens. Antigens tell the immune cells not to destroy the cells that are part of that person's body. Somehow HLAs incorrectly identify the beta cells as "non-self" and destroy the insulin-producing cells of the pancreas. Thus the body can no longer make insulin. Every person has many different types of HLA genes that have been inherited from both parents. Therefore, each HLA has multiple variations thus making it impossible to link all Type 1 diabetes to genetics.

Viruses

Today many scientists have made a link between viruses and Type 1 diabetes.[2] People have been documented to develop Type 1 diabetes after a viral infection or after viral epidemics. It is suspected that the same virus that causes mumps, German measles and the Coxsackie family of viruses, which cause polio, may be causing Type 1 diabetes. When a virus enters the body, it might change the structure of the antigens on the surface of the islet cells. This will alter the appearance of the cell to make it appear to be an invader to the immune system. Gian Franco Bottazzo, a diabetes researcher, believes that diabetes is caused by a slow-acting virus that causes the immune system to attack proteins in the pancreas.[3]

Word Power

Mycotoxins
Pronunciation: \mī-kə-täk-sən\
Function: *noun*
Date: 1962
: a toxic substance produced by a fungus and especially a mold

Food

Other researchers believe food may play a role in the development of Type 1 diabetes. It was found that children newly diagnosed with Type 1 diabetes have higher amounts of antibodies that recognize a specific protein in cow's milk. Auto-antibodies bind to a protein that appears on the surface of the insulin-producing beta cells in the pancreas after an illness. The immune system response is to attack the beta cells leading to the destruction of the cells that are responsible for insulin. Current science indicates that it is the fat cells of the milk that may be the cause of Type 1 diabetes. Livestock feed is allowed to contain up to 300 parts per billion of aflatoxin, a carcinogenic chemical secreted by the fungus *Aspergillus*. Other studies show that withholding wheat and soy, which may also contain mycotoxins from fungus, will help prevent or delay diabetes.[4] The mycotoxin, ochratoxin, is typically found in corn, barley and wheat. This mycotoxin is 10 times more toxic than aflatoxin and can afflict extreme damage on the human body.[5]

---

1 "Pancreatic autoimmunity and HLA antigens" Bottazzo GF, Doniach D (1976) Lancet 2: 800
2 "Diabetes and Hypoglycemia" Michael T. Murray, N.D., Prima Publishing, Roseville, CA, 1994.
3 "β-Cell damage in diabetic insulitis: are we approaching a solution?" Bottazzo GF, Diabetologia, Volume 26, Number 4 / April, 1984.
4 "The Control of Mold and Mycotoxins in Ruminant Foods" Kemin.com. Kemin Armericas, Inc. Dec. 2002.
5 "Mycotoxins: Risks in Plant, Animal and Human Systems" Council for Agricultural Science and Technology. Task Force Report Number 139. CAST.Ames, IA. Jan. 2003.

Free Radicals

Oxygen-free radicals, which are formed as a by-product of many chemical reactions in the body, destroy systems throughout the body. In the past the body had ways of stopping that action, but air pollution, diet, water, smoke and petrochemicals have led to excessive amounts in the human body; so the immune system is finding it impossible to contend with everything. These free radicals overwhelm the body and may easily attack the islet cells, which are at a disadvantage because of their very low levels of the enzymes that break down free radicals.

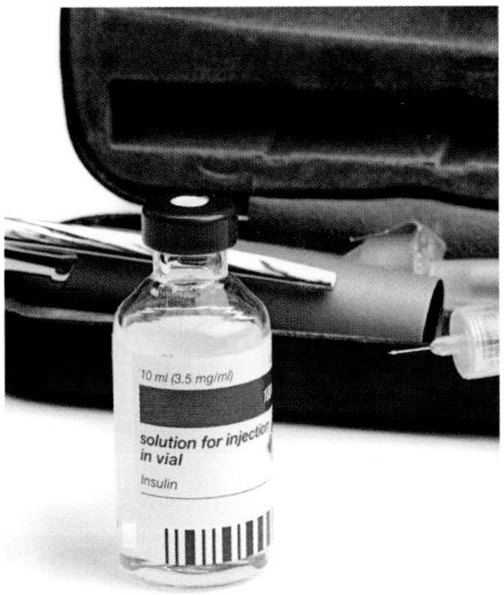

Type 2

Type 2 diabetes accounts for about 90 to 95 percent of all diagnosed cases of diabetes. It usually begins with insulin resistance, a disorder in which the cells do not use insulin properly or there is not enough insulin to go around the body. This leads to high levels of glucose in the blood. All cells in the body contain special proteins called receptors that bind to insulin. Insulin acts like a key to open the gates or receptor sites on the cell. In Type 2 there is either a faulty lock or a malfunctioning insulin receptor. The key doesn't open the lock and the glucose is shut out. Type 2 diabetics' cells are starving even though the person may be eating constantly. In some diabetics the beta cells in the pancreas do not produce enough insulin. It is thought that after many years of working overtime to overproduce insulin, the pancreas begins to burn out.

Genes

Many of the same factors that are attributed to Type 1 diabetes are the same for Type 2. Diabetic families seem to pass down diabetes from generation to generation. Researchers have identified a protein that shuts down the insulin receptor that creates insulin resistance and is found in most people with Type 2 diabetes. Recent research indicates that genes leading to obesity may also play a role in diabetes. Obesity is the most common trigger that leads to Type 2. It is defined as weighing more than 20 percent over a desirable body weight. Three-fourths of all people with Type 2 diabetes are or have been obese. The latest 2008 health statistics reveal that 38 million Americans are obese. Other factors are age, specifically the elderly, and lifestyle.

Chemical Exposure

Recent research has linked chemical exposure and the use of man-made drugs to Type 2 diabetes. There are studies that have linked dioxin, a deadly chemical used in pesticides and the defoliant Agent Orange to diabetes. Another study links dioxin to the worldwide increase of diabetes in children. Researchers are speculating that a connection exists between dioxin, obesity, diabetes and the body's storage of chemicals in fat cells. The side effect of some drugs for HIV and heart disease is diabetes. A study at the University of Southern California Medical School found that those who have gestational diabetes with a family history of diabetes and take certain birth control pills after delivery may triple their risk of developing diabetes later in life.

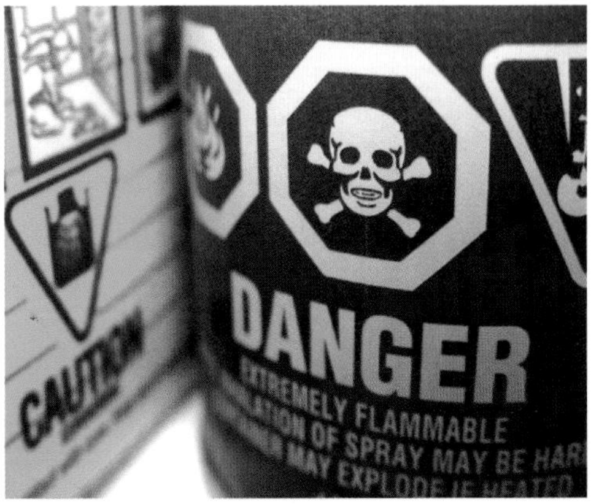

As research continues, it is highly unlikely that either genetics or environmental factors are the only causes for diabetes, but if a person with genetic susceptibility is exposed to a virus, an environmental chemical or drugs with a compromised immune system, then diabetes is likely to occur. Refer to Appendix S for more information on toxins and household chemicals.

The History of the Diabetes and Microscopic Fungi Link[6]

"Fungal toxins in the food we eat represent the number one worry we face as a human race." Simon Shane, Louisiana State University Press, 1991[7]

The following is an excerpt from "Infectious Diabetes" by Doug Kaufman.

1954 - Griffiths discovers that uric acid can lead to diabetes in laboratory animals.

1963 - Svlhia notes that *Sacchromyces* yeast produce uric acid.

1976 - Isogai reports finding *Cryptococcus* fungi in the islets of Langerhans cells of two children dying from diabetes. In later studies, when researchers injected *Cryptococcus* into the pancreatic arteries of laboratory animals, necrosis (cell death) of the islet of Langerhans resulted. *Cryptococcus* produces alloxan, a uric acid by-product.

1990 - Moody successfully uses cyclosporine A, an antifungal medication, to treat *Cryptococcus* fungi.

1990 - Chase reports that Type 1 diabetes can be cured if treated with cyclosporine-A within four months of the disease's onset, but the anti-fungal medicine has serious multiple side effects.

1973 - Escher et al. finds that cured mutton is loaded with mycotoxins.

1981 - Helgason and Jonasson report that a dramatically disproportionate number of Icelandic women who ate cured mutton, a holiday dish, close to the time they became pregnant eventually gave birth to babies with diabetes.

1980 - Pojo demonstrates that alloxan, a mycotoxin, damages the insulin-producing beta cells in the pancreas's islets of Langerhans.

1981 - Hayes induces diabetes in laboratory animals by injecting them with streptozotocin, a mycotoxin produced by *Strptomyces* mold.

1990 - Coleman et al. feed mice a 10 percent brewer's yeast diet. The animals develop diabetes.

1973 - Varsano et al report on the consistent occurrence of diabetes in cancer patients who have been treated with a mycotoxin called L-asparaginase. Asparaginase is a cancer-fighting drug used in chemotherapy. It is produced by the soil fungus *Cylindrocarpon obtusisporum*.[8]

1990 - Raha induces diabetes in lab animals by injecting them with L-asparaginase.[3]

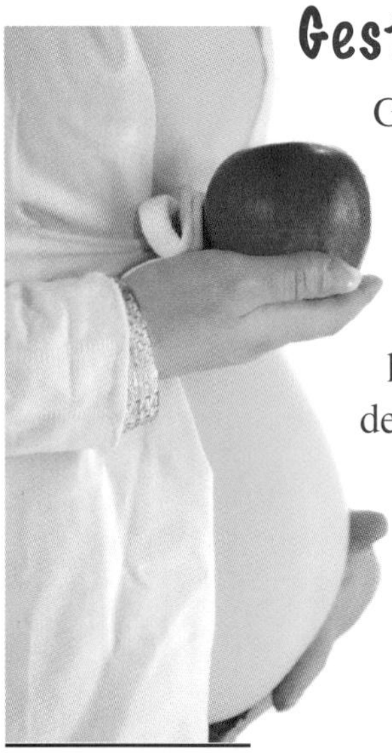

Gestational Diabetes

Gestational diabetes is not unlike the other types. The cause is not known, but some researchers are suggesting that hormones are the contributing factor. The placenta produces large amounts of various hormones and some of them have been linked to blocking insulin action. It has been discovered that all pregnant women have some degree of insulin resistance. Therefore gestational diabetes is associated more with the genes responsible for Type 2 diabetes. Women who have had gestational diabetes have a 40 to 60 percent chance of developing diabetes in the next five to ten years.

Word Power

Gestation

Pronunciation: \je-stā-shən\

Function: *noun*

Etymology: Latin *gestation-, gestatio,* from *gestare* to bear, frequentative of *gerere* to bear, Date: 1615

1: the carrying of young in the uterus : pregnancy 2: conception and development especially in the mind — ges·ta·tion·al \-shnəl, -shə-nᵊl\ *adjective*

6 "Infectious Diabetes" Doug Kaufman and David Holland, M.D., Triton Media Group

7 "Economic Significance of Mycotoxicoses" Pennington Center Nutrition Series. Vol. 1: Mycotoxins, Cancer and Health. LSU Press. Baton Rouge. 1991.

8 "Unraveling the cause of diabetes" Marx, Jean. Science, Vol.296. 26 April, 2002.

In all forms of diabetes the symptoms are similar and the result is too much sugar, or glucose, in the blood. The body is unable to remove glucose from the blood and deliver it to the cells. The sugar accumulates in the blood causing damage to the many different body systems. All forms of diabetes are treatable, but according to the ADA there is no cure. Today, even though scientific research continues to look for a drug to cure diabetes, many are turning to natural remedies and looking at food as the main factor in curing diabetes.

Fun Fact

On May 21, 1922, James Havens became the first American to receive insulin successfully.

Diagnosing Diabetes

(Mg/dl = milligrams per deciliter.)

Diagnosis	Fasting Glucose	Random Glucose
Normal	Less than 110 mg/dl	Less than 140 mg/dl
Impaired glucose tolerance	Greater than or equal to 100 mg/dl and less than 126 mg/dl	Greater than or equal to and less than 200 mg/dl
Provisional diabetes	Greater than or equal to 126 mg/dl	Greater than 200 mg/dl

Criteria for Diagnosis of Type 2 Diabetes

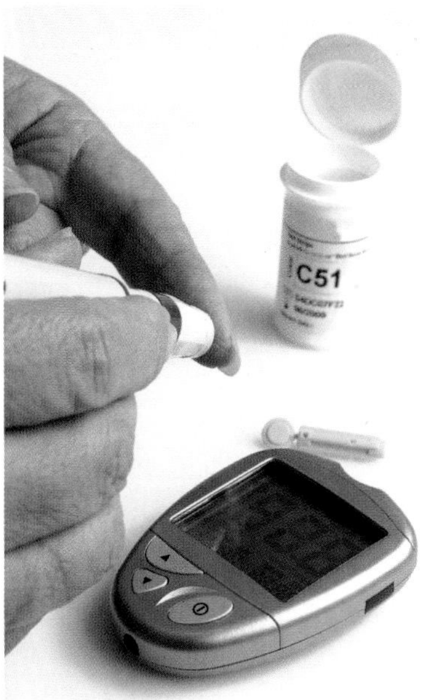

- Symptoms of diabetes plus casual plasma glucose, or blood sugar, concentration greater than or equal to 200 mg/dl. Casual is defined as any time of day without regard to time since last meal.
- Fasting plasma glucose (FPG) greater than or equal to 126 mg/dl. Fasting means no food for a minimum of eight hours.
- Or two hour plasma glucose greater than or equal to 200 mg/dl during an oral glucose tolerance test.

Symptoms of Type 2 Diabetes

- Unusual thirst
- Frequent desire to urinate
- Blurred vision
- Frequent, prolonged fatigue with no apparent cause
- Leg pain
- Unexplained weight loss

Risk Factors of Developing Diabetes[9]

- I had a baby weighing more than 9 pounds at birth or had diabetes during my pregnancy
  If yes, score 6. If no, score 0.

- I have a parent, sister, or brother with diabetes.
  If yes, score 3. If no, score 0.

- I am Hispanic, African American, Native American, Asian American or Pacific Islander.
  If yes, score 3. If no, score 0.

- I am overweight.
  If yes, score 3. If no, score 0.

- I have been told I have a high blood sugar level.
  If yes, score 6. If no, score 0.

- I am between 45 and 64.
  If yes, score 1. If no, score 0.

- I am under 65 and I get little or no exercise during the usual day.
  If yes, score 3. If no, score 0.

- I am 65 or older.
  If yes, score 3. If no, score 0.

Those who score 1 to 5 points are at a low risk of developing diabetes. Scores of 6 or more, indicate a high risk of having or getting diabetes.

Diabetes and Carbohydrates

Blood sugar levels are affected by the dietary intake of carbohydrates and fiber. Understanding the cause, prevention and treatment of diabetes is directly connected to this group of foods that are crucial to provide energy for body functions.

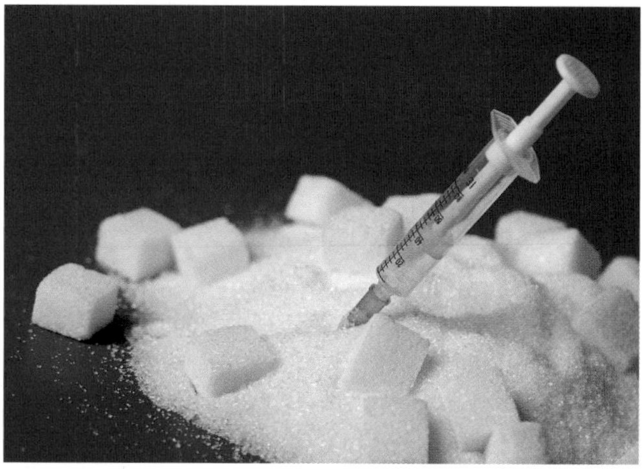

Simple carbohydrates are sugars that are quickly absorbed by the body for energy. The natural simple sugars in fruits and vegetables are accompanied in foods by a wide range of nutrients that aid in the utilization of the sugars. When carbohydrates like white sugar and other sources are refined, they are stripped of these nutrients. When high-sugar foods are eaten alone, the blood sugar level rises quickly. Currently, more than one half of the carbohydrates being consumed are in the form of sugars, added to processed foods as sweetening agents; sucrose, glucose, maltose, lactose, fructose, corn syrup or white grape concentrate.

It is impossible to control blood sugar levels without medication while eating a constant source of high-sugar foods. To absorb the sugar, the pancreas has to release insulin. The more sugar in the system the more insulin is

9 Developed by the University of Washington.

needed for the cells to absorb it. Cells throughout the body respond to insulin by absorbing the sugar and causing the bloodstream to drop in sugar levels, which causes the pancreas to taper off the production of insulin. The lower the blood sugar, the less insulin needs to be produced. The less insulin produced by the body, the less energy and enzymes needed for metabolism and work of all body organs. This equals a longer lifespan for the body.

A healthy individual secretes approximately 31 units of insulin daily.
An obese Type 2 diabetic secretes an average of 114 units daily, nearly four times the normal amount.
A lean Type 2 diabetic secretes about 14 units.
Type 1 diabetics secrete only four units of insulin daily.

It is speculated that the average diabetic cuts 15 years off his or her lifespan.

Fruit and Fructose

In extreme cases of diabetes in which blood sugar levels remain over 200 mg/dl with medication, fruits and fructose from raw fruits should be avoided until blood sugar levels are controlled and within safety guidelines. For other diabetics, recent research has revealed that fructose from certain raw fruits such as green apples, berries, avocados, grapefruit, lemons and limes does not cause a rapid rise in blood sugar level. When fed to **non-insulin** dependent diabetics over four weeks, fructose has actually been shown to enhance the sensitivity to insulin by 34 percent.[10] Because the liver must change fructose into the glucose, the blood level raises more slowly than after consumption of other simple sugars. Sucrose is not tolerated by most diabetics, but moderated amounts of fructose from these raw fruits can be consumed without losing blood sugar control. The only exception is if there is any liver damage; in this case even fructose should be avoided until a liver detoxification is done.

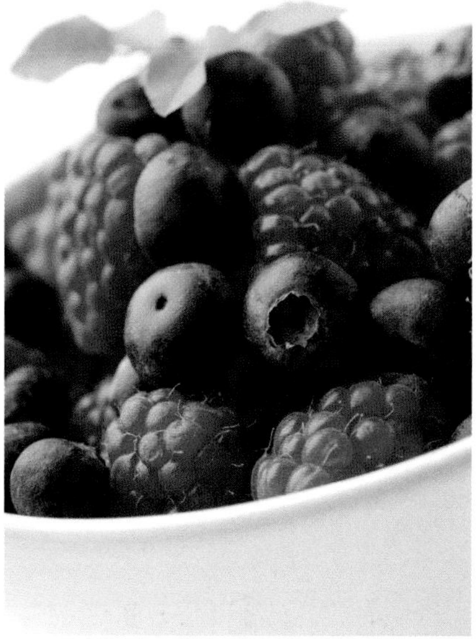

A surprising result of regular fruit consumption is that it also may help control sugar cravings, decrease the amount of calories and fat consumed, and promote weight loss in overweight individuals.

Since fruit contains fructose in a natural form, consuming a serving of fruit 30 minutes before dinner may result in fewer calories being consumed. Consuming fruit in-between meals may help stabilize blood sugar and may help with weight loss while consuming less calories. Regular fruit consumption offers a great source of natural health promoting nutrients that lead to significant protection from chronic degenerative diseases.

Fructose from Corn and HFCS

Warning! Not all fructose is the same. Fructose from raw fruit is present in the fruit with fiber that helps the body metabolize the fructose into glucose much slower, thus keeping the blood sugar levels from rising too rapidly. Fructose from corn is metabolized differently by the body because corn is a starch. It causes blood sugar levels to raise much quicker than the fructose from raw fruit. High fructose corn syrup (HFCS) is not natural and is made chemically from corn. Its molecular structure is altered during processing, which causes blood sugar levels to spike when consumed. HFCS should be completely avoided by diabetics and even by those who are not diabetic.

10 "Fructose and insulin sensitivity in patients with Type 2 diabetes" Koivisto VA and Yki-Jarvinen H, J Intern Med 233:145, 1993.

The Glycemic Index

The glycemic index reveals the rise of blood glucose after eating a particular food. The standard value of 100 is based on the rise of blood sugar after ingesting glucose. The index ranges from 20 for fructose and barley to about 98 for a baked potato. The insulin response to carbohydrate containing foods is similar to the rise in blood sugar.

Foods with a high glycemic value should be avoided by people with diabetics and hypoglycemia. Food high in bad fat such as ice cream and sausage also should be avoided because it has been proven to impair glucose tolerance. Refer to the Glycemic Index chart in Unit 5 Chapter 4.

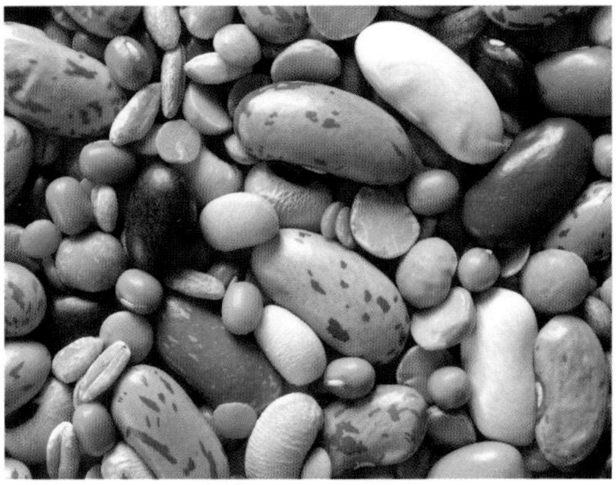

The Importance of Fiber

Water-soluble fiber has the most beneficial effects on blood sugar. Water-soluble fiber is able to slow down digestion, help absorb carbohydrates, prevent rapid rises in blood sugar and increase the sensitivity of tissues to insulin. Fiber prevents the excessive secretion of insulin and improves the uptake of glucose by the liver and other tissues, preventing a sustained elevation of blood sugar. Complex carbohydrates rather than simple processed carbohydrates should be included in moderation. Vegetables, legumes and grains are excellent sources of complex carbohydrates. Daily intake of 50 grams of dietary fiber from plant foods is recommended to help diabetics.

Good Food for Diabetics

All **vegetables** should be raw or slightly steamed. It is important for diabetics to make sure that the enzymes in their food are not denatured or destroyed. Fighting a disease over time may deplete the store of enzymes in the body.

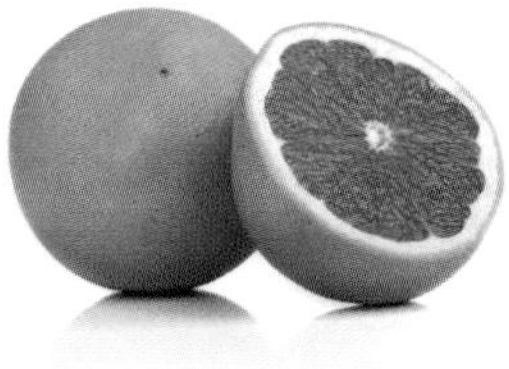

Fruits that are acceptable if the blood sugar is below 200 mg/dl include: green apples, berries, avocados, grapefruit, lemons and limes in limited quantities. Other citrus fruit can be added once blood sugar levels drop. It is important to test the blood sugar to determine what fruit can be added to the diet.

Use raw blue agave nectar or organic Grade B maple syrup as **natural sugar substitutes** in limited quantities with blood sugar testing.

Low levels of insulin can prevent the accumulation of plaque in the arteries of the heart, legs and neck and also is believed to prevent some cases of Alzheimer's disease. Rather than carbohydrate snacking to maintain proper insulin levels, **protein** rich snacks are preferred. Fifty-eight percent of proteins can be converted by the body to blood glucose as needed without raising insulin levels.

Fish and chicken are good choices along with raw cheese and nuts. Vegetables such as steamed peas or steamed carrots allow the body to receive a small amount of carbohydrates and stimulate it to use the protein for muscle building. Low-carbohydrate fruit such as raspberries, strawberries, blueberries or green apples also serve as small carbohydrate stimulants. Other good protein sources are raw soaked nuts, especially almonds, legumes, eggs and limited quantities of lean grass-fed meat.

Other Beneficial Foods

Unpasteurized apple cider vinegar
Filtered water
Organic teas
Olive oil
Coconut oil
Low glycemic foods can be added with testing of blood sugar.

Bad Foods for Diabetics

Sugar, especially refined, white and corn fructose
All artificial sweeteners
Bananas and melons, until blood sugar levels are in a safe range without medication
All processed food, especially juices
Dried fruits
Meat that is grain-fed or corn-fed
All breads and crackers
Dairy, which is hard to digest
All corn and corn products
Sodas
Coffee and non-herbal teas
Alcohol
Peanut products
Mushrooms
Fermented soy products
Egg substitutes
Margarine
Partially hydrogenated oils
Corn and peanut oil

Refer to Appendix DD for details about how contributing author Karen Hopkins, B.S. used nutrition, supplements and exercise to overcome diabetes.

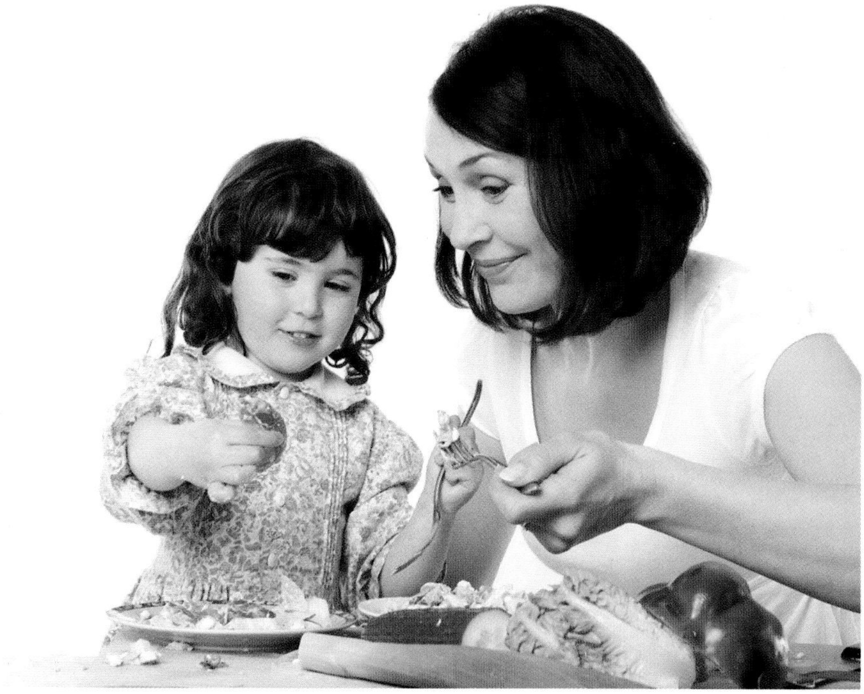

Unit 6 Chapter 3 Discussion Questions

1. Do you know anyone who has diabetes?
2. Based on what you have learned, how can protect your body from diabetes?
3. What are some scriptures you could pray over someone who has been diagnosed with diabetes?
4. What are your favorite raw vegetables? Fruits? Needs and seeds?

Activities - plus the Veggie Linguine with Fresh Tomato Sauce "Power" Recipe and activities.

Elementary

1. Find out the names of the two German physiologists who accidentally discovered in 1889 that the pancreas was involved in diabetes.
2. Interview a person who has diabetes. How does diabetes affect his or her daily life? What dietary changes has this person made since the diagnosis?
3. Go the cereal isle of the grocery store and find all the popular brand name cereals that tout being high in fiber. Look at the ingredients label and list all the different kinds of sugars and sugar substitutes listed for each cereal. Refer to Unit 5 Chapter 4 to re-familiarize yourself with the different names for sugars and sugar substitutes. Does the list surprise you? What other ingredients are listed that are bad for the body?
4. Look at the list of natural sugar substitutes in Appendix P and list all the safe and healthy sugar alternatives for diabetics. (Hint: They should have a low glycemic level.)
5. Revisit the fiber index in Appendix K to assure that you are maintaining a healthy balance of fiber. Encourage other family members to do the same.

Secondary

Choose any from above plus

1. Research the meaning of mg/dl.
2. What are the differences between Type 1, Type 2 diabetes and gestational diabetes?
3. Research gestational diabetes to learn what dangers are associated for the baby and mother.
4. Plan a healthy dinner and dessert with an overall low glycemic level for your family that would include a variety of recommended foods that are beneficial to diabetics. Make sure this meal also is high in fiber. You may refer to Appendix K for a list of foods high in fiber. Compare that list to the list of foods good for diabetics to find the best high fiber foods for diabetics.
5. What is the difference between leaven and unleavened bread?
6. Read Exodus 12:29-34. Based on this, what is the symbolism of unleavened bread used during Passover?

Additional Resources

Books:

"Infectious Diabetes" Doug A. Kaufman, Trition Media Group

Endocrine System Power

Raw Vegetables

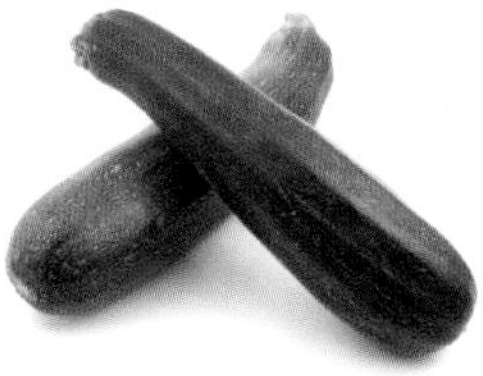

Raw vegetables are high is fiber, which is important in helping maintain normal blood sugar levels. They are also high in enzymes, vitamins and other nutrients vital to those overcoming diabetes.

Veggie Linguine with Fresh Tomato Sauce

This is a great raw vegetable recipe with lots of health support, especially for diabetics.

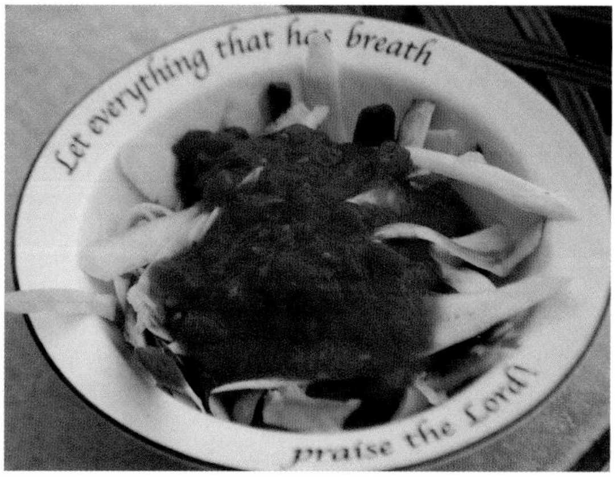

4 medium zucchini
4 medium yellow squash
Extra virgin olive oil
2 small cans or 1 large can whole peeled tomatoes
1 Tbs. fresh basil, minced
1 tsp. fresh thyme, minced
1 clove garlic, crushed
Sea salt and pepper to taste

Wash and cut off ends of squash. Using a vegetable peeler, slice the squash end to end in long strips. For strips wider than one inch, slice lengthwise to have ½ inch wide strips. Place strips in a bowl and drizzle with olive oil.

For the sauce, add tomatoes, basil, thyme, garlic, salt and pepper into blender. If the ends are on the tomatoes, you may remove them before blending. Blend until pureed. Pour over the Veggie Linguine, toss and serve. This makes a great side dish.

Activities

Elementary

1. What is linguine and what does it mean in Italian?
2. Look at linguine at the grocery store, in a cookbook or online before helping to preparing the vegetables.
3. What does it mean to drizzle?
4. Have your family rate this dish on a scale of 1 to 5, with 1 being bad and 5 being great. Then, tabulate the votes. If it scores below a 5, discuss what changes you want to make and set a date when everyone will be home to try the recipe again.

Secondary

Choose any from above plus

1. What is the difference between summer and winter squash?
2. To what botanical family do the squash and zucchini belong?
3. Why is substituting the pasta for vegetables good for diabetics?
4. Typically linguine is served with pesto or seafood. What is pesto? Why should we limit our intake of seafood?

Chapter 4

Emotions

Society is filled with emotional turmoil. Currently, there is more focus on emotional behavior and psychological conditions of the body than in the past. Many doctors are recognizing that a number of diseases are tied to emotional problems of childhood. So many people are taking anti-anxiety or anti-depression medications. Children as young as three years old can be prescribed anti-depressant medication.[1] Is this really necessary? Is there a better answer?

Do emotions really affect physical wellbeing? It is easy to see how emotions affect mood and attitude and how a person feels mentally, but can they make one physically sick? Many people would definitely say, "yes." Chronically ill people have often observed improved health once the emotional root to the health challenge was addressed.

The Bible has many references to our physical health being tied to our emotional health. The King James Version of the Christian Bible uses the word fear 39 times. Twenty-seven of them or 72 percent of these references say, "Do not fear." The twelve remaining references say to "Fear God." There is no mention in the Bible that we are to fear any thing or person, yet many people are controlled by fears and phobias.

What do thoughts produce?

A person should ask himself:

- Do my thoughts produce mental clarity, focus and peace, or confusion, judgment and criticism of self or others?
- Do I jump to conclusions? Do I chew on my thoughts?
- Am I willing to hear the other side of the story or am I closed-minded?
- Am I quick to believe the bad or negative comments about someone or are they innocent until proven guilty?

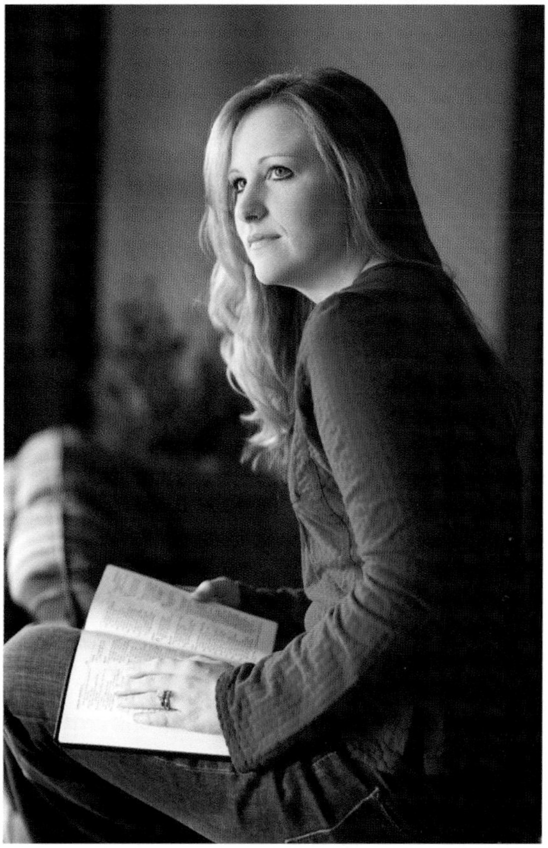

What about will power?

- Am I able and willing to make changes for a healthier lifestyle?
- Do I settle in and say, "That is just my lot in life. There is nothing I can do about it. God made me that way."

We cannot blame God when wrong decisions more than likely brought ill health. Choosing diet soda filled with artificial sweeteners, sugar-filled pastries and refined grains can create an unhealthy body and poor mental state.

Isaiah 55:1-3 asks the following:
"Ho, everyone that thirsteth, come ye to the waters and he that hath no money, come ye buy and eat; yea, come buy wine and milk without money and without price. **Wherefore do ye spend money on that which is not bread?** And you labor for that which staisfieth not? Hearken diligently unto me and eat ye that which is **good**, and let your soul delight in fatness."

1 "Trends in the prescribing of psychotropic medications to preschoolers" Zito JM, Safer DJ, dosReis S, Gardner JF, Botes M, Lynch F. Journal of the American Medical Association, 2000; 283(8): 1025-30.

Proverbs 23:7 states, "For as he thinketh in his heart, so is he." This is not to say, a person says "Today I will be a millionaire," and <poof> millions are deposited into her bank account. Rather we should ask:

- What does my heart dwell on?
- How do I see myself?

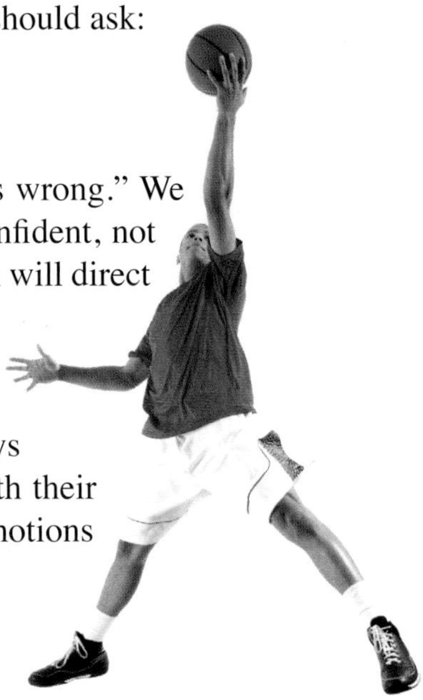

Do not say "Woe is me. I'll never have much. I'm always right. Everyone else is wrong." We should say what the Word of God says about us, "I live an abundant life. I'm confident, not arrogant. I'm blessed, so I can be a blessing to others." The thoughts we dwell upon will direct our lives.

Professional athletes don't just dream of being a star player. They practice and perfect their skills to the best they can be. Highly successful people are always learning and trying new things. Some will fail and make mistakes, but people with their eyes on a goal look at mistakes as learning opportunities. They do not let their emotions regarding past failures stop them from achieving.

Emotions and the Body

Have you ever been nervous about taking a test, speaking in public or meeting someone new only to experience butterflies in the stomach? Have you ever suffered the loss of someone close to you and your heart actually ached? Has your blood pressure elevated only while visiting the doctor? Have you ever watched a scarry movie or been in a near car accident and your heart rate soared? The brain senses a situation and the body responds.

Medical research shows that there is definitely a connection between emotions, physical response, health and even disease.[2] The most destructive of all emotions are fear, anger and grief.

Pastor Henry Wright, author of "A More Excellent Way" has worked with people all over the world helping them to understand the emotions behind many diseases. Once the people learned to deal with their emotions, many of the diseases went away, such as high blood pressure, cancer, allergies of all sorts, head aches, digestive issues and more.

Fear

The Hebrew meaning of the word fear is "to see the hand, activity and deeds of God." God intended fear to be a positive experience. We are to have a worshipful fear of God. Psalms 139:14 says we are "fearfully and wonderfully made."

However, today people understand fear in a much different light – a painful emotion marked by alarm or anticipation of danger, fright or dread. While having a healthy fear of fire or true danger is not bad, the fear that is destructive is fear without a cause. God tells us not have this type of fear. The real root of this type of fear is abandonment – the fear that someone of significance will leave or did so in the past, and the fearful person has not moved on from it.

The organ most affected by fear is the heart[3] – both physically and spiritually. The number one killer in America is heart disease. God instructs us to not fear because fear kills. Fear can manifest itself in anxiety, bitterness, blame,

2 "Emotion, behavior pattern and disease progression" Dan L. Dumitrascu, International Congress Series,Volume 1287, April 2006, Pages 128-134.

3 "Prospective study of phobic anxiety and risk of coronary heart disease in men" I Kawachi, GA Colditz, A Ascherio, EB Rimm, E Giovannucci, MJ Stampfer and WC Willett Department of Nutrition, Harvard School of Public Health, Boston, MA 02115. Circulation, Vol 89, 1992-1997, Copyright © 1994 by American Heart Association

confusion, doubt and panic. To overcome fear a person needs the healing responses of security, approval, positive words, honor, certainty, care, trust, confidence and love. Those who do not hear these words from others should say them aloud to themselves. We also should affirm these to those who we know who need to hear these positive words. The definition of the word affirmation is "something declared to be true; a positive statement." Gather Bible verses to repeat aloud on a daily basis.

Fear and love cannot live in the same house. The apostle John says in 1 John 4:18, "There is no fear in love, perfect love casts out all fear." Gary Young, world renowned essential oil expert, said this of fear, "Fear is a **f**alse **e**motion **a**ppearing **r**eal." Many people have fears of germs, dying, flying, accidents, cancer and other things. Other conditions like constipation, irritable bowel syndrome and diarrhea are often fear based.[4]

Anger

God's instruction on anger is to not let the sun go down on wrath, or anger. Angry people tend to carry grudges and remember everything that anyone else has done to them. They tend to be unforgiving, revenge seeking and get the most angry at the person wanting to help them.

The organ most affected by anger is the liver.[5] The liver is the most significant detoxification organ in the body. It cleanses the body and the blood. It is interesting that the gallbladder is most impacted by bitterness and resentment as the gall bladder is attached to the liver, and these emotions are so attached to anger. Anger is very destructive to a person and to their body. The number two killer in America is cancer, which most naturopathic practitioners agree has it has beginnings in the liver.

Grief

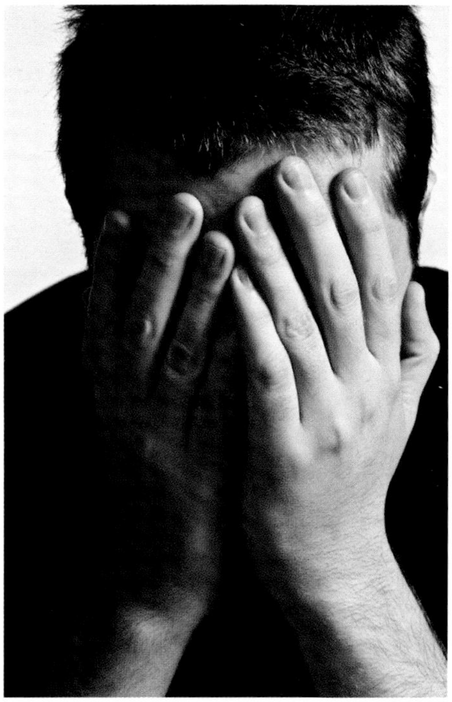

Grief or sorrow also is known as lack of sweetness and usually is tied to those close to us. Sorrow expects hurt, rejection and loneliness.

The organ most affected by grief is the pancreas,[6] which may be part of the reason diabetes and other blood sugar problems are now epidemic in this country as the third leading causes of death. From the beginning, God said in Genesis 2:18, "It is not good that the man should be alone." We are designed for relationship and fellowship. Aloneness often brings sorrow. While it is okay to express deep grief or sadness upon the passing of a loved one, this time should be short. In the Bible it was 30 days. Depending on the person and circumstances, the timeframe may be different, but grief should not last a lifetime. Proverbs 15:13 says, "A merry heart maketh a cheerful countenance: but by sorrow of the heart the spirit is broken."

When life is not sweet, many people seek out food to fill the void. After the death of someone dear or a divorce, many turn to food for comfort resulting in weight gain and even damage to the pancreas.

---

4 "Anger and ego-defence mechanisms in non-psychiatric patients with irritable bowel syndrome" Zoccali R, Muscatello MR, Bruno A, Barillà G, Campolo D, Meduri M, Familiari L, Bonica M, Consolo P, Scaffidi M. Dig Liver Dis. 2006 Mar;38(3):195-200. http://www.ncbi.nlm.nih.gov/pubmed/16500602

5 "Anger experiences among hepatitis C patients: relationship to depressive symptoms and health-related quality of life" Dan AA, Crone C, Wise TN, Martin LM, Ramsey L, Magee S, Sjogren R, Ong JP, Younossi ZM. Psychosomatics. 2007 May-Jun;48(3):223-9.

6 "The role of affiliative loss in the recruitment of helper cells among insulin-dependent diabetics." McClelland DC, Patel V, Brown D, Kelner SP Jr., Boston University Center for Applied Social Science, Behav Med. 1991 Spring;17(1):5-14.

Emotional Links

The body's immune system can be adversely affected by thoughts through two pathways - the **central nervous system** and the **limbic system**. The limbic system includes the hypothalamus, which connects the nervous system to the endocrine system. It also includes the hippocampus and amygdala. The endocrine system and its array of hormones are managed by the limbic system, which also controls emotions. As the limbic system is directly connected to the parts of the brain that control heart rate, breathing, blood pressure, stress, memory and hormone levels, the wrong hormones produced with certain negative thoughts or emotions can suppress the immune system, setting up the body for disease and ill health.

The **thalamus** makes the decisions in our emotional minds. It can be likened to the hard drive of the brain. Everything that has ever happened to a person is recorded in the thalamus, whether consciously remembered or not. It determines whether a person is safe or not safe. If an event occurs that resembles the first time something traumatic happened in the past, the thalamus reacts. After a few times of reacting in the same way, it becomes an automatic response not even thought about. The body turns to autopilot and reactions are made to triggers and not to reality.

For example, if a person has been told he is allergic to cats he can walk into a home, see a cat and immediately experience a swollen throat and shortness of breath. In reality, the physical body has not had the time to really react to the allergens, but the thalamus has, and the response is the same.

During traumatic events, the thalamus collects sensory information and sends messages to the **hippocampus**. This is the part of the brain that seems to paralyze a person during such an event. A person cannot seem to run, cannot make decisions, cannot fight back and cannot even think of what to say. Emotionally, a person can get stuck at the age of their earliest wound.

The hippocampus then sends quick, high voltage signals to the **amygdala**. The amygdala is very important for storing and releasing trauma memories. The amygdala sets off adrenaline in the fight-or-flight response by signaling to the hypothalamus, which then stimulates the sympathetic nervous system responsible for the actual physical fight-or-flight response. If the traumatic event is not dealt with in a positive way, a person can revert to their old habits of negative response and freeze or retreat.

The **hypothalamus** is the facilitator and originator of all expressions of fear including fast heart rate, sweat, pain, anxiety, stress, body temperature, tension, panic, phobias, rage, anger and aggression. It is the brain of the endocrine system, sending out various types of chemical messengers, or hormones, to the endocrine system. It is negative hormones, such as the stress hormone cortisol, released during traumatic events with negative emotions that end up causing the diseases related to those emotions. When a negative emotion is continually played out and the hormones continue to flow, diseases can result.

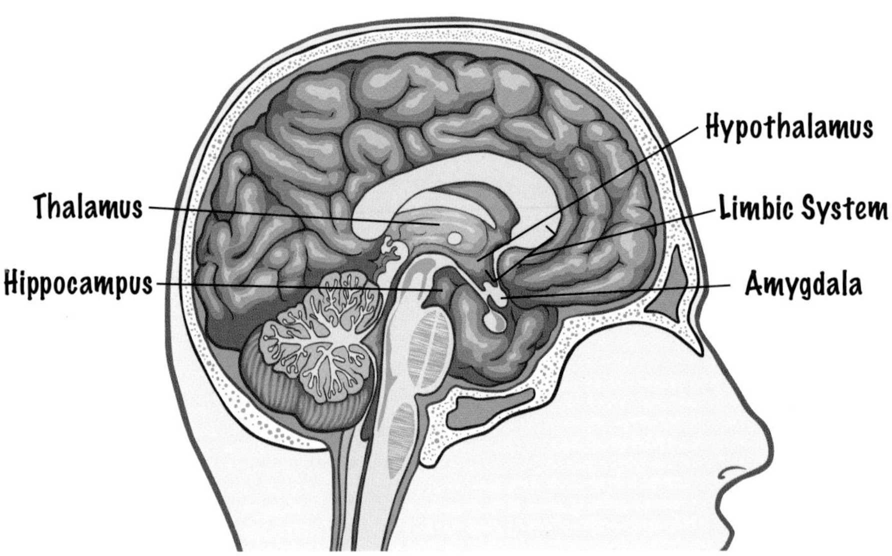

Stress and Cancer

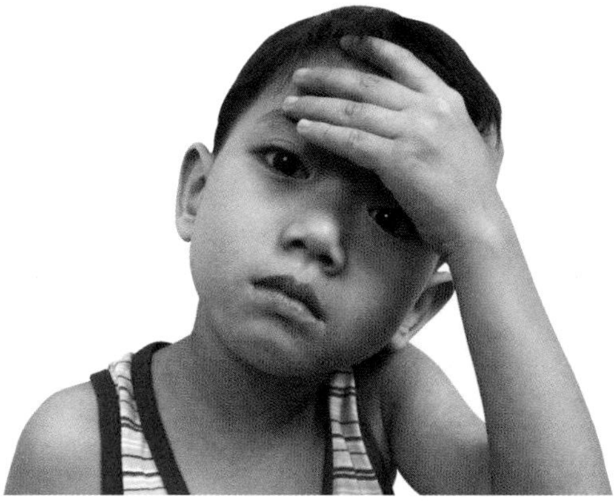

What about daily stress? In the book "The Official Anti-aging Revolution" by Ronald Klatz, M.D. and Robert Goldman, M.D., they list 34 stressful events and assign a value. The lower the score, the less effect the event has on a person's health. For example:

Death of a spouse - 100
Serious injury or illness - 53
Begin or end school - 26
Change school – 20

They suggest that anyone with a score greater than 150 is in real danger and are at "genuine risk for premature illness and accelerated aging." Even if someone experiences stressful events, it is the way in which the person handles it that can make a difference in his or her physical health.

Cortisol is considered to be the stress hormone. Abnormal fluctuations in cortisol have been linked to a decreased survival time with advanced breast cancer.[7] The American Cancer Society states that 30 percent of all cancers are of unknown etiology. In other words they do not know the cause. The same can be said for diseases ending in the word syndrome. While the symptoms are real, there is no known cause.

Pastor and author Henry W. Wright[8] believes the Bible teaches that bad thinking causes disease and good thinking can prevent disease – cancer included. He also believes that all diseases that end with the word syndrome, have a spiritual root.

Emotional Frequency

Every living thing, such as plants, animals, humans and essential oils, has a frequency. This includes thoughts and the expressions of those thoughts – or emotions – can raise or lower the body's frequency. These changes in frequency caused by emotions can even be seen in dark field microscope analysis of the blood.

A high frequency level is life to the body. A low frequency leads to disease and eventual death. Feelings should not be confused with emotions. Feelings are our sensory data – I see ... I feel ... I hear … – whereas our emotions are the result of what we believe about that sensory data.

Frequency of Food

According to Tainio Technology and Technique, Inc., currently the originator of the most accurate instrument for measuring food frequencies, the following foods contain these vibration measurements:

Fresh fruits (organic and picked when ripe) 80 MHz, raw green vegetables (organic) 65-72 MHz, wild fish 50-55 MHz, farmed fish 40-45 MHz, wine 40-50 MHz, chicken (organic, free range) 40-45 MHz, beef (organic, grass fed) 40-45 MHz, sprouted grains 35-45 MHz, chicken (caged) 20-25 MHz, pork 15-20 MHz, beef (commercial) 15-20 MHz. raw non-green vegetables (organic) 13-21 MHz, processed sprouted-grain products 10-15 MHz, cooked inorganic vegetables 7-25 MHz, cheeseburger 5-10 MHz, nuts (raw) 5-7 MHz, grains (refined, processed) <1 MHz, fast food French fries <1 MHz

7 "Diurnal Cortisol Rhythm as a Predictor of Breast Cancer Survival", Sandra E. Sephton, Robert M. Sapolsky, Helena C. Kraemer, David Spiegel, Journal of the National Cancer Institute, Vol. 92, No. 12, 994-1000, June 21, 2000.
8 www.beinhealth.com

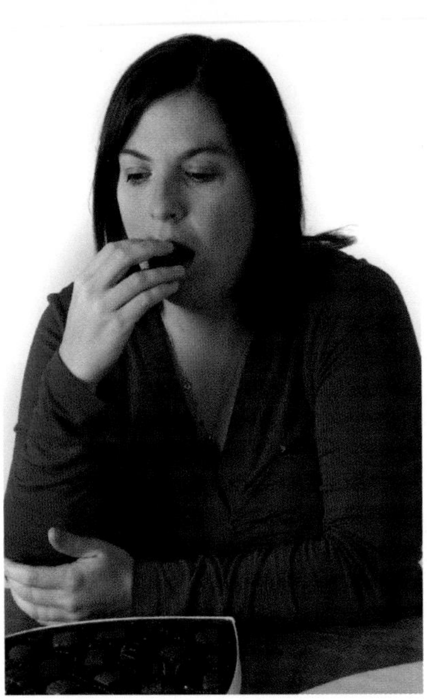

Can food affect emotions?

Abolutely! From Unit 1, we learned that the brain needs critical nutrients like Omega-3 fatty acids, B vitamins, amino acids and others to function properly. The brain is so very complex and controls every part of the body including emotions. The chemicals in the brain must maintain a delicate balance for optimal performance. Any time the brain is deprived of critical nutrients or is bombarded with food toxins like additives and preservatives, the hormone and chemical balance is disrupted and brain function is affected including emotional stability.

The National Institute of Mental Health cites that about one in four Americans suffer with some sort of diagnosable mental disorder in a given year.[9] With the 2004 U.S. census population estimate applied, it correlates to about 57.7 million people. With so many people lacking adequate brain nutrition, it is no wonder that the numbers are so very high.

Emotional Eating and Comfort Food

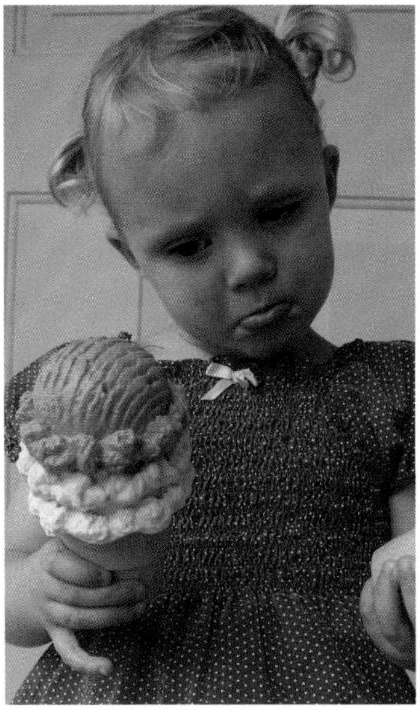

In times of sadness or depression, many often turn to their favorite comfort food. While foods like ice cream and chocolate candy provide temporary satisfaction and even a sense of euphoria, they are definitely not a cure all for emotional distress.

Once the sugar high wears off and the blood sugar levels drastically drop, a person is still left dealing, or not dealing, with the negative emotions. Besides being a hinderance to brain function, comfort foods laiden with sugar and excess fat and calories may also lead to weight gain.

Healthier Options

Healthier versions of comfort food are much better options for those who have emotional eating habits. See the recipe at the end of this chapter for an example of a healthier comfort food recipe. Following the dietary suggestions laid out in **Nutrition 101: Choose Life!** and adding more nutritious, brain foods will help promote better emotional health.

Sowing and Reaping

From business owners to stay-at-home moms, we all have the power to change another person's life with every smile or frown, kind word or critical word. Emotions can signal success or failure. If a person is happy, energetic and positive, people will see that and respond to her in like fashion. The same goes for if those who are always complaining, grumbling and whining. They won't be resonating a frequency other people want to be around. However, those who we admire and are always upbeat, wear a smile and are positive about life are the people we want to be around.

The law of sowing and reaping resonates with emotions. Whether positive or negative emotions are sown even within oneself, both will have determined outcomes.

---

9 "Prevalence, severity, and comorbidity of twelve-month DSM-IV disorders in the National Comorbidity Survey Replication" (NCS-R) Kessler RC, Chiu WT, Demler O, Walters EE. Archives of General Psychiatry, 2005 Jun;62(6):617-27

Releasing Emotions and Reclaiming Life

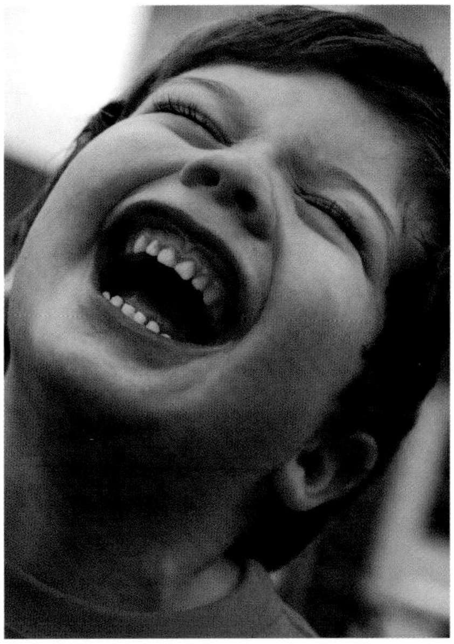

Other than a miracle from God, the only known way to release emotions is through the **sense of smell**. The olfactory system is the only one of five senses that is wired directly to the seat of our emotions and hormones – the limbic system.

Emotions and Essential Oils

Some people say certain smells trigger fond memories of eating dinner at their grandmother's house when they were children while other smells remind them of their favorite season or holiday. Some smells can even trigger bad memories and the release of the emotions related to them. Some say smelling an essential oil makes them feel happy or sad or causes them to cry. Essential oils when smelled have an instant impact on a person's mental and emotional life.

Unadulterated essential oils from plants that God made are His tools to help us release the negative emotions that hold us back and allow us to reach our highest potential.[10] When inhaled, therapeutic-grade essential oils enter the limbic region of the brain through the olfactory system and into the hypothalamus releasing stored negative emotions. This is the science of aroma-therapy.

Emotions can control us and keep us from reaching our highest potential. However, essential oils, which God has graciously given us from the plants that He made, are part of the answer to emotional freedom.

To learn about which essential oils are used for emotional wellbeing, please refer to Appendix DD.

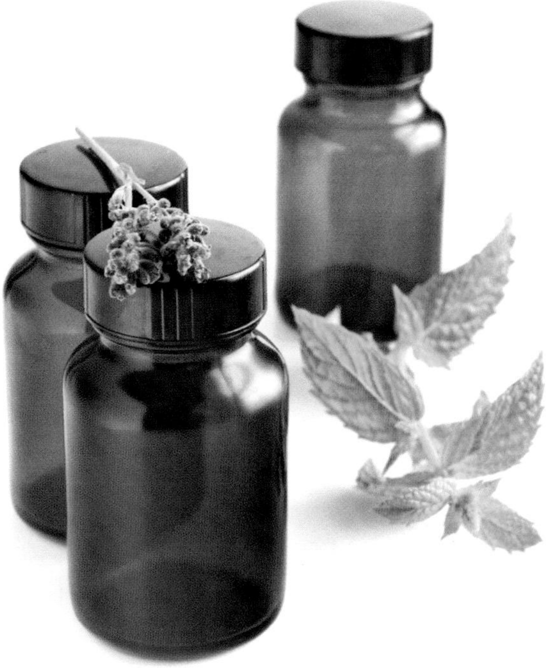

10 "Chemistry of Essential Oils Made Simple: God's Love Manifest in Molecules" David Stewart, Ph.D., D.N.M., Care Publications, 2006.

Unit 6 Chapter 4
Discussion Questions

1. What do you think Isaiah 55:1-3 means?
2. How is the joy of the Lord our strength?
3. How are the heart, tongue and mind connected?
4. What songs do you about emotions that can encourage and uplift you?

Activities - plus the Tropical Vanilla Ice Cream "Power" Recipe and activities.

Elementary

1. Read Psalm 126 and identify all of the words associated with emotions.
2. Use several different pieces of colored paper to draw seven different fruit and label them with the characteristics of the Spirit, found in Galatians 5:22. Display the fruit in your home for the family to see and to help you memorize the scripture.
3. Demonstrate how emotions are like magnets, by gathering several magnets so the positive and negative sides are exposed. What happens when the positive sides are facing one another? What about a negative and a positive? What about two negatives? How are these like emotions? Share your findings with your family and describe how positive and negative emotions attract and repel others.
4. Think of three some specific smalls that you relate with good or bad emotions. Example, the scent of pine may remind you of Christmas trees.
5. What kind of professionals help people deal with negative emotions?

Secondary

Choose any from above plus

1. Using scriptural references for, describe the relationship between the mind and the heart. Now, find scriptures that connect the heart and the tongue. Then, the tongue and the mind. Using these, create a prepare a written or oral report to support
2. If science has proven that every living thing has a frequency, find evidence supporting frequencies of certain foods. Do raw foods have a higher frequency than cooked foods? How does this effect the types of foods you want to eat? How can the combination of food and emotions affect the frequency of your body?
3. Who coined the term aromatherapy and when?
4. What is the difference between psychology and psychiatry?
5. How do you believe the treatment of emotional issues would differ from a Christian professional versus a non-Christian?

Additional Resources

Books:

"Reverse The Curse In Your Body And Emotions" and mini-book "Quantum Faith" Annette Capps, available at www.charlescapps.com

Web sites:

http://www.tsbvi.edu/Outreach/seehear/summer05/smell.htm

Endocrine Sytem Power

Healthy Comfort Foods

In times of emotional stress, people often turn to comfort foods, such as chocolate candy and ice cream. While food should never act as an emotional crutch, healthy versions of comfort foods are better options and may provide needed nutritional support.

Tropical Vanilla Ice Cream Shake

While packed with healthy fat and nutrients from coconuts, this shake is dairy and refined sugar free and is a much better dessert option than regular ice cream.

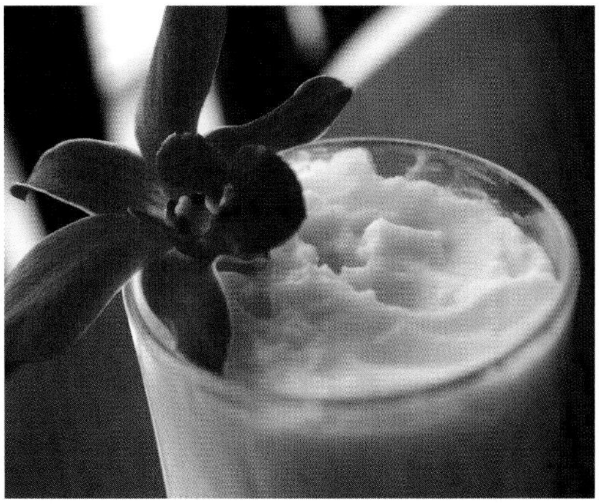

1 can organic coconut milk
½ cup Blue Agave Nectar
2 ½ tsp. organic vanilla extract
3 cups ice

Add coconut milk, blue agave, vanilla and ice in blender. Blend until thick and smooth. Add more ice if necessary. Add strawberries, pineapple or carob powder for different flavor options.

Activities

Elementary

1. What makes this recipe tropical?
2. Experiment with other tropical fruits, various berries or citrus fruits to add color and flavor to this recipe.
3. Check the agave you are using to verify that it is raw, blue agave nectar. What is its glycemic index?
4. Make this recipe for someone you know who has diabetes.
5. What kind of emotional response do you have while eating this with your family? Ask other members to share what they are feeling.

Secondary

Choose any from above plus

1. What happens to this shake if you put it in the freezer for 15 minutes? How does it change?
2. Why does this recipe call for coconut milk rather than raw or pasteurized milk?
3. What have you learned about milk that you did not know before you started this program?
4. Smell each ingredient in the recipe separately and then smell the finished product. Are these pleasant or unpleasant? Do they recall any memories? Have other members of your family do this and see if any smells trigger emotions.
5. Using this recipe as a base, find a way to make ice cream.

Unit 6 Additional Recipes

Use organic ingredients when possible.

Maple Toasted Walnuts

2 cups raw walnuts
Grade B maple syrup
Pinch of sea salt

Place walnuts in skillet and drizzle with Grade B maple syrup. Add a pinch of sea salt. Toast walnuts until warm and maple syrup is caramelized. Spread out onto a baking sheet to cool. Serve 1/3 cup portions as a quick snack or light dessert. For a low glycemic version, substitute raw blue agave for the maple syrup.

Sesame Wedges

Wax paper
Sesame seeds
Almond butter

Spread ¼ almond butter on wax paper, press flat. Place another sheet of wax paper on top of almond butter and using a rolling pin spread into an 1/8 inch thin sheet. Carefully remove the top sheet of was paper. Sprinkle a generous amount of sesame seeds on the almond butter and press. Be sure to cover the entire surface. Place a new sheet of wax paper on top, flip the flat sheet over so sesame seeds may be pressed into the other side. If enough sesame seeds are pressed onto both sides, it will not be sticky. These make great snacks. Prepare several at a time and store with wax paper between each and store in refrigerator.

Cucumber Salad

2 large cucumbers, partially peeled, sliced very thin
½ red onion sliced very thin
4 tablespoons olive oil
2 teaspoons Apple cider vinegar
1 drop tarragon Young Living essential oil
Salt and pepper to taste

Toss and let sit one hour before serving.

Cold Pea Salad

1 cup frozen green English peas
1 cup shredded carrots
2 tablespoons organic Ranch style dressing

Combine in a bowl and let sit until peas begin to thaw, but still cold.

Tortilla Soup

¼ cup olive oil
¼ cup chicken stock or broth
1 cup diced white or yellow onions
1 tsp. ground cumin
1 tsp. chili powder
1 tsp. granulated garlic
¼ tsp. cayenne pepper
1 cup Masa Harina
2 qt. water (divided)
1 cups crushed Tomatoes
1 lb. cooked, cubed chicken
2 ripe avocados, sliced into wedges
Handful of organic, non-GMO corn tortilla chips crumbled

In large pot, place oil, chicken base, onion and spices. Sauté until onions are soft and clear, about 5 minutes. In another container, combine Masa Harina with 1 quart of the water. Stir until all lumps dissolve. Add to sautéed onions and bring to boil. Once mixture starts to bubble, continue cooking 2-3 minutes, stirring constantly. This will eliminate any raw taste from Masa Harina. Add remaining 3 quarts water to pot. Add tomatoes; let mixture return to boil stirring occasionally. Add chicken; heat through. Spoon into bowls, top with chips and avocado slices.

Energy Soup

1 lb. fresh green beans
1 cup chopped celery
1 summer squash, chopped
1 zucchini squash, chopped
1 medium onion, diced
1 cup chopped Roma tomatoes
1 cup water
1 cup vegetable or chicken broth
Season with a pinch of salt and pepper.

Combine in a pot, simmer one hour. Serve with a green salad.

Creamy Garlic and Rosemary Mashed Potatoes

8 organic Red Russet potatoes
2 Tbs. of organic unsalted butter
1 clove of garlic
Spring of rosemary
1 egg
Salt and pepper

Wash and quarter the potatoes. If the potatoes are not organic, peel them before quartering. Put the potatoes in a pot and fill it with water until the potatoes are covered. Bring to a boil and reduce heat to simmer. Mince the garlic and pull the rosemary from the sprig. When the potatoes are soft or easily pierced with a knife, turn off the heat. Before draining the water from the potatoes, reserve a ladle full of the water in a small bowl. Once the potatoes are drained, crack the egg into the reserved water, which should still be hot. Whisk the egg for 20 seconds. Immediately add this and the butter to the potatoes, combining with a potato masher or hand mixer. Once the desired creaminess is attained, blend in the remaining ingredients and serve.

Hearty Chili

1 lb. ground lean meat – beef, turkey or chicken
½ cup yellow onion, chopped
½ cup celery, chopped
½ cup red bell pepper, chopped
2 cloves garlic, minced
2 Tbs. chili powder
1 Tbs. cumin
¼ tsp. cayenne pepper (optional)
1 tsp. black pepper (or to taste)
Sea salt to taste
1 can organic black beans
1 can organic kidney beans
1 can organic tomato sauce
1 can organic diced tomatoes, not drained
1 small can of green chiles, chopped and drained (optional)

While browning meat, add onions, celery, red bell pepper, garlic, and spices. In a separate large pot, combine beans, tomatoes, tomato sauce and optional green chiles. Once meat is browned, add meat, veggies and spices to large pot. Stir and simmer 30 minutes. For a vegetarian version, omit meat and add double the beans. For even more kick, add some chopped and seeded jalapenos.

Orange Fluff Dessert

2 medium oranges, peeled and separated into segments in bowls for each person
½ tsp. grated orange rind
1 drop Young Living lemon oil
3 Tbs. low fat yogurt, vanilla
2 Tbs. creamed honey

Whisk lemon oil, honey, and rind until combined. Fold in yogurt. Spoon mixture on top of orange segments.

Final Thoughts

Congratulations! You've just finished a remarkable journey of health, wellness and longevity through nutrition. We hope that along the way your families' taste buds were delighted with delicious and nutritious recipes and your collective appetite for learning more about whole health is insatiable.

You now know the body in a whole new light, how the foods we eat heal it, help it or tear it down. You can continually use and review this information. Hopefully you'll look at food in a whole new light – as tools for health and wellness. God's creation includes a multitude of foods, all given for us to enjoy. How we process and prepare these foods can enhance their goodness or remove nutritional value.

In the World, But Not of It

Be encouraged in your journey and mindful that your new habits are different from many of your friends and extended family members. Remember that the Holy Spirit is gentle, not forceful. If friends or extended family turn a deaf ear to your findings, just keep showing them love. True change comes to those who are receptive or have revelation of the truth. Those who are in Christ Jesus are not condemned because they walk in the Spirit, not in the flesh (Romans 8:1).

If your family eats outside of the home, there are many ways to stay on track. If you go to another friend's home, and the hostess is not preparing a meal, eat beforehand or bring your own snacks. During special occasions and holidays, there are times to partake in moderation.

However, you should protect your bodies by taking enzymes and applying essential oils before and after going out. Teach your children what you want them to say beforehand when confronted with an offer of an unhealthy option. Usually a simple "no thank you" accomplishes the goal without offending the person offering.

If you do not want your child to partake during a special occasion, like a birthday party, you can eat beforehand or ask the hostess if you can bring a treat for your child to eat at the same time as other party goers. This is more common as so many children have food allergies. When your friends show an interest in your healthy lifestyle, you will be there with the information they want and need.

At restaurants beware that many healthier options are on the menu are not as good as they sound. Some places provide menus and nutritional information online to review before venturing out. This is especially helpful in planning for a vacation.

Our Prayer for Your Family is That ...

God will satisfy your mouth with good things that nourish the body. That you'll not spend your money on that which is not food. That you'll think on things of a good report. That you'll delight yourself in Him. That you live out all your days with energy, vitality, health and happiness from the top of your head to the soles of your feet and you will use God's food and medicine (essential oils) when needed to balance and restore health. Beloved, we wish above all things that you prosper and be in health, even as your soul prospers.

Activity Guide

Unit 1 Chapter 1

Elementary

1. Explain to the children that these activities are designed to exercise the brain and make it do things it doesn't routinely do. This creates new neurol connections in the brain and improves brain power.
2. Self explanatory.
3. Establish guidelines for selecting items, such as nothing sharp and highly valuable or irreplaceable objects.
4. Examples: Philippians 2:5, Luke 10:27 and I Corinthians 2:16.
5. Self explanatory.

Secondary

1. Self explanatory.
2. Lobe is derived from the Latin word lobus and the Greek word lobos.
3. Careers associated with the brain include neurologists, psychologists, teachers, safety gear designers to name some.
4. Self explanatory.

Unit 1 "Power" Recipes Activity Guide

If necessary, refer to the "Power" Recipe instrucion page.

Kitchen Talk

1. Recap the discussion questions from each corresponding chapter and review what you learned.
2. Talk about the "Power" food in the recipe.
3. While preparing the dish, talk about the preparation methods used, and, if needed, demonstrate techniques for them such as chopping and mincing. For children old enough, allow them to help.
4. Choose one or more of the activities in the appropriate grade levels for children to do.

Guacamole

Elementary

1. Self explanatory.
2. Self explanatory.
3. Put the avocado and apple in a small paper bag. Leave the bag closed overnight or up to 24 hours.
4. To grow an avocado plant you will need: a soft avocado, toothpicks, a glass, water, potting soil and a pot. To germinate the seed, stab the seed with three toothpicks around the middle. Place it on top of the glass. Fill the glass with water so half an inch of the seed is submerged. Place the seed in a warm location with indirect light, but not too much direct light. In one to two weeks, you will see a root growing at the bottom and a shoot coming out the top. Make sure you keep the same level of water in the glass. When the green shoot has grown six inches, plant it in a pot keeping the soil damp by watering every few days. Make sure the pot has at least one drainage hole at the bottom. In a year or so, when the roots are sturdy enough, you can plant it in the ground. Also, check out www.kidsgardening.com for more tips and information.

Secondary

1. The ethylene gas emitted from the apple actually speeds the ripening process. To find out more about this process, check out www.mindfully.org/Plastic/Ethylene-Gas.htm.
2. The banana probably won't ripen the avocado as fast as the apple, but it will brown quickly.
3. If a serving size of an avocado is half of the avocado and a whole avocado has about 22.5 grams of fat, then a serving has about 11.25 grams of fat. For older children, let them look up this information. You can go to www.avocado.org to find out more. Click on "Healthy-living".
4. An avocado contains mono unsaturated fat.

Unit 1 Chapter 2

Elementary

1. Self explanatory.
2. Self explanatory.
3. Fish, chia seed and flaxseed.
4. Self explanatory. You will need fast food French fries, a plastic, sealable bag and a permanent marker.
5. Self explanatory.
6. Self explanatory.

Secondary

1. Self explanatory.
2. The highest Omega-3 plant source is Evening Primrose and the highest fish source is salmon.
3. Omega is the first letter in the Greek alphabet.

4. Self explanatory.
5. Self explanatory.
6. Self explanatory.
7. Self explanatory.
8. Self explanatory.

Greek Salad

Elementary

1. Olive oil, vinegar, glass bowl
2. The olive oil is a mono unsaturated fat, so it will go rancid. All of the food in the recipe will eventually go rancid because whole, fresh, unprocessed, live food immediately begins to oxidize.
3. Self explanatory.

Secondary

1. As vinegar and oil do not mix, you will observe them separate and "bead" on the other ingredients.
2. Make a list of the green leafy vegetables at the market and then do a search on the internet or research at the library to find their nutritional values.
3. Refer to the good/bad brain foods chart.

Unit 1 Chapter 3

Elementary - All self explanatory.

Secondary

1. For example, 1. Sensory - Eyes see an apple. 2. Integrative - Brain says, "That's an apple. I want to eat that apple". 3. Motor - Stomach and salivary glands start producing secretions, and arms and hands reach out to grab the apple and put it in the mouth.
2. Self explanatory.
3. Self explanatory.
4. Self explanatory.

Potato Salad with Flaxseed Oil - Hold the Mayo

Elementary

1. Self explanatory.
2. True. Nut is a general term for the dry seed or fruit of some plants. Nuts are both the seed and the fruit, and cannot be separated. Seeds come from fruit, and can be removed from the fruit, like almonds, cashews and pistachios, which were once inside fruit.
3. For more information on where flax grows and harvesting it, go to www.plantmanagementnetwork.org/pub/cm/management/2003/flax/.
4. Self explanatory. Find conversion charts for tablespoons to ounces in most cookbooks or through online sources.

Secondary

1. Self explanatory.
2. Self explanatory.
3. A dry ounce is a measure of weight, and a fluid ounce is a measure of volume.

Unit 1 Chapter 4

Elementary

1. Self explanatory.
2. For example, use categories such as: from a plant, from an animal, color grouping and must be refrigerated.
3. Self explanatory
4. Refer to the list of amino acid plant sources.
5. Self explanatory.
6. Self explanatory.
7. Self explanatory.
8. Self explanatory.
9. Refer to Appendix F.

Secondary

1. Self explanatory.
2. Self explanatory.
3. Check www.usda.gov and do a search for RDA.
4. Self explanatory.
5. Refer to Appendix D. This is a relatively new word and may not be in the dictionary.

Stuffed Eggs - Hold the Mayo

Elementary - All self explanatory

Secondary

1. Self explanatory.
2. Self explanitory.
3. You will need to do more research on flaxseed oil and olive oil to find out what happens to them when they are heated. For example, do they maintain their chemical structures and their nutritional values? Find answers online or at the library.

Unit 2 Chapter 1

Elementary

1. Self explanatory.
2. Self explanatory.

3. Self explanatory.
4. The stomach can hold two to four liters. There are four liters in a gallon.

Secondary
1. Self explanatory.
2. Self explanatory.
3. Self explanatory.
4. A regulation-size tennis court is 78 feet wide by 36 feet long. The square footage is 2,808.
5. Self explanatory.
6. Self explanatory.
7. Self explanatory.

Unit 2 "Power" Recipes Activity Guide

If necessary, refer to the "Power" Recipe instruction page.

Kitchen Talk

1. Recap the discussion questions from each corresponding chapter and review what you learned.
2. Talk about the "Power" food in the recipe.
3. While preparing the dish, talk about the preparation methods used, and, if needed, demonstrate techniques for them such as chopping and mincing. For children old enough, allow them to help.
4. Choose one or more of the activities in the appropriate grade levels for children to do.

Fruit Salad

Elementary
1. Self explanatory.
2. An antioxidant is defined as a substance (as beta-carotene or vitamin C) that inhibits oxidation or reactions promoted by oxygen, peroxides or free radicals. Antioxidants are known to contain disease-fighting compounds.
3. Organic refers to food produced with the use of feed or fertilizer of plant or animal origin without chemically formulated fertilizers, growth stimulants, antibiotics or pesticides. Depending on the source, the definition can vary.
4. Self explanatory.

Secondary
1. Blueberry, strawberry, apple, peach and nectarine are good antioxidant rich fruits. Fruits and vegetables that are purple, blue, red and orange typically are the highest in antioxidants. However, some of the antioxidants cannot be absorbed by the body based on a theory called bioavailability. According to researcher Ronald Prior, PhD, a chemist and nutritionist with the U.S. Department of Agriculture's Arkansas Children's Nutrition Center in Little Rock, Ark. "Bioavailability has to do with absorption or metabolism in the gut. What's absorbed will be impacted by the mechanical structure of different antioxidants in food -- if they're tied up with fiber or if they have sugar molecules attached." Dr. Prior, who authored a landmark study on bioavailability, admits that researchers still are learning more about this subject and learning more about cooking and drying such foods. For example, they believe that lightly steaming blueberries enhances the antioxidant level. The key is having a variety of these types of antioxidant foods, especially berries.
2. The most chemically treated fruits and vegetables are peaches, apples, sweet bell peppers, celery, nectarines, strawberries, cherries, pears, grapes (imported), spinach, lettuce and potatoes. The least chemically treated fruits and vegetables are papaya, broccoli, cabbage, bananas, kiwi, frozen sweet peas, asparagus, mangoes, pineapples, frozen sweet corn, avocado and onions.
3. Self explanatory.

Unit 2 Chapter 2

Elementary
1. Self explanatory.
2. Self explanatory.
3. Cruciferous vegetables have excellent cancer fighting properties. Research suggests that these cruciferous vegetables contain a kind of phytochemical, known as isothiocyanates, which stimulate our bodies to break down potential cancer-causing agents.
4. Self explanatory.
5. Self explanatory.
6. Self explanatory.
7. Self explanatory.

Secondary
1. Scriptures about food preparation and mealtime include Genesis 18:1-8, 25:29-34, 27:1-40; Exodus 11; Lev.iticus11; Deuteronomy 16; Ruth 2:2-48; I Samuel 2:12-17, 21:1-6; Esther 5:3-8; Psalm 23:5; Daniel 1; Matthew 12:1-8,14:14-21; 15:32-38, 26-29; Mark 6:30-44, 8:1-10, 14:12-25; and Luke 5:1-11. 6:1-11 and 22:1-30.
2. Digestive glands in the stomach lining produce the

acid and an enzyme that digests protein. A thick mucus layer coats the lining and helps keep the acidic digestive juice from dissolving the tissue of the stomach itself. In most people, the stomach mucus is able to resist the juice, although food and other tissues of the body cannot.

3. Self explanatory.
4. Self explanatory.
5. pH test strips may be purchased online or at some pharmacies. Instructions for homemade strips are in the Teacher's Guide under Secondary activity #2 of the of the Green Bean Apple Salad.

Green Apple Bean Salad

Elementary

1. Julienne is means to cut into narrow, fine sticks that can measure from two to three inches long and 1/8 inch square. A finer julienne measures 1/16 of an inch square. Blanching is the scalding of vegetables in boiling water or steam. Blanching slows or stops the action of enzymes. The most convenient way to blanch vegetables is in a large kettle of boiling water. Allow one gallon of water per pound of vegetables. Bring the water to boil and lower vegetables into the water, allowing the water to continue boiling. Cover and start counting the blanching time.
2. The Granny Smith apple originated in Australia in 1868 from a seedling propagated by Maria Ann Smith (Sherwood), also know as Granny Smith. They are found wild in New Zealand. Originally introduced to the United Kingdom around 1935 and the United States about 1972, Granny Smith apples are crisp, juicy, and tart. This makes them perfect for either baking in pies, stewed in sauces or eating out of hand. They're also great in salads because once cut, they keep their color longer than other apples.
3. As onions are sliced, cells are broken, allowing enzymes to break down amino acid sulfoxides and generate sulfenic acids. Sulfenic acids are unstable and spontaneously rearrange into a compound called propanethial-s-oxide, which is released in a vapor when onions are cut. The gas dissipates through the air and eventually reaches the eye, where it reacts with the water to form a dilute solution of sulfuric acid. This acid irritates the nerve endings in the eye, making them sting. Tear glands produce tears to dilute and flush out the irritant.

Secondary

1. Lemon juice is acidic in its natural state, but turns alkaline after being metabolized in the body. A variety of health problems can occur when the body is either too alkaline or acidic, but the typical American diet is too acidic. When the body fluids become too acidic, a condition called acidosis develops. On the other hand, when the body fluids become too alkaline, alkalosis may develop. Foods are determined to have either an alkaline or acid-forming potential based on their pH values. The word pH (power of Hydrogen) comes from the chemistry formula for calculating the concentration of hydrogen ions present in a substance. A pH of 7 is neutral. Foods that are more alkaline have pH values above 7. Foods that are more acidic have pH values below 7. Pure water has a neutral pH of 7.
2. You can purchase pH testing strips, but this homemade project also is fun. This experiment will tell you whether a substance is an acid or base, but not the exact value of pH; the pH scale ranges from acid (zero to six), through neutral (seven) to alkaline or base (eight to 14). If you want to calibrate your cabbage juice pH indicator, you will have to test your substances with another quantitative indicator (e.g. litmus paper) and compare those results to the colors of the cabbage juice pH indicator in those solutions; litmus paper can be obtained from several scientific suppliers or from your local swimming pool store.

To prepare the test strips or indicators, follow these instructions. For more information, search Internet sites such as www.wikihow.com or www.howstuffworks.com.

You will need:

- A head of red cabbage
- A stove
- A pot
- Distilled water
- A funnel or coffee filter basket
- Coffee filters
- A set of eyedropper bottles (e.g., clean infant medicine bottles)
- A medicine cup with teaspoon or milliliter markings
- Several small paper cups
- Some clear test substances (e.g., lemon juice, clear sports drink, lemon-lime soda, window cleaner, vinegar)
- Eye protection and pot holders

Follow these instructions to prepare your pH indicator:

- Put ½ cup of distilled water in the pot.
- Shred some red cabbage leaves and add to the pot.
- Bring the pot to a boil on the stove, and boil for five to 10 minutes. (Note - You should wear some form of eye protection and use pot holders when handling boiling solutions.)
- While waiting for the mixture to boil, prepare the clean glass jar and place the funnel on top of it and the coffee filter inside the funnel.
- Pour the water with the boiled leaves through the filter to remove the pieces of cabbage, collecting the filtered juice in the clean glass.
- Let the mixture cool; it should appear purple.
- Once cool, pour the juice into the eyedropper bottles for use and storage.
- This filtered juice is your pH indicator. Note that the concentration of the indicator solution depends upon the amount of cabbage and the volume of water used; the more cabbage in the smallest possible volume of water will yield a high concentration of indicator molecules.
- To use your pH indicator, pour about two teaspoons (10 ml) of each test substance into a separate paper cup. To each cup, add approximately ½ teaspoon (2 ml) of cabbage juice indicator. Now watch for the color changes.
- If the substance is an acid (pH below 7), the indicator should turn bright pink. If the substance is neutral (pH of 7), then the indicator should remain reddish-purple. Finally, if the substance is alkaline or base (pH above 7), then the indicator should turn greenish yellow.

3. Self explanatory.

Unit 2 Chapter 3

Elementary

1. Self explanatory.
2. Self explanatory.
3. Self explanatory.
4. Bread, wine, fish and lamb are examples.

Secondary

1. Self explanatory.
2. Self explanatory.
3. The fermenting of new wine builds up pressure in its container. This effect is illustrated when a bottle of wine is uncorked. In Bible times, new wineskins would stretch as new wine was put in them and continued to ferment. Then, the wineskins would harden. If new wine was put into a hardened wineskin, the continued fermentation risked bursting the skin. In this parable, Jesus also refers to new, unshruken cloth being used to patch already-shrunken cloth.
4. Fermentation is the conversion of a carbohydrate, typically a sugar into an acid or alcohol. Fermentation also can refer to using yeast to change sugar into alcohol or using bacteria to create lactic acid. Because it occurs naturally in different foods given the right conditions, humans have used the fermenting process for thousands of years in food preparation.
5. Self explanatory.

Quinoa Vegetable Risotto

Elementary

1. When referring to fresh foods, such as fruits and vegetables, raw means being in the natural state, not processed or diluted and full of enzymes that aid in digestion.
2. Enzymes in fresh, raw fruits and vegetables are full of enzymes that promote healthy digestion in the body.
3. Quinoa (pronounced KEEN-wah or KEE-no-uh) is an amino acid-rich (protein) seed that has a fluffy, creamy, slightly crunchy texture and a somewhat nutty flavor when cooked.
4. Self explanatory.
5. The following is provided by The George Mateljan Foundation through "The World's Healthiest Foods, Essential Guide for the Healthiest Way of Eating" online at www.whf.com. Quinoas are indigenous to South America, but have been grown in the United States since 1980. If you cannot find it in your local supermarket, look for it at natural foods stores throughout the year or order online. Quinoa is generally available in prepackaged containers, as well as bulk bins. Whether purchasing quinoa in bulk or in a packaged container, make sure that there is no evidence of moisture. When deciding upon the amount to purchase, remember that quinoa expands during the cooking process to several times its original size. Not only is quinoa high in protein, but the protein it supplies is *complete protein*, meaning that it includes all nine essential amino acids. Not only is quinoa's amino acid profile well balanced, making it a good choice for vegans concerned about adequate protein intake, but quinoa is especially

well-endowed with the amino acid *lysine*, which is essential for tissue growth and repair. In addition to protein, quinoa features a host of other health-building nutrients. Because quinoa is a very good source of manganese as well as a good source of magnesium, iron, copper and phosphorus, this *grain* may be especially valuable for persons with migraine headaches, diabetes and atherosclerosis.

6. Self explanatory.

Secondary - All self explanatory.

Unit 2 Chapter 4

Elementary - All self explanatory.

Secondary

1. Self explanatory.
2. Self explanatory.
3. Beans or legumes contain a sugar, oligosaccharide, which the body cannot digest. Unlike other sugars, oligosaccharides are not broken down and absorbed by the lining of the small intestine. The body does not produce the enzyme that breaks down oligosaccharides. Oligosaccharides are large molecules and make it all the way to the large intestine, nearly the end of the alimentary canal, still intact. Since the sugar has not been broken down at earlier stages of the digestive process, these bacteria seize upon it as a source of nutrition, consuming it and quickly multiplying. The resulting gas is a byproduct of the digestive process of the bacteria. This gas must eventually leave the body through the rectum. By the same principal, other foods that come into the large intestine without being properly absorbed in the small intestine will cause gas. Emotional issues, such as stress, can cause food to move through the intestinal tract too quickly to be properly digested, with the end result being gas in the large intestine. We will discuss this further in Unit 6.
4. Ezekiel 4:9 says "Take also unto thee Wheat, and Barley, and beans, and lentils, and millet, and Spelt, and put them in one vessel, and make bread of it..." When these six grains and legumes sprout and are combined, they create a complete protein that resembles the protein found in milk and eggs. It contains all nine essential amino acids with 18 amino acids present – from easily digestible sources.

Spice Cookies

Elementary

1. To calculate necessary water consumption, take the person's weight and divide it by two. This number is the amount in ounces of pure, clean water that person should drink each day.
2. Refer to the "Fiber requirements by age" chart in Appendix K.
3. Honey, applesauce and the prunes add sweetness without spiking the blood sugar like regular white sugar or even organic sugar.
4. Refer to the chart in Appendix K.
5. Self explanatory.

Secondary

1. Follow the directions for the first and second answers in the Elementary section.
2. Same as previous answer.
3. Self explanatory. The experiment was intended to extend for a month to emphasize the importance of water and fiber, but also because repeating an activity for 21 and 30 days will help it become a habit.

Unit 3 Chapter 1

Elementary

1. Athletes, firemen, swimmers, opera singers, mountain climbers, astronauts, etc.
2. Doctors, air conditioning manufacturers, perfumers, household cleaner manufacturers, respiratory therapists, Environmental Protection Agency (EPA) workers, etc.
3. Self explanatory.
4. Self explanatory.
5. Self explanatory.
6. Self explanatory.

Secondary

1. Self explanatory.
2. Foods rich in beta- cryptoxanthin include: cilantro, citrus fruits, oranges, papaya, red bell peppers, watermelon and winter squash
3. Foods rich in magnesium include: broccoli, pumpkin seeds, spinach, summer squash and Swiss chard.
4. Self explanatory.

Unit 3 "Power" Recipes Activity Guide

If necessary, refer to the "Power" Recipe instruction page.

Kitchen Talk

1. Recap the discussion questions from each corresponding chapter and review what you learned.
2. Talk about the "Power" food in the recipe.
3. While preparing the dish, talk about the preparation methods used, and, if needed, demonstrate techniques for them such as chopping and mincing. For children old enough, allow them to help.
4. Choose one or more of the activities in the appropriate grade levels for children to do.

No Dairy No Chocolate "Chocolate" Pudding

Elementary

1. Self explanatory.
2. Ripe fruit is fully grown and developed. If the fruit is not ripe, it is not ready to eat and will taste different from fruit that is ripe and ready.
3. Carob is a tropical pod that contains a sweet, edible pulp and inedible seeds. After drying, the pulp is roasted and ground into a powder that resembles cocoa powder, but does not have the same flavor and texture of chocolate. Cocoa powder and chocolate also come from a tropical pod. The pods hold cacao beans that are processed to make cocoa powder and chocolate. Unsweetened carob powder is higher in carbohydrates and has more calories than unsweetened cocoa powder. However, carob is caffeine free and contains three times the calcium of carob powder. The sugar added during processing is usually the other difference. In general, cocoa powder has more sugar, which is mucus forming.
4. Self explanatory.

Secondary

1. Coconut milk is used rather than traditional dairy products that are mucus forming. In addition to providing flavor, the coconut milk helps blend the other ingredients. Rice milk and almond milk would also serve as good substitutes. Be sure to note the amount of sugar in these non-dairy substitutes.
2. Self explanatory.
3. Self explanatory.

Unit 3 Chapter 2

Elementary

1. Self explanatory.
2. Self explanatory.
3. Self explanatory.
4. Certain breeds of dogs and bats, pigs, deer, rhinos, bears, shrews and moles. It has been theorized that some animals with poor eyesight more than compensate for this problem with keen sniffers.

Secondary - All self explanatory.

Basil and Garlic Pesto

Elementary

1. According to Merriam-Webster Dictionary, an herb (the "h" is silent) is a seed-producing annual, biennial, or perennial that does not develop persistent woody tissue but dies down at the end of a growing season or a plant or plant part valued for its medicinal, savory or aromatic qualities. Legend quotes King Charlemagne referring to herbs as "the friend of physicians and the praise of cooks." This response might seem odd to some in modern times, but Charlemagne's answer was certainly indicative of his era. From Scripture and historical documents, we know that people had been using herbs for medicinal value since Creation. Herbalism and medicine were essentially the same practice.
2. Herbs come from the leaves of plants. Fresh basil leaves are more potent that the dried basil because the dried herb is dead. The smell is from the essential oil, also known as the aromatic oil or the life blood of the plant.
3. The recipe yields six servings. Double the ingredients to feed 12 and multiply by five to feed 30.

Secondary

1. Basil can be grown in pots or in a typical garden with other plants as long as it has adequate light, good water drainage and favorable temperatures.
2. Follow the instructions for growing basil that come with the plant or follow instructions at http://www.gardeningpatch.com/herbs/growing-basil.aspx.
3. Among others, basil has been used medicinally as an antidepressant, antiseptic, anti-inflammatory, antimicrobial, antispasmodic, expectorant, to prevent vomiting, to stimulate the adrenal cortex, to soothe itching, to lower blood pressure and blood sugar levels, to reduce fever and in tonics.
4. The fresh herbs are alive and the dried herbs are dead. When it comes to cooking, the topic of whether herbs are the most flavorful when they

are fresh or dry, is largely a matter of taste, but it will take more dried herbs than the fresh herbs. Taste however, can be affected by both storage and cooking techniques. When substituting dry herbs for fresh, use this conversion: one tablespoon of fresh equals one teaspoon of dry. If you are cooking something for several hours, avoid cooking out the flavors and wait until the dish is almost ready before adding either fresh or dried herbs. For foods you are chilling, such as pasta salads, you'll need to do the opposite, since adding herbs several hours in advance gives the flavors a chance to meld.

Unit 3 Chapter 3

Elementary

1. Self explanatory.
2. Frequencies are measured in hertz, which means cycles per second and is abbreviated Hz. The frequency of a sound is also known as its pitch. The higher the frequency, the higher the pitch and the shorter its wavelength.
3. A normal human can hear between 20 Hz and 20,000 Hz. Twenty Hz is a very low pitch sound or very deep tones. 20,000 Hz is a high pitch. Dogs and some other animals can hear sounds at higher frequencies than 20,000 Hz. That is why people can't hear a special dog whistle, while the dog will react to it. Being able to hear the higher frequencies may be useful in hunting for the animal. It is believed that cats probably can hear higher frequencies also, but most are too independent to respond to such a whistle.

   On the other end of the spectrum, elephants can hear frequencies much lower than the range of humans. Some researchers who were studying elephants in Africa discovered this. The story goes that a herd of elephants they were observing suddenly perked up their ear and ran off in a direction, as if they heard someone calling them. The researchers said they didn't hear anything, but some said they felt something strange in their bodies, just before the elephants ran off. After studying this situation, they found that elephants could make a very low frequency sound that humans can't hear. Elephants are able to hear this sound coming from up to five miles away. It is amazing the distances from while they can communicate with each other.
4. Self explanatory.
5. Self explanatory.
6. Self explanatory.

Secondary

1. Self explanatory.
2. Self explanatory.
3. Bartolomeo Eustachi (1500 or 1514 – August 27, 1574), also known by his Latin name of Eustachius, was one of the founders of the science of human anatomy. He also is believed to be the legendary Christian martyr known as Eustachius or Eustace or Saint Eustace.
4. Self explanatory.
5. Self explanatory.
6. Self explanatory.

Spinach Salad

Elementary

1. Spinach contains vitamin E and folate, and minerals fluorine and iodine,
2. Fungi (plural of fungus) are a group of organisms and micro-organisms that are classified within their own kingdom, the fungal kingdom, as they are neither plant nor animal. Fungi draw their nutrition from decaying organic matter, living plants and even animals. They do not photosynthesize as they totally lack the green pigment chlorophyll, present in green plants.
3. Self explanatory.

Secondary

1. There is much debate on this in the culinary world. Mushrooms are absorbent, meaning that they will soak in the water. The most common way to clean mushrooms is to just brush off any dirt with a damp cloth. If your mushrooms are very dirty, it is OK to quickly rub the dirt off under running water. One thing chefs do agree on: don't wash mushrooms until you are ready to cook or eat them and don't let them sit in water.
2. Self explanatory.
3. Like the heart, a tomato has four chambers and is red. Research shows that tomatoes are loaded with lycopene and are indeed pure heart and blood food.

Unit 3 Chapter 4

Elementary

1. Self explanatory.
2. To find the percentage, divide the number of people with corrective lenses by the total number of family members included in the experiment.

3. Self explanatory.
4. See the "Power" Recipes or the additional recipes for the chapter to provide ideas.
5. Self explanatory.

Secondary
1. Self explanatory.
2. Smoking causes cancer, specifically in the lungs, which are part of the respiratory system. Emphysema is another illness directly associated with smoking. People who smoke have weaker immune systems, making them more susceptible to germs. Viral and bacterial infections may be prolonged due to a person's smoking habit.
3. Ophthalmology is the study of the diseases and surgery of the visual pathways, including the eye, brain and areas surrounding the eye, such as the lacrimal system and eyelids. Optometry is a health care discipline focusing on the examination, diagnosis, treatment and management of disorders of the visual system, the eye, and associated structures as well as the diagnosis of related systemic conditions.

   Ophthalmologists must acquire a Doctor of Medicine (M.D.) degree, a broad knowledge of general medicine, and clinical training. If a person requires medical or surgical care for an eye disease or an eye injury, he or she will seek the assistance of an ophthalmologist.

   Optometrists have received a Doctor of Optometry (D.O.) degree are doctors who perform annual examinations to treat any vision problems and detect signs of disease and abnormal conditions. Examinations may also include testing for glaucoma, color perception, depth, and the ability to focus and coordinate the eyes. Optometrists must be licensed and pass a state board examination.

   Ophthalmologists and optometrists both can diagnose and manage eye problems, but ophthalmologists specialize in surgical procedures, while optometrists are more likely to specialize in optical corrections (glasses and contact lenses).
4. Self explanatory.

Fresh Carrot and Fruit Juice or Smoothie

Elementary
1. A sliced carrot looks like the human eye with a pupil, iris and radiating lines. Eye health and eating raw carrots is not just a myth. Science now shows that carrots greatly enhance blood flow to and function of the eyes
2. Apricots, berries and canteloupe.
3. Juicers separate the pulp from the juice so that the body can immediately take in the nutrients and not spend energy trying to breakdown the fiber. Blenders don't separate the pulp from the juice, resulting in the juice being very thick and usually not drinkable.

Secondary
1. With processed juices, most of the nutrients from fresh fruits and vegetables are long gone. In order to distribute juice, manufacturers include preservatives, giving the juice a longer shelf life and negating the need to refrigerate. This preservation also alters the structure of the food and makes it harder for the body to recognize, use and digest it. Also, many manufacturers include artificial sweeteners to make the juice more palatable for those who are accustomed to sugary drinks. Products that are "Not From Concentrate" mean the fruit is squeezed, and the juice is often then pasteurized or heated and packaged. Products "From Concentrate" mean the fruit is squeezed, and water is extracted to produce a concentrated form; then at a later time the water is added back in, the juice is then pasteurized or treated with ultra-violet heat and packaged.
2. Juiced pulp is high in dietary fiber and can add bulk and help retain moisture in other recipes. Fruit pulp can be added in muffins, cakes and smoothies, as well as added to salads or homemade desserts. Vegetable pulp can be added in many kinds of dishes. Experimentation with pulp us fun, but many recipes can be found online. Pulp can be frozen for later use by placing in a freezable container until ready to use it. The nutritional properties of freshly made juice are at their peak straight away, and the nutritional value rapidly declines due to oxidation of enzymes. The fibrous nature of juiced pulp on the other hand will not rapidly decline. Fresh pulp also can be used in garden composts.
3. Self explanatory.
4. Research on the Internet to find out how much vitamin A is in a serving of each of the fruit and carrots used in your juice or smoothie. One good Web site is www.whfoods.org. Calculate how much of each ingredient you used to find the total amount of Vitamin A.

Unit 4 Chapter 1

Elementary

1. Joseph's bones were carried out of Egypt. Verse 19 states, "And Moses took the bones of Joseph with him: for he had straightly sworn the children of Israel, saying, God will surely visit you; and ye shall carry up my bones away hence with you."
2. Having a hollow center allows the paper to support more weight and made it stronger. The large bones in the human body also are hollow. In addition to being stronger, the bones are lighter, so it takes less energy to move them.
3. After the frame is built, the walls are added and then the roof. Without the frame, the walls and roof could not be secured nor would they provide adequate support for the building to stand.
4. Self explanatory.
5. Self explanatory.
6. Self explanatory.
7. Self explanatory.

Secondary

1. Orthopedicsurgeons,chiropractors,rheumatologists, neurologists/neurosurgeons and physiatrists (doctors who specialize in physical rehabilitation) are trained to treat bones and the spine.
2. Self explanatory.
3. The small spools at the top represent the cervical vertebrae, the medium spools represent the thoracic vertebrae and the larger bottom spools represent the lumbar vertebrae. The vertebrae, like the spools, are not permanently attached together the human body can bend and lean in different directions. Between each pair of vertebrae is a disk of cartilage that acts as a shock absorber, just as the cardboard circle between the spools keeps them from knocking together. Without this flexible disc the vertebrae would grind together and the body would be able to twist, turn, or bend the torso without pain and damage.
4. Vinegar contains an acid, which dissolves the calcium phosphate in the bones. Without calcium bones will lose their hardness and will become weaker.
5. Self explanatory.
6. Self explanatory.
7. Self explanatory.

Unit 4 "Power" Recipes Activity Guide

If necessary, refer to the "Power" Recipe instruction page.

Kitchen Talk

1. Recap the discussion questions from each corresponding chapter and review what you learned.
2. Talk about the "Power" food in the recipe.
3. While preparing the dish, talk about the preparation methods used, and, if needed, demonstrate techniques for them such as chopping and mincing. For children old enough, allow them to help.
4. Choose one or more of the activities in the appropriate grade levels for children to do.

Nut Balls

Elementary

1. Drupes are fruit that have an outer fleshy part that surrounds a hard shell with a seed inside.
2. Sesame seeds are seeds. Almonds, walnuts and pecans are nuts and drupes. Dates and coconut are fruit and drupes.
3. Pulsing is a term used when cooking with a food processor. It means to turn the blade on and off to mix and chop the ingredients without blending them entirely.
4. The Middle East grows and consumes the majority of dates in the world. In the United States, commercial date growing is limited to states with high temperatures, low humidity and an abundant supply of water for the roots, such as California, Arizona, Florida and Texas.
5. Self explanatory.

Secondary

1. Self explanatory.
2. Crushed nuts, ground cinnamon and small shaving of other dried fruits are examples of substitutes.
3. The coconut has been and is a nutritious source of meat, juice, milk and oil for people around the world for generations. Nearly one-third of the world's population depends on coconut to some degree for their food and their economy. Among these cultures the coconut has a long and respected history. Highly nutritious and rich in fiber, vitamins, and minerals, coconut provides many health and medicinal benefits beyond its nutritional content.
4. Allergies to other tree nuts such as almonds, walnuts and pecans have been recorded, but are not as commonly known as peanut allergies. This may be because of the inexpensive methods of commercial

peanut production in the U.S. and their inclusion in many food products.

5. Find the amount of protein and calcium on the Internet. The following page www.whfoods.org/foodstoc.php will be helpful. To determine the amount of protein and calcium in each nut ball, divide the total numbers of protein and calcium by the number of nut balls made in the recipe.

Unit 4 Chapter 2

Elementary

1. Self explanatory.
2. Self explanatory.
3. As fun as this activity is, there is more to learn. Once the participants are paired up, time them to see how fast they can eat the bowl of grapes. The goal is for the participants to learn about team work. If there are more than one pair, have a race and see which team eats all their grapes the fastest. Have fun!
4. Doctors, nurses, physical therapists and trainers, and physiology teachers.
5. Self explanatory.
6. Gorillas, elephants and oxen (non-artic breeds) are a few examples.

Secondary - All self explanatary.

Traditional Hummus Dip with Basil

Elementary

1. Self explanatory.
2. The Latin name for garbanzo beans, Cicer arietinum, means "small ram," reflecting the unique shape of this legume that somewhat resembles a ram's head. Garbanzo beans are also referred to as chickpeas, Bengal grams and Egyptian peas. The name chickpea traces back through the French chiche to Latin cicer (from which the Roman cognomen Cicero was taken). The word garbanzo comes from Old Spanish (perhaps influenced by Old Spanish garroba or algarroba) through arvanço which may be linked to the Greek erebinthos.
3. Baking mainly refers to flour-based foods in which the heat of an oven sets their structures. This includes breads, cakes, muffins, and loaves and dishes that firm while cooking and brown on the outside. Roasting traditionally indicated meat cooked on an open fire. In modern times, it includes meats, vegetables and fish cooked in the enclosed space of an oven. Oven roasting generally means a dry-heat method of cooking without water-based liquids. In contrast, the terms pot roasting and braising mean oven-cooking in with added broth or liquid. Such techniques may be used for tougher cuts of meat as moisture helps dissolve their more plentiful connective tissues, increasing tenderness and adding flavor.

Secondary

1. Self explanatory.
2. Gluten is a type of protein that is commonly found in rye, wheat and barley and is found in most types of cereals and bread. Gluten-free grains include wild rice, corn, buckwheat, miller, amaranth, quinoa, teff, oats, soybeans and sunflower seeds.
3. Self-explanatory.

Unit 4 Chapter 3

Elementary

1. Self explanatory.
2. Self explanatory.
3. Braille is a code which enables blind people to read and write. It was invented by blind Frenchman Louis Braille in 1829.
4. Self explanatory.
5. Self explanatory.
6. Self explanatory.

Secondary - All self explanatory.

Cabbage Slaw

Elementary

1. Self explanatory.
2. Cabbage is a dietary staple in cultures around the world and is widely available around the global because it stores well.
3. Sauerkraut is a dish traditionally made with fermented cabbage.
4. Self explanatory.
5. Apple cider vinegar is a sour liquid produced from the fermentation of diluted alcohol products. Sometimes known simply as cider vinegar, it is made from cider or apple must, and is often sold unfiltered, with a brownish-yellow color.

Secondary

1. Cabbage contains 16 minerals: boron, calcium, chloride, chromium, copper, fluorine, iodine, iron, magnesium, manganese, molybdenum, phosphorus,

potassium, selenium, sodium and zinc. For additional details go to www.whfoods.com.
2. Self explanatory.
3. Made from fermented cabbage sauerkraut has a history. Although typically associated with Germany because early German settlers introduced cabbage and the traditional sauerkraut recipe in the United States, variations of the dish were used throughout Europe. It was even consumed by Dutch sailors during extended voyages to prevent scurvy.
4. Self explanatory.

Unit 4 Chapter 4

Elementary - All self explanatory.

Secondary

1. To determine heart rate intensity, a person must first determine his heart rate. Do this by following the guidelines in Chapter 4. Heart rate intensity should be measure immediately following intense aerobic activity. Use the chart in Chapter 4 to determine what the rate should be for the corresponding age. A higher rate could indicate a more regular exercise routine is needed. A body conditioned for exercise will have a rate at or below the level for its age.
2. Self explanatory.
3. Self explanatory.
4. Self explanatory.
5. Self explanatory.
6. Self explanatory.

Chicken Nuggets

Elementary

1. Self explanatory.
2. Self explanatory.
3. Salmonella is a bacteria that is most commonly associated with intestinal infections, specifically Salmonellosis, in the United States. More information can be found at www.about-salmonella.com.
4. Guidelines are available at http://www.about-salmonella.com/salmonella_prevention.

Secondary - All self explanatory.

Unit 5 Chapter 1

Elementary

1. Self explanatory
2. Self explanatory.
3. Self explanatory.
4. A sphygmomanometer is used to take the blood pressure. The cuff of the sphygmomanometer is placed around a patients arm above the elbow. The sphygmomanometer's squeezable bulb is used to inflate the cuff, and its valve is used to measure the systolic and diastolic blood pressure in millimeters of mercury.
5. CPR stands for Cardiopulmonary Resuscitation. Medical professionals, emergency response professionals, certified childcare providers and teachers are some of the professionals required to be trained in CPR.
6. Self explanatory.
7. Self explanatory.
8. Self explanatory.

Secondary

1. Self explanatory.
2. Like eye color, blood type is passed genetically from parents to children. The following chart illustrates the blood type possibilities for children based on their parents' blood types.

	Parent 1	AB	AB	AB	AB	B	A	A	O	O	O
	Parent 2	AB	B	A	O	B	B	A	B	A	O
Possible blood type of child											
	O					X	X	X	X	X	X
	A	X	X	X	X		X	X		X	
	B	X	X	X	X	X	X		X		
	AB	X	X	X			X				

3. The auscultatory method is the most common and non-invasive method of measuring/monitoring blood pressure using a sphygmomanometer and a stethoscope. The cuff of the sphygmomanometer is placed on a patient's arm above the elbow, while the person taking the blood pressure places a stethoscope at the elbow, just below the cuff. The person taking the blood pressure then pumps the squeezable bulb to inflate the cuff with air until the valve on the pump reaches just above 180 millimeters of mercury (mm Hg). When the first sound is heard through the stethoscope, the patient's blood pressure should be noted; this is the systolic blood pressure. When the sound disappears, that will be the diastolic blood pressure. Systolic blood pressure for most healthy adults is between 90 and 120 mm Hg, while normal diastolic blood pressure is between 60 and 80 mm Hg. Blood pressure measurements over 130/80 are

considered high.

4. Blood can be used in several ways and can be separated into platelets, plasma, red cells, white cells or a combination of these. The process to separate these components is known as apheresis (ay-fur-ee-sis), from the Greek "to take away." The primary difference between a whole blood donation and an apheresis donation is that the whole blood donation takes about seven to 10 minutes for the collection, while the apheresis donation requires an appointment because it can last between 1 ½ to 2 ½ hours. The uses of the blood depend on the donors' blood type and the needs of his or her community. According to the American Red Cross, approximately five million people in the U.S. receive blood transfusions each year, five percent of the eligible U.S. population donates blood in any given year.
5. According to the American Red Cross, "To give blood for transfusion to another person, you must be healthy, be at least 17 years old or 16 years old if allowed by state law. You must weigh at least 110 pounds, and not have donated whole blood in the last 8 weeks (56 days) or double red cells in the last 16 weeks (112 days) … Other aspects of each potential donor's health history are discussed as part of the donation process before any blood is collected. Each donor receives a brief examination during which temperature, pulse, blood pressure and blood count (hemoglobin or hematocrit) are measured. Making donations for your own use during surgery (autologous blood donation) is considered a medical procedure that requires a written prescription and the rules for eligibility are less strict than for regular volunteer donations." People with type O blood can donate to anyone. People with type A can donate to types A, B and AB. People with type B can donate to types B and AB. People with type AB can only donate to type AB. Immediately after donating the body starts to replace the donated blood with new blood.
6. Self explanatory.

Unit 5 "Power" Recipes Activity Guide

If necessary, refer to the "Power" Recipe instruction page.

Kitchen Talk

1. Recap the discussion questions from each corresponding chapter and review what you learned.
2. Talk about the "Power" food in the recipe.
3. While preparing the dish, talk about the preparation methods used, and, if needed, demonstrate techniques for them such as chopping and mincing. For children old enough, allow them to help.
4. Choose one or more of the activities in the appropriate grade levels for children to do.

Heart Healthy Oatmeal with Fruit

Elementary

1. Arrowroot powder is a fine, powdery white food and is easily digested. It resembles cornstarch, which is highly processed, and can be used in many traditional recipes as a thickening agent in place of cornstarch.
2. Arrowroot powder is extracted from the dried root stalk of the fleshly tropical arrowroot plant.
3. Staple foods are common components of an average diet that can be stored for long periods of time. Typically, these are starches that provide high energy in the form of carbohydrates.
4. A few examples: Cornstarch and arrowroot powder; refined sugar and organic, raw blue agave; quick oats and steel-cut rolled oats; bleached flour and unbleached organic flour or whole wheat flour; brown sugar and unsulphured blackstrap molasses.
5. Self explanatory.

Secondary

1. Arrowroot is the only starch that contains calcium ash. The calcium content in arrowroot powder, which is in the form of calcium chloride, is critical for the proper acid and alkaline balance in the human body.
2. Self explanatory.
3. Most pure vanilla extracts contain water, glycerin and vanilla bean extract. Imitation vanilla is more processed and typically contains synthetic substances, such as corn syrup and propylene glycol.
4. Self explanatory.

Unit 5 Chapter 2

Elementary

1. Self explanatory.
2. Self explanatory.
3. The leaves of the celery pull the water up for nourishment, highlighting the veins in the celery.

4. Self explanatory.
5. Self explanatory.
6. Self explanatory.
7. Self explanatory.

Secondary
1. Learn more at www.framinghamheartstudy.org.
2. Self explanatory.
3. Self explanatory.
4. Based on revenues, the top five companies at the time of publishing were: Johnson & Johnson (www.jnj.com), Pfizer (www.pfizer.com), GlaxoSmithKline or GSK (www.gsk.com), Novartis (www.novartis.com) and Sanofi-Aventis (www.sanofi-aventis.us).
5. Self explanatory.
6. Self explanatory.

Rice Stuffed Tomatoes

Elementary
1. Some possible answers: red, four chambers, fluid, squishy flesh and delicate.
2. Self explanatory.
3. Self explanatory.
4. Self explanatory.

Secondary
1. There are hundreds of varieties of tomatoes, so many that they are categorized: plum (for eating fresh or cooking), beefsteak (for sandwiches, grilling and cooking), salad (fresh with greens, vegetables and fruits), cherry (for salads and snacking) and paste or drying tomatoes (with minimal seeds for drying or boiling into paste).
2. The top 12 foods to buy organic are apples, cherries, grapes, nectarines, peaches, pears, raspberries, strawberries, bell peppers, celery, potatoes and spinach.
3. Self explanatory.
4. Self explanatory.

Unit 5 Chapter 3

Elementary
1. Cyte means cell and is a New Latin word derived from the Greek kytos, meaning hollow vessel.
2. Peyer's patches are a collection of large oval lymph tissues located in the mucous lining of the small intestine. These lymph nodules are especially abundant in the ileum, the lowest portion of the small intestine. This condition is named for the Swiss anatomist, Hans Conrad Peyer.
3. Anaphylaxis is a serious allergic condition that requires immediate medical attention and may cause death. The most common causes of allergy are related to food, medicine, insect stings or chemicals, such as latex.
4. Self explanatory.
5. Self explanatory.
6. Self explanatory.
7. Self explanatory.
8. Self explanatory.

Secondary
1. Self explanatory.
2. Self explanatory.
3. It is believed that all cells in the body have memory.
4. Self explanatory.
5. Vaccine exemptions are allowed in most all states based on reasons of conscience including a religious belief or for medical reasons. Interestingly enough, vaccinations are NOT mandatory in ANY state. There are no laws mandating vaccinations.
6. Self explanatory.

Mixed Berry Salad

Elementary
1. Blackberries, raspberries and strawberries are all members of the Rosoideae family, a subfamily of roses. Flowers in this group usually have at least 10 ovaries, often many more.
2. Keifer is raw or unpasteurized milk drink, from goat or cow's milk, filled with organisms that may boost the immune system. It is similar to yogurt.
3. More people consume goat milk than cow milk. Most third world countries and quite a few European countries prize goats and goat milk over cow milk. Goats are less expensive to raise and require less space than cows. Also goats produce more milk pound-for-pound than cows, with the capability to produce up to 10 percent of their body weight.
4. Hybrid seeds are the first-generation offspring of two distant and distinct parental lines of the same species. A seed taken from a hybrid may be sterile or fail to breed. Farmers began using hybrid seeds for large, commercial production because of their high yields, which typically are attained with fertilizers, herbicides, pesticides and high volumes of water.
5. Non-hybrid seeds also are known as heirloom.

Secondary
1. Self explanatory.
2. Self explanatory.
3. Blackberries, blueberries, strawberries and raw milk/yogurt are more acidic. Raspberries are more alkaline.
4. Self explanatory.

Unit 5 Chapter 4

Elementary
1. According to the Merriam-Webster Dictionary online, vilify means "to lower in estimation or importance" and "to utter slanderous and abusive statements against" and "defame."
2. When the sweet potato plant was growing with its roots in the water and its leaves in the sun, it produced food through photosynthesis and the stored carbohydrates in the potato. This stored food in the sweet potato provided the energy needed to grow a new plant.
3. You should see a difference in color.
4. Self explanatory.
5. Self explanatory.

Secondary
1. Self explanatory.
2. Self explanatory.
3. Self explanatory.
4. Some inconsistencies on www.sweetsurprise.com: Although the home page states that HFCS is made from corn, it provides a brief synopsis on the refining process, wherein HFCS becomes a chemical; The site states that HFCS and table sugar are comparable nutritionally and in sweetness; The site delves into glycemic index information, but states that the GI of HFCS has not been measured, just that it would rank around honey and sucrose (60-75); HFCS is presented as a minor contributor to the overall GI of a normal, note it does not say healthy, diet; according to the site, HFCS does not cause diabetes or obesity, nor does it state that it shouldn't be used by diabetics, contrary to the estimated GI.
5. Self explanatory.
6. Self explanatory.

Almond Butter Chip Bars

Elementary
1. Almonds in the U.S. most commonly are grown in California.
2. Generally, there are 96 teaspoons in a pound for dry ingredients, which is different than for wet ingredients. This also may vary with the type of dry ingredient. One way to figure this out is that there are three teaspoons in a tablespoon and 32 tablespoons to a pound (3 x 32 = 96). Because some dry ingredients have a different density than others, this may vary by ingredient. Look on the nutritional label of a pound of flour, sugar, etc., it should say how many teaspoons or tablespoons are in that pound.
3. Typically they come in a dozen, but sometimes are sold in half dozen or in cases of 18 or 24.
4. Eggs are classified as Grade AA, Grade A or Grade B. Grades AA and A are the grades most commonly marketed at retail. Size classifications, based on the minimum net weight per dozen without the carton, are: jumbo (30 ounces), extra large (27 ounces), large (24 ounces), medium (21 ounces) and small (19 ounces).
5. The color of the shell is determined by the breed of hen that produced the egg. Unless noted on the carton, color does not affect the egg's nutritive value, cooking properties, flavor or quality.

Secondary
1. Other nut and seed butters include cashew, pistachio, macadamia, hazelnut, pumpkin, sunflower, Brazil, pecan and walnut.
2. Self explanatory.
3. Self explanatory.
4. Self explanatory.

Unit 6 Chapter 1

Elementary
1. Self explanatory.
2. Self explanatory.
3. The skin.
4. Self explanatory.

Secondary
1. Self explanatory.
2. Self explanatory.
3. There are three common types of jaundice experienced by adults. Haemolyptic jaundice is caused by destruction of red blood cells, increasing bilirubin formation and anaemia. Obstructive jaundice is a result of blockage in the pathway where bilirubin is made in the liver cells and where bile

goes into the duodenum. Hepatocellular jaundice is caused by damage from viral infection or toxins to liver cells. In babies, there are five types of jaundice. Physiological (normal) jaundice occurs in most newborns and is due to the immaturity of the baby's liver. Jaundice of prematurity occurs frequently when the body of a premature baby is less ready to excrete bilirubin effectively. Breastfeeding jaundice happens when a breastfeeding baby is not getting enough breast milk, but is not caused by a problem with the breast milk itself. In rare cases, Breast milk jaundice may be caused by substances produced in their mother's breast milk that can cause the bilirubin level to rise. Blood group incompatibility (Rh or ABO problems) occurs if a baby has a different blood type than the mother. In these cases the mother might produce antibodies that destroy the infant's red blood cells, creating a sudden buildup of bilirubin in the baby's blood. For more about jaundice in healthy babies, go to http://kidshealth.org/parent/pregnancy_newborn/common/jaundice.html

4. The hormones involved in digestion are polysaccharides (salivary glands and pancreas), maltose (intestinal cells), glucoseproteins (stomach and pancreas), peptides (intestinal cells) and amino acids (pancreas).

Unit 6 "Power" Recipes Activity Guide

If necessary, refer to the "Power" Recipe instruction page before the "Power" Recipes.

Kitchen Talk

1. Recap the discussion questions from each corresponding chapter and review what you learned.
2. Talk about the "Power" food in the recipe.
3. While preparing the dish, talk about the preparation methods used, and, if needed, demonstrate techniques for them such as chopping and mincing. For children old enough, allow them to help.
4. Choose one or more of the activities in the appropriate grade levels for children to do.

Ultimate Pizza

Elementary

1. Fresh herbs are preferred over the dried form because of superior in flavor and less is needed in food preparation. Fresh oregano leaves be a vibrant green in color with firm stems and free from darks spots or yellowing. Wrap fresh oregano in a damp paper towel and store it in the refrigerator. It also may be frozen, either whole or chopped, in airtight containers. Dried oregano should be kept in a tightly sealed glass container in a cool, dark and dry place where it will keep fresh for about six months.
2. Warm water activates the yeast.
3. Self explanatory.
4. Tomato pies are built the opposite of pizza pies - first the cheese, then the toppings, and then the sauce.
5. Self explanatory.

Secondary

1. At the height of the Persian Empire, it is said that the soldiers of Darius the Great (521-486 B.C.), accustomed to lengthy marches, baked a kind of bread flat upon their shields and then covered it with cheese and dates.
2. Self explanatory.
3. Active forms of yeast, like the kinds bakers, brewers and winemakers use, can continue to grow in your intestine, robbing your body of valuable nutrients. Too much yeast will result in many health challenges. Deactivated yeast, such as nutritional yeast, are popular with vegans and health buffs who use it to make cheese substitutes, as a topping for popcorn, gravies and many other dishes. Available at health food stores, fortified nutritional yeast is taken as a source of vitamin B12.
4. Self explanatory.

Unit 6 Chapter 2

Elementary

1. Self explanatory.
2. Some examples are blueberries, NingXia wolfberries, cranberries, flaxseed, sesame seed and chia seed.
3. Kidney beans resemble the kidney. The tomato resembles the heart. Walnuts are similar to the brain. A sliced carrot looks like an eye. Celery and rhubarb look like bones. Some sweet potatoes resemble the pancreas.
4. Self explanatory.
5. Self explanatory.

Secondary

1. Human growth hormone or HGH is natural in the body, however it takes effort to produce it. So scientists created a synthetic version that is

used to treat things such as anti-aging issues and weight gain, making it is popular in modern society's dream of magic, no-effort, miracle cures. The food industry uses it with animals grown for consumption. Synthetic HGH can rapidly increase the development of animals and provide more meat for processing.
2. Self explanatory.
3. Self explanatory.
4. The leading causes of liver failure are: overdose of acetaminophen or exposure to a toxin or a viral infection. Visit www.liverhope.com.
5. Some activities may include meals that highlight a kidney-supporting food or choosing a cleanse in which the entire family can participate.
6. Self explanatory.

Brussels Sprouts with Lemon Pepper Dressing

Elementary

1. The cruciferous, or brassica, family of vegetables are called this because they known to botanists as Cruciferae or Brassicaceae. They have it all: vitamins, fiber, and disease-fighting phytochemicals.
2. Other vegetables in this family include, but are not limited to: broccoli, cauliflower, kale, cabbage, collard greens and bok choy.
3. Brussels sprouts have been traced to the late 16th century. They are named for the capital of Belgium, where they were a local crop in the region until their use spread across Europe during World War I. Now they are grown all over Europe and the United States.
4. Goitrogens are naturally-occurring substances in certain foods that can interfere with the functioning of the thyroid gland. Brussels sprouts contain goitrogens. Although cooking the sprouts may help to inactivate the goitrogenic compounds, people with pre-existing and untreated thyroid problems may want to avoid them. It is not clear from the research exactly what percent of goitrogenic compounds are inactivated by cooking or the risk is involved with the consumption of Brussels sprouts by those with thyroid problems.

Secondary

1. Self explanatory.
2. The phytonutrient sulforaphane. (http://www.juicing-for-health.com/phytochemical-phytonutrient.html)
3. The phytonutrients indoles and isothiocyanates. (http://www.juicing-for-health.com/phytochemical-phytonutrient.html)
4. The October 1996 issue of the Journal of the American Dietetic Association showed that 70 percent or more of the studies found a link between cruciferous vegetables and protection against cancer. Scientists know that chopping or chewing raw cruciferous vegetables causes the formation of bioactive glucosinolate to breakdown products, such as isothiocyanates and indole-3-carbinol.

Unit 6 Chapter 3

Elementary

1. Joseph von Mering and Oscar Minkowski. Their accidental discovery was made after they removed the pancreas from a healthy dog in order to study the role of the pancreas in digestion. Several days after the dog's pancreas was removed, the doctors happened to notice a swarm of flies feeding on a puddle of the dog's urine. On testing the urine to determine the cause of the flies' attraction, the doctors realized that the dog was secreting sugar in its urine, a sign of diabetes. Because the dog had been healthy prior to the surgery, the doctors knew that they had created its diabetic condition by removing its pancreas and thus understood for the first time the relationship between the pancreas and diabetes. With more tests, von Mering and Minkowski concluded that a healthy pancreas must secrete a substance that controls the metabolism of sugar in the body. Though many scientists tried in vain to isolate the particular substance released by the pancreas after von Mering and Minkowski's accidental discovery, Frederick G. Banting, a young Canadian doctor, and Professor John J.R. MacLeod of the University of Toronto established that the mysterious substance was insulin. They shared a Nobel Prize in 1923 for their isolation and clinical use of insulin against diabetes.
2. Self explanatory.
3. Many of these "high fiber" cereals will list many different sugars and hide them by using different names. Look for these words – sugar, honey, brown sugar, barley malt, maltitol, high fructose corn syrup, high maltose corn syrup, corn syrup, glycerine, sucralose (or Splenda), sucrose, glucose, fructose, natural flavors, etc.
4. The best choices are grade B maple syrup and blue agave nectar.
5. Self explanatory.

Secondary

1. Mg/dl is a measure of concentration (mass per unit volume) using milligrams per deciliter.
2. Type 1 is absolute deficiency of insulin. Type 2 is relative deficiency of insulin. Type 1 means the body's islet cells were destroyed, typically attributed to the body's own immune system, while Type 2 is due to overworking of the islet cells. Gestational diabetes only occurs during a woman's pregnancy. Modest elevation of blood sugar after meals is normal during pregnancy, but the danger of gestational diabetes is that the rising placental hormones increase the blood sugar to levels that can affect the growth and development of the baby. Although any woman can develop gestational diabetes, some are at a higher risk than others.
3. Self explanatory.
4. Self explanatory.
5. Leavened bread contains yeast and unleavened bread does not.
6. In Exodus 12, the Hebrews had to leave Egypt quickly. They did not have the time to allow their bread to rise, so they took the raw dough on their journey and baked it in the hot desert sun into a hard unleavened cracker called matzoh. The Passover refers to God passing over the houses of the Jews, as he was slaying the first borne of Egypt. Matzoh bread is used by Jewish families in Seder services, commemorating the Passover and exodus of the Jews from Egypt.

Veggie Linguine with Fresh Tomato Sauce

Elementary

1. Linguine is a form of Italian pasta. It is flat and narrow and its name means "little tongues."
2. Self explanatory.
3. To drizzle is to pour a very fine stream or sprinkle drops of a liquid over food.
4. Self explanatory.

Secondary

1. Although both varieties are available year round, they are called summer and winter squash because those were the seasons they were harvested and are at the peak of their goodness.
2. Both zucchini and squash are members of the Cucurbitaceae family and relatives of the melon and cucumber.
3. The raw vegetables contain enzymes that are good for everyone to eat. Replacing the pasta reduces the sugar in the recipe, making it a diabetic-friendly meal.
4. Pesto is a simple Italian sauce that utilizes a few basic ingredients and dates back to the Roman Empire. There are two forms of pesto sauce, pesto alla genovese and pesto alla siciliana, which originated in Genoa and Sicily, respectively. The first, which is widely recognized as the original recipe, contains a few basic ingredients: garlic, salt, extra virgin olive oil, Pecorino Sardo cheese and basil. The latter has tomatoes and uses less basil. Regarding seafood, certain types are valuable for their Omega-3 fatty acids. However, due to pollution consumers should limit their intake to avoid mercury contamination. Shellfish, such as lobster, crab, shrimp, oysters, scallops, mussels, clams, are contaminated by environmental factors at an alarming rate. This contamination is passed along to those who consume them. These known scavengers, which eat things that die in water, have been found to have mercury, lead, arsenic and thousands of synthetic and chemical contaminants.

Unit 6 Chapter 4

Elementary

1. Psalm 126 contains the following words associated with emotions: laughter, singing, glad, tears, joy, weeping and rejoicing. Your answers may vary based on the translation of your Bible.
2. Self explanatory.
3. Self explanatory.
4. Self explanatory.
5. Professionals that help people deal with negative emotions include pastors, counselors, psychologists, psychiatrists, wellness chiropractors, naturopaths and aromatherapists, among others.

Secondary

1. Scriptural references describing the relationship between the mind and the heart: Deuteronomy 11:18, 28:65; I Samuel 2:35; I Chronicles 28:9; Job 10:12-13, 38:36; Psalm 7:9; Psalm 26:2; Psalm 64:6, 73:7; Isaiah 46:8; Jeremiah 11:20, 17:10, 20:12, 31:33; Matthew 22:37; Mark 12:30; Luke 10:27; Acts 4:32; Romans 8:27; Philippians 4:7; and Hebrews 8:10 and 10:16. Scriptural references describing the relationship between the heart and

the tongue: Deuteronomy 30:14; I Samuel 2:1; Job 22: 21; Psalm 5:9, 16:9, 17: 13-10, 19:14, 39:3, 45:1, 49:3, 62:4; Proverbs 10:20, 15:4, 16:1 and 23, 17:20; Ecclesiastes 5:2, Isaiah 29:13, Jeremiah 9:8, Ezekiel 33:31, Matthew 12:34, 15:18; Luke 6:45, Romans 10:8-10, 15:6; and Acts 2:26. Scriptural references describing the relationship between the tongue and the mind: Numbers 30:4; II Samuel 14:19; Job 7:11, 31:30; Psalm 57:4, 63:5, 120:2; Proverbs 13:2, 18:7, 21:23; Isaiah 32:4; Ezekiel 4:14; I Corinthians 14:4; and James 3:5-6.

2. Self explanatory.
3. French chemist René-Maurice Gattefossé is credited with coining the term aromatherapy in 1928 in an article he wrote supporting the use of using essential oils in their whole without breaking them down into their primary constituents. Gattefossé conducted experiments with essential oils on wounded soldiers during World War 1 and found that essential oils were antiseptics that detoxified better than the chemical compounds that were currently being used.
4. Both psychiatrists and psychologists counsel patients, perform various forms of therapy and conduct research studies. The suffix "-iatry" means medical treatment, and "-logy" means science or theory. Basically, psychiatry is the medical treatment of the psyche, and psychology is the science of the psyche. Psychiatrists attend medical school and earned a doctor of medicine degree (M.D.), and can prescribe medications, while psychologists hold a doctorate degree in philosophy (Ph.D.), psychology (Psy.D.) or education (Ed.D.), and are not licensed to prescribe medications.
5. Self explanatory.

Tropical Vanilla Ice Cream Shake

Elementary

1. Coconut is a tropical fruit, so that is why it is titled a tropical ice cream shake.
2. Self explanatory.
3. The glycemic index of raw, blue agave nectar from the agave tequilana plant is 11.
4. Self explanatory.
5. Self explanatory.

Secondary

1. Self explanatory.
2. Dairy products cause mucus, while coconut milk does not. There also is a huge difference between raw and pasteurized milk. For more information see Appendix O.
3. Self explanatory.
4. Self explanatory.
5. Some suggestions to transform this into an ice cream recipe: Omit the ice and consider heating the liquid in a saucepan. Arrowroot powder, which is only activated by heat, can be used as a thickening agent. Consult other recipes in this program or other healthy living cookbooks.

Appendix A: Health Statistics in the United States

Arthritis

- **46 million people, including children, have arthritis.** http://www.cdc.gov/arthritis/data_statistics/arthritis_related_statistics.htm

Asthma

- **Approximately 20 million Americans have asthma. Nine million U.S. children under 18 have been diagnosed with asthma.** http://www.aaaai.org/media/resources/media_kit/asthma_statistics.stm

Cancer

- **12 million cancer cases will be reported for 2007 worldwide, with 7.6 million deaths.** http://www.cancer.org/docroot/MED/content/MED_2_1x_New_Report_Estimates_12_Million_Cancer_Cases_Worldwide.asp, http://www.cdc.gov/cancer/npcr/uscs/2004/facts_major_findings.htm

Cardiovascular Disease

- **652,091 deaths recorded from cardiovascular disease 2005*.** http://www.cdc.gov/nchs/fastats/heart.htm

- **24.1 million people diagnosed with cardiovascular disease 2006*.** http://www.americanheart.org/presenter.jhtml?identifier=4478

- **Worldwide 3.8 million men and 3.4 million women die each year from coronary heart disease.** http://www.who.int/cardiovascular_diseases/en/cvd_atlas_14_deathHD.pdf

Cholesterol

- **50 million Americans have significantly elevated cholesterol.** http://www.pslgroup.com/dg/1FB6F6.htm

- **107 million Americans have cholesterol between 200 and 239, which is considered elevated, putting them at risk for heart disease.** http://healthcare.utah.edu/healthtools/articles/cholesterol.html

Diabetes

- **23.6 million Americans are diabetics and 57 million are pre-diabetic.** http://www.diabetes.org/diabetes-statistics.jsp

Obesity

- **58 million Americans ages 50-74 are overweight (BMI greater than 30 percent).** http://www.health-goods.com/Education/Nutrition_Information/Weight_Control/overweight_obesity_facts.htm

- **55 percent of Americans are overweight, 23 percent are considered obese.** http://www.rense.com/general/obese.htm

- **32 percent of American children are obese, up from just 20 percent a few years ago, and it is con sidered an epidemic in Western countries.** http://en.wikipedia.org/wiki/Childhood_obesity

** The Center for Disease Control and various governmental agencies compile data from all across the country to document these statistics. Generally, the statistics available to the public are two to three years later.*

Appendix B: Nutrition 101: Choose Life! Food Pyramid

History of Nutritional Guidelines in the U.S.

Even before vitamins and minerals were discovered, the U.S. Department of Agriculture (USDA) published dietary recommendations to the nation in 1894. For over 100 years, these recommendations have been modified because of the changes that have occurred in the way food is grown and processed and consumed during times of war and peace, as well as the improvement of technology and science that analyzes the components of food – vitamins, minerals, amino acids, fiber, fats, etc.

USDA nutritionist Caroline Hunt, was the first to categorize foods into groups in 1916. By 1941, the USDA established Recommended Dietary Allowances (RDA) for Americans to follow. Two years later, it announced the Basic Seven, a special modification of the nutritional guidelines to account for the shortage of food supplies during World War II. It was later simplified as the Basic Four and used for the next 20 years. In the 1970s, the USDA added a fifth category: fats, sweets and alcoholic beverages.

Since the 1980's the USDA has distributed its Pattern for Daily Food Choices, but it wasn't until 1988, that there was a graphic to represent the food groups. The Food Guide Pyramid was issued in 1992. Then, the Nutrition Labeling and Education Act, enacted in 1994, required all foods to contain nutritional labels. Although the USDA Food Guide Pyramid is undoubtedly one of the best known, there are hundreds of versions that have been produced over the years that are based on a variety of theories.

Many Americans are perplexed by this issue. The USDA conducted a survey in 1996 and found that over 40 percent of people agreed with this statement: "There are so many recommendations about healthy ways to eat, it's hard to know what to believe."

The **Nutrition 101: Choose Life! Food Pyramid** is based on the nutritional guidelines presented in this curriculum. Many people have followed these guidelines and have had great success at improving their health.

Historical attribution: Davis, Carole A., and Etta Saltos. "The Dietary Guidelines for Americans - Past, Preent, Future," Family Economics and Nutrition Review, Vol. 9, No. 2, Spring 1996.ent, Future," Family Economics and Nutrition Review, Vol. 9, No. 2, Spring 1996.

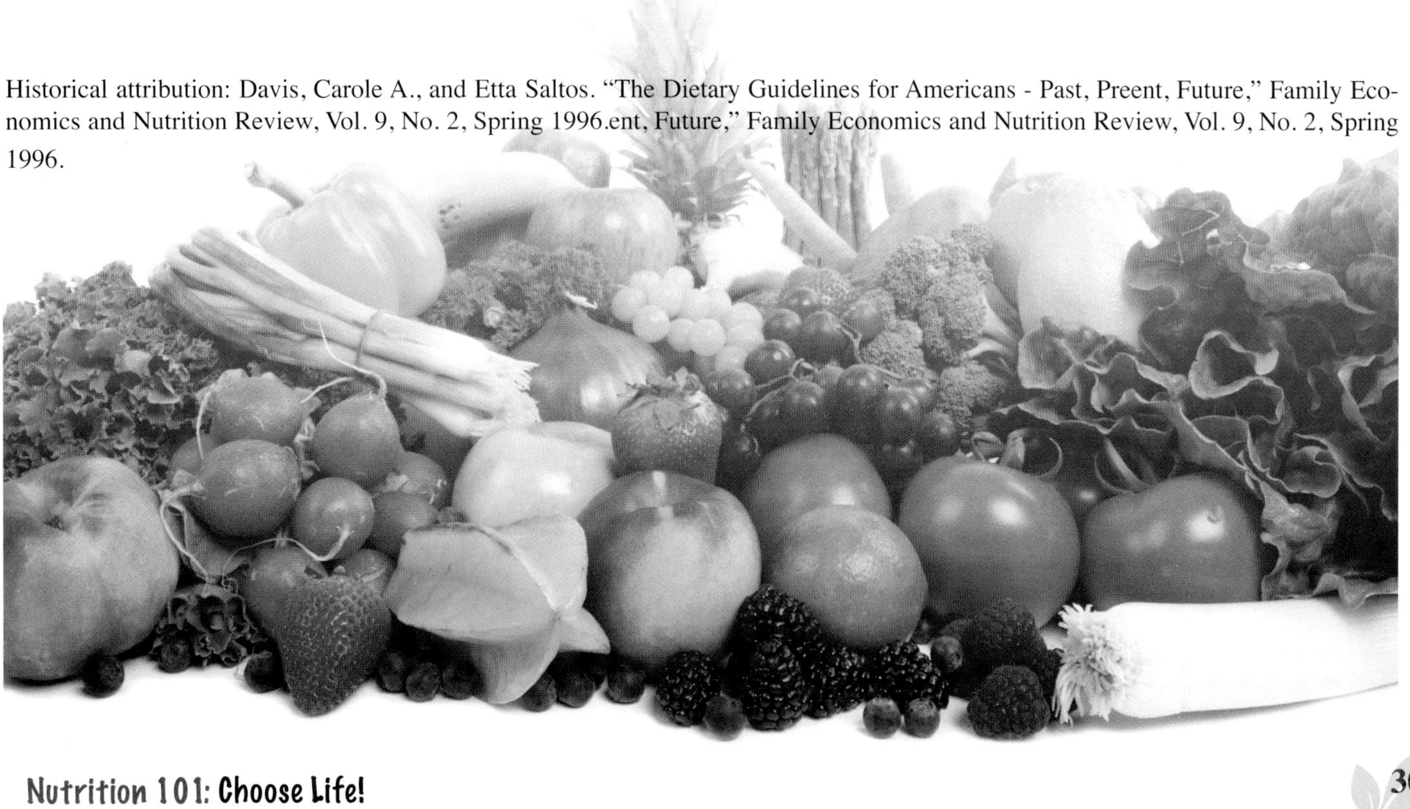

Nutrition 101: Choose Life! Food Pyramid

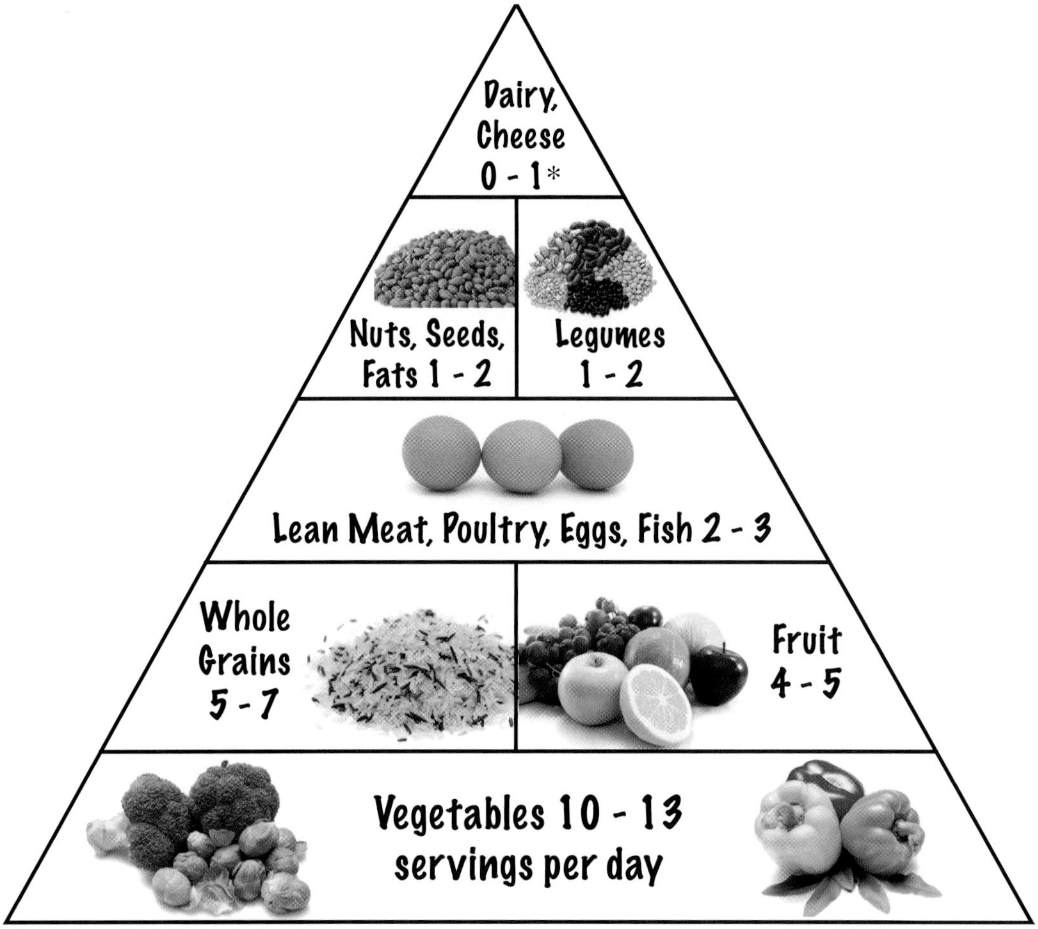

* Numbers indicate recommended servings per day.

How much is a serving?

Vegetables
½ cup cooked or raw
1 cup leafy
¾ cup juice

Fruit
1 medium apple
½ grapefruit
1 small banana
¼ cup dried fruit
¾ cup juice
½ cup berries

Legumes
¼ cup cooked

Nuts, Seeds
1/3 cup
2 tablespoon nut butter

Fats
2 Tbs.

Grains
½ cup cooked cereal
1 slice whole grain bread
1 cup cooked whole grain pasta
½ bun
1 roll
½ English muffin
3 to 4 small crackers
1 ounce ready to eat cereal
½ cup rice

Lean Meat, Poultry, Eggs
2 to 3 ounces cooked
1 egg

Fish
6 ounces raw
4 ounces cooked

Dairy, Cheese, Yogurt
1 cup milk or yogurt
1 ½ ounces cheese

Sample daily menu base, non vegetarian:

Breakfast: 2 cup assorted fruit salad (2), 2 slices whole grain bread (2), 1 egg
Snack: 1 banana (2), ½ cup dried fruit (1), 10 nuts (1)
Lunch: 2 cups leafy green salad base (2), 1 cup assorted raw julienne vegetables (2), ½ sliced avocado (1) or 2 tablespoons olive oil for dressing
Snack for afternoon: 1 cup assorted raw vegetables (2)
Dinner: 1 cup cooked pasta (1), 2 cups steamed or sautéed vegetables (4)
Dessert: 1 cup popcorn (1), 1 cup mixed berries (2) with ½ cup yogurt (½)

Serving totals:
Vegetables 10
Whole grains 4
Fruit 5
Nuts, seeds, fats 1 ½
Meat, Eggs, Poultry or Legumes 2
Dairy, cheese ½

Sample daily menu base, vegetarian

Breakfast: 2 cup assorted fruit salad (2), 1 slice whole grain bread (1), 2 Tbs. nut butter (1)
Snack: 1 banana (2), ½ cup dried fruit (1), 10 nuts (1)
Lunch: 2 cups leafy green salad base (2), 1 cup assorted raw julienne vegetables (2), ½ sliced avocado (1) or 2 tablespoons olive oil for dressing (1)
Snack for afternoon: 1 cup assorted raw vegetables (2)
Dinner: 1 cup cooked pasta (1), 1 cups steamed or sautéed vegetables (3), ½ cup cooked garbonzo beans (1)
Dessert: 1 cup popcorn (1), 1 cup mixed berries (2) with ½ cup wheat germ (½)

Serving totals:
Vegetables 10
Whole grains 4
Fruit 5
Nuts, seeds, fats 2 ½
Meat, Eggs, Poultry or Legumes 2
Dairy, cheese 0

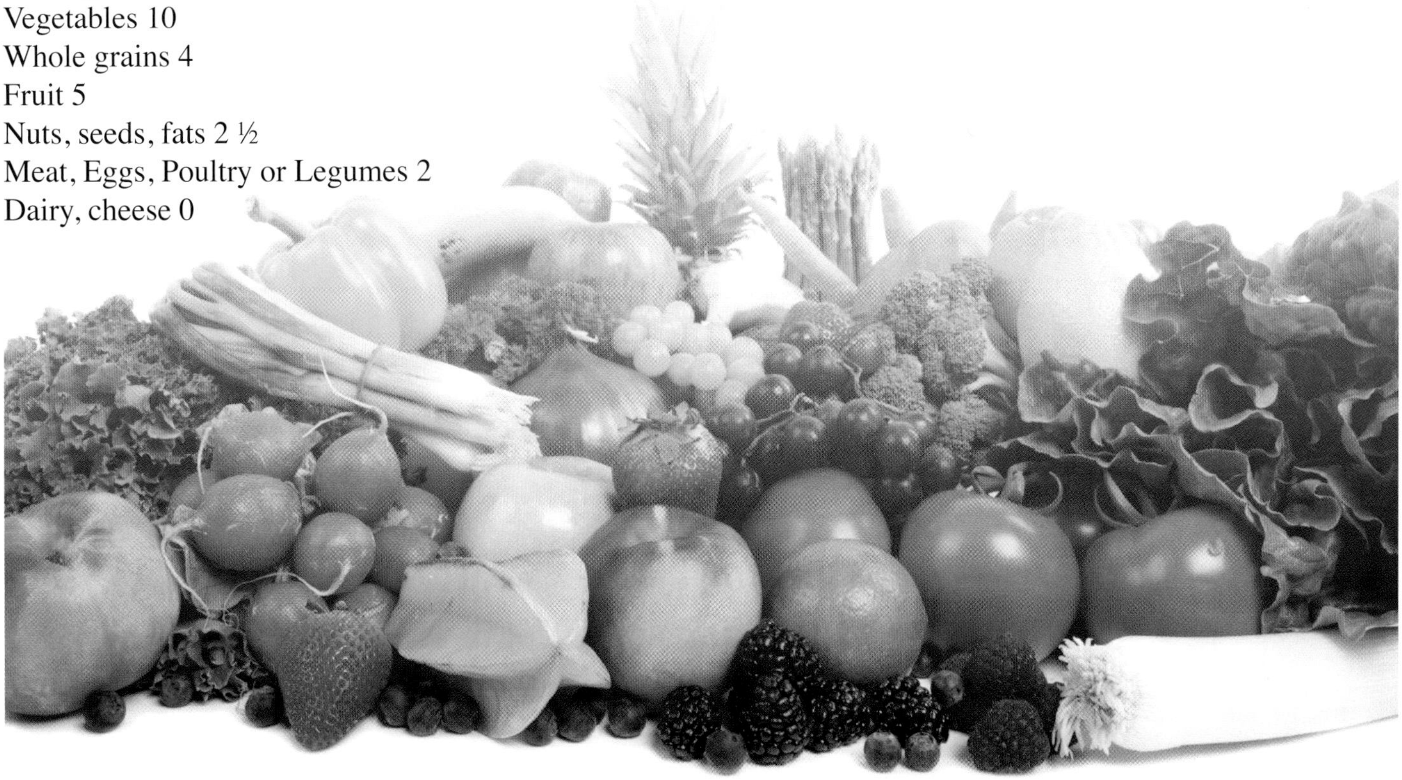

Nutrition 101: Choose Life! Food Pyramid Serving Checklist

Use this checklist to help keep track of daily food servings. For optimal health, try to consume as many of the recommended servings from each food category as possible.

Thanks to Beverly Boytim, homeschool mom, for creating this wonderful checklist!

Food	Sunday	Monday	Tuesday	Wednesday	Thursday	Friday	Saturday
Vegetables ½ cup cooked/raw 1 cup leafy ¾ cup juice Asparagus, broccoli, cabbage, cucumber, green beans, greens, kale, okra, peppers, potatoes, spinach	☐☐☐☐☐☐☐☐☐☐☐☐☐	☐☐☐☐☐☐☐☐☐☐☐☐☐	☐☐☐☐☐☐☐☐☐☐☐☐☐	☐☐☐☐☐☐☐☐☐☐☐☐☐	☐☐☐☐☐☐☐☐☐☐☐☐☐	☐☐☐☐☐☐☐☐☐☐☐☐☐	☐☐☐☐☐☐☐☐☐☐☐☐☐
Fruit 1 med apple ½ grapefruit 1 small banana ¼ cup dried fruit ¾ cup juice ½ cup berries Apples, cherries, dates, kiwi, melon, oranges, pineapple	☐☐☐☐☐	☐☐☐☐☐	☐☐☐☐☐	☐☐☐☐☐	☐☐☐☐☐	☐☐☐☐☐	☐☐☐☐☐
Grains ½ c. cooked cereal 1 slice WG bread 3-4 small crackers ½ cup rice Amaranth, oats, quinoa, rice, rye, wheat	☐☐☐☐☐☐☐	☐☐☐☐☐☐☐	☐☐☐☐☐☐☐	☐☐☐☐☐☐☐	☐☐☐☐☐☐☐	☐☐☐☐☐☐☐	☐☐☐☐☐☐☐
Meats/Eggs 4 oz. fish 1 egg 2-3 oz. other meat Beef, bison, chicken, mackerel, salmon, tuna, turkey, venison	☐☐☐	☐☐☐	☐☐☐	☐☐☐	☐☐☐	☐☐☐	☐☐☐
Nuts/Fats 1/3 cup 2 Tbs. nut butter 2 Tbs. fat or oil Almonds, Brazil, cashews, coconut oil, flaxseed, olive oil, pumkin, sunflower, walnuts	☐☐	☐☐	☐☐	☐☐	☐☐	☐☐	☐☐
Legumes ¼ cup cooked black, garbanzo beans, lentils, black eyed peas	☐☐	☐☐	☐☐	☐☐	☐☐	☐☐	☐☐
Dairy 1 cup milk or yogurt 1 ½ oz. cheese	☐	☐	☐	☐	☐	☐	☐

*This page may be duplicated as needed.

Appendix C: Nutrition 101: Choose Life! Shopping List

Purchase organic when available. Those items listed as organic are strongly recommended. Add these items, especially the staples, when the best quality is available and as budget allows.
This Shopping List and the following single-paged mini Alkaline/Acid Food Chart may be duplicated as needed to aid in your grocery shopping

Vegetables

- ☐ Artichoke
- ☐ Asparagus
- ☐ Avocado
- ☐ Bell peppers, red, orange,yellow
- ☐ Broccoli
- ☐ Brussels sprouts
- ☐ Cabbage, green
- ☐ Cabbage, red
- ☐ Carrots
- ☐ Cauliflower
- ☐ Celery
- ☐ Crimini mushrooms
- ☐ Cucumber
- ☐ Garlic
- ☐ Green beans
- ☐ Kale
- ☐ Lettuce, green or red leaf
- ☐ Lettuce, romaine
- ☐ Onions, green
- ☐ Onions, red, white, yellow
- ☐ Olives
- ☐ Peas
- ☐ Potatoes, red russet
- ☐ Potatoes, Yukon
- ☐ Romaine lettuce
- ☐ Spinach
- ☐ Squash, summer or winter
- ☐ Sweet potatoes
- ☐ Swiss chard
- ☐ Yellow squash
- ☐ Zucchini

Grains

- ☐ Buckwheat
- ☐ Millet
- ☐ Oats
- ☐ Quinoa
- ☐ Rice, brown or white
- ☐ Rice, black or purple
- ☐ Rice, wild
- ☐ Rye
- ☐ Wheat

Beans/legumes

- ☐ Dried peas, split peas
- ☐ Kidney. red, light red, white
- ☐ Garbanzo/chickpea
- ☐ Lentils
- ☐ Lima
- ☐ Pinto
- ☐ White navy

Fruits

- ☐ Apples
- ☐ Apricots
- ☐ Bananas
- ☐ Blackberries
- ☐ Blueberries
- ☐ Cantaloupe
- ☐ Cranberries
- ☐ Dates
- ☐ Figs
- ☐ Grapefruit
- ☐ Grapes
- ☐ Kiwi
- ☐ Lemons
- ☐ Limes
- ☐ Oranges
- ☐ Mangoes
- ☐ Papaya
- ☐ Peaches
- ☐ Pears
- ☐ Pineapple
- ☐ Plums
- ☐ Prunes
- ☐ Raisins
- ☐ Raspberries
- ☐ Strawberries
- ☐ Tomatoes
- ☐ Watermelon

Nuts and Seeds

- ☐ Almonds
- ☐ Brazil
- ☐ Cashews
- ☐ Chia
- ☐ Flax
- ☐ Hazelnuts
- ☐ Pecan
- ☐ Pine nuts
- ☐ Pumpkin seeds
- ☐ Sesame seeds
- ☐ Sunflower seeds
- ☐ Walnuts

Proteins

- ☐ Beef, grass fed
- ☐ Cheese, feta and mozzarella, from organic milk
- ☐ Chicken
- ☐ Cod
- ☐ Eggs
- ☐ Salmon
- ☐ Tuna
- ☐ Turkey

Spices

(Fresh or dried)

- ☐ Allspice
- ☐ Basil
- ☐ Cayenne pepper
- ☐ Cilantro
- ☐ Cinnamon
- ☐ Oregano
- ☐ Nutmeg
- ☐ Paprika
- ☐ Rosemary
- ☐ Sage
- ☐ Tarragon
- ☐ Thyme

Staples

- ☐ Apple cider vinegar
- ☐ Applesauce
- ☐ Arrowroot powder
- ☐ Baking powder, aluminum free
- ☐ Baking soda
- ☐ Balsamic vinegar
- ☐ Blue Agave Nectar
- ☐ Broth powder, vegetable or beef
- ☐ Carob chips
- ☐ Carob powder
- ☐ Celtic salt
- ☐ Chicken stock
- ☐ Cocoa powder, organic
- ☐ Coconut flakes
- ☐ Coconut flour
- ☐ Coconut milk
- ☐ Coconut oil, extra virgin
- ☐ Cream of tartar
- ☐ Crispy rice cereal
- ☐ Flaxseed oil
- ☐ Grade B maple syrup
- ☐ Grapeseed oil
- ☐ Honey, raw unfiltered
- ☐ Mustard
- ☐ Olive oil, extra virgin
- ☐ Peanut butter, organic
- ☐ Pumpkin seed oil
- ☐ Rice milk
- ☐ Rolled oats
- ☐ Sesame oil
- ☐ Sesame seeds
- ☐ Sweet pickle relish, organic
- ☐ Unbleached all-purpose flour, organic
- ☐ Walnut oil
- ☐ Whole wheat flour, organic
- ☐ Vanilla extract, organic

Mini Alkaline/Acid Food Chart

Use this chart along with the Shopping List when on grocery trips to help with choosing the healthiest food possible. See Appendix H: Alkaline/Acid Food chart for a bigger, more detailed chart.

* NOTE: This chart may be duplicated as needed.

Most Alkaline	Alkaline	Lowest Alkaline	Food Category	Lowest Acid	Acid	Most acid
asparagus, broccoli, cucumber, garlic, kale, onions, parsley, radish, spinach (raw), sprouts, most vegetable juices	beets, beet greens, celery, cilantro, collard greens, endive, green beans, lettuce, mustard greens, okra, sorrel, squash, sweet potato, Swiss chard greens, soy and radish sprouts, zucchini	artichokes, cabbage, carrots, cauliflower, eggplant, horseradish, kohlrabi, mushrooms, parsnips, peas, peppers, potato skins, pumpkin, turnip, rutabaga, watercress	**FRESH, RAW VEGETABLES**	cooked vegetables	corn, frozen vegetables, canned vegetables, potatoes (no skins)	fermented (pickled) vegetables
avocado, lemons, limes, mangoes, papayas	apples, dates, grapes, honeydew melon, kiwi, musk melon, raisins, raspberries, tomatoes	bananas (unripe), cherries (sour), coconut, oranges, peaches, wolfberries	**FRESH, RAW FRUITS**	blackberries, cherries (sweet) figs, grapefruit, nectarines, plums, processed fruit juices, strawberries, watermelon	apricots, cantaloupe, currant, pear, rhubarb, tangerines	blueberries, canned fruits, cranberries, glazed fruits, pineapple, prunes
barley, kamut grasses, oat straw, soy and radish sprouts, wheat grass	other sprouted grains, wheat	alfalfa, amaranth, millet, quinoa, wild rice	**GRAINS and CEREALS**	brown rice, hemp seed flour, rice milk, spelt, sprouted wheat bread,	corn products, crackers, buckwheat, oats, rye, white rice	pastries, pasta, wheat bread, white flour
			MEATS and EGGS	cold water fish (such as fresh herring, rainbow trout, salmon, sardines, tuna, etc.), eggs, venison	buffalo, chicken, duck, lamb, organ meats, rabbit, turkey	beef, pork, shellfish, veal
		horseradish, kohlrabi, lentils, lima beans, mung beans, navy beans, peas, soybeans	**BEANS and LEGUMES**	kidney beans, string beans	black beans, chickpeas, pinto beans	chocolate beans
almonds	hazelnuts	caraway, chestnuts, cumin, fennel, sesame	**NUTS and SEEDS**	Brazil nuts, flaxseed, filberts, pumpkin seeds, sunflower seeds, tahini	cashews, pecans	peanuts, pistachios, walnuts
Evening primrose	borage oil, flaxseed oil	olive oil	**OILS**	butter, safflower oil, sesame oil	canola oil, sunflower oil	margarine
	breast milk	buttermilk, goat cheese, soy cheese, soy milk, whey	**DAIRY**	butter, cottage cheese, yogurt	raw milk	cheese, homogenized milk, ice cream
potassium, sodium	calcium	magnesium	**MINERALS**			
	cayenne, chili pepper, cinnamon, curry, dandelion, ginger, herbs (all), miso, sea salt, tamari	carob, horsetail, dandelion,	**HERBS, SPICES and SEASONINGS**		cocoa	
herbal teas, lemon water	green tea, teccino (coffee substitute)	ginger tea	**BEVERAGES**	black tea	coffee	beer, liquor, soft drinks
agave, stevia	blackstrap molasses, maple syrup, rice syrup	honey (raw), sugar (raw)	**SWEETENERS**	honey (processed), molasses	brown sugar, white sugar	aspartame, corn syrup, Equal, NutraSweet, Splenda, Sweet 'N Low
			OTHER		ketchup, mayonnaise, soy sauce	chips, fast food

Appendix D: How to Select Fresh Produce

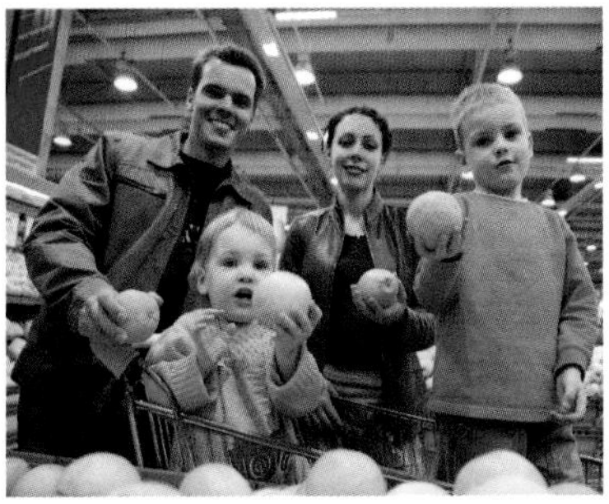

It is best to have a diet full of fresh, raw fruits and vegetables. Based on your location, interest and commitment, there are many ways to achieve this balance in your diet.

Many people choose to grow their own produce. This requires a lot of time and planning. Consult your local library, local agricultural cooperative or Master Gardner's association for tips about ph soil testing and crops appropriate for your area. Check the course schedule at the local community college or a continuing education program for a class that will offer more hands-on instruction or go to www.kidsgardening.com. Those who do not have the land, means or ability to manage a garden, must find a trusted source from which to purchase produce.

Organic and Non-GMO

Choose organic when at all possible. Please note that the USDA organic seal includes three subcategories: 100% organic, 95% Organic and Made with Organic Ingredients. Organic is defined as food and fiber that is grown without relying on toxic, synthetic chemical pesticides. This does not mean that the seed has not been altered or genetically modified, also known as GMO. **Choose non-GMO foods whenever possible.**

As USDA organic certification is expensive, some local farmers grow their produce and raise their animals without any pesticides, herbicides, growth hormones or antibiotics, yet do not go through the expensive process of having their food officially certified as "organic". The best way to know whether or not local farmers follow organic practices is to talk with the farmers and visit their farms to see how their food is grown and raised.

A locavore or localvore is someone who exclusively – or at least primarily – eats foods from his or her local foodshed or a determined radius from his or her home. Commonly, the distance is either 100 or 250 miles, depending on location. By eating locally, most locavores hope to create a greater connection between themselves and their food sources, resist industrialized and processed foods, and support their local economy. For more information about buying locally from local growers, visit www.localharvest.org and www.pickyourown.org.

Vegetable	In Season	Appearance/texture	Storage
Asparagus 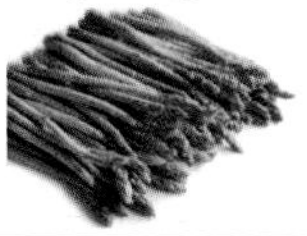	March through June, peak in April and May; available year round in some areas.	Look for straight, firm, bright-green stalks. Avoid very thick or very thin stalks because they may be stringy.	Use wet paper towels to wrap the bases of fresh spears and keep them tightly sealed in a container up to four days.
Beans, green 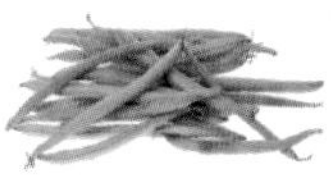	April through September; available year round in some areas.	Select bright-colored and crisp beans that are free of bruises, scarring, brown streaks or spots. Bulging or leathery beans are old.	Keep covered in a container in the refrigerator up to five days.
Beets 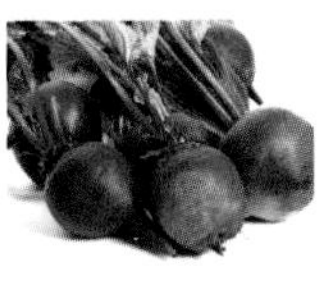	Available year round, peak from June to October.	Choose firm beets small to medium size that are attached to red stems and have fresh green tops. Loose beets without their tops are typically older than those that are attached to their green tops. Large beets can be tough and less sweet.	Trim the tops, leaving one to two inches of stem. Do not cut the root. Store up to a week in the refrigerator without washing or covering.

Vegetable	In Season	Appearance/texture	Storage
Broccoli 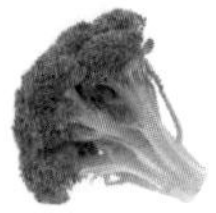	July to October; available year round in some areas.	Choose buds with dark green or purplish hues. The heads should be tightly budded. Avoid light green or yellow heads.	Keep covered in a container in the refrigerator up to four days.
Brussels sprouts 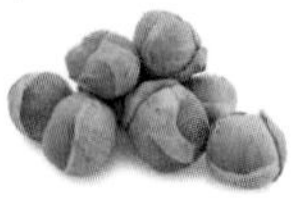	Available year round, peak from August through April.	Choose smaller, vivid green sprouts. Larger sprouts tend to be bitter.	Keep covered in a container in the refrigerator up to two days.
Cabbage 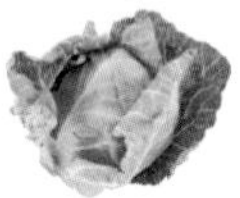	Available year round with peak from June to November.	Select a heavy head, for the size, with unwithered, brightly colored leaves free of spots.	Keep covered in a container in the refrigerator up to five days.
Carrots 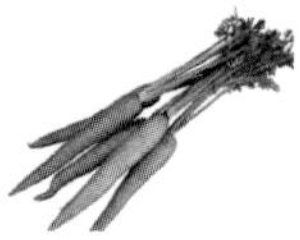	Available year-round, but best from July to September	Avoid thick carrots, as they often have tough centers. Choose firm roots with relatively smooth skin.	Keep refrigerated in a sealed container or plastic bag for up to two weeks.
Cauliflower 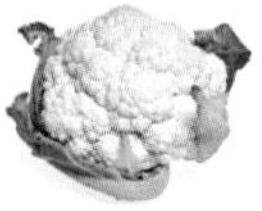	Available year round with peak from September to December	Select a solid, heavy head with bright green leaves . Avoid any with brown bruises or yellow leaves.	Keep covered in a container in the refrigerator up to four days.
Celery 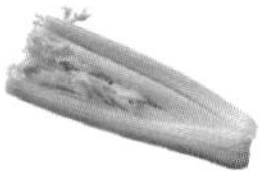	Available year round.	Choose crisp, firm unwilted and unblemished ribs.	Keep tightly wrapped in the refrigerator up to two weeks.
Collards 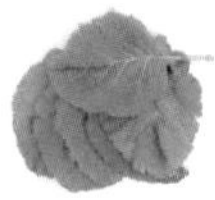	Available year round with peak from January to April	Choose large, flat, dark green leaves that are crisp and upright and are not yellow or wilted.	Keep refrigerated in a sealed container for up to five days.
Cucumbers 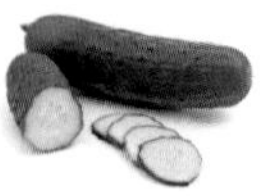	Available year-round, but best from June to September	Select dark green, firm and generally unblemished cucumbers.	Keep salad cucumbers in the refrigerator up to 10 days. Pickling cucumbers should be picked and used the same day.
Eggplant 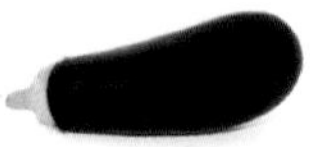	Available year round with peak from August to September	Choose eggplants that are heavy for their size with smooth skin free of scarring and bruising and a cap that is free of mold.	Keep refrigerated whole up to two days.
Garlic 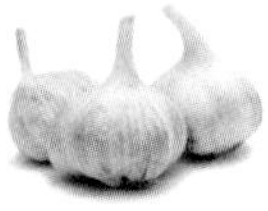	August to October	Select plump and firm bulbs that are completely surrounded by their tissue-like covering. Avoid any with green sprouts.	Store in a cool, dry location or refrigerate for up to eight weeks. Individual cloves can be stored for eight to 10 days.
Leeks 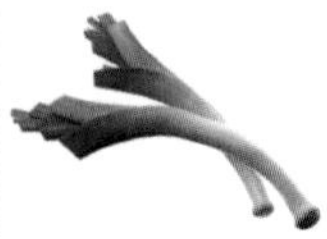	Available year round with peak from August to November	Look for leeks that have dark green leaves and clean, white bulbs. Leaves that have yellow and brown spots usually are overripe.	Keep tightly wrapped in the refrigerator up to five days.

Vegetable	In Season	Appearance/texture	Storage
Lettuce, leaf 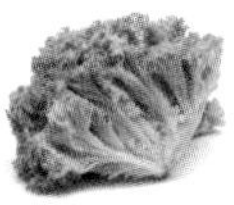	Available year round, but best from mid-May to late November	Choose heads that are loosely packed, but not withered with brightly colored leaves free of dark streaks and torn leaves.	Refrigerate in a sealed container for up to five days.
Lettuce, butterhead (Bibb or Boston) 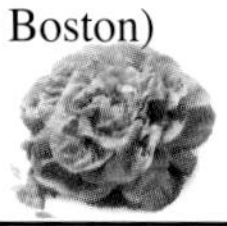	Available year round, but best from mid-May to late November	Choose heads that are loosely packed, but not withered with brightly colored leaves free of dark streaks and torn leaves.	Refrigerate in a sealed container for up to five days.
Lettuce, romaine 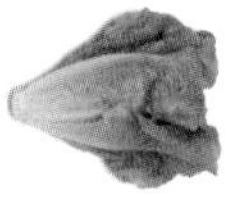	Available year round, but best from mid-May to late November	Choose heads that are loosely packed, but not withered with brightly colored leaves free of dark streaks and torn leaves.	Refrigerate in a sealed container for up to five days.
Mushrooms (all varieties) 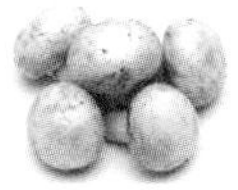	Available year round; morel variety available from April through June.	Should not be slimy or have bruises or blemishes. Fresh mushrooms are not wrinkled. Size is only a matter of personal preference	Keep unwashed in the refrigerator for up to two days. Using a paper bag or damp cloth bag allows mushrooms to breathe so they stay firmer longer.
Okra 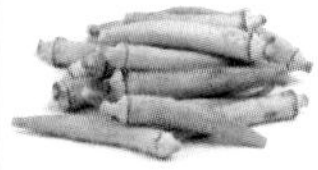	July to October	Choose small, crisp, unshriveled and brightly colored pods free of brown spots or blemishes.	Keep tightly wrapped in the refrigerator up to three days.
Onions, dry 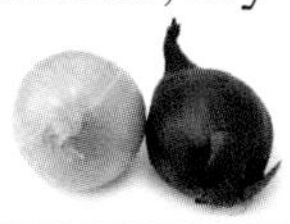	Available year round	Look for firm, dry bulbs without soft spots, blemishes or sprouts.	Store in a cool, dry, well-ventilated location for several weeks.
Onions, green 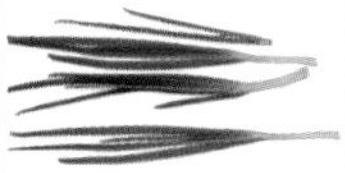	July to September	Choose bright green leaves that are not slimy.	Store in a cool, dry, well-ventilated location for several weeks.
Parsnips 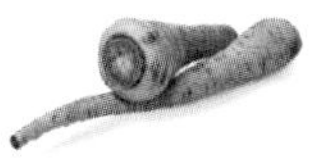	Available year round with peak from November through March	Select smooth-skinned parsnips that are heavy for their size.	Refrigerate for up to two weeks.
Peas 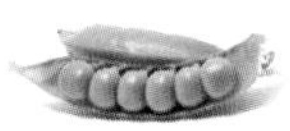	January through June with peak from March through May. Pea pads are available from February through August	Choose crisp and brightly colored pods that are free of brown spots and unshriveled.	Keep tightly wrapped in the refrigerator up to three days.
Peppers 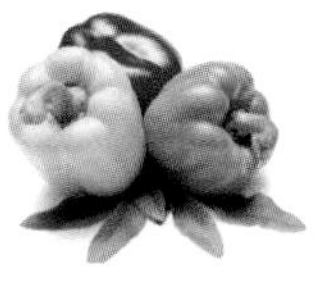	Available year round	Choose peppers that have thick, brightly colored smooth skin and a good shape. Avoid one with shriveled spots or breaks in the skin.	Keep refrigerated in a covered container for up to five days.

Vegetable	In Season	Appearance/texture	Storage
Potatoes 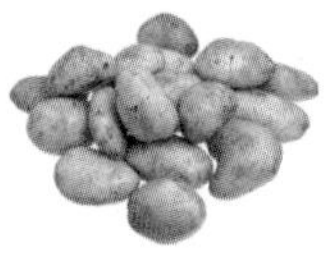	September to January	Choose firm potatoes that are free of bruises, cracks, sprouts, green spots, soft spots and shriveled spots.	Store in a cool, dry, well-ventilated, slightly humid location for several weeks. Avoid refrigeration as cold temperatures result in overly sweet one that darken when cooked.
Pumpkins 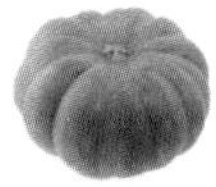	Mid-September to late October	Select firm and well-rounded gourds.	Use fresh pumpkin within 24 hours.
Rutabaga 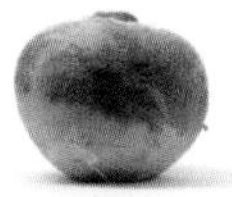	Available year round with peak from September through March	Select smooth-skinned rutabagas that are heavy for their size.	Refrigerate for up to two weeks.
Spinach 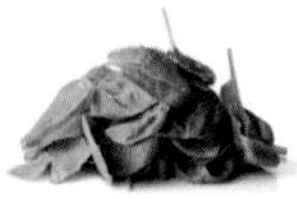	June to October	Choose spinach that is dark green with no signs of yellowing, sliminess, or wilting.	Refrigerate in a sealed container for up to three days.
Squash, summer 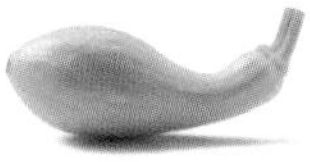	Available year round in some places with peak from June through September	Select small, firm squash that are free of cuts and soft spots. Due to tender skin, it is hard to find squash completely blemish free.	Refrigerate tightly wrapped for up to five days. Store it fresh from the garden for up to two weeks.
Squash, winter 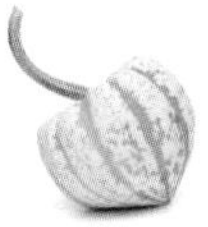	Available year round in some places with peak from September through March	Look for hard, smooth skin with no cracks or bruising.	Store whole in a cool, dry place for up to two months. Refrigerate cut pieces and keep wrapped tightly for up to four days.
Sweet potatoes 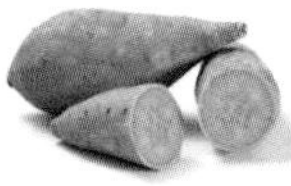	October to March	Choose small to medium, firm and smooth skinned sweet potatoes that do not have any cracks or soft spots.	Store whole in a cool, dry place for up to one week.
Turnips 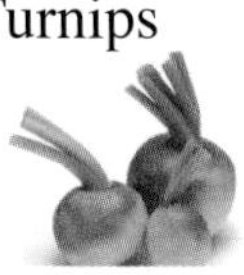	Available year round with peak from October through March	Select smooth-skinned turnips that are heavy for their size.	Refrigerate for up to two weeks.
Yams 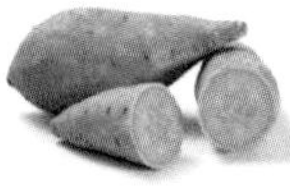	October to March	Choose small to medium, firm and smooth skinned yams that do not have any cracks or soft spots.	Store whole in a cool, dry place for up to one week.
Zucchini 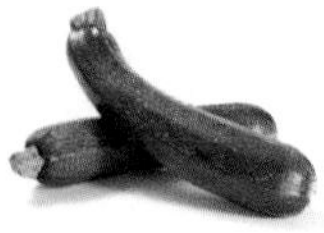	Available year round in some places with peak from June through September.	Look for firm, dark green skin. Old zucchini are soft and wrinkly. The smaller, the more likely to be free of cuts. Due to tender skin, it is hard to find completely blemish-free zucchini.	Refrigerate tightly wrapped for up to five days. Store it fresh from the garden for up to two weeks.

How to Select Fresh Produce - Fruit

To ripen fruit, place it in a clean paper bag and close it. To speed up the ripening process, put an apple or ripe banana in the bag with under ripe fruit. The ethylene gas in the apple or banana will help ripen the fruit. The banana will ripen (brown) quickly, so using an apple is preferred.

Fruit	In Season	Appearance/Texture	Storage
Apples 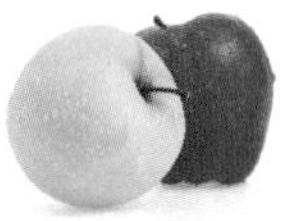	Available year round with peak from September through November	Firm and free of bruises. For red-colored varieties, look for apples that are mostly red. For yellow-colored apples, look for apples that are mostly bright yellow. Red and yellow apples that have several patches of green color are generally not as tasty as bright red and yellow apples.	Store in bulk in a cool, moist place for up to two weeks. Refrigerate up to six weeks.
Apricots 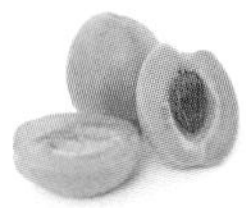	May through July	Select plump, fairly firm fruit with deep yellow or orange-yellow tinted skin.	Keep refrigerated ripe fruit, when it yields to gentle pressure and is golden in color, up to two days.
Avocado (Hass) 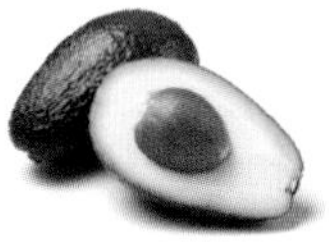	Available year round.	If left at room temperature, avocados that are any shade of green should eventually ripen. Avocados are ready to eat when their skins are dark and they give a little to slight pressure. Choose avocados that have roughly-textured skin; those that are relatively smooth skinned tend to have less flavor.	Store ripened fruit for up to four days. To maintain freshness of cut fruit or guacamole, leave the pit with the fruit.
Bananas 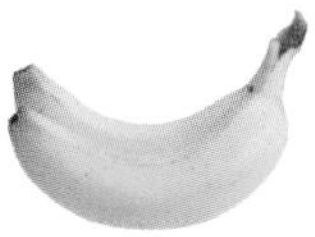	Imported year-round	Look for bananas that do not have bruises or soft spots, especially along the undersides of the bottom-most row. If left at room temperature, bananas that are any shade of green should eventually ripen. Extra-ripe bananas can be peeled and stored in a container in the freezer for smoothies or banana ice cream	Ripen at room temperature until the fruit is bright yellow. Brown bananas are overripe.
Blackberries 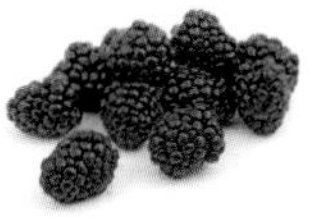	July to August	If picking them fresh, choose berries that separate easily from the stem.	Keep refrigerated berries in a single layer, loosely covered, for up to two days.
Blueberries 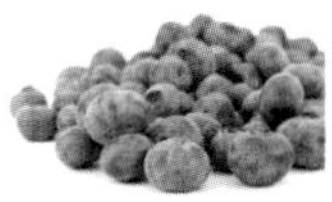	Mid-June to late August (Frozen wild blueberries are available year-round)	Firm in various shades of blue. If picking them fresh, choose berries that separate easily from the stem.	Keep refrigerated berries in a single layer, loosely covered, for up to two days.
Boysenberries 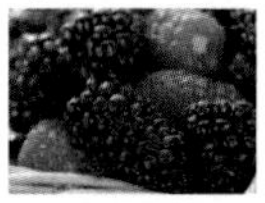	Late June through early August.	If picking them fresh, choose berries that separate easily from the stem.	Keep refrigerated berries in a single layer, loosely covered, for up to two days.

Fruit	In Season	Appearance/Texture	Storage
Cantaloupe 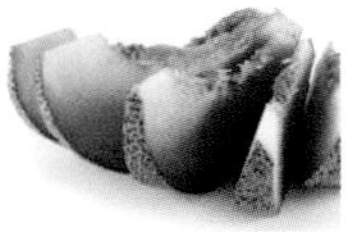	Available year round with peak from June through September.	Choose a sweet smelling cantaloupe that is heavy for its size. Avoid wet, dented, bruised or cracked fruit. A strong scent may indicate over ripeness.	Keep refrigerated whole melon up to four days. Refrigerate cut fruit in a covered container or tightly wrapped for up to two days.
Carambolas (Starfruit) 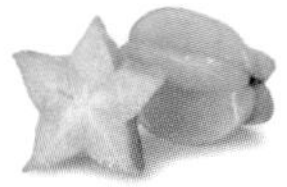	Late August through February	Choose firm, shiny-skinned golden fruit. Minimal browning on the edge of the fins is natural and should not affect the taste.	Keep refrigerated ripened fruit in a covered container or tightly wrapped for up to one week.
Cherries 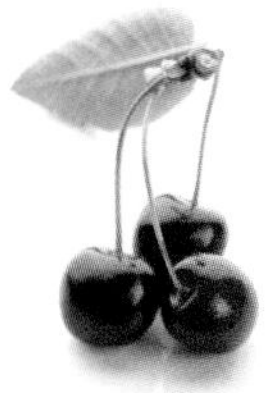	Sweet variety available from May to August with peak in June; Tart variety available from June to August with peak in June and July.	Select firm, brightly colored fruit.	Keep refrigerated in a covered container for two to three days.
Cranberries 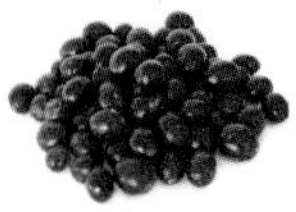	Available from October through December with peak in November	Look for firm fruit free of shriveling and bruises. It is ripe when solid.	Keep refrigerated for up to four weeks or freeze for up to one year.
Figs (fresh, not dried) 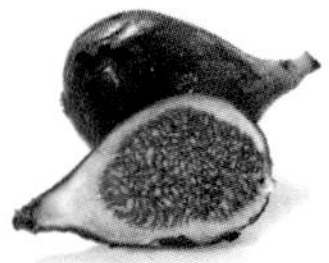	Available year round with peak from June through July.	Be sure to pick ones that smell nice; old figs tend to smell a tad sour because the sugar in the fruit begins to ferment. Plump and heavy for their size. As they ripen, they soften to the touch.	Refrigerate fresh figs. Dried figs can be stored in the refrigerator or at room temperature or several months. Either way, wrap them tightly in an air- and moisture-proof container to keep them from losing moisture and becoming hard.
Grapefruit 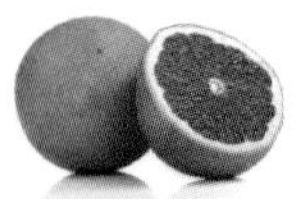	Available year round	Select fully colored grapefruit that is well rounded and heavy for its size.	Keep refrigerated for up to two weeks.
Grapes 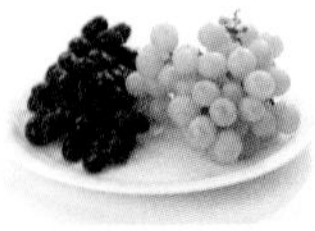	Available year round	Green grapes tend to be more sour than red grapes. Grapes can be purchased as seedless or with seeds. Choose grapes that are firm; soft grapes or those that feel like little water balloons tend to be too ripe.	Keep refrigerated in a covered container for up to one week.
Honeydew melon 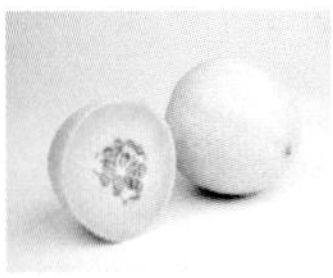	Available year round with peak from June through September.	Leave at room temperature until they give ever so slightly to heavy pressure. Their skins may wrinkle slightly and may give off a mild melon fragrance when they are ripe. Free of bruises and no areas of broken skin/rind.	Keep whole melon refrigerated up to four days. Keep refrigerated cut fruit in a covered container or tightly wrapped for up to three days.

Fruit	In Season	Appearance/Texture	Storage
Kiwi 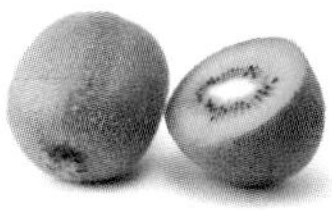	Available year round in some areas with peak October through May	Select plump-looking fruit that is free of bruises. Firm fruit requires additional ripening time at room temperature. Ripe, ready-to-eat fruit yields to gentle pressure when squeezed in the palm of the hand.	Keep ripe kiwi refrigerated up to four weeks or at room temperature up to three days. Refrigeration retards its ripening, so unripe kiwi may last over a month in the fridge.
Lemons 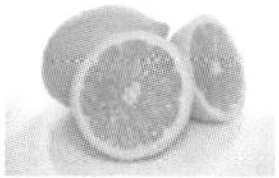	Available year round.	Choose firm, well shaped fruit with smooth, even yellow skin that is free of bruising and wrinkling.	Keep refrigerated for up to two weeks.
Limes 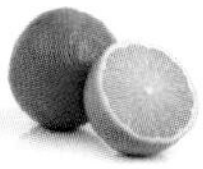	Available year round.	Choose firm, well shaped fruit with smooth, even yellow skin that is free of bruising and wrinkling.	Keep refrigerated for up to two weeks.
Nectarines 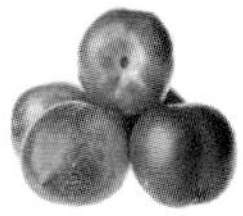	May through September with peak from July through August.	Ripe fruit should yield slightly to gentle pressure. Choose fruit with golden-yellow skin and no tinges of green.	Keep refrigerated for up to five days.
Oranges 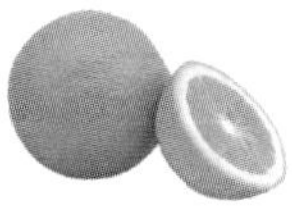	California navel oranges are in season from about mid-November to late spring. They are sweetest from about January to early March.	For eating out of hand, choose California navel oranges that are heavy for their size and without obvious blemishes.	Keep refrigerated for up to two weeks.
Peaches 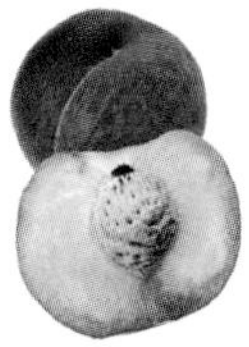	May through September	Choose peaches that have smooth skin without bruises, and that give a bit to pressure. Peaches that do not give to pressure can ripen, but often do not get as soft and sweet as those that are already somewhat ripe at the market.	Keep refrigerated for up to five days.
Pears 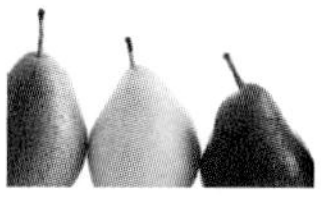	Available year round	Various shades of yellow, brown, red and green. Smooth skin and no bruises.	Keep refrigerated for several days.
Pineapple 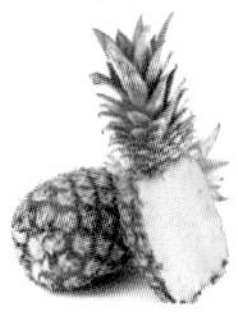	Available year round with peak from March through July	Select a plump, sweet smelling fruit that is slightly soft to the touch, heavy for its size and has deep green leaves.	Keep whole fruit refrigerated for up to two days. Cut fruit lasts a few more days if refrigerated in a tightly sealed container.
Plantains 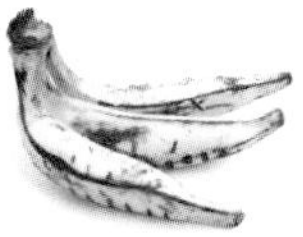	Available year round	Depending on intended use, choose from green (under ripe) to dark brown or black (fully ripe). Some bruising is acceptable as the skin is very tough.	Fruit will ripen at room temperature. This must be cooked before eating.

Fruit	In Season	Appearance/Texture	Storage
Plums 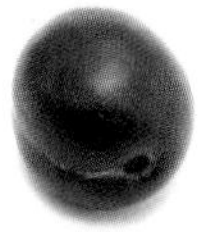	Available May through October with peak from June through July	Choose firm, plump, well-shaped fruit that gives slightly when pressed gently. The light gray cast on the skin, called bloom, is natural and does not change taste.	Keep refrigerated for up to three days.
Raspberries 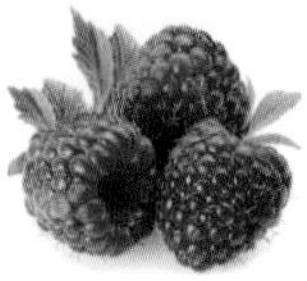	Available year round with peak from May through September.	Choose raspberries that are bright red. Look carefully to be sure that there are no signs of mold, the most common one being the presence of white, cotton-like strands in and around the berries. If picking them fresh, choose berries that separate easily from the stem.	Refrigerate berries in a single layer, loosely covered, for up to two days.
Rhubarb 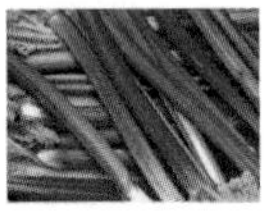	Available from February through June with peak from April through June.	Select crisp stalks that are tender, but not bendable. Avoid thick and wilted stalks.	Keep refrigerated and wrapped tightly for up to five days.
Strawberries 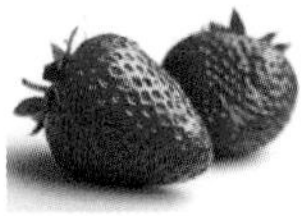	Available year round with peak from June to early July.	Plump, dark red, and without bruises. Fresh berries carry a distinct strawberry fragrance. If picking them fresh, choose berries that separate easily from the stem.	Refrigerate berries in a single layer, loosely covered, for up to two days.
Tomatoes 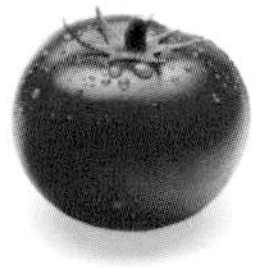	Available year round with peak from June through September.	Bright red, firm, and free of bruises. Like strawberries, fresh tomatoes will carry their own distinct fragrance.	Store at room temperature for up to three days. Do not store whole tomatoes in the refrigerator as they lose flavor. Sliced tomato should be refrigerated.
Watermelon 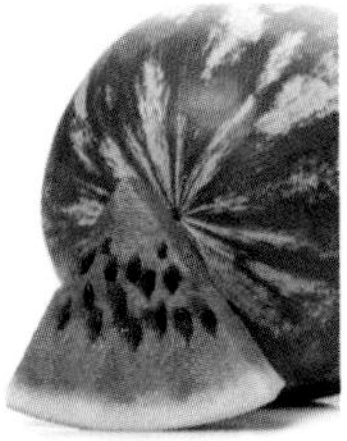	Mid-May to late August	Firm, dark green rind. A slight hollow sound upon tapping with your knuckles is often a sign of a full and juicy melon. Choose a hard, smooth rind that is free of cracks, bruises and dents. The fruit should be heavy for its size. Watermelon does not ripen after picking.	Keep whole melon refrigerated up to four days. Cut fruit should be kept in a covered container or tightly wrapped for up to three days.

Appendix E: Kitchen Safety

- Small children may use plastic serrated knives, kitchen shears, spoons and even melon-ballers as opposed to real knives.
    - Plastic knives work well for tasks like spreading and icing.
    - Kitchen shears can be used for everything from chopping herbs to cutting lean meat.
    - Spoons and melon-ballers can be used for cutting fruit, scraping seeds out of cucumbers and even peeling ginger.
- Knives should be sharp; dull knives can lead to accidents.
- Older children should learn to hold knives properly with the fingers of their dominant hand securely gripping the knife handle and the fingers of their other hand curled under as they hold the food. Curling the fingers under ensures they are free from the danger of the blade.
- Remember, graters, zesters, microplanes and peelers are sharp, too. Children should not use these utensils until they are old enough (usually around age 9 or 10) to learn to use them properly. And no matter how old your child is or how adept he seems to be at cooking, you should always be there in the kitchen with him when he's cooking.
- Never leave food cooking on your stove or in your oven when you leave home and stay in the kitchen whenever anything is cooking. Turn off stoves and appliances promptly when you're finished using them and unplug electrical appliances when they are not in use.
- Keep appliances clean to avoid grease fires. Wipe appliance surfaces after spills and clean stove surfaces and ovens regularly.
- Be alert and no horse play.
- Wear close-fitting sleeves that do not dangle too close to hot stove burners and catch fire. Don't store things on or above your stove.
- Keep flammable objects clear of the stove.
- Do not overload electrical outlets.
- Prevent burns and stovetop fires by always turning pot handles in toward the back of the stove.
- Never pour water on a cooking fire. If a pan of food catches fire, carefully slide a lid over the pan and turn off your stove burner. Keep the lid on until completely cooled. If a fire starts in your oven, close the oven door and turn off the heat source. If the flames do not go out immediately, call the fire department.
- Use pure, therapeutic-grade lavender oil (not lavandin) over a burn. This will minimize skin damage and ease the pain. Never apply butter or other grease to a burn. If the burned skin is blistered or charred, see a doctor immediately.
- Stop, drop and roll if your clothing catches fire. If someone else's clothes catch fire, push him to the ground and roll him over and over, or smother the flames with a flame-resistant blanket or carpet.

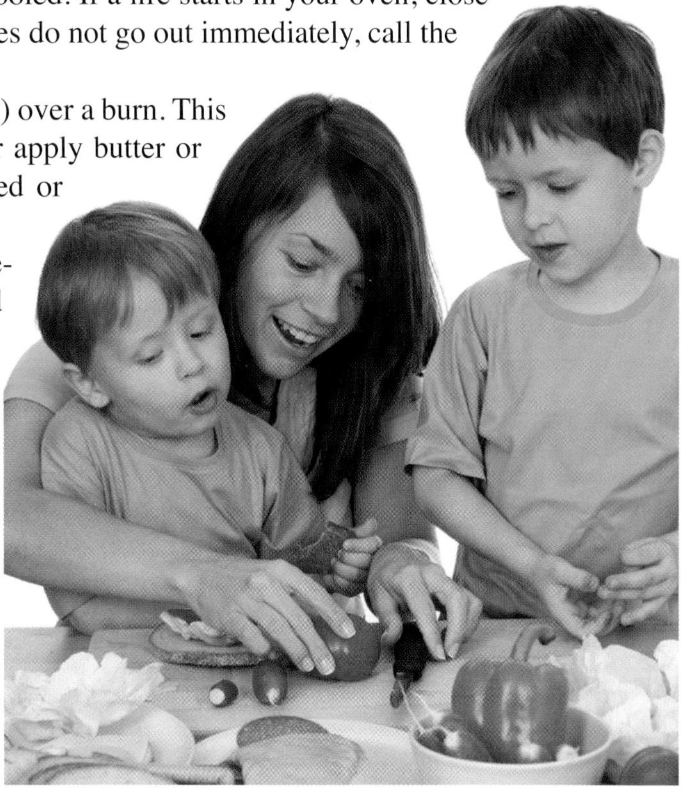

Resources

Kitchen Safety for Kids - Knife Skills, Knowing the Proper Way to Use Kitchen Utensils is Key to Cooking Safe with Kids, by Stephanie Gallagher, About.com

Fire Prevention for Kids www.westcov.org/kids/kitsafe.html

Appendix F: Vitamin Chart

Vitamin Nutrient	Food Sources	Stability in Foods	Metabolism	Use in Body	Effect of Deficiency
Vitamin A	apricots, asparagus, broccoli, butternut squash, cantaloupe, carrot, chlorella, cod, collards, dandelion, dock, paprika, parsley, pimento, pumpkin, red hot peppers, spirulina, sweet potatoes.	Insoluble in water. Soluble in fats. Stable to low heat. Destroyed by during, oxidation, very high temperatures	Bile necessary for absorption.	Promote growth and reproduction. Stored in liver, eyes, skin, lungs, gallbladder and kidneys.	Slow growth, poor bone and tooth development. Night blindness. Reduce ability to resist infection, keratosis, xerophthalmia.
B_1 Thiamine	Rice bran, wheat germ, sunflower seeds, pinon nut, peanut, kidney beans, peas, whole grains, molasses, chickpeas, spirulina, asparagus, coriander.	Highly soluble in water. Stable in dry form and acid solution. Destroyed by heat in neutral or alkaline solution, sulfites	Limited storage in body. Part of enzyme system. Depleted by sugar and smoking.	Builds energy and appetite. Aids digestion. Proper function of heart, liver	Lack of appetite, nervous instability, depression, fatigue, constipation, Beriberi, polyneuritis, cardiac failure, edema
B_2 Riboflavin	alfalfa, almond, asparagus, barley, mushroom, peppermint, red hot pepper, safflower seed, wheat germ, wild rice.	Slightly soluble in water. Resistant to heat in acid solution. Sensitive to alkali. Decomposed by light.	Limited storage in body. Part of enzyme system. Transfers hydrogen from one metabolite to another.	Raises resistance to disease, delays degeneration, improves skin and eye conditions. Liver, kidneys and heart.	Cracks at lip corners. Inflammation of lips and tongue. Burning, itching eyes, Photophobia, blurred vision
B_3 Niacin	beets, peanuts, rice bran, wheat germ.	Slightly soluble in water; stable to heat, oxidation, light, acid, and alkali.	Active part of enzyme system-transfers hydrogen	Builds mental health. Aids nervous system. Helps maintain appetite. Adrenal glands.	Pellagra, canker sores, gastrointestinal, skin problems, neurological changes.

Vitamin Nutrient	Food Sources	Stability in Foods	Metabolism	Use in Body	Effect of Deficiency
B_5 Pantothenic acid, also known as Pantethine	brewer's yeast, buttermilk, corn, lentils, egg yolks, mushrooms, peanut butter, peanuts, pecans, rice bran, royal jelly, salmon, sunflower seeds, tahini, whole grains.	Destroyed when heated with acids, alkali or dry heat: 33 percent lost during cooking meat and 50 percent lost in the milling of flour.	Occurs in all living cells, found in blood, excreted in urine, vital role in cellular metabolism. Aids in its assimilation. Most effective when combined with royal jelly.	Highest concentration in the brain. Boosts energy, speeds wound healing, prevents hair loss and graying of hair. Thought to slow the aging.	Vomiting, burning feet, cramps, upper respiratory infections, skin disorders, adrenal exhaustion, rheumatoid arthritis, sleep disturbances.
B_6 Pyridoxine	almonds, avocados, bananas, Brazil nuts, brown rice, carrots, chicken, lentils, oats, salmon, sunflower seeds, tuna, walnuts, whole grains.	Destroyed by heat and light.	Essential for RNA and DNA synthesis. Maintains potassium and sodium balance.	Excreted in urine, found only in muscles. Only take as a B-complex, unless directed by a doctor.	Nausea, low blood sugar, hair loss, anemia, dermatitis, headaches, cracks on mouth and sore tongue.
B_7 Biotin	brewer's yeast, cauliflower, egg yolk, rice, royal jelly, whole grains.	Inactivated by rancid fats and choline.	Produced in intestines by bacteria, excreted in urine, stored in liver, kidney, brain, and adrenals.	Builds healthy hair and skin.	Loss or thinning hair, gray skin color and rash around lips.
B_9 Folate, Folacin (natural form) Folic Acid (synthetic form)	asparagus, beans, brewer's yeast, broccoli, lettuce, oranges, spinach, rice, romaine.	Destroyed by high heat, light, and being left at room temperature for long times.	Part of B-complex functioning as an enzyme - utilization of proteins. Active in cell division.	Prevents some birth defects and protective against skin cancer.	Anemia, poor growth, gray hair and mental illness.
B_{12} Cobalamin, Cyanocobalamin	red meat, eggs, cheese, Plant sources not readily absorbed: devil's claw, dulse, goldenseal, nettle, red peppers.	Destroyed by heating with strong acids or alkali.	Stored in liver, aids in formation of healthy blood cells. Vegans should supplement.	Stimulates metabolism, restores appetite, prevents mental deterioration.	Anemia, impaired blood cell reproduction. Soreness and weakness in limbs and jerky or diminished reflexes.

Vitamin Nutrient	Food Sources	Stability in Foods	Metabolism	Use in Body	Effect of Deficiency
Choline - recently accepted into the family of B vitamins	Found in foods rich in lecithin. egg, cabbage, rice bran, oat bran, turnips.	Highly soluble in water. Stable in dry form and acid solution. Destroyed by heat in neutral or alkaline solution	Co-enzyme in action. Functions with insotol. Keeps fats in solution, essential for myelin sheath of nerves.	Memory enhancer, improves mood.	Alzheimer's, fatty deposits in liver, kidney and heart problems, nerve related diseases.
Vitamin C	acerola cherry, acerola juice, black currant, broccoli, Brussels sprouts, cantaloupe, citrus fruits, collards, coriander leaf, guava, kale, kiwi, mango, papaya, parsley, red cabbage, red hot peppers, rose hips, sago palm, strawberry, sweet pepper, watercress.	Highly soluble in water; easily destroyed by heat, air, alkali, enzymes; acid inhibits destruction; copper accelerates destruction.	Little storage in body; greatest concentrations in most active tissues; aids in metabolism of some amino acids. Aids absorption of iron.	Forms and maintains intercellular substance; aids teeth and gums.	Cutaneous hemorrhages, poor bone development, weakened cartilage, muscle degeneration, anemia, stunted growth and susceptibility to infection, scurvy
Vitamin D	Only found in beef, dairy, egg, fish and lamb. Also synthesized by sun exposure.	Fat soluble; stable heat and oxidation.	Synthesized in skin by activity of ultra-violet light, stored in liver.	Promotes normal bone and tooth development. Regulates absorption and fixation of calcium and phosphorous.	Rickets; soft, fragile bones enlarged joints, bowed legs; titanic convulsions, Osteomalacia
Vitamin E	almonds, barley, brown rice, cabbage, egg yolk, green leafy vegetables, hazelnuts, legumes, nuts, rice germ, rye, salmon, spinach, sunflower seeds, spinach, tuna, wheat germ.	Soluble in fat, oil. Stable to heat and alkalies in absence of oxygen. Also acid at low temperature. Oxidized in rancid fats, presence of iron, lead, silver, salts and ultraviolet light.	Not stored in body. Reduces oxidation of Vitamin A and carotene.	Prevents liberation of hemoglobin from red blood cells; aids heart, reproduction and utilization of fatty acids.	Sterility, muscle degeneration.

Vitamin Nutrient	**Food Sources**	**Stability in Foods**	**Metabolism**	**Use in Body**	**Effect of Deficiency**
Inositol	brewer's yeast, citrus fruits, liver, molasses, whole grains.	Highly soluble in water. Stable in dry form and acid solution. Destroyed by heat in neutral or alkaline solution	Aids in proper nervous system function and helps body produce lecithin.	Aids in cell growth. Depleted by caffeine.	Eczema, constipation, poor sight, hair loss and high blood cholesterol.
Vitamin K	alfalfa, asparagus, cauliflower, cheese, egg yolk, green leafy vegetables, green tea, kelp, lettuce, molasses, oats, safflower oil, watercress.	Fat-soluble. Destroyed by radiation, air pollution, aspirin and rancid fats.	Absorbed in upper intestines. Body can manufacture with yogurt or kefir, Bile required for absorption.	Normal blood clotting.	Celiac disease, colitis, hemorrhaging, bruising

Appendix G: Mineral Chart

Mineral Nutrient	Food Sources	Metabolism	Uses in the Body	Effects of Deficiency
Calcium	almond, basil, Brazil nuts, broccoli, celery seed, citrus fruit, dill weed, dulse, figs. filbert, green leafy vegetables, oregano, parsley, prunes, sunflower seed, thyme, kelp, sesame seed, sage, molasses, whole grains	Absorption aided by vitamin D, ascorbic acid, lactose; interfered by oxalic acid. Use regulated by parathyroid hormone and vitamin D. Stored in bone, acid-binding.	Builds bones and teeth. Used for muscle contraction, normal heart action, nerve irritability. Activates some enzymes. Used for blood coagulation, normalize metabolism. Most abundant mineral in the body.	Retarded bone and tooth development, fragile bones, stunted growth, rickets, osteomalacia, osteoporosis, nervosity, muscle sensibility, muscle spasms.
Chloride	avocado, celery, coconut, dates, kelp, kale, lettuce, tomato, turnips.	Excretion in urine, acid-forming.	Aids digestion and elimination, normalizes osmotic pressure in blood and tissues, sustains normal heart activity, acid-base balance, blood, epithelium nerves.	Disturbed digestion, weak water retention, weight decrease.
Chromium	Herbs and spices are best source: nettle, horseradish, red clover and stevia. Also black pepper, brewer's yeast, broccoli, corn, chicken, egg, rice polishings, spirulina, whole grains	Absorption rate is poor as it competes with other minerals like zinc. Primarily stored in spleen and kidneys. Used in metabolism of carbohydrates.	Essential for the production of glucose tolerance factor which is necessary for production of insulin. Also involved in digestion and metabolism of fats and proteins.	
Copper	barley, black pepper, beets, Brazil nuts, cocoa, dried coconut, green olive, legumes, molasses, nuts, raisins, sage, whole grains.	Stored in liver and central nervous system. Excreted by bile into small intestine. Acid-forming.	Liver, gallbladder, blood, lungs and heart. Absorption and metabolism of iron. Oxidation of fatty acids, of tyrosine to melanin pigments. Metabolism of ascorbic acid.	Retarded hemoglobin production. Defective respiration, general debility, limited growth.
Fluorine	Almond, black tea, beet greens, carrot, dandelion, spinach, turnip greens.	Acid-forming	Bones, teeth, blood, skin, nails and hair.	Decay of teeth, spinal curvature, weakened eyesight

Mineral Nutrient	Food Sources	Metabolism	Uses in the Body	Effects of Deficiency
Iodine	asparagus, black walnut, blueberry, dulse, garlic, kale, kelp, lima beans, spinach, Swiss chard, turnip greens, watermelon.	Stored in thyroid gland. Excreted in urine. Acid-forming	Constituent of thyroxine which regulates rate of energy exchange. Aids oxidation of fats and proteins. Stimulates circulation.	Goiter or enlarged thyroid gland. Cretinism or subnormal basic metabolism. Sensitivity to infection, general weakness. Low body and mental activity. Nervous disturbances.
Iron	almonds, beef, blackstrap molasses, dulse, kelp, green vegetables, pistachios, sesame seed, squash seed, yellow dock.	Aided by gastric acidity, ascorbic acid, copper essential, stored in liver, bone marrow, spleen, kidneys. Absorption hindered by excess phosphorous, (soft drinks, red meat)	Hemoglobin, myoglobin, oxidative enzyme, bones, brain, muscle.	Anemia, Chlorosis, paleness limited growth, inferior vitality.
Magnesium	almonds, banana, cocoa powder, dark green vegetables, date, dried fruit, kelp, legumes, potato, turmeric seed, whole grains.	Acid-binding, over 300 enzymes require magnesium as a cofactor. Aids in intracellular mineral transport, hormone synthesis, digestive enzyme synthesis.	Strengthen nerves and muscles, conditions liver and glands, stimulate elimination, activates enzymes in carbohydrates, metabolism, blood albumen, bones, teeth.	Soft bones and teeth, digestive disorder, exhaustion, irritability, nervosity and spasticity, heartbeat acceleration, convulsions, poor complexion.
Manganese	beet, blueberries, blackstrap molasses, carrot, celery, chives, cloves, cucumber, ginger, lima beans, navy beans, parsley, raw potatoes, red raspberry leaf, rice bran, sunflower seeds, walnuts, whole grains.	Absorption is limited. Liver is most active organ of metabolism. Main elimination is by intestine. Acid-binding.	Thyroxine formation, formation of urea, Lipotropic activity of choline. Utilization of thiamine, metabolism of carbohydrates. Strengthen tissue and bones, kidneys, liver, pancreas, spleen, brain heart, lymph.	Weak tissue respiration, restricted growth, glandular disorders. Defective reproduction functions.

Mineral Nutrient	Food Sources	Metabolism	Uses in the Body	Effects of Deficiency
Phosphorus	asparagus, broccoli, cabbage, cranberry, cocoa, dried fruit, egg yolk, grains, green vegetable leaves, legumes, nuts, pumpkin seed, rice bran, seaweed, squash seeds.	Absorption aided by Vitamin D, excreted in urine. Acid-forming. Major energy transfer catalyst.	Builds bones, teeth, blood and hair. Activates some enzymes, nervous tissue. Metabolism of fat and carbohydrate. Transport of fatty acids.	Poor mineralization of bones, poor growth, rickets, decrease in weight, general weakness.
Potassium	avocado, banana, beet, blackstrap molasses, broccoli, carrot, cauliflower, cabbage, celery, coriander leaf, dates, dried fruits (apricot, peaches), green vegetables, horseradish, kelp, legumes, butter beans, lemongrass, nuts, parsley, peppermint, radish, raisins, seaweed-dulse, Swiss chard, winter squash.	Second most abundant mineral in plants. Excreted in urine. Acid-binding. Potassium is the principle catalyst in intracellular fluids, aids in carbohydrate metabolism, protein synthesis, muscle contraction and nerve impulse conduction.	Intercellular fluid balance, regular heart rhythm, regulates nervous and muscular irritability. Aids elimination. Aids formation of glycogen from glucose, fats from glycogen, proteins from peptones and proteases	Affected growth, incomplete digestion, nervous disorders, insomnia, constipation, irregular heat beat, muscle damage.
Selenium	apple cider vinegar, Brazil nuts, butter, cinnamon, garlic, nutmeg, radishes, Swiss chard, turnips, whole grains.	Nature's most important cancer-blocking agent. Strengthens immunity. Essential for reproduction. Found in non-fat tissue.	Immune system booster.	Premature aging, mental retardation, diminished vision, nerve disorders.
Silicon	bell peppers, cucumber, dandelion, dulse, lettuce, strawberry, sunflower seed, thyme, well water, whole grains.	Acid-forming	Blood, muscles, skin, nerves, nails, hair, connective tissue, pancreas, tooth enamel, antiseptic action	Reduced resistance to infectious disease.
Sodium	beet greens, carrot, celery, dried fruit, dulse, grapefruit, kale, kelp, radish, raisin, real salt.	Readily absorbed. Excretion through kidneys. Controlled by adrenal cortical hormone. Acid-binding	Aids formation of digestive juices, aids elimination of carbon dioxide, regulates osmotic pressure. Maintains water balance. Nerve irritability	Nausea, diarrhea, muscular cramps, digestive disorders, general debility and decreased weight.

Mineral Nutrient	Food Sources	Metabolism	Uses in the Body	Effects of Deficiency
Sulfur	garlic, kale, kelp, lettuce, onion, raspberry, turnip.	Excess excreted in urine. Acid-forming	Hair, nails, insulin, cartilage, blood. Aids digestion and elimination. Oxidizing agent in hemoglobin	Restricted growth, eczema, dermatitis, poor growth of nails and hair.
Zinc	alfalfa seeds, almonds, bilberry, buchu, cardamon, carroway, chevil, chickpeas, celery seed, dried basil, hot peppers, maple syrup, mustard seeds, onions, poultry, pumpkin seed, sage, sesame seed flour, skullcap, thyme, wheat germ and bran.	Excreted mainly from intestine, immune system strengthener.	Effects transfer of carbon dioxide from tissue to lungs, constituent of digestive enzyme for hydrolysis of protein, aids healing of wounds. Brain, genital organs, thyroid, liver, kidneys.	Defective intestinal absorption Restrictive growth

Appendix H: Alkaline/Acid Chart

To maintain health, the diet should consist of 60 percent alkaline-forming foods and 40 percent acid-forming foods. To restore health, the diet should consist of 80 percent alkaline-forming foods and 20 percent acid-forming foods.

Most Alkaline	Alkaline	Lowest Alkaline	Food Category	Lowest Acid	Acid	Most acid
asparagus, broccoli, cucumber, garlic, kale, onions, parsley, radish, spinach (raw), sprouts, most vegetable juices	beets, beet greens, celery, cilantro, collard greens, endive, green beans, lettuce, mustard greens, okra, sorrel, squash, sweet potato, Swiss chard greens, soy and radish sprouts, zucchini	artichokes, cabbage, carrots, cauliflower, eggplant, horseradish, kohlrabi, mushrooms, parsnips, peas, peppers, potato skins, pumpkin, turnip, rutabaga, watercress	**FRESH, RAW VEGETABLES**	cooked vegetables	corn, frozen vegetables, canned vegetables, potatoes (no skins)	fermented (pickled) vegetables
avocado, lemons, limes, mangoes, papayas	apples, dates, grapes, honeydew melon, kiwi, musk melon, raisins, raspberries, tomatoes	bananas (unripe), cherries (sour), coconut, oranges, peaches, wolfberries	**FRESH, RAW FRUITS**	blackberries, cherries (sweet) figs, grapefruit, nectarines, plums, processed fruit juices, strawberries, watermelon	apricots, cantaloupe, currant, pear, rhubarb, tangerines	blueberries, canned fruits, cranberries, glazed fruits, pineapple, prunes
barley, kamut grasses, oat straw, soy and radish sprouts, wheat grass	other sprouted grains, wheat	alfalfa, amaranth, millet, quinoa, wild rice	**GRAINS and CEREALS**	brown rice, hemp seed flour, rice milk, spelt, sprouted wheat bread,	corn products, crackers, buckwheat, oats, rye, white rice	pastries, pasta, wheat bread, white flour
			MEATS and EGGS	cold water fish (such as fresh herring, rainbow trout, salmon, sardines, tuna, etc.), eggs, venison	buffalo, chicken, duck, lamb, organ meats, rabbit, turkey	beef, pork, shellfish, veal
		horseradish, kohlrabi, lentils, lima beans, mung beans, navy beans, peas, soybeans	**BEANS and LEGUMES**	kidney beans, string beans	black beans, chickpeas, pinto beans	chocolate beans

Most Alkaline	Alkaline	Lowest Alkaline	Food Category	Lowest Acid	Acid	Most acid
almonds	hazelnuts	caraway, chestnuts, cumin, fennel, sesame	**NUTS and SEEDS**	Brazil nuts, flaxseed, filberts, pumpkin seeds, sunflower seeds, tahini	cashews, pecans	peanuts, pistachios, walnuts
Evening primrose	borage oil, flaxseed oil	olive oil	**OILS**	butter, safflower oil, sesame oil	canola oil, sunflower oil	margarine
	breast milk	buttermilk, goat cheese, soy cheese, soy milk, whey	**DAIRY**	butter, cottage cheese, yogurt	raw milk	cheese, homogenized milk, ice cream
potassium, sodium	calcium	magnesium	**MINERALS**			
	cayenne, chili pepper, cinnamon, curry, dandelion, ginger, herbs (all), miso, sea salt, tamari	carob, horsetail, dandelion,	**HERBS, SPICES and SEASONINGS**		cocoa	
herbal teas, lemon water	green tea, teccino (coffee substitute)	ginger tea	**BEVERAGES**	black tea	coffee	beer, liquor, soft drinks
agave, stevia	blackstrap molasses, maple syrup, rice syrup	honey (raw), sugar (raw)	**SWEETENERS**	honey (processed), molasses	brown sugar, white sugar	aspartame, corn syrup, Equal, NutraSweet, Splenda, Sweet 'N Low
			OTHER		ketchup, mayonnaise, soy sauce	chips, fast food

Appendix I: Nutritional Recommended Daily Allowances (RDA) for Children, Women and Men

Nutrient	Infants 0-6 mo	Infants 7-12 mo	Children 1-3 yrs	Children 4-8 yrs
Carbohydrates	60 grams	95 grams	130 grams	130 grams
Dietary Fiber	N/A	N/A	19 grams	21 grams
Fats	31 grams	30 grams		
Omega-3	0.5 grams	0.5 grams	0.7 grams	1.1 grams
Omega-6	4.4 grams	4.6 grams	7 grams	14 grams
Minerals				
Calcium	210 mg	270 mg	500 mg	
Chloride	180 mg	570 mg	1,500 mg	1,200 mg
Chromium	0.2 mcg	5.5 mcg	11 mcg	2,000 mg
Copper	200 mcg	220 mcg	340 mcg	20 mcg
Fluoride	N/A	N/A	N/A	900 mcg
Iodine	110 mcg	130 mcg	90 mcg	150 mcg
Iron	0.27 mg	11 mg	7 mg	8 mg
Magnesium	30 mg	75 mg	80 mg	320 mg
Manganese	0.003 mg	0.6 mg	1.2 mg	1.8 mg
Molybdenum	2 mcg	3 mcg	17 mcg	45 mcg
Phosphorus	100 mg	275 mg	460 mg	700 mg
Potassium	400 mg	700 mg	3,000 mg	4,700 mg
Selenium	15 mcg	20 mcg	20 mcg	55 mcg
Sodium	120 mg	370 mg	1,000 mg	1,200 mg
Zinc	2 mg	3 mg	3 mg	8 mg
Protein	9.1 grams	13.5 grams	13 grams	46 grams
Vitamins				
Biotin	5 mcg	6 mcg	8 mcg	30 mcg
Choline	125 mg	150 mg	200 mg	425 mg
Folic Acid	65 mcg	80 mcg	150 mcg	400 mcg
Vitamin A	400 mcg	500 mcg	300 mcg	700 mcg
Vitamin B1	0.2 mg	0.3 mg	0.5 mg	1.1 mg
Vitamin B2	0.3mg	0.4 mg	0.5 mg	1.1 mg
Vitamin B3	2mg	4 mg	6 mg	14 mg
Vitamin B5	1.7mg	1.8 mg	2 mg	5 mg
Vitamin B6	0.1mg	0.3 mg	0.5 mg	1.5 mg
Vitamin B12	0.4mg	0.5 mcg	0.9 mg	2.4 mcg
Vitamin C	40mg	50 mg	15 mg	75 mg
Vitamin D	5 mcg, (200 IU)	5 mcg, (200 IU)	5 mcg, (200 IU)	10 mcg (400 IU)
Vitamin E	4 mg	5 mg	6 mg	15 mg
Vitamin K	2 mcg	2.5 mcg	30 mcg	90 mcg

Nutrient	Females 9-13 years	Females 14-18 years	Females 19-30 years	Females 31-50 years	Females 51-70 years	Females 70+ years	Pregnancy	Lactation
Carbohydrates	130 grams	130 grams	130 grams	130 grams	130 grams	130 grams	175 grams	210 grams
Dietary Fiber	26 grams	26 grams	25 grams	25 grams	21 grams	21 grams	28 grams	29 grams
Fats								
Omega-3	1 gram	1.1 grams	1.1 grams	1.1 grams	1.1 grams	1.1 grams	1.4 grams	1.4 grams
Omega-6	10 grams	11 grams	17 grams	17 grams	14 grams	14 grams	13 grams	13 grams
Minerals								
Calcium	1,300 mg	1,300 mg	1,000 mg	1,000 mg	1,200 mg	1,200 mg	1,000 mg	1,000 mg
Chloride	2,300 mg	2,300 mg	2,300 mg	2,300 mg	2,000 mg	1,800 mg	2,300 mg	2,300 mg
Chromium	21 mcg	24 mcg	25 mcg	20 mcg	20 mcg	20 mcg	30 mcg	45 mcg
Copper	700 mcg	890 mcg	900 mcg	900 mcg	900 mcg	900 mcg	1 mg	1.3 mg
Fluoride	N/A	N/A	N/A	N/A	N/A	N/A	N/A	N/A
Iodine	120 mcg	150 mcg	150 mcg	150 mcg	150 mcg	150 mcg	220 mcg	290 mcg
Iron	8 mg	15 mg	18 mg	18 mg	8 mg	8 mg	27 mg	9 mg
Magnesium	240 mg	360 mg	310 mg	320 mg	320 mg	320 mg	360 mg	320 mg
Manganese	1.6 mg	1.6 mg	1.8 mg	1.8 mg	1.8 mg	1.8 mg	2 mg	2 mg
Molybdenum	34 mcg	43 mcg	45 mcg	45 mcg	45 mcg	45 mcg	50 mcg	50 mcg
Phosphorus	1,250 mg	1,250 mg	700 mg	700 mg	700 mg	700 mg	700 mg	700 mg
Potassium	4,500 mg	4,700 mg	4,700 mg	4,700 mg	4,700 mg	4,700 mg	4,700 mg	5,100 mg
Selenium	40 mcg	55 mcg	55 mcg	55 mcg	55 mcg	55 mcg	60 mcg	70 mcg
Sodium	1,500 mg	1,500 mg	1,500 mg	1,500 mg	1,200 mg	1,200 mg	1,500 mg	1,500 mg
Zinc	8 mg	9 mg	8 mg	8 mg	8 mg	8 mg	11 mg	12 mg
Protein	34 grams	46 grams	46 grams	46 grams	46 grams	46 grams	71 grams	71 grams
Vitamins								
Biotin	20 mcg	25 mcg	30 mcg	30 mcg	30 mcg	30 mcg	30 mcg	30 mcg
Choline	375 mg	400 mg	425 mg	425 mg	425 mg	425 mg	450 mg	550 mg
Folic Acid	300 mcg	400 mcg	400 mcg	400 mcg	400 mcg	400 mcg	600 mcg	500 mcg
Vitamin A	600 mcg	700 mcg	700 mcg	700 mcg	700 mcg	700 mcg	770 mg	1,300 mcg
Vitamin B1	0.9 mg	1 mg	1.1 mg	1.1 mg	1.1 mg	1.1 mg	1.4 mg	1.4 mg
Vitamin B2	0.9 mg	1 mg	1.1 mg	1.1 mg	1.1 mg	1.1 mg	1.4 mg	1.4 mg
Vitamin B3	12 mg	14 mg	14 mg	14 mg	14 mg	14 mg	18 mg	17 mg
Vitamin B5	4 mg	5 mg	5 mg	5 mg	5 mg	5 mg	6 mg	7 mg
Vitamin B6	1 mg	1.2 mg	1.3 mg	1.3 mg	1.5 mg	1.5 mg	1.9 mg	2 mg
Vitamin B12	1.8 mcg	2.4 mcg	2.4 mcg	2.4 mcg	2.4 mcg	2.4 mcg	2.6 mcg	2.8 mcg
Vitamin C	45 mg	75 mg	75 mg	75 mg	75 mg	75 mg	85 mg	120 mg

Nutrient	Females 9-13 years	Females 14-18 years	Females 19-30 years	Females 31-50 years	Females 51-70 years	Females 70+ years	Pregnancy	Lactation
Vitamin D	5 mcg (200 IU)	5 mcg (200 IU)	5 mcg (200 IU)	5 mcg (200 IU)	10 mcg (400 IU)	15 mcg (400 IU)	5 mcg (200 IU)	5 mcg (200 IU)
Vitamin E	11 mg	15 mg	15 mg	15 mg	15 mg	15 mg	15 mg	19 mg
Vitamin K	60 mcg	75 mcg	90 mcg	90 mcg	90 mcg	90 mcg	90 mcg	90 mcg

Nutrient	Males 9-13 years	Males 14-18 years	Males 19-30 years	Males 31-50 years	Males 51-70 years	Males 70+ years
Carbohydrates	130 grams	130 grams	130 grams	130 grams	130 grams	130 grams
Dietary Fiber	31 grams	38 grams	38 grams	38 grams	30 grams	30 grams
Fats						
Omega-3	1.2 grams	1.6 grams	1.6 grams	1.6 grams	1.6 grams	1.6 grams
Omega-6	12 grams	16 grams	17 grams	17 grams	14 grams	14 grams
Minerals						
Calcium	1,300 mg	1,300 mg	1,000 mg	1,000 mg	1,200 mg	1,200 mg
Chloride	2,300 mg	2,300 mg	2,300 mg	2,300 mg	2,000 mg	1,800 mg
Chromium	25 mcg	35 mcg	35 mcg	35 mcg	30 mcg	30 mcg
Copper	700 mcg	890 mcg	900 mcg	900 mcg	900 mcg	900 mcg
Fluoride	N/A	N/A	N/A	N/A	N/A	N/A
Iodine	120 mcg	150 mcg	150 mcg	150 mcg	150 mcg	150 mcg
Iron	8 mg	11 mg	8 mg	8 mg	8 mg	8 mg
Magnesium	240 mg	410 mg	400 mg	420 mg	420 mg	420 mg
Manganese	1.9 mg	2.2 mg	2.3 mg	2.3 mg	2.3 mg	2.3 mg
Molybdenum	34 mcg	43 mcg	45 mcg	45 mcg	45 mcg	45 mcg
Phosphorus	1,250 mg	1,250 mg	700 mg	700 mg	700 mg	700 mg
Potassium	4,500 mg	4,700 mg	4,700 mg	4,700 mg	4,700 mg	4,700 mg
Selenium	40 mcg	55 mcg	55 mcg	55 mcg	55 mcg	55 mcg
Sodium	1,500 mg	1,500 mg	1,500 mg	1,500 mg	1,300 mg	1,200 mg
Zinc	8 mg	11 mg	11 mg	11 mg	11 mg	11 mg
Protein	34 grams	52 grams	56 grams	56 grams	56 grams	56 grams
Vitamins						
Biotin	20 mcg	25 mcg	30 mcg	30 mcg	30 mcg	30 mcg
Choline	375 mg	550 mg	550 mg	550 mg	550 mg	550 mg
Folic Acid	300 mcg	400 mcg	400 mcg	400 mcg	400 mcg	400 mcg
Vitamin A	600 mcg	900 mcg	900 mcg	900 mcg	900 mcg	900 mcg

Nutrient	Males 9-13 years	Males 14-18 years	Males 19-30 years	Males 31-50 years	Males 51-70 years	Males 70+ years
Vitamin B1	0.9 mg	1.2 mg	1.2 mg	1.2 mg	1.2 mg	1.2 mg
Vitamin B2	0.9 mg	1.3 mg	1.3 mg	1.3 mg	1.3 mg	1.3 mg
Vitamin B3	12 mg	16 mg	16 mg	16 mg	16 mg	16 mg
Vitamin B5	4 mg	5 mg	5 mg	5 mg	5 mg	5 mg
Vitamin B6	1 mg	1.3 mg	1.3 mg	1.3 mg	1.7 mg	1.7 mg
Vitamin B12	1.8 mcg	2.4 mcg	2.4 mcg	2.4 mcg	2.4 mcg	2.4 mcg
Vitamin C	45 mg	75 mg	90 mg	90 mg	90 mg	90 mg
Vitamin D	5 mcg (200 IU)	5 mcg (200 IU)	5 mcg (200 IU)	5 mcg (200 IU)	10 mcg (400 IU)	15 mcg (600 IU)
Vitamin E	11 mg	15 mg	15 mg	15 mg	15 mg	15 mg
Vitamin K	60 mcg	75 mcg	120 mcg	120 mcg	120 mcg	120 mcg

Appendix J: Fats and Omega Essential Fatty Acids

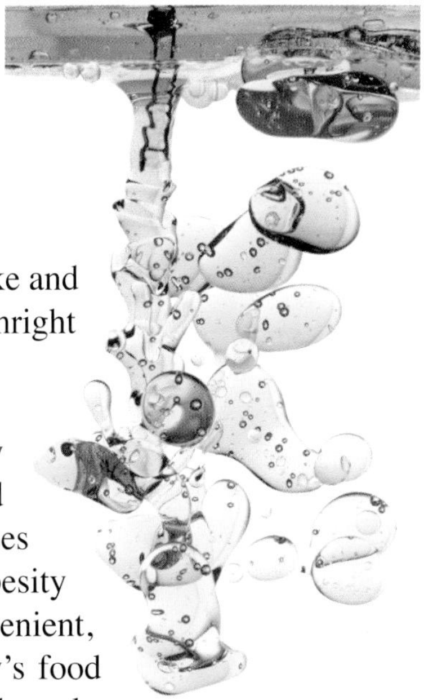

Vegetable Fats

In recent years, nutritionists have concentrated on the connection between fat intake and degenerative disease. So which fats are good, which are bad and which are downright ugly?

One hundred years ago, the diseases that affected children and adults were mostly infectious disease, which for the most part, are greatly controlled and reduced through better hygiene. Today, Americans are plagued with degenerative diseases that were once rare but are now rampant and on the rise. Cancer is out of control, obesity is skyrocketing, and high blood pressure and heart disease are soaring. Convenient, over-processed, canned, frozen, enriched and preserved to last for years – today's food supply has dramatically changed. Tomatoes no longer come from the backyard garden but from hundreds of miles away, picked green, ripened in a truck and sprayed with some unpronounceable chemical. Fats are over processed. For example, an olive is pressed not once or twice but several times, heated and then hydrogenated. Consuming nutritionally deficient food has health consequences, and the more we consume refined foods the more likely we will endure health concerns.

It is widely known that cultures untouched by modernization and food refinement are much healthier than industrialized cities. We can take a page from their books on fats. Nut, seed and vegetable oils are more than just tasty; they also are healthy and have the ability to help with cardiovascular and immune system issues.

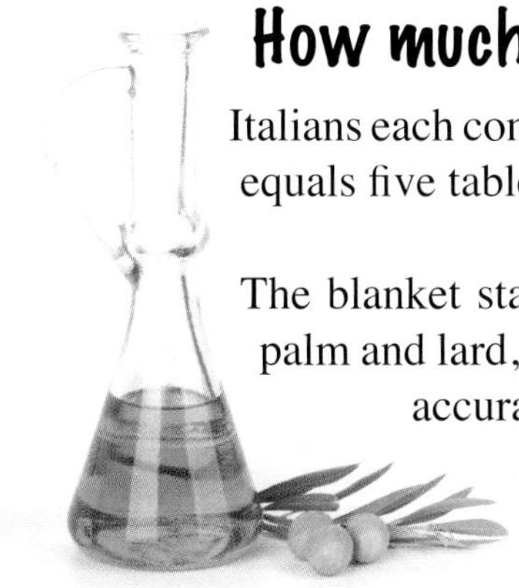

How much olive oil is consumed per year?

Italians each consume 10 liters annually. Libyans consume 20 liters. Greeks consume 23 liters, which equals five tablespoons per day. Greeks have the lowest incidence of heart disease in Europe.[1]

The blanket statement to avoid all saturated fats (hard at room temperature) like coconut, butter, palm and lard, and eat only poly or mono-unsaturated fats (liquid at room temperature) is no longer accurate. While saturated oils are linked to some forms of heart disease, tropical oils are heart healthy. Some fats are essential for our health. Some supply the body with hormone-like substances called prostaglandins and other fats give us lignans known to be active in cancer prevention.

Saturated Fats

Butter, though not a vegetable oil, is better than margarine, which has its beginnings as a vegetable oil, typically corn. According to health pioneer Dr. Alfred Vogel, a healthy liver can metabolize only up to two tablespoons of butter daily. So use butter in moderation and not even daily. If using to sauté, be careful as butter burns and once it burns it is no longer healthy.

Dr. William P. Castell, director of the renowned Framingham Study of 1992 concluded, "The more saturated fat one ate, the more cholesterol one ate, the more calories one ate, the lower people's serum cholesterol." Through that study, it became evident that something other than cholesterol and saturated fat were causing coronary disease.

---

1 "Mediterranean diet and prevention of coronary heart disease in the elderly" Anastasios S Dontas, Nicholas S Zerefos, Demosthenes B Panagiotakos, and Dimitrios A Valis. Clin Interv Aging. 2007 March; 2(1): 109–115.

A study in "Preventative Medicine" reported that "Very low total cholesterol, less than 160ml/dl, has been shown to increase the risk of mortality from lung cancer by 1.75 times for men and 3.29 times for women."[2]

"Margarine correlates with the risk of heart disease more strongly that any other food, including butter". Lancet, 1993, VOL. 341

Timeline of dietary fat intake in the U.S. food supply from 1909 to 1993[3]

1909 – Average American ate less than two grams of liquid vegetable oil.
1910 – Proportion of animal fats in diet; 83 percent.
1911 – Crisco went on sale.
1920 – Butter consumption is 18 pounds per person annually.
1930 – Heart attack deaths: 3,000.
1940 - Hydrogenated margarines introduced.
1950 – Butter consumption: 10 pounds per person annually.
1960 - Heart attack deaths: 500,000.
1970 - Proportion of animal fats in diet; 62 percent.
1970 - Butter consumption: four pounds per person annually.
1993 - Average American consumes more than 30 grams of liquid vegetable oil
2004 – Heart disease deaths: 876,000.

Fun Fact

Trans fats are processed fats that are designed to turn an oil into solid product.
Crisco was the prototype first marketed in 1912.
Artificially hardened fats are listed on labels as hydrogenated, modified, fractionated or partially hydrogenated. Always avoid these trans fats.

Oh, So Good Olive Oil

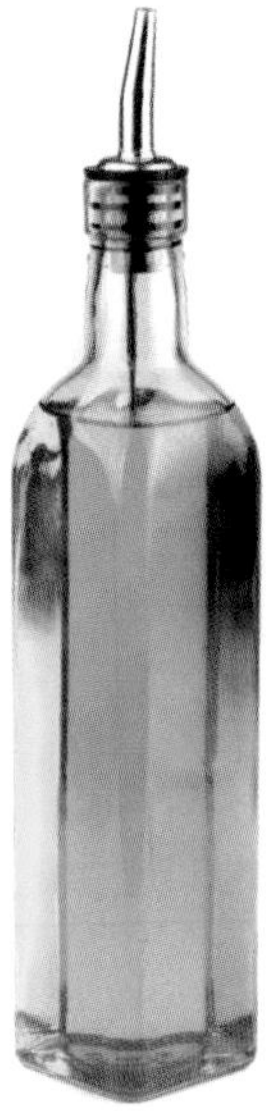

Praised by health enthusiasts, nutritionists, alternative health professionals worldwide and a staple of the Mediterranean diet, olive oil (unrefined, extra virgin, cold pressed) affectionately called EVOO, is loaded with health benefits. Since EVOO consists mostly of Omega-9 fats it can be used in cold dishes and cooking. Olive oil may be heated to 215° F with no change in its profile.

Crazy For Coconut Oil

Once labeled taboo, coconut oil is now becoming a rising star in the oil world. Listed as a saturated fat, it was lumped together with other unhealthy saturated fats for many years. But today research is continuing to emerge on the health benefits of coconut oil. As we have seen earlier, many health cultures consume large quantities of fat. The Polynesian people consume up to 60 percent of their total calories in coconut oil, yet live a remarkable long, healthy life.

Coconut oil may[4]:

Reduce risk of atherosclerosis and heart disease.
Reduce risk of cancer and other degenerative diseases.
Help prevent bacterial, viral and fungal infections.
Support immune system function.
Help control diabetes.

2 Preventative Medicine, 1995; 24:557-62
3 "21 Days to a Healthier Heart" Alan L. Watson, Diet Heart Publishing, 2002.
4 "The Healing Miracles of Coconut Oil," Bruce Fife, N.D., HealthWise Publications, 2003.

Provide and immediate source of energy.
Support healthy metabolic function.
Improve digestion and nutrient absorption.
Supply important nutrients necessary for good health.
Supply fewer calories than other fats.
Promote weight loss.
Help prevent osteoporosis.
Has a long shelf life.
Heat resistance making it a healthy choice for cooking.
Prevent premature aging and wrinkling of the skin.
Help protect again skin cancer and other blemishes.
Function as a protective antioxidant.

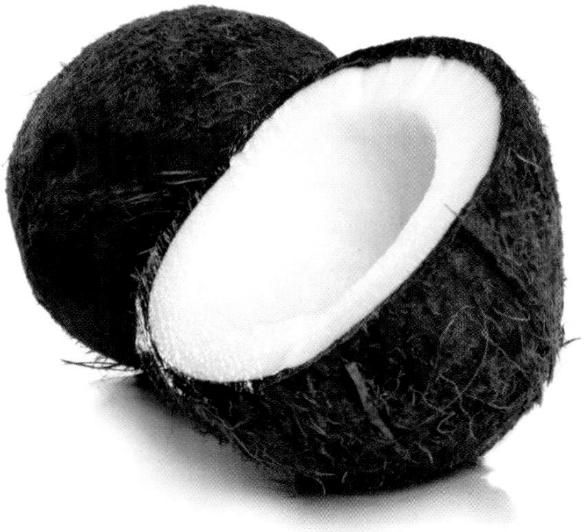

Coconut does not:

Increase blood cholesterol levels.
Promote platelet stickiness.
Contribute to atherosclerosis or heart disease.
Make you gain weight.

Coconut oil is not the watery liquid that runs out from a fresh coconut when cracked, but rather the oil is pressed from the fresh coconut meat. Consuming three and a half tablespoons of coconut oil daily is considered to be very beneficial to health. Coconut oil can be used in baking muffins, cakes, breads, cookies, added to pancake and waffle recipes, added to smoothies, used in salad dressings and used in frying vegetables or meat.

Fabulous Flax

Flaxseed oil is made from the linseed plant and is in a class by itself because it is the only oil comprised almost entirely of good, polyunsaturated essential fatty acids. Flaxseeds are approximately 42 percent oil and a rich source of linolenic acid (48 to 64 percent) or Omega-3. The rest of the oil is lenoleic acid (16 to 34 percent) or Omega-6 and oleic acid (18 percent) or Omega-9.

Flaxseed oil goes rancid quickly, so purchase it in small bottles and always chose cold or expeller pressed oil. Flaxseed oil is best used cold in salads and dips and should not be used in cooking or heated for frying.

Some observed benefits of consuming flax oil are:

- Normalized blood fat levels, lowering of low-density lipoprotein or LDL, increased blood flow and preventing blood platelets from sticking together.
- Rebalance prostaglandins elevating blood estrogen levels which may elevate symptoms of PMS and menopause.
- Help burn body fat.
- Support healthy liver function.
- Stimulates immune system function.

Corn Oil was the first cooking oil making its debut in 1911 under the name Mazola®. Corn oil is cholesterol free and rich in vitamin E. Its high smoke point has made it a favorite for frying. Processing removes free fatty acids and phospholipids from the crude corn oil. Corn oil is founds in most processed foods and is a main component of margarine. Economically friendly, corn oil has downsides. Being high in Omega-6 polyunsaturated fatty acids, corn oil may increase the likelihood that post menopausal women will develop breast cancer.[5] A similar effect was

5 The International Journal of Cancer, http://www.interscience.wiley.com/journal/120780752/abstract

seen with prostate cancer.[6] As most corn oil comes from genetically modified corn (GMO), it should be avoided.

Almond Oil is skin friendly and has been used in massage for many years, but it was not until some 20 years ago that its nutritional value was known. Almond oil pressed from sweet almonds yields a pleasant smelling, mild tasting oil similar to olive oil and contains mainly Omega-9 essential fatty acids making it tolerant of heat. It may be used in baking or grilling.

Walnut Oil is rich in Omega-6 essential fatty acids and has been used historically by women wanting to increase fertility. It has been observed to lower LDL levels, reduce hypertension and normalize blood fat levels. Walnut oil is best used cold in cold in salads and dips and should not be used in cooking or heated for frying.

Chia Seed Oil contains a rich source of non-fish Omega-3 essential fatty acids for health and wellness. Some reports indicate that chia oil may even have a higher concentration of essential fats as compared to flaxseed oil, which is generally considered to be the best plant source of Omega-3 fatty acids. The essential fatty acids in chia oil contribute to the health of the heart, nerves and immune system. Chia oil is pressed from seed of the chia (Salivia hispanica) plant and contains 60 percent minimum Omega-3.

Hazelnut Oil is a heart healthy choice. The hazelnut is high in the amino acid arginine which relaxes blood vessels and has one of the highest concentrations of folate (folic acid) among tree nuts. Hazelnuts contain 12 percent Omega-6 with the same benefits of the other Omega-6 nut oils. It is used for both culinary and cosmetic purposes. Hazelnut oil can withstand moderate heat without compromising quality.

Avocado Oil is not pressed, but is made from a mixture of the ripe fruit and water placed in a centrifuge to produce the oil. Avocado oil contains 7 percent mono-unsaturated, 16 percent saturated and 5 percent polyunsaturated oils. It may be used in cooking and makes a great mayonnaise substitute. Sometimes varieties of avocados are called vegetarian butter. They are highly nutritious and rich in valuable fats.

Sesame Seed Oil must be purchased cold-pressed because refined sesame oil is processed with hexane. Roasted sesame seed oils are full of trans fats. Cold pressed sesame seed oil can be used cold or in cooking. It is a staple in Asian stir-fry. Sesame seed oil contains 46 percent polyunsaturated (oleic acid) oil and 35 percent polyunsaturated (linoleic) oil.

Pumpkin Seed Oil is a treasure among chefs for its distinct color and nutty flavor. High in protein, the pumpkin seed's unrefined oil has been used by many people suffering from bladder weakness and to prevent hormonal buildup in the prostate gland, which may lead to an enlarged prostate. It has many of the same healing properties as flax seed oil and should also be cold or expeller press and used cold or at room temperature.

Butter gets a bad rap. Before WWII margarine was homemade from natural, unrefined palm and coconut oils with a touch of salt and then blended with sunflower oil. The end product was solid yet still soft at room temperature and was a naturally healthy alternative to butter. Then came the age of hydrogenation and unhealthy mass-produced margarine.

Butter is a fat from cow or goat milk and is easily digested. It was the margarine and shortening industry that duped the consumer into thinking butter was unhealthy especially for the heart, when actually the opposite is true.

---

6 The Journal of Clinical Investigation http://pubmedcentral.nih.gov/articlerender.fcgi?artid=1890998

Fats and Omega Essential Fatty Acids

Amount of Omega-3 in four ounces of fish

Fish	Omega-3 – grams
Salmon	2.1
Sardines	1.4
Scallops	1.1
Shrimp	0.4
Tuna	0.3
Cod	0.03

Vegetable Oils – Omega-3, Omega-6 and Saturated Fat percentages

Food	Omega-3%	Omega-6%	Sat %
Almond oil	-	26	9
Chia oil	64	22	3
Corn oil	-	59	17
Coconut oil	-	3	91
Evening Primrose	-	81	8
Flaxseed oil	57	18	9
Hazelnut oil	-	15	7
Olive oil	-	8	10
Pumpkin oil	15	42	9
Safflower oil	-	79	8
Sesame oil	-	41	13
Sunflower oil	-	69	13
Walnut oil	8	51	16
Wheat germ oil	5	50	18

Percentages and types of fats in food

Food	% Polyunsaturated	% Monounsaturated	% Saturated	% Fat
Butter	10	29	61	100
Margarine	55	20	25	98
Cod	57	16	27	8
Haddock	45	21	34	7
Tuna	40	40	20	32
Mackerel	32	41	27	63
Salmon	30	43	27	42
Sardines	22	57	21	62
Brazil nuts	40	35	25	85
Peanuts	30	50	20	73
Almonds	74	20	72	8
Sunflower seeds	67	21	12	73
Avocados	8	80	12	80
Cottage cheese	63	11	25	40
Cheddar cheese	33	21	47	74
Milk, Whole	5	30	65	49
Milk, Skim	5	30	65	5
Chocolate, Milk	3	34	63	36
Olive oil	10	13	61	100
Beef	17	48	35	71
Pork	10	48	42	65
Bacon	9	48	43	80
Chicken	6	49	45	32
Lamb	7	41	52	76

Appendix K: Fiber-Rich Foods

The average American's daily intake of fiber is about five to 14 grams per day. This may account for a significant number of health issues families face, such as constipation, diabetes (Type 2), obesity, some cancers and heart disease. The current recommendations from the National Academy of Sciences Institute of Medicine are to achieve an adequate intake of fiber based on your gender and age. This recommended amount is expected to meet or exceed the average amount needed to maintain a defined nutritional state of health.

Food	Amount to eat for 10 grams of fiber
Almonds	1/8 cup
Apple	3-4 apples
Apricots, dried	1 cup
Baked Beans	1 cup
Baked Potato with skin	1 large
Bananas	3 medium to large bananas
Broccoli, raw or cooked	1 large head
Cabbage	1 medium head
Carrots	3 carrots
Cauliflower	1 large head
Chia seed	6 tsp.
Chickpea/Hummus dip	¾ cup
Figs, dried	1/3 cup
Flax seed	1 cup
Grapes	40 grapes
Lentils, cooked	2 cups
Oats	1 cup
Oranges	3 oranges
Peaches	6 peaches
Peanuts	1 cup
Pears	2 ½ pears
Peas, green	1 cup
Prunes	1 cup
Sunflower seeds	1 cup
Wheatbran	½ cup
White Bread, store bought	15 slices
Whole Grain Bread, store bought	5 slices
Whole Grain Bread, homemade	3 slices

Fiber requirements by age:

Females	Grams per day	Males	Grams per day
2-14 years	Age plus 5*	2-14	Age plus 5*
15-50 years	25 grams	15-50 years	38 grams
51+ years	21 grams	51+ years	30 grams

* For younger children take their age and add the number five for the total number of grams of fiber per day. Example: A five-year-old would need 10 grams of fiber; an eight-year-old would need 13 grams.

Some helpful tips about adding fiber to your diet.

1. **Increase slowly:** The best way to begin is to figure out how much fiber is currently consumed each day. Once the number is known, slowly increase how much is eaten until the recommended amount is reached. Increasing too quickly can lead to gas, bloating, and/or diarrhea.

2. **Drink water:** Without enough pure, clean water in a high-fiber diet, constipation may result. The fiber will swell, peristalsis (the wave like motion of the intestines) will not ocurr, and bowel movements will be hard. Drink at least 16 ounces of pure water between meals.

3. **Don't add too much too quickly:** More is not always better, so fiber should be increased a little at a time. There is no limit on how much fiber can be consumed, and there are no reported problems with excess fiber intake. We should listen to our bodies and pay attention to how our health challenges and bowel movements are responding to fiber intake.

4. **Creative Ways to add fiber to Meal Time**

   a. Add flaxseeds, chia seeds, seeds, or nuts to your salad, soup, cereal, or yogurt.
   b. Keep fresh and frozen fruit such as peaches, blueberries, strawberries, and raspberries to add to cereal, dessert, shakes or yogurt.
   c. Use pre-cut-up vegetables, stored in small baggies, available to take for snacks and to quickly add to a soup or salad.
   d. Choose a whole grain cereal with a minimum of four grams of fiber in each serving. It may serve as a meal, or alone as a snack.
   e. Lentils, beans and peas go with everything. Add them in salad or soup or have them with your meals or as snacks.
   f. Select breads and pastas made from whole grain flour. The off-white color is easy to cover with a fresh tomato sauce until everyone is used to the color. Vegetable powders often are often added to pasta for unique natural colors, which are great for summer pasta salads.
   g. Have vegetables with meals whenever possible.
   h. Use fruit with, or in between, meals. Set a minimum number of servings to have each day and be sure to reach it. Always go for the fruit with the skin and/or seeds for the fiber.

5. **Gas and bloating:** Taking an enzyme with specific starch and fiber components will greatly reduce bloating and gas from the extra fiber in the raw vegetables and/or beans and make eating much more pleasurable.

Appendix L: Baking with 100% Whole Grains

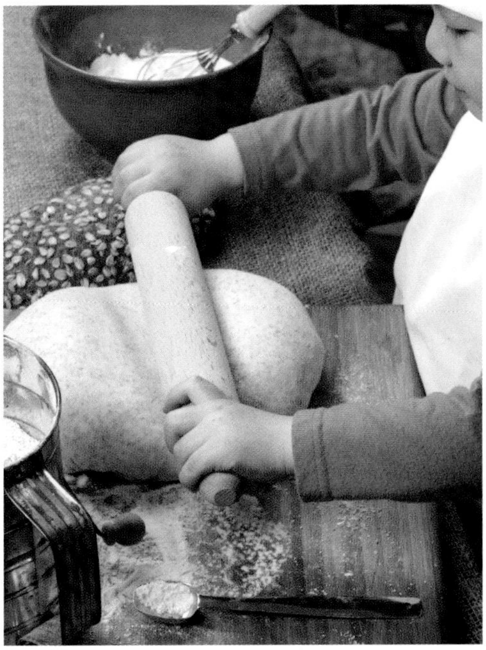

Grains have long been the staple in food storage plans. In nearly every culture grains provide the bulk of nutrition needed by people and livestock. If properly packaged and kept dry, grains will last indefinitely. When archeologists uncovered the tomb of King Tutankhamun in Egypt they discovered wheat among the artifacts. The wheat was planted, and it sprouted – in good condition and full of nutrition. It had been kept dry and free from bugs and was still good after many hundreds of years.

The most familiar grains include wheat, rye, oats, millet, rice, barley and corn. The bread grains (wheat, barley and corn) require some type of processing before they can be eaten, such as milling into flour for bread, pasta, cereal and chips. The dish grains (oats, millet and rice) can be cooked and served in their whole state. Grains contain a number of essential vitamins and minerals. Most grains also can be soaked, sprouted, and then prepared using low heat to retain their full complement of live enzymes. Wheat grass juice – a powerhouse of nutrition – is gaining popularity as a healthy beverage,.

Wheat is high in vitamin E, folate and the B-complex vitamins. In fact, of the 44 known nutrients essential to humans, only four are lacking in the wheat berry. Sprouting the wheat berry provides three of these nutrients, leaving only iodine to obtain elsewhere. These nutrients are lost when the outer bran layer is removed during commercial processing and then stored for long periods before using.

Wheat looses 75 percent of its nutrients within 48 hours after being milled into flour. Once the grain is milled the germ is exposed. This contains the vitamin E, which begins to turn rancid within 72 hours.

To get optimum freshness and the most nutrition from your grains they should be bought whole and processed just prior to using.

Having a hand or electric mill allows you to mill fresh whole grains and thus serve the most delicious and nutritious bread, pancakes, pastas, rolls, pizza and desserts possible. A mill will pay for itself very quickly in savings over store-bought flour products. Medical problems due from eating over processed and nutritionally depleted bread flour products will often times vanish after eating 100 percent whole-grain bread products.

Bread made from whole grain flour has eight times the fiber of ordinary store bought whole wheat bread and all of the essential vitamins and minerals are still present. An increase in fiber has been shown to decrease a host of diseases including, heart disease, hemorrhoids, constipation and some cancers.

All whole wheat flour sold commercially retains some of the bran for color, but the wheat germ and germ oil have been removed as they will turn rancid in less than a week. These two elements contain the life force of the grain and are essential for good health. Whole wheat flour should be ground fresh daily as needed.

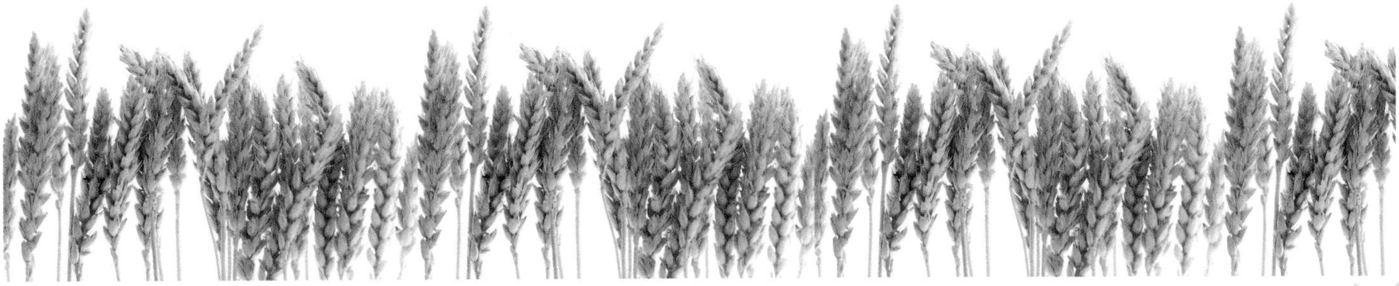

Wheat comes in several varieties: Hard Spring Red and White, Hard Winter Red and White, and Soft White. Spring wheat's are grown in the extreme northern states and Canada and have the highest gluten content. Winter wheat is often grown in warmer winter climates and has slightly less gluten content than Spring wheat, though this will vary due to climate and growing conditions. Dough enhancers or conditioners are sometimes added to low gluten flours to assist in the texture and rise of the bread. This can be in the form of added wheat gluten or a commercial dough enhancer.

Some winter wheat and all soft wheat is lower in gluten content and better suited for pastries and pasta. The red grains impart a darker color to the finished product, and the white grains produce a product looking more like store-bought breads, cakes, cookies, etc. Some families like bread with half red and half white wheat. The only other ingredients needed for great bread are honey, salt, oil, yeast and water.

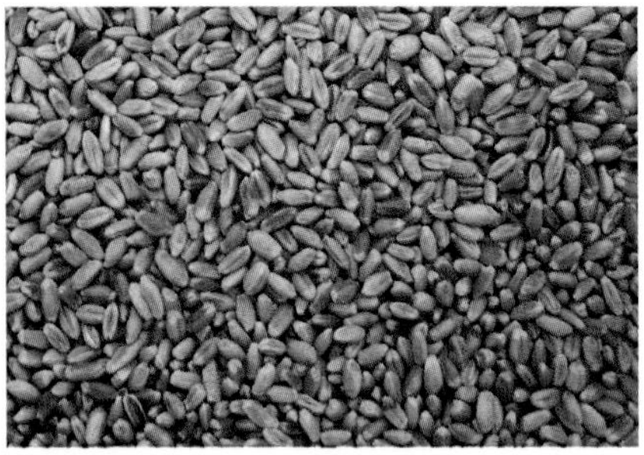

Hard Spring Wheat is planted in the spring, mostly in the northern plains states with extremely cold winters where winter wheat is prone to winter kill. It is grown without irrigation or watering, except by natural rain and snow. It yields a high protein and low moisture wheat berry. This type of grain is usually more expensive than its winter wheat counterpart and is endorsed by both home and professional bakers nationwide.

Hard Winter Wheat is planted in the fall. It also is grown without irrigation or watering, except by rain or snow. The extreme northern states are too cold for this type of wheat, but it grows well across Kansas and states south of the hard freeze line. Dry climate during the winter and spring make for a good protein content and low moisture. Hard winter wheat is a favorite of farmers as it produces high yields, making it less expensive to grow.

The color of the wheat berry – either red or white – makes very little difference in the protein and moisture content of the wheat. The difference is only in the color of the finished product. The red varieties produce a heartier, darker bread, while the white wheat varieties produce a slightly milder loaf, less coarse and much lighter in color.

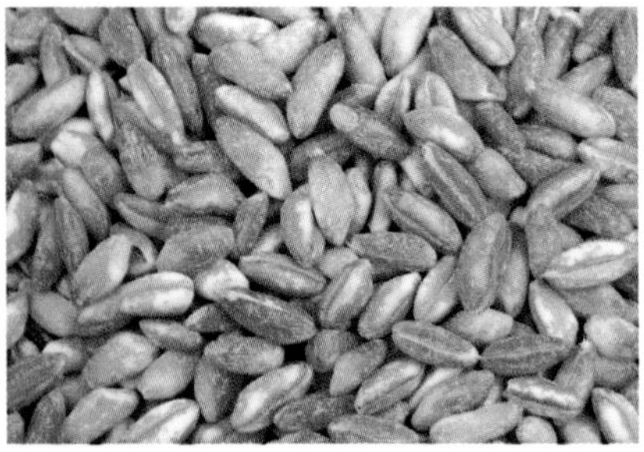

Soft Spring Wheat is planted in the spring and is irrigated. It usually has a higher yield than hard wheat, but is lower in protein. Soft wheat is best when used in cakes, cookies, pastries and other baked goods that use baking powder, baking soda or shortening as leavening.

Durum Wheat is used for making macaroni, noodles and all forms of pasta. In 1996 the disease Kamal Bunt nearly wiped out the entire Durum wheat crop. The remaining crop was quickly sold off to commercial producers. This resulted in the home pasta makers being forced to purchase already milled durum flour rather than buying the whole berry and milling fresh flour.

Other cereal and bread grains include barley, oats and rye. These can be ground into flour and added to bread and pastry recipes. The also can be eaten in the whole state boiled for cereals or pilafs.

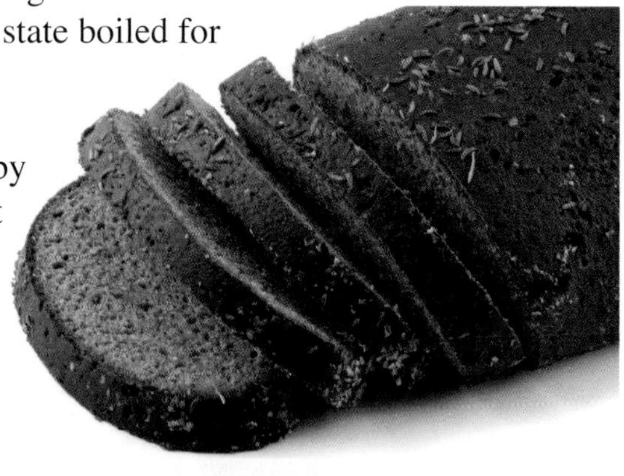

Rye was brought to America by the Dutch settlers. It also is know by the name black cumin, a seed used in cooking. Although rye is not as versatile as the aforementioned grains, it is a welcome addition to food storage plans as its hardy flavor adds variety to your meals, especially in breads and muffins. Rye can be used in pilafs, casseroles and as a cereal. It is generally mixed with wheat in bread making as rye flour by itself is very heavy and dark.

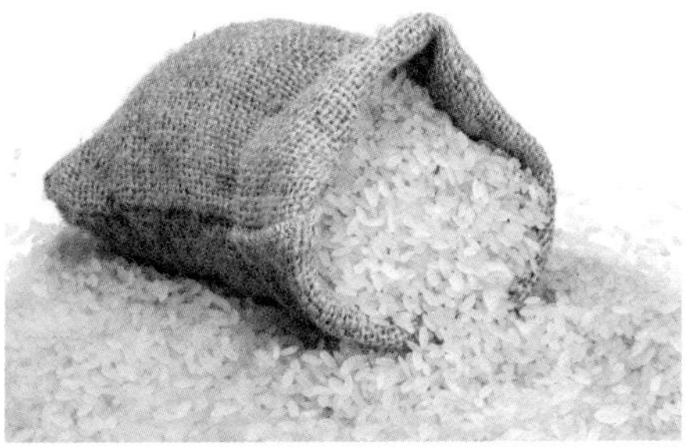

Rice has long been a staple grain for much of the Asian countries. It thrives in a moist climate and was not introduced to North America until 1686. Once rice is milled and the white kernel is exposed, little nutrition is left. As with all grains, the most nutrition is derived from eating the whole grain. With rice, the outer hull and a small amount of bran is removed, resulting in brown rice. Polished rice is the term for white rice. White rice keeps better than its brown counterpart, storing for many years under proper conditions. Brown rice must be vacuumed sealed and frozen to last longer than six months without becoming rancid.

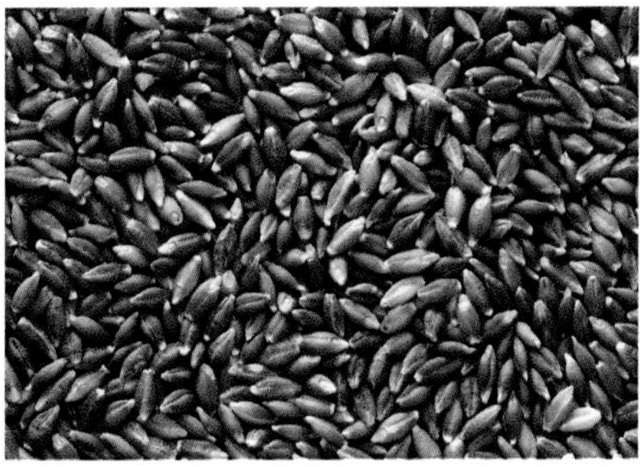

Barley is exceptionally well suited to cakes and cookies as it imparts a lighter color and texture than wheat alone. For every cup of flour used in a recipe substitute two table- spoons barley flour for two tablespoons of the whole wheat flour. Barley flour is interchangeable in recipes calling for arrowroot powder or cornstarch. Barley also is used in soups, stews and pilaf recipes. Barley is a non-gas forming grain (alkaline) making it easy to digest. It contains the same amount of carbohydrates as corn, but with slightly more protein. Barley also is high in the amino acid Lysine and should be part of your grain storage program.

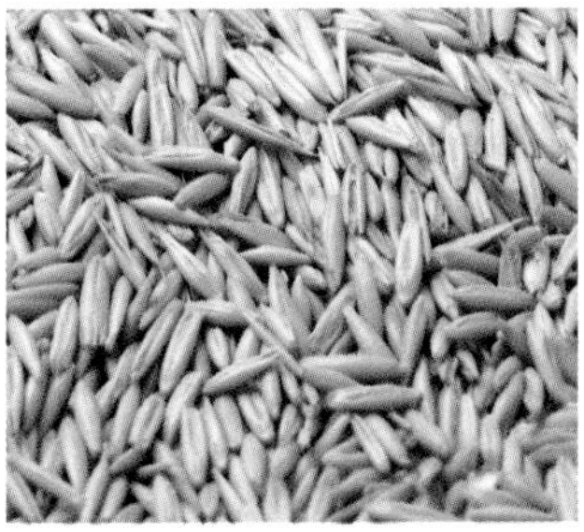

Oat groats can be cooked in their whole state into cereal or rolled with the use of an oat roller to produce traditional oatmeal flakes for hot cereals, oatmeal cookies, breads and homemade granola. Higher in protein than any other cereal grain, oats also are very high in fiber, easy to digest and are an excellent addition to grain storage because of their versatility. Oats do not grind easily in stone mills, as they are soft and the pores of the stones may become clogged with the flour.

Gluten Intolerance

Many people suffer from occasional to very serious complications when consuming gluten or grains, chiefly wheat. Gluten is the protein found in wheat, rye and barley. The following is a list of gluten-free grains, flours and starches and may be substituted for traditionally gluten containing items:

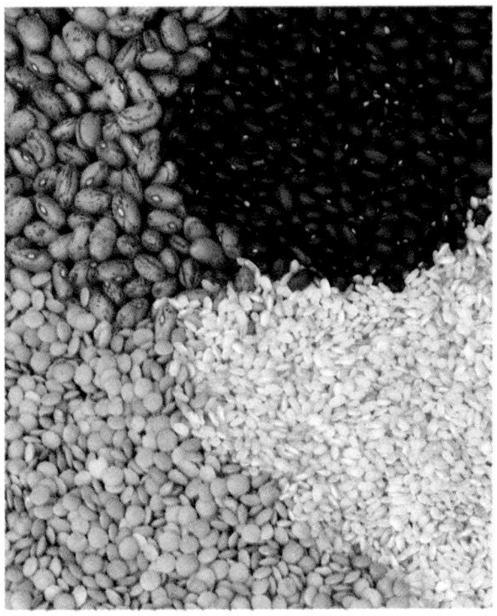

Almond
Artichoke
Arrowroot
Beans
Black Gram
Buckwheat
Chickpea (Besan)
Corn
Garbanzo
Garfava
Lentil
Millet
Nut Flours
Pea
Pinto
Potato
Quinoa
Rice
Sorghum
Soy
Sweet Potato
Tapioca (Manioc)
Teff

Despite being wheat free and well tolerated by individuals seeking to avoid wheat Kamut, Spelt and Tritical contain gluten and must be avoided to ensure a gluten-free meal. Other grains containing gluten and/or wheat include barley, bulgur, couscous, durum, farina, graham, Matzoh meal, rye, semolina and wheat germ.

People with severe intolerance to gluten are diagnosed with Celiac disease. It is believed to be brought about by intestinal damage that has occurred over many years causing poor nutrient absorption. One also must note that some people with symptoms of gluten intolerance have no symptoms when they change from over-processed, refined grains to whole grains. Persons with intestinal damage would do well to incorporate a probiotic supplement and enzymes with meals. See Appendix DD for information on selecting a probiotic.

The Web site of the Celiac Sprue Foundation contains helpful information for people with gluten intolerances including recipes and flour substitutes. http://www.csaceliacs.org/gluten_grains.php

Debra's Famous Whole Grain Bread

(This recipe was used by one of Debra's students to win first prize at a county fair. It contains her secrets to making great bread.)

This recipe is for three loaves and five loaves of bread using the Bosch Universal Mixer.

Ingredients	Three loaves	Five loaves
Oil	1/3 cup	2/3 cup
Honey	1/3 cup	2/3 cup
Salt	¾ tsp.	1 tsp.
Dough Enhancer	2 Tbs.	4 Tbs.
Hot Water	3 1/3 cups	5 ½ cups
Flour	9 cups	15 cups
Yeast	2-3 Tbs.	3 ½ - 4 Tbs.

Combine oil, honey, salt, gluten (dough enhancer), half the flour and the water. Turn Bosch to setting one. While mixing, sprinkle in yeast. After one minute turn off mixer and let rest for one to two minutes to allow the flour to absorb the water. This is the first secret to great bread.

Turn the mixer back on to number one and begin adding the flour one cup at a time until the dough begins to pull away from the sides of the bowl. When it does, **do not add any more flour**. This is secret number two! Turn the setting to knead for eight minutes.

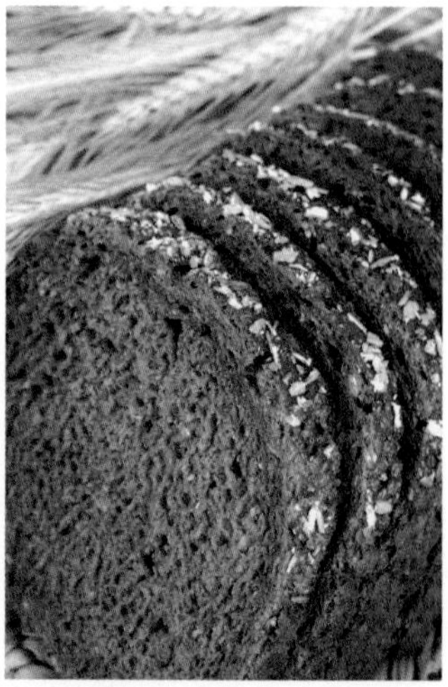

Remove from bowl, shape into desired loaves, breadsticks, rolls, buns, pizza crust, etc. Let rise for about 30 minutes or until double in size. Cooler house temperatures will require longer rise times. An alternative is to turn the oven to 200° F, turn off when temperature is reached, open oven door and place bread pans on the door to warm. Place in pre-heated 350° F oven. Let bake for 25 to 30 minutes. Remove from oven, let sit five minutes and remove from pans onto a cooling rack to keep the bread from sweating in the hot pans. You can use this dough for pizza crust, dinner rolls, sandwich buns, bread sticks and cinnamon rolls.

Good For You Cookies

By Ann Howard

Feel free to double, triple or further multiply this family favorite recipe.

1 ¼ cup whole wheat flour ground fine (soft white wheat works well)
½ stick soft butter
¼ cup Blue Agave Nectar (may substitute 1 cup Sucanat)
1 egg
1 tsp. vanilla
1 tsp. baking soda
½ tsp. salt
1-1 ½ cup rolled oats (oatmeal)

Optional (add any of the following for an extra treat): ½ cup each: copped dates, currents, raisins, coconut and carob chips.

Mix butter and agave or sucanat well. Add egg and vanilla and whisk. In a separate bowl, stir flour, soda and salt. Add to the liquid ingredients. Add in oatmeal and optional ingredients.

Bake in a pre-heated 350° F oven for 14 minutes.

Oatmeal Cookies

A healthy twist to a cookie that has stood the test of time.

1 cup butter, room temperature
2 cups Sucanat (may substitute ½ cup Agave, if you do you will need an additional ¼ cup flour – best choice would be barley flour)
2 eggs
½ tsp. vanilla
1 tsp. baking soda
½ tsp. salt
½ tsp. cinnamon
1 ¼ soft white wheat ground fine
3 cups rolled oats (oatmeal)
1 cup raisins

Preheat oven to 375° F. Lightly oil a cookie sheet or line it with parchment paper. Cream butter, Sucanat or Agave together. Add in eggs and vanilla. Mix dry ingredients in a separate bowl, then slowly add to creamed ingredients. Drop by spoonfuls onto cookie sheet. Bake for 12 to 15 minutes. Remove from cookie sheet onto drying racks. The longer they are baked the crispier they become.

Wolfberry Cookies

NingXia wolfberries have the highest antioxidant level of known fruit on the planet.

1/3 cup diced, dried apricots
1/3 cup wolfberries
1 egg
1 ½ cup rolled oats (oatmeal)
1 ½ cup whole wheat flour, ground fine (we like using soft white wheat)
3 Tbs. unsweetened apple juice or water
½ cup Blue Agave Nectar
¼ cup olive oil or coconut oil
¼ cup butter (salted or unsalted)
¼ tsp. salt
½ tsp. baking powder

Optional: ¼ cup carob chips

Preheat oven to 350° F. Lightly oil a cookie sheet or line it with parchment paper. Soak apricots and wolfberries in apple juice and ½ cup warm water. Cream butter and oil, then add egg, blue agave and salt. Cream until fluffy. Add dry ingredients and mix well. Drain liquid off soaking fruit and reserve. Add fruit, carob chips and add three tablespoons of the reserved liquid, stir until mixed. Place in spoonfuls on greased baking sheet. Bake 8 to 10 minutes, until cookies melt and are light brown.

Whole Wheat Breakfast or Dessert Crepes

Enjoy these French staples with fruit for a sweet treat.

½ cup whole wheat flour, ground fine
2 eggs
1 cup milk (may be raw cow, goat, almond or rice milk)
1 Tbs. melted butter
Pinch of sea salt
Baking Powder

In a lightly buttered omelet pan, pour two tablespoons of the crepe batter and allow it to roll around the pan so the batter coats the entire bottom of the pan. Cook until golden brown on the bottom, flip and cook other side if necessary. Roll cooked crepes and store between two plates or pie pans until all are cooked.

Breakfast: Place two to three crepes on plate and top with fruit. For a citrus topping, squeeze the juice of one lemon in a bowl and whisk in one teaspoon of Agave and drizzle over the top.

Dessert Filling: Puree fresh fruit (strawberries, peaches, blueberries, etc.). Unroll the crepe, spoon in the puree filling, roll and drizzle with honey. For those who choose to consume dairy, blend cream cheese with honey orAgave and/or fruit for a delicious filling.

Gluten-Free Pumpkin Pancakes

This tempting flapjack batter can also be used for waffles.

1/2 cup sorghum flour
1/2 cup rice flour
1/4 cup tapioca flour
2 tsp. baking powder
1 tsp. pumpkin pie spice
1/2 tsp. salt
1Tbs. Blue Agave Nectar
6 heaping Tbs. of pumpkin puree
2 Tbs. melted butter or olive oil
1 cup milk or water
1 egg

In a medium bowl, whisk together dry ingredients. In a separate bowl, stir together wet ingredients. Mix wet ingredients into dry ingredients. Cook pancakes in a skillet or on a griddle with butter or oil. Use about 1/4 cup of batter for each pancake.

Appendix M: Protein-Rich Plant and Animal Sources

The RDA for protein in adults is equal to 0.8 g of protein per kilogram of body weight per day which translates to about 60 grams, and for children it is 0.5 grams per kilogram of body weight daily or about 35 grams. The average American diet provides from one to two times the RDA for protein. This may lead you to think that a protein deficiency is unlikely in the U.S. However, the RDA for protein has been derived from research studies performed on healthy individuals. Growing children, pregnant and lactating women, the elderly, and anyone undergoing severe stress (trauma, hospitalization, surgery), disease, disability or someone recovering from an injury, needs more protein.

Food source	Serving size	Grams of protein
Asparagus	1 cup	5
Baked beans	1 cup	12
Black beans	1 cup	15
Lima Beans	1 cup	15
Pinto beans	1 cup	14
Carrots raw	1 cup	1
Carrots cooked	1 cup	1.74
Cauliflower raw	1 cup	1.9
Cauliflower cooked	1 cup	2.9
Romain lettuce	1 cup	0.9
Okra	1 cup	3.8
Onion raw	1 cup	1.28
Onion cooked	1 cup	2.8
Pumpkin canned	1 cup	3.79
Spinach raw	1 cup	0.86
Spinach cooked	1 cup	5.97
Sweet potato	1 cup	4.21
Buckwheat	1 cup	15
Oat bran raw	1 cup	16
Brown rice	1 cup	5
Whole wheat bread	2 slices	5
Beef	per ounce	7
Chicken	4 ounces	35
Fish	3.5 ounces	22
Turkey	1 cup	39
Whole Milk	1 cup	8
Eggs	1 large	6
Pumpkin seeds	1/4 cup	19
Flax seeds	1/4 cup	8

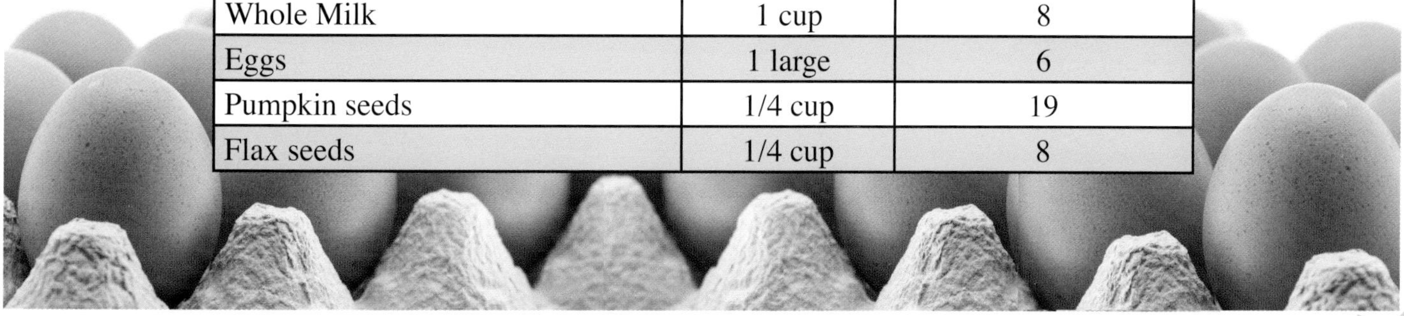

Appendix N: Calcium-Rich Foods

In 1998, the Institute of Medicine at the National Academy of Sciences issued new Adequate Intake (AI) levels for calcium.[1] The recommendations are as follows:

- 0-6 months: 210 mg
- 6-12 months: 270 mg
- 1-3 years: 500 mg
- 4-8 years: 800 mg
- 9-13 years: 1300 mg
- 14-18 years: 1300 mg
- 19-30 years: 1000 mg
- 31-50 years: 1000 mg
- 51+ years: 1200 mg
- Postmenopausal women not taking hormone replacement therapy: 1500 mg
- Pregnant and lactating women (younger than 18 years): 1300 mg
- Pregnant and lactating women (older than 18 years): 1000 mg

So are milk or dairy products really the best choice? Many other foods are higher in calcium and other nutrients beneficial to the body. See the chart below for many good foods high in calcium, and for more information about milk, see Appendix 0: Milk - The Big Debate.

Food	Serving	Amount of Calcium (mg)
Cow's milk	1 cup (8 oz.)	296.70
Goat's milk	1 cup (8 oz.)	325.74
Sesame seeds	¼ cup	351.00
Spinach, boiled	1 cup	244.80
Collard greens, boiled	1 cup	226.10
Turnip greens, boiled	1 cup	197.28
Kale, boiled	1 cup	93.60
Broccoli, steamed	1 cup	74.72
Green beans, boiled	1 cup	57.50
Garlic	1 oz-wt	51.31
Oranges	1 each	52.40
Basil, dried, ground	2 tsp.	63.40
Thyme, dried, ground	2 tsp.	54.16
Cinnamon, dried, ground	2 tsp.	55.68
Blackstrap molasses	2 tsp.	117.53

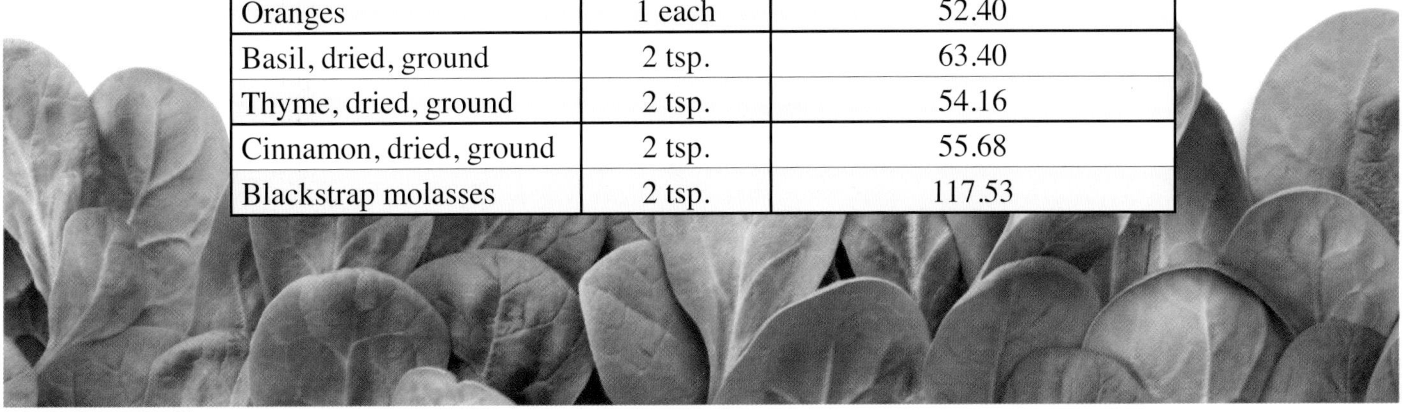

1 http://ods.od.nih.gov/factsheets/calcium.asp

Appendix O: Milk - The Big Debate

Of all the foods we consume, none evokes more controversy than milk. Should we drink milk? Aren't there other sources of protein and calcium? If we drink milk, does it make a difference if it comes from a cow or a goat? What about pasteurization or raw? Lots of questions. Are there clear answers?

As stated several times in **Nutrition 101: Choose Life!**, we suggest avoiding dairy products, especially for those with a propensity for any type of respiratory health concerns, such as allergies, asthma, chronic cough, chronic runny nose, etc. Seven percent of U.S. children show symptoms of cow milk allergy as wheezing, congestion, frequent ear infections, eczema, skin rashes and digestive troubles.

However, medical doctors and the dairy industry tout the benefits of increased milk/dairy consumption. Here is a closer look at milk, including the benefits or hazards. **This will allow each family to decide whether or not milk is right for them.**

More and more people are not just including milk in their diet, but have changed to raw or unpasteurized milk, instead of the traditional pasteurized, homogenized store bought milk. The U.S. Food and Drug Administration warns that raw milk can carry disease-causing bacteria, while advocates say raw milk is healthy because it contains good bacteria, enzymes and fats that help to boost your immune system and aid digestion.

Dairy products have always been seen as the optimal source of calcium for its benefit in bone health and preventing osteoporosis. Yet, the United States consumes more dairy than most other countries and still has the highest osteoporoses rate.

Overloading the body with too much of any nutrient even in natural food form,
can be just as unhealthy as too little.

To build strong healthy bones (as discussed in Unit 4) takes way more than just calcium. According to much research, the recommended daily supplementation of calcium – 1,500 to 2,000 mg – may be too high. Between 500 and 1,000 mg of calcium daily seems to be the norm for adults with good nutrition. Excess calcium – that which cannot be used by the body – may contribute to other health concerns, such as bone spurs. Getting all of your calcium from heavy milk consumption also increases the amount of sugars and mucus in the body. Calcium is found abundantly in green leafy vegetables, nuts and seeds.

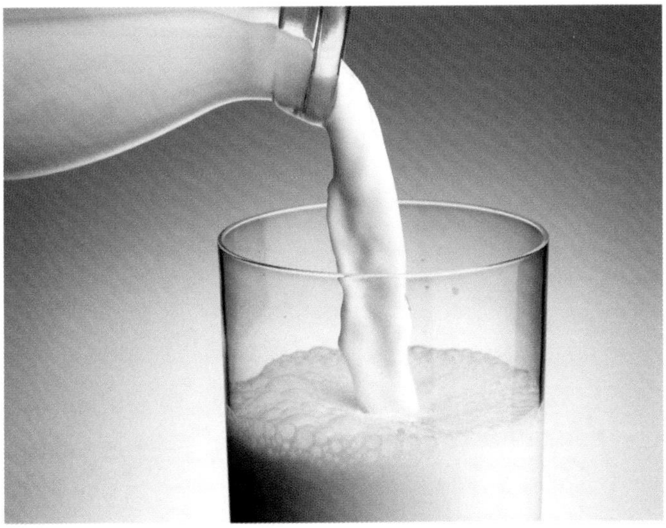

Today we don't go to the barn each morning and milk the family cow and consume fresh milk. Rather we buy pasteurized, homogenized and sterilize milk from the store in bottles or cartons with lengthy shelf life. This processing destroys the natural enzymes and good bacteria that allow milk to be more easily digested. This may be why thousands of people who suffer with constipation, allergies, asthma and many other health concerns gain significant benefits from excluding milk and other dairy products from their diets.

Processing is, at least in part, the reason behind the mucus-forming nature of milk in many individuals. This can simply be from consuming too much or their body's inability to properly break down the components of milk. For some people this excess mucus that contributes to nasal congestion, coughing, poor breathing or allergies, is simply an allergic reaction. This allergic reaction is caused by a histamine response. Once milk and dairy products are eliminated and the respiratory nutrition discussed in Unit 3 is incorporated, individuals with such health concerns may find the problems under control naturally or better yet, eliminated. At that point, then it is a personal choice to add raw dairy products back into the diet.

Pasteurization

Pasteurization began when people went away from family farming and instead relied on large commercial farms to produce milk. Possibly due to unhealthy farming practices, people were getting sick. Based on the work of Louis Pasture – from which the word pasteurization comes – pasteurization uses high heat to kill bacteria. Now, there is even ultra pasteurization processing for extended shelf life. Of course, it also kills all of the good bacteria – acidophilus/bifidus – we know to be helpful in digestion and elimination. These bacteria also are called probiotics.

Unless labeled raw, all milk sold in stores is pasteurized. The heat used in pasteurization to destroy supposed harmful bacteria actually alters the milk. This process is what makes many people, who otherwise wouldn't be affected, intolerant to milk. People who are lactose intolerant cannot digest the sugars in milk. Lactose intolerance is not a milk allergy, nor does it mean milk is not good for them; it simply means that the milk sugar, which is called lactose, cannot be assimilated properly by the body because the lactase enzyme is either not there or is in an insufficient amount and causes a problem. Also remember that pasteurization may kill bacteria, but does not remove dead bacteria from the milk. This means that pasteurized milk contains the dead bacteria, giving the body another thing with which to deal.

Milk straight from the cow is loaded with lactase – the lactose digesting enzyme – so it wouldn't cause a problem. However, during pasteurizing the lactase enzymes are destroyed. Many people who are lactose intolerant can handle raw milk as long as they don't use it to cook with because cooking temperatures also destroy these enzymes.

Other people have a problem with the protein in the milk, which also does not occur until it is heated. More and more we see whey (milk protein) powders for smoothies and protein drinks using undenatured whey protein for better digestion and assimilation.

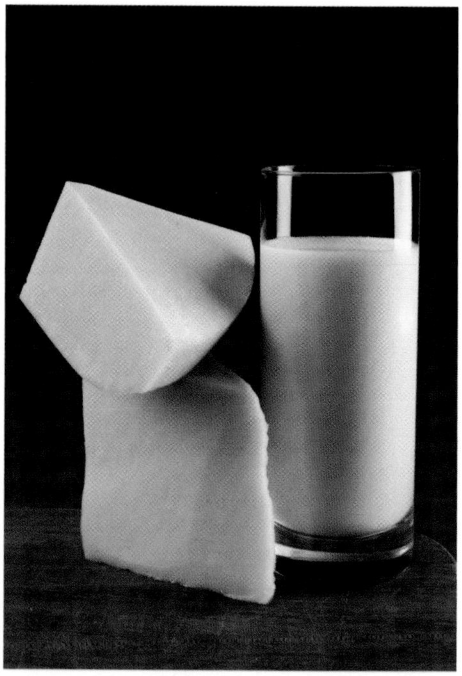

Homogenization

What about homogenization? Milk is supposed to naturally separate so the fat or cream comes up to the top. Not that long ago, before milk was homogenized, people always shook the milk bottle or carton before using it.

Ever had to stir your peanut butter? If you are buying natural peanut or other nut butter from the store there is often a section of oil at the top of the jar that must be stirred in. If you poured off this oil, the remaining nut butter would be very dry and not as tasty as with the nuts natural oils. Peanut butter often is homogenized with partially hydrogenated (artery-clogging, cancer-causing) fats so it won't separate and the oils won't come up to the top anymore. That is exactly what homogenization does to milk. Homogenization breaks the molecules up into smaller particles to make them so small that they will no longer separate.

Raw Milk

Both anecdotal and scientific reports support the health benefits of raw milk. One study by researchers at the Institute of Social and Preventive Medicine at the University of Basel in Switzerland found that children who drank raw milk had a lower risk of asthma and allergies. Raw milk can be sold for human consumption in 28 states, but only eight states allow it to be sold in stores. As a result, many people have begun to form buying clubs that buy raw milk directly from the dairy. If you choose to drink milk, try to find a milk co-op in your area.

Raw dairy farmers predominantly grass feed their animals, meaning the animals are feeding on more of what God wanted them to eat. This grass feeding practice is more costly, as the cows must be moved from pasture to pasture. Therefore you can expect to pay a little more for raw milk, but the cost is well worth it for your health. A good quality, raw dairy cow will eat mostly grass and may supplement with alfalfa hay, but not grains. Grass fed cows generally do not have as many health problems as over crowded, large commercial dairy cows. An interesting note – most dairy farmers consume their milk straight from the cow!

To Drink or Not to Drink

Frank A. Oski, M.D., is the former physician-in-chief of John Hopkins Children's Center and Professor and Chairman of the Department of Pediatrics at John Hopkins University School of Medicine and author of "Don't Drink Your Milk". If you have questions concerning your families' milk consumption, this book is an excellent eye opener to the myths and facts concerning milk in America.

"Among physicians, so much concern has been voiced about the potential hazards of cow milk that the Committee on Nutrition of the prestigious American Academy of Pediatrics, released a report entitled, 'Should Milk Drinking by Children Be Discouraged?' Although the Academy's answer to this question has been a qualified 'maybe,' the fact that the question was raised at all is testimony to the growing concern about this product. Does drinking milk help prevent osteoporosis because of the calcium it contains? ... both Africans and African-Americans consume less calcium and milk, and yet have greater bone density and less osteoporosis than Caucasians in America. While Americans get 807 mg of calcium each day from drinking milk, the average citizen of Ghana gets but 8 mg. As Dr. Oski points out, this low amount has made them 'neither toothless nor lying about immobilized because of repeated bone fractures'."
- excerpted from page three of "Don't Drink Your Milk"

Goat Milk

In the United States, over 10 million cows are maintained to provide milk and dairy products to our country, producing more than 125 billion pounds of milk annually. Yet on a worldwide basis, there are more people who drink the milk of goats than from any other single animal. Over 440 million goats (worldwide) produce an estimated 4.8 million tons of milk that is predominantly consumed locally or processed into various types of cheeses.

Properties of goat milk include smaller fat molecules with thinner, more fragile membranes, and more acid buffering capacity than cow milk, soy infant formula and nonprescription antacid drugs. Goat milk has a higher content of short and medium fatty acids, such as capric and caprylic, known to inhibit candida (yeast) infections. Goat milk may be more suitable for human consumption because it is non-allergenic and its nutrients are more readily accessible. Children fed goat milk tend to surpass those on cows milk for weight gain, stature, skeletal strength and density, blood plasma, vitamin A, thiamine, riboflavin, niacin and hemoglobin concentrations. Goat milk is considered non-allergenic as it does not have the protein that is the main stimulant of allergenic reactions, b-lactoglobulin.

Respiratory Health Concerns

Naturopath and Certified Nutrition Counselor Debra Raybern asks her nutrition clients with any type of respiratory health concern to stop all milk (raw or pasteurized, goat or cow) and dairy products[1] for three months. Incorporating better nutrition and proper cleansing can then restore and heal the body. After three months, raw cow or goat milk and dairy may be re-incorporated into the diet *if* the health concern is gone and if the client wishes, but the dairy must be reintroduced in very small amounts to see if it is well tolerated.

Is cow and goat milk just for baby cows and goats, and not for humans? That debate is for you and your family to decide. One of the major concepts in **Nutrition 101: Choose Life!** is to get families eating foods in their most natural form. Milk, like vegetables, can be changed when processed. People do not have to consume milk or dairy products to be healthy, but if they choose to "Get Milk" – be sure it is the right *RAW* choice!

1 Dairy products include anything made from cow or goats milk – butter, yogurt, milk, ice cream, cheese, etc. Some people think that eggs are dairy, but they are classified as a protein in the meat category, not a diary food.

Appendix P: Sugar Alternatives - Artificial vs. Natural

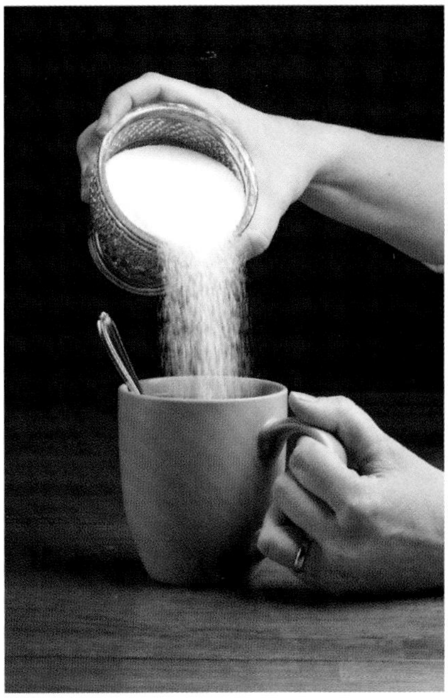

With the average person consuming over 140 pounds of sugar a year, sweets have become an everyday and every meal part of the American diet. For most, it is hard to imagine life without daily indulging in some sort of sweet morsel whether it is made with sugar, an artificial sweetener or even fruit. In 1852, the average person only consumed 10 pounds of sugar a year[1], and before that most people were constrained to eating the sweets straight from nature around them like honey and fruit from plants and trees indigenous to their land.

But now, Americans have a plethora of sweets in which to indulge at any time, in every meal and in nearly every processed food. It is not a wonder that Americans deal so greatly with major health issues such as obesity and diabetes. One out of three people in America is obese,[2] while 23.6 million Americans are diabetic and 57 million pre-diabetics.[3]

The statistics are overwhelming. So with Chapter 4 of Unit 5 clearly covering all the dangers and effects of sugar, what if anything can be used in place of sugar in our diets. Are artificial sweeteners safe? Are there alternatives to both sugar and artificial sweeteners? Do we really need to curb the sweet tooth?

Artificial Sweeteners

Artificial sweeteners were created in an effort to avoid sugar, lose weight and allow diabetics to indulge in something sweet. With the rate of diabetes soaring and sugar now being more publicly demonized, more kinds of artificial sweeteners are being used in more and more food products.

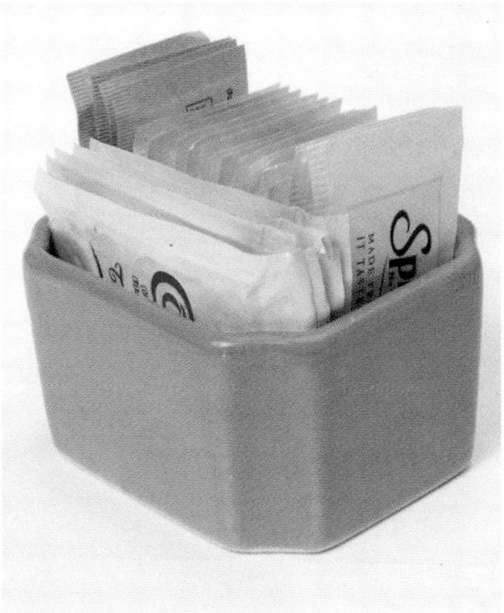

While artificial sweeteners once were commonly seen only in diet sodas and sugarless gum, they now are showing up in cereals, juice, flavored milk, ketchup, snack foods, bread, cookies, pasta sauce and more commonly consumed items. In 2004, 11 percent of the new food products introduced contained artificial sweeteners, double that of the two years pervious.[4] Sales in granulated sugar have dropped due to the public perception that natural is somehow not as good as artificial. With such an infiltration into so many food sources, there is great concern with the safety of artificial sweeteners.

There are many forms of artificial sweeteners, which include Splenda (sucralose), Sweet'N Low (saccharin), Equal and NutraSweet (aspartame), acesulfame K and neotame.

1 "The Crazy Makers: How the Food Industry is Destroying Our Brains and Harming Our Children" Carol Simontacchi, Jeremy P. Tarcher/Penguin, 2000.

2 "Obesity among adults in the United States – no change since 2003—2004." Ogden CL, Carroll MD, McDowell MA, Flegal KM. NCHS data brief no 1. Hyattsville, MD: National Center for Health Statistics, 2007.

3 "Total Prevalence of Diabetes and Pre-diabetes" American Diabetes Association, www.diabetes.org.

4 "Sugar is Latest Super Market Demon" Melanie Warner, The New York Times, May 15, 2005.

Splenda®

Splenda currently is by far the most popular artificial sweetener. It came out onto the market during a time when concerns were rising about the dangers of artificial sweeteners. Once the public heard that Splenda® was different than the rest and made from sugar, everyone thought that at last they could have their cake and eat it, too.

Splenda is the patented brand name for sucralose. According to the manufacturer's Web site, it is not natural and is chemically made through a multistep process that begins with sugar, or sucrose. Scientists replace the three hydrogen-oxygen groups on the sugar molecule with three chlorine atoms.[5] The resulting sucralose cannot be identified or broken down by the body for fuel, making Splenda a non-caloric sweetener.

There are many concerns about the safety of sucralose. According to a recent study conducted on rats at Duke University, Splenda "suppresses beneficial bacteria and directly affects the expression of the transporter P-gp and cytochrome P-450 isozymes that are known to interfere with the bioavailability of drugs and nutrients. Furthermore, these effects occur in Splenda doses that contain sucralose levels that are approved by the FDA for use in the food supply.[6]"

Dr. Susan Schiffman, a sweetener specialist and a professor of medical psychology at Duke University Medical Center, is among the many doctors and nutritionists that have safety concerns about sucralose. In a *New York Times* article, she noted that in the Food and Drug administration's 1998 report giving approval for sucralose they said it is "weakly mutagenic in a mouse lymphoma mutation assay." That means that it caused minor genetic damages in mouse cells, and further tests said sucralose is a possible carcinogen.[7]

Dr. Schiffman said, "The sucralose people keep saying, 'It's just a little bit of a mutagen.' Well, I don't want a little bit of a mutagen in my food supply. How do you know what happens in a long life span or to the next generation or to your eggs and sperm? I don't feel like the issues have been answered.[8]"

Aspartame

Aspartame, the main ingredient in Equal® and NutraSweet®, is responsible for the most serious cases of poisoning due to the fact that the body can actually digest it. European university studies have shown that aspartame breaks down into several dangerous components including formaldehyde, which accumulates in the brain and can damage the central nervous system and immune system and cause DNA damage.[8] Dr. H. J. Roberts has collected more than 1,300 reports of aspartame issues, and he calls it an "an ignored epidemic."

In 1980, a public board of inquiry composed of physicians unanimously determined that aspartame should not go on the market and provided their findings to the FDA. However, the sweetener was approved for use in 1981. Many proponents, among them researchers and doctors, indicate that the decision was based on politics, not science.

Aspartame has had the most complaints of any food additive available to the public. It's been linked with multiple sclerosis, lupus, fibromyalgia and other central nervous disorders. Possible side effects of aspartame include headaches, migraines, panic attacks, dizziness, irritability, nausea, intestinal discomfort, skin rash and nervousness. Some researchers have linked aspartame with depression, manic episodes and even male infertility. Aspartame should be avoided by most women, especially those with neuropsychiatric concerns.

5 www.splenda.com

6 "Splenda Alters Gut Microflora and Increases Intestinal P-Glycoprotein and Cytochrome" P-450 in Male Rats, Mohamed B. Abou-Donia; Eman M. El-Masry; Ali A. Abdel-Rahman; Roger E. McLendon; Susan S. Schiffman, Journal of Toxicology and Environmental Health, Part A, Volume 71, Issue 21 January 2008.

7 "Sugar is Latest Super Market Demon" Melanie Warner, The New York Times, May 15, 2005.

8 "Formaldehyde derived from dietary aspartame binds to tissue components in vivo" Trocho C, et al. Life Sciences 1998;63:337-349.

Saccharin

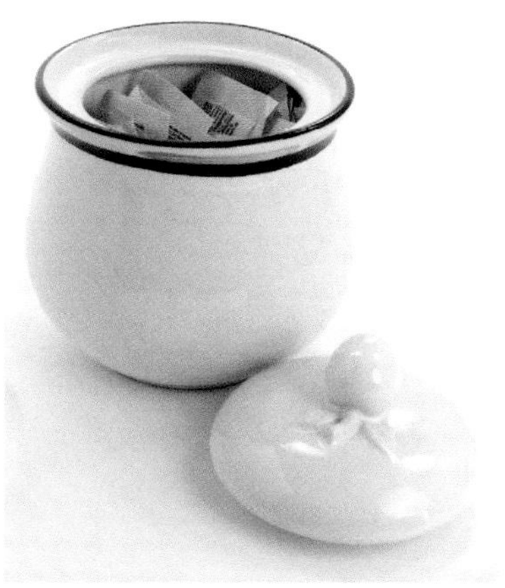

Discovered in 1879, saccharin, also known as Sweet 'N Low®, was the first chemical sweetener to gain popularity but is hardly referred to any more in the U.S. Derived from petroleum, it maintains a strong European presence.

While NutraSweet took its place in almost every diet soda, saccharin is still an ingredient in some prepared foods, gum and over-the-counter medicines. Years ago, there were carcinogen warnings on the side of products that contained saccharin. However, industry testing showed that saccharin only caused bladder cancer in rats, so the labels were removed. Contrary to industry findings, many researchers agree that in sufficient doses saccharin is carcinogenic in humans.

Neotame

A new version of aspartame called neotame was approved by the FDA in 2002. Neotame is chemically related to aspartame without the phenylalanine dangers for individuals with pheylketonuria, also known as PKU. It is much sweeter than aspartame with a potency of approximately 7,000 to 13,000 times sweeter than sucrose. The problem with neotame is that it discreetly entered the market without any studies performed to address its long-term health effects.

Additional artificial sweeteners are being introduced to the market and are awaiting FDA approval. Consumers must be wise to discern what products truly are healthy and which are being marketed for those who are not educated on the subject. For that reason, it is best to avoid products that contain an unknown ingredient and choose the sweeteners that are natural and defined below.

Artificial sweeteners are chemicals and act as toxins in the body! They are never a good idea to consume for anyone, especially pregnant and lactating women, children and teenagers. Despite the reduced sugar content, the possible link to irreversible cell damage is not worth the risk.

Natural Sugar Substitutes

Sweeteners made naturally tend to be less refined than white table sugar and contain small to generous amounts of vitamins and minerals. White sugar is refined to 100 percent sucrose. It is a refined carbohydrate that the body has a hard time using without the associated vitamins and minerals that were present in the plant, beet or sugar cane before refining. Below is a list of sugar substitutes. Some are low on the glycemic index (GI), while others are high. Also some have nearly as many calories as refined sugar. Refer to the chart at the end of this Appendix for more caloric information.

Raw blue agave nectar is an organic liquid sweetener made from the Mexican blue agave plant (agave tequilana) that is sweeter than sugar. It has a GI of just 11 compared to honey at 55 and table sugar at 68. Raw blue agave nectar is an ideal choice for anyone wanting to maintain healthy blood sugar levels and still enjoy a sweet treat once in a while. Blue agave is a great sweetener for hot tea, baked goods, coleslaw, salad dressings, topping for pancakes, waffles, grapefruit and more. There are many species of the agave plant and many different types of agave syrup which differ in glycemic values ranging up to 32. For this reason, it is important to select raw blue agave nectar from the agave tequilana plant if possible. It is available at health food stores and online.[9]

Stevia is derived from the leaves of the South American shrub called stevia rebaudiana. A good quality leaf is estimated to be 300 times sweeter than cane sugar, so a little bit of stevia goes a long way. Pure stevia extract has a slightly licorice flavor, is essentially non-caloric, and has been reported to possess antiviral activity. It also may

9 Authors recommend Young Living® Blue Agave Nectar.

help maintain proper blood sugar levels, making it a great aid for those with diabetes and hypoglycemia.

Beware of the new branded stevia based sweeteners. While they all tout that they are made with stevia or derivatives of stevia, they do contain other ingredients including flavorings. As with most new-on-the-market sweeteners, long term effects are not known, so try to stick with pure stevia extracts that contain no added ingredients.

Stevia is available in health food stores and some grocery stores.[10]

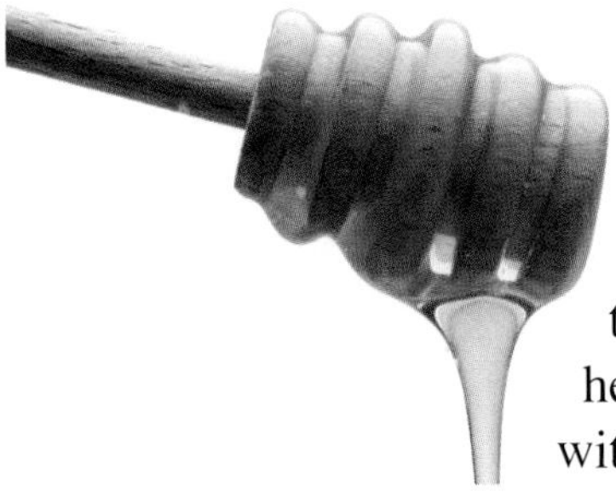

Honey is a sweet substance that honey bees make from plant nectar and has a GI of 55. However, locally harvested raw honey can differ in GI, such as a GI of 32 in Romania and 87 in Canada. Alfalfa and wild flower are the most common types of honey, and the source of the nectar determines the color and texture of the honey. Darker honey has more mineral content and has a stronger taste. Some health experts believe that consuming local honey will decrease allergic responses with pollen allergies.

Honey is available raw or pasteurized. Commercial honey is pasteurized, or heated, to prevent crystallization and yeast fermentation. Organic or raw honey has not been heat treated, so when it is kept in the refrigerator or has been exposed to extreme temperature fluctuation, crystallization may occur. Honey should be stored at room temperature away from direct sunlight as refrigeration and extreme temperature fluctuation cause crystallization. Honey that has crystallized can still be used by simply scooping out the honey and warming it gently in a double boiler to return it to its liquid state. Do not microwave crystallized honey to return it to its liquid state as microwaves will destroy the nutrients and disrupt the electrochemistry.

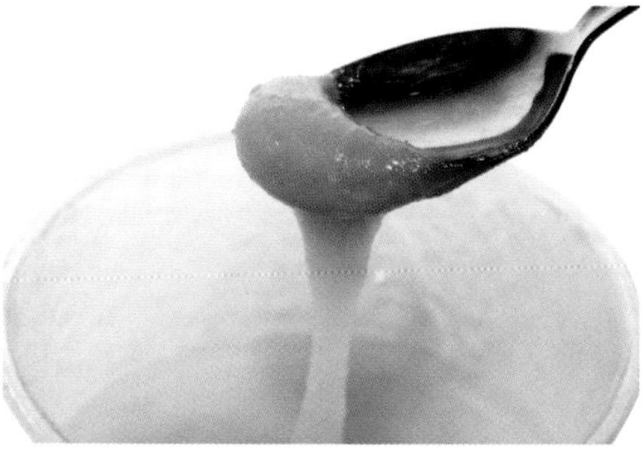

Honey is not recommended in any form for infants under the age of two as it can contain clostridium botulism spores, the bacteria that causes botulism. Heat treatment is not sufficient to destroy the bacteria, but the high sugar content of the honey prevents the spores from germinating, preventing the risk of deadly botulism in children and adults. However, the gastrointestinal tract of young infants can promote spore germination. Organic, raw honey is best purchased locally from a health food store or farmers market.

Maple syrup is made from the boiled down sap of the maple tree. It is graded by color and flavor strength. Grade A is the lightest color with a delicate flavor. Grade B is a darker color with a stronger flavor. Grade C has the highest vitamin and nutritional content with minimal processing and the strongest flavor. Its GI is listed at 55. The flavor in grade C syrup can change from batch to batch and can be hard to locate. Some syrup producers use formaldehyde pellets in the tree sap holes to prolong sap flow. Some will even inject the tree with it. Since formaldehyde is a known carcinogen, it is important to make sure that the syrup purchased has not been extracted in this manner. Choosing the right syrup is not only a matter of flavor, but also quality. Grade B maple syrup can be found in some grocery stores and in health food stores. Grade C maple syrup is harder to find.

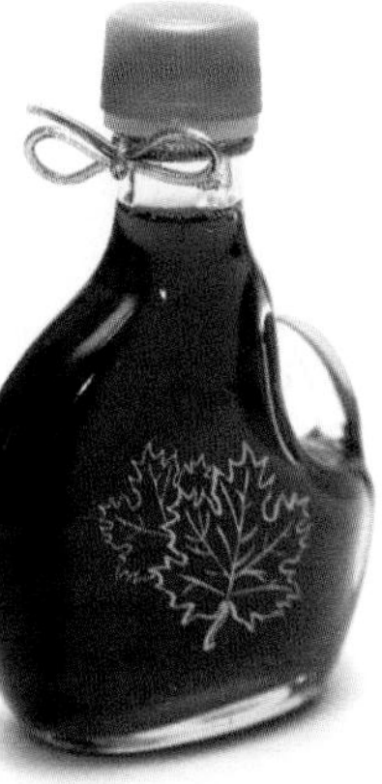

Molasses is a boldly flavored, thick syrup that is mainly used in cooking recipes. Unsulfured molasses is made from the juice of sun-ripened sugar cane. Sulfured molasses is a byproduct of refined sugar. Barbados molasses is made from the first press of the sugar cane and has a light flavor. Robustly flavored blackstrap molasses is made from the last pressing of the sugar cane and is very dark and very nutritious with high levels of calcium, iron,

10 Authors recommend Young Living® Stevia Extract.

and potassium. It also contains selenium, a known anti-inflammatory. However, molasses is 65 percent sucrose and has a GI of 47, so it can spike blood sugar levels.

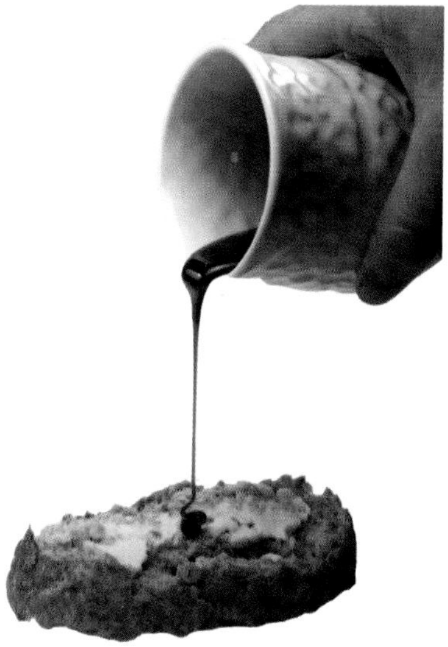

Molasses is generally used in the preparation of ginger bread, pecan pie, baked beans and spiced cookies. For an extra mineral boost in the morning, molasses tea can be made using one teaspoon of unsulfured blackstrap molasses to one cup boiling water and a squeeze of lemon. This is great a great drink for those with anemia. Five or six drops of cayenne tincture also can be added for a pick me up morning hot beverage. Blackstrap molasses is available in most grocery stores and health food stores.

Barley malt is a thick, dark, boldly flavored, slow-digesting sweetener made from sprouted barley. In dehydrated form, it is known as maltrose. It has a malt-like flavor and is not as sweet as honey, having a GI of 20. It is great over pancakes and can be delicious with roasted or baked sweet potatoes and winter squash. Barley malt syrup makes cakes and muffins moist and is a great addition to sweet breads such as squash and pumpkin. You can also make a wonderful glaze for sweet potatoes with barley malt. This sweetener contains trace amounts of eight different vitamins and minerals including potassium. Barley malt must be stored in a cool dark place and may begin to ferment if stored for more than one year. Refrigeration will extend its life. Signs of fermentation include bubbles coming through the malt and an unpleasant odor; such signs mean that it has fermented beyond use and should be discarded. Barley malt can be found at health food stores.

Brown rice syrup is a very thick, surly sweetener made from cooking sprouted brown rice. With a slightly butterscotch flavor, it is the mildest of the liquid sweeteners and sometimes is overpowered by other flavorings in baked goods. It can be used like honey, but more might be needed to match honey's sweetness. It also makes a excellent topping for waffles or as a spread for fresh bread. Rice syrup has long shelf life, requires no refrigeration and also will not crystallize like honey. Brown rice syrup is available at health food stores.

Sucanat® is a branded ingredient whose name stands for "sugar cane natural." It is made from evaporated sugar cane juice. The syrup is dehydrated and then milled into a medium grain powder. Water is the only additional ingredient. It is not as crystalline in appearance as raw sugar and is slightly less sweet. Sucanat retains more vitamins and minerals than ordinary sugar cane sugar. It is considered less refined than raw sugar and should only be mixed with dry ingredients in baked goods, since it does not blend well with creamy ingredients. Because it dissolves easily, it is ideal for use in hot drinks. Sucanat is available at most health food stores.

Unrefined sugar is sugar in its natural state – naturally milled cane sugar. One brand, Florida Crystals®, may be used one-for-one in any recipe, cereal, tea, coffee or with any food as a substitute for refined white sugar. It is natural but still high on the GI at 65. The sugar cane used in Florida Crystals is organically grown. It is available at most health food stores.

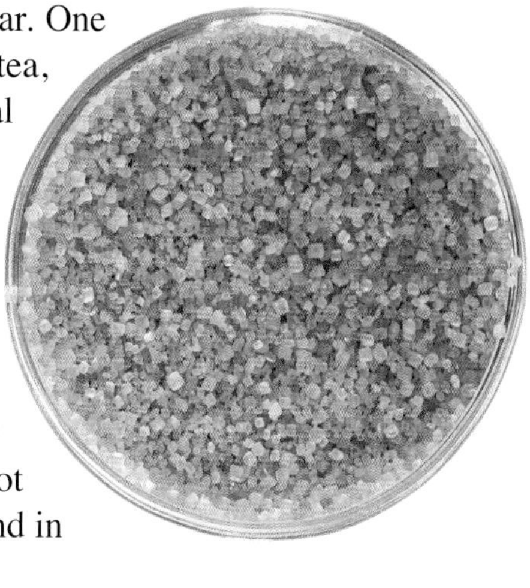

Turbinado sugar also is called raw sugar or turbinated sugar. It is made by steaming unrefined raw sugar. A common brand is "Sugar in the Raw." It has a light brown color and larger grains than refined white sugar. It is 96 percent sucrose whereas white table sugar is bleached and refined to 99 percent sucrose. Turbinado does have a higher GI of 68 and the fact that it is not highly processed is the main advantage it has over white sugar. It can be found in health food stores and some grocery stores.

Rapadura, Portuguese for a form of sugar cane, is a sweetener popular in Brazil and known throughout Latin America and South America by several other names: raspadura (Panama), Tapa dulce (Costa Rica), panela (Colombia), piloncillo (Mexico) and chancaca (Peru). Rich in silica and iron, rapadura is dried sugar cane that is sold in brick form as an easier method of distributing it in warm, tropical regions. It can be purchased as crystals and is a good choice for those who choose a vegan diet. Despite these positive attributes, rapadura does have a higher GI, around 65. It can be found predominantly online.

Polyols, or sugar alcohols that occur naturally, are found in commercial products. The most common include **maltitol, mannitol, sorbitol** and **xylitol**. Sweeter than sugar, these are used by health food manufacturers and the international confectionary industry because they are digested easier by the body. They may used to sweeten a variety of products, but should be consumed in moderation as more than 45 grams may cause upset stomach or diarrhea.

Besides sweeteners, **carob chips** can be used interchangeably with the traditional chocolate chips found in many holiday treats. Carob chips are all vegetarian and created by combining Mediterranean carob with an all natural malted grain sweetener, usually barley or corn. They are naturally sweet and make an ideal baking ingredient. They can be used to make a chocolate style pie, traditional chocolate chip cookies, oatmeal cookie bars and more. Carob powders also are available for baking needs.

Note** Many of the sweeteners on the market today used as sugar substitutes come in liquid form. When using a liquid sweetener in place of white table sugar, reduce the liquid content in the recipe by one quarter cup. If the recipe does not call for any liquid, then add three to five tablespoons of organic flour for each ¾ cup of liquid sweetener used.

Sugar Substitutes for Baking

For one cup of granulated sugar:

½ cup Blue Agave Nectar (when substituting Blue Agave sweetener in recipes, reduce your liquid slightly – sometimes by as much as 1/3 less and reduce oven temperature by 25 degrees).
½ teaspoon Stevia
1/8 teaspoon Stevia extract
1/3 to ½ cup honey
1/3 to ½ cup maple syrup
1/3 cup molasses
1 ½ cups barley malt
One cup of either sucanat or organic sugar or rapadura

Curbing the Sweet Tooth

"Watch and pray so that you will not fall into temptation. The spirit is willing, but the body is weak." Matthew 26:41

One of the keys to optimal health lies not only in just finding a natural sugar substitute to oblige the sweet tooth, but also it lies in curbing the sweet tooth. Refer to Appendix B to the **Nutrition 101: Choose Life! Food Pyramid**. Notice how vegetables are the predominant food in the daily diet with fruit being a smaller portion. Notice how sugary sweets are not located anywhere on the food pyramid.

Curbing a sweet tooth may seem like a daunting task, but once changes in the diet have been made, such as adding more fresh vegetables and limiting sweets, the body will begin to acclimate itself. With discipline and dedication over time, curbing a sweet tooth can be accomplished.

Sugar, Natural Sugar Substitutes and Artificial Sweeteners Table

Type	Source	Recommendations	Common Uses	Comments	Calories/ tsp	Glycemic index (GI)
Aspartame	Laboratories (NutraSweet® and Equal®)	Avoid completely.	Diet beverages and foods labeled sugar free.	Heat makes it lose sweetness. May cause allergic reactions and toxic effects on fetal brain.	0	14
Barley malt syrup	Sprouted barley	Use organic, 100 percent barley malt.	Primarily breads.	Half as sweet as honey. Resembles molasses in consistency and flavor. Can ferment.	20	20
Barley, wheat syrups	Barley, wheat	Not recommended, especially gluten-free diets.	Empty calories.	Use brown rice syrup instead.		
Blackstrap molasses	By-product of sugar refining process	Organically produced unsulphured is best to avoid chemicals and additives.	Most nutritional type of molasses providing iron, calcium, copper, magnesium, phosphorus, potassium, selenium and zinc.	Sweeter than sugar, less is required for cooking. Sulfured molasses is a byproduct of refined sugar.	45	47
Blue agave nectar	Mexican blue agave plant (Agave Tequilana)	Organic	To substitute for sugar in about anything.	Regular agave nectars differ in GI up to 30, but blue agave has the lowest.	20	11
Brown rice syrup	Sprouted brown rice.	Organic	Makes an excellent topping for waffles and cereal or as spread for fresh bread.	Butterscotch flavor. Long shelf life, no refrigeration required and will not crystallize.	19	Low
Brown sugar, packed	White sugar dyed with molasses, 95 percent sucrose.	Not recommended.	Empty calories.	Use sucanat or molasses instead.	15	68

Type	Source	Recommendations	Common Uses	Comments	Calories/ tsp	Glycemic index (GI)
Confectioner's sugar	White sugar finely powdered, 99.9 percent sucrose	Not recommended.	Empty calories.	Use rapadura powder instead.	31	68
Dried fruit puree	Dried fruits (apricots, cranberries, dates, figs and prunes)	Organic, unsulphured.	Baked goods such as cakes, scones, cookies and cakes.	Used finely chopped or soak in juice and puree in food processor.	Depends on fruit.	
Fructose	Corn syrup	Highly processed and corn that is possible genetically modified organisms	Empty calories, widely used in soft drinks and manufactured foods.	Look for products with agave or other alternative with low GI.	54	19
Fruit juice	Fresh fruit such as grape, peach or apricot.	Organic fresh juices with no added sugar.	Baked goods such as cakes, scones, cookies and cakes.	Apple and pear juices are considered junk juice due to sugar content and caloric load. Avoid concentrated juices as they don't have the same nutritional value as fresh fruit.	Depends on fruit.	
Honey	Bees extract it from flower nectars (glucose and fructose)	Organic, raw and unfiltered from a single type of alfalfa or wild flower.	Substituted for sugar in most instances, but recipe modification required due to liquid increase.	Not vegan. Sweeter, lower in calories and more nutritious than sugar. Gastrointestinal tract of young infants can promote spore germination. For this reason, infants under two years of age are not recommended to consume honey in any form.	64	55
Maple sugar	Dehydrated maple syrup (sucrose)	Organic pure 100 percent maple sugar, expensive.	Anything that calls for sugar.	Very sweet and distinct strong flavor	32	55

Type	Source	Recommendations	Common Uses	Comments	Calories/ tsp	Glycemic index (GI)
Maple syrup, Grade A	Sap of maple tree	Organic pure 100 percent maple syrup, expensive, purchase locally.	Contains twice as much calcium as milk.	Lightest color with a delicate flavor.	17	55
Maple syrup, Grade B	Sap of maple tree	Organic pure 100 percent maple syrup, expensive, purchase locally.	Great for baking cakes but reduce other liquids about 1/4 cup.	Darker color with a stronger flavor.	17	55
Maple syrup, Grade C	Sap of maple tree	Organic pure 100 percent maple syrup, expensive, purchase locally.	Great for baking cakes but reduce other liquids about 1/4 cup.	Highest vitamin and nutritional content with minimal processing and the strongest flavor. Hard to locate.	17	55
Unrefined sugar	Minimally processed sugar cane	Organic	Used exactly as white sugar--no noticeable change in flavor.	A better version of white table sugar.	15	65
Rapadura	Dried from sugar cane juice	Organic	Anything that calls for sugar.	Very sweet, resembles a slight molasses and caramel flavor	15	65
Raw sugar	Sugar cane juice	Better than refined sugar, but agave, sucanat or rapadura are healthier alternatives.	Empty calories.	Very sweet and offers no nutritional benefits,	15	68
Saccharin	Laboratories	Avoid completely as may cause cancer and has bitter taste.	Widely used in diet beverages and sweet sugar free foods.	Use agave or unrefined sugar instead.	1	14

Type	Source	Recommendations	Common Uses	Comments	Calories/ tsp	Glycemic index (GI)
Stevia liquid or powder	Dried stevia rebaudiana leaves	Organic powder or liquid, expensive	Any food or drink that calls for sugar. An excellent replacement for artificial sweeteners. Suitable for diabetics and weight loss dieters. Contains no calories and zero GI.	Strong, distinct flavor that is 300 times sweeter than sugar and highly concentrated. Cannot be used for baking above 389° F.	0	0
Sucralose	Laboratories (patented name for Splenda®)	Avoid completely	Diet beverages, foods labeled sugar free and as a sugar substitute.	Many safety concerns about the use.	0	14
Sucanat	Sugar cane juice	Organic	Anything that calls for sugar, good replacement for brown sugar.	Very sweet, resembles molasses flavor. Granule form, not crystals.	15	50
Turbinado sugar	Steamed unrefined sugar.	Better than refined sugar, but sucanat is a healthier alternative.	Empty calories	Very sweet. A more refined version of raw sugar. Like brown sugar, it hardens when exposed to air.	11	68
White table sugar	Made from sugar cane and beets.	Avoid completely.	Empty calories, commonly used in manufactured and fast convenience foods.	Sweet without any benefits.	45	68
Xylitol	Derived from fruits and vegetables, making it 100 percent carbohydrate.	Consume in commercial products, no more than 15 grams per day.	Entered market as a sweetener that promoted dental health. Is often used in gums, breath mints and dental hygiene products. Used in candy making in Asia and parts of Europe.	May cause upset stomach or diarrhea when consumed in excess. Do not allow animals to consume.	5	7

Appendix Q: Asthma - Taking a Deep Breath

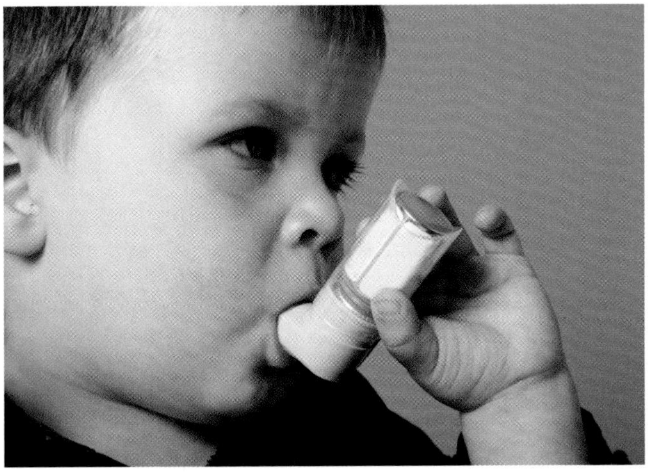

Asthma is rare in many countries and was virtually unheard of until 100 years ago. If it is a relatively new disease, what has happened that nearly 20 million American's suffer from asthma today? Why have nine million U.S. children under the age of 18 been diagnosed with asthma? In 2002, children from five to 17 years of age missed 14.7 million school days due to asthma. Every day in America 40,000 people miss school or work, 30,000 people have an asthma attack, 5,000 people visit the emergency room, 1,000 people are admitted to the hospital, and 11 people die due to asthma.[1]

The answer is simple. Profound changes have occurred in our diets, lifestyle and environments. Incidents of asthma in children are greater in urban areas than rural areas, even though rural areas generally have more plants, trees, grasses and shrubs that can trigger many asthma related symptoms.

So what exactly is asthma? Asthma is described as a chronic inflammatory condition, not a respiratory disease. People with asthma have inflamed, hyper-reactive airways and produce excessive bronchial mucus. Over the long term, asthma permanently damages the airway, making it more prone to inflammation and less functional. Repeated allergy attacks thicken the airway making it even more inflexible.

Long term use of asthma and allergy control drugs, specifically containing steroids, affects many more organ systems than just the lungs and bronchial airways. Side effects include weight gain, obesity, fluid retention, osteoporosis, diabetes, yeast infections and glaucoma.

Identifying and then eliminating asthma triggers is essential in keeping asthma under control. There are two types of bio-chemicals responsible for most asthma chronic bronchial and lung inflammation: free radicals and leukotrienes.

Free radicals can irritate and inflame tissues all over the body. Leukotrines keep inflammation running once triggered.

Food allergies also can be asthma triggers. Common triggers include eggs, soy, dairy, wheat and some citrus fruits. Another trigger is histamine, which is produced when special connective tissue cells called mast cells are activated. Mast cells are activated by circulating immune system cells when they sense danger from a toxin or foreign invader.

Prescription and over-the-counter remedies lose their effectiveness over time, so what can be done for a person with asthma?

A. Environment changes

1. Carpets, upholstery in furniture, drapes and curtains, bedding and mattresses all harbor of dust and dust mites. Cleaning carpets two to three times per year and vacuuming with an advanced HEPA or water filtration cleaner will dramatically cut down on the number of allergens floating within a home.
2. Dust with a slightly damp cloth (see the Dusting Recipes in Unit 3 Chapter 1), so that dust does not just float around to land somewhere else.

1 http://www.aaaai.org/media/resources/media_kit/asthma_statistics.stm

3. Air conditioning filters should be changed regularly and upgraded to allergen trapping models.
4. Mattresses should be covered with dust mite protective covers. Stay away from foam mattresses or pads as they breakdown over time and emit small particles of chemical foam into the air. Replace mattresses over ten years old.
5. No smoking for anyone in an asthmatic household.
6. Use chemical-free products throughout the home for cleaning, bathing, skin care etc.
7. Change out landscaping for non-pollinating plants and shrubs.
8. Deep clean closets and shelving at least twice per year, as dust can collect, especially on books.
9. Clean the air in the home by diffusing therapeutic-grade essential oils. Please do not think that the air fresheners bought at the store have anything but detrimental effects with allergies as they contain many synthetic and even toxic substances.

B. Diet and nutrition

Immediately stop eating corn, dairy, soy and sugar, the main triggers for asthma.

Corn

This includes chips, tortillas, fresh corn, and anything packaged that has the word corn, include corn syrup or high fructose corn syrup.

Dairy

All dairy is mucus forming. Dairy products made from cow's milk are very mucus forming. This includes milk, ice cream, cheese, sour cream and yogurt. It will take about three months of absolutely no dairy to completely cleanse the lungs of mucus and therefore show positive results in asthma-related symptoms, but the person will begin to realize relief much sooner. Lemon, anise and fennel are foods known to reduce bronchial mucus. Eating a more alkaline diet also is helpful.

Are you concerned with calcium intake? Milk is not the best choice. It is possible to get the calcium you need without dairy products, contrary to the statements by the milk and dairy industry. Nuts are an amazing powerhouse of useable calcium.

One cup of sesame seeds gives 1,404 mg of calcium. In contrast, one cup of whole milk delivers just 296 mg. Sesame seeds can be used as nut butter, sprinkled over vegetables, ground and used in casseroles. The uses are endless and with such a mild taste, everyone is sure to enjoy them.

Many vegetables even contain calcium, particularly green leafy vegetables like spinach, turnip greens, mustard greens and collard greens.

Sugar

Sugar suppresses the immune system function and is very acid (inflammatory) and mucus forming. Don't just switch to raw sugar, maple syrup, agave or honey; instead curb your sweet tooth with fresh fruit. An occasional treat is not the offender, but the problem is daily consumption of sugar from food and drink.
Food in general should be made from scratch using only whole food ingredients. Eat as close to the way God created the food as possible. Fresh, raw or lightly steamed fruits and vegetables are more beneficial than when processed or cooked.

"My ten-year-old son, Duncan has always joined whoever has been sick, and all his asthma problems are soon to follow. The doctors told me there was no cure for asthma, but to keep him on his "safe" medications (Prednisone, Albuterol, Singulair and Advair) and that one day, he may outgrow his asthma. For the last three or four years, he was getting worse during the cold/flu season and winter months. He had one attack that was so severe, he had to go to the hospital right before Christmas in 2007. It felt like his asthma was out of control.

Shortly thereafter, I discovered therapeutic-grade essential oils. We began using the essential oil ravensara from Young Living® (YL). He was 80 percent over his asthma except when he'd get allergies or a cold and then we were forced to rely again on his asthma prescriptions. Then, Duncan met with Debra Raybern, N.D., who explained to him the importance of staying away from dairy and sugar, increasing his fiber intake and using Inner Defense™ to bolster his immune system. After that he wasn't sick for two months, something that has never happened in his 10 years. He especially had never gone that long without sickness and asthma problems during the winter months. By April, he continued to watch his diet and remained healthy! We are nearing one year of him being off of his medications completely, and now it looks like he's over his asthma forever!

A doctor was irate with me when she found out I was no longer giving Duncan maintenance meds. I tried their way, and I saw no difference. All the meds were doing was rescuing him from the present attack, not preventing anything. Medicine and doctors have their place, but most of what we rely upon them for is unnecessary if we would just take responsibility for ourselves and if the truth was more readily available.

These oils have saved us so much money on prescriptions. Because of the essential oils and other YL products, we went with higher deductible insurance this year and are no longer paying for something we no longer use. The money we save goes to purchase essential oils and other YL products. They keep us from having to pay co-pays and prescriptions, plus we are healthy!"

I thank God for Young Living Essential oils and everything I have been learning about them and nutrition from Debra Raybern." – Mia, Texas

Natural Support and Relief

First of all, a person already using a prescription drug or inhaler should not stop. As he supports his body and makes changes to his diet and environment and incorporates herbs and essential oils, his dependence for these medicines will diminish over time and soon thereafter may no longer be necessary.

Vitamin C – Vitamin C is the primary antioxidant for the lungs and is a powerful antihistamine. Suggested doses are 1 gram of vitamin C, three times per day. Asthmatics do better on ascorbic acid or naturally derived vitamin C supplements.[2] Smelling the essential oil lemon also may be beneficial.

Magnesium – Possibly the most overlooked nutrient for asthma sufferers is magnesium. Asthma attacks drain the body of magnesium at an alarming rate, and the condition will only worsen if not supplemented. Magnesium is found in abundance in dark green leafy vegetables. A person with asthma who does not consume large amounts of magnesium-rich vegetables must supplement 400 to 800 milligrams (mg) daily. The form magnesium glycinate will not cause loose stools in those prone to having them with additional magnesium.

Multi-vitamin and minerals – A complete whole foods multi-vitamin and mineral supplement also is very beneficial. Be sure it includes the B-complex vitamins and all the major macro-minerals. Zinc should be 15 to 20 mg.[3]

Probiotics – Studies reveal that lowered intestinal bacteria equate to an increase in asthma attacks. Asthmatics often take antibiotics for asthma-related illness, thus killing off the good, friendly bacteria in the gut. Restoring the proper balance makes perfect sense. Also, lowered good gut flora weakens the immune system.[4]

2 The authors recommend Young Living® vitamin C supplements: Super C™ and Super C™ Chewable. Super C™ contains 1.2 grams for each 2 tablets.

3 The authors recommend Young Living's True Source™, which is a great whole food vitamin and mineral supplement at a cost comparable to conventional store bought synthetic vitamin/mineral tablets.

4 The authors recommend Life 5™ capsules, from Young Living®, which contains five strains of bacteria, three of which are

Quercetin -- A bioflavanoid found in some fruits and vegetables, quercetin has been known to block the release of histamine. Foods with high sources of quercetin are garlic, onions and cayenne.

Herbs – Herbal products aid asthma sufferers due to the naturally occurring chemicals they contain called phytochemicals that directly reduce inflammation without harmful side effects. Some herbs have anti-histamine and decongestant properties and others can act as bronchial relaxants.

Colsus forskoli is a safe dilator of bronchial tubes. It is used in inhalers in Europe and available in capsule and patch form in the United States. 100 to 150 mg capsules taken three times daily or up to 10 mg daily of a standardized forskolin extract is suggested.

Ginkgo biloba is an herb known for its ability to block the release of histamines. The suggested dose is 120 to 240 mg of a standardized product daily.

Stinging nettle has a long history as a tea or in capsules to reduce asthma attacks, especially those triggered by plants and flowers.

Essential oils -- The most potent part of the plant is captured as an essential oil. Daniel Pénoël, M.D., in his book, "Natural Home Health Care Using Essential Oils," describes his success in treating mild and serious respiratory complaints, including asthma, with essential oils. He used these topically, in reflexology (massage on the feet), inhaled and as a nasal wash.

Dr. Pénoël's two main guidelines:

1. The secret to success lies in frequent repetition of the application, at very close intervals at first (every 10 minutes), and then spacing according to the relief.

2. Above all, remember that the essential oil must be available immediately so you can start at the first sign of an infection or attack. The oils he used included: eucalyptus radiate, eucalyptus globules, eucalyptus polybractea, tea tree, rosemary, ravensara, lavender, sage, thyme and myrtle. [5]

Other suggested oils from the "Essential Oils Desk Reference" and the "Reference Guide to Essential Oils"[6] include: cypress, frankincense, Evergreen Essence™, pine, and tsuga to open respiratory tract. Avoid steam inhalation. Drop on pillow at night. Inhaling, wearing on the back of the neck, on the chest and on the lung point of the foot have all shown great success. Inhalers for essential oils can be found at www.abundanthealth4u.com. Another fast and direct route to the lungs is via the rectum. Mix one teaspoon Young Living's V-6™ oil with five to 10 drops RC™ or Raven™ and insert into the rectum at bedtime.

Remember Mia's testimony? She combined both diet and essential oils for her son and he became asthma free in three short months. Asthma is a serious condition and is nothing with which to play around. But it is also not a health challenge that must be endured for life. The sooner a person begins making changes, the sooner he or she will lessen the use of drugs and breathe more freely.

---

considered super strains – Howaru™ Bifido (Bifidobacterium lactis), Howaru™ Rhamnosus (Ld. rhamnosus) and L. acidiophulis (LA-14).

5 Use only Young Living therapeutic-grade essential oils, which are pure, unadulterated and most can be ingested, applied topically and inhaled.

6 These books can be purchased through www.abundanthealth4u.com.

Appendix R: Mold

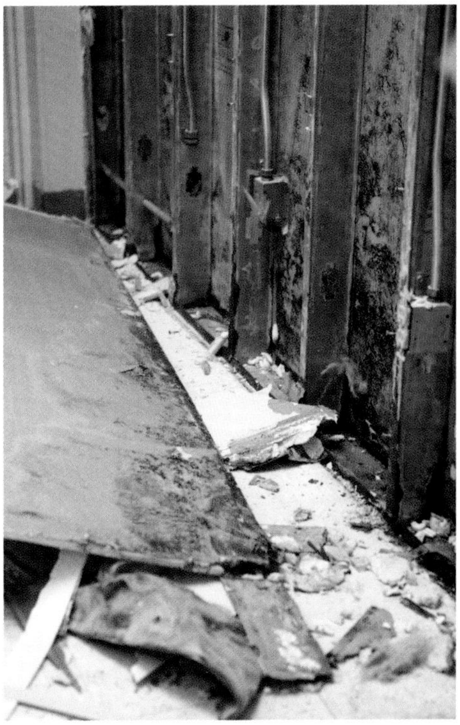

What can destroy a home, cause mild to severe respiratory discomfort, flu-like symptoms, nosebleeds, brain fog, headaches, ear infections, sinusitis, and even death? Mold! Mold is not as visible until it creates a super-colony of fruiting structures. Even when there are over 50,000 spores in a cubic meter of air, they are not visible to the human eye.

A 1999 study by the Mayo Clinic found that 96 percent of the some 37 million Americans who suffer with sinusitis symptoms do so because of mold exposure. About 4.6 million cases of asthma may be attributed to dampness and mold exposure in the home.[1] There is virtually no place on earth where mold is not found.

Since mold can be a major contributor in respiratory health, is there a way we can get control over mold in our environments? The answer is yes. Twenty thoroughly documented, field-tested case studies provide proof that a blend of carefully selected therapeutic-grade essential oils eliminates mold in as little as 24 hours and keeps it from coming back. In his book, "Nature's Mold Rx - the Non-Toxic Solutions to Toxic Mold," environmental engineer Edward Close, Ph.D., reveals the problems and remedies for the growing mold problem.[2]

Cleaning with the Young Living® exclusive Thieves® Blend Household Concentrated Cleaner and diffusing with the Thieves® oil blend along with proper sampling, cleaning and repair is part of the ten step program Dr. Close has developed and proven to be effective in ridding indoor environments of mold.

Illnesses Associated with Mold Exposure

- Allergies
- Allergic rhinitis
- Asthma
- Bleeding lungs
- Breathing difficulties
- Cancer
- Central nervous system problems
- Chronic coughing
- Dandruff not remedied with special shampoos
- Death
- Dermatitis
- Diarrhea
- Digestive disorders
- Earaches
- Eye and vision problems
- Fatigue
- Flu-like symptoms
- Headaches
- Hearing impairment
- Hemorrhagic pneumonitis
- Hives
- Irritability
- Itching
- Kidney failure
- Learning difficulties
- Mental dysfunction
- Memory loss
- Personality changes
- Peripheral nervous system effects
- Redness of the sclera (part of the eye)
- Runny nose
- Seizures
- Sinus congestion
- Skin sores
- Sleep disorders
- Sneezing fits
- SIDS
- Tremors
- Verbal dysfunction
- Vertigo
- Vomiting

1 Lawrence Berkely National Department, International Journal of Indoor Environment and Health. 2007.
2 "Nature's Mold Rx - the Non-Toxic Solutions to Toxic Mold" Edward Close, PhD and Jacquelyn Close, RA. 2007.

Appendix S: Labels and Household Toxins

Courtesy of "The Poison Control Team"

We go to great lengths to select the right education, toys, friends and experiences to nurture our children, but then expose them to a myriad of dangerous and toxic chemicals. We set off a bug bomb in the room where they sleep, clean the toilets and tubs with bleach, have toxic air fresheners to mask smells, wash dishes and clothes in chlorine detergents, use anti-bacterial soaps, and then wonder why our families are sick.

It isn't that we don't care. We really do, but we have been programmed by what our mothers did, what the magazine ads and television commercials say will help us lead a better quality of life and by convenience. Our homes should be a clean, sanitary, safe haven, not a toxic dump. It's time to slow down a bit and detoxify our homes. We are exposed to more toxins in a day than our grandparents where in a lifetime. We have no control over some of this exposure, but we can control many things in our living environments.

Chemical Cocktail

The U.S. Environmental Protection Agency (EPA) has estimated that there are over 80,000 chemicals present in our environment today and less than two percent of those have been tested for human safety. Over 3,000 chemicals are added to the foods we eat found in any supermarket, and over 700 different chemical compounds are found in common drinking water, not to mention the thousands of chemicals used in cleaning and personal care products and construction materials.

With such a chemical cocktail invading our bodies every day, imagine what the long-term effects could be, especially to children. Research reveals that toxic chemicals entering the body by inhalation, skin absorption, and ingestion stay in the body long after they enter it. Stored in the body, they continue to cause adverse effects years later, lowering the immune system and promoting disease. They may even cause weight gain and inhibit weight loss.

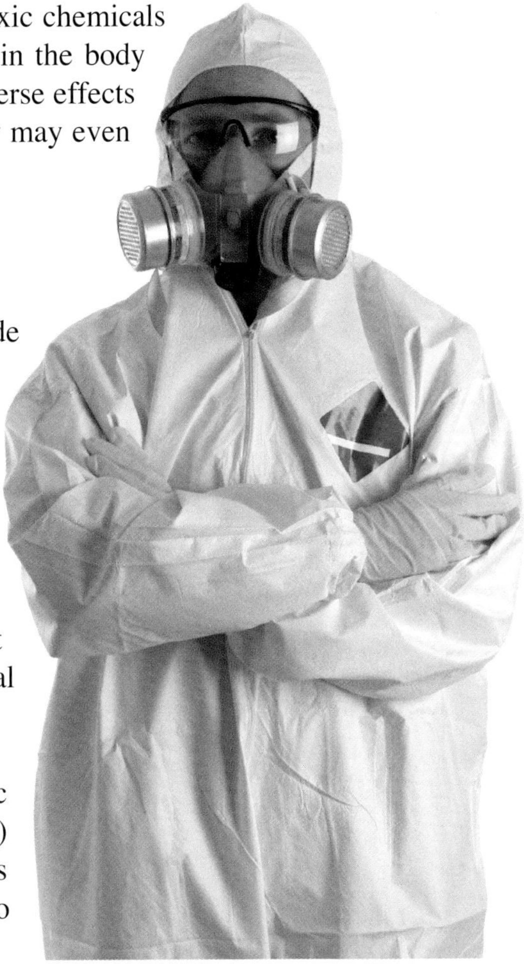

More Cause for Concern

The U.S. Bureau of Labor Statistics report 127 janitors died nationwide between 1993 and 2001 as a result of cleaning products they were using[1]. It is estimated that 37 percent of the population suffer from allergies and rashes due to chemicals. In 2000, poison control centers reported 18,863 injuries to children from chlorine products. Chlorine ranks first in industrial injuries and deaths in the U.S. Autistic spectrum disorders now affect one in 166 children, up from one in 10,000 ten years ago[1]. Chemicals are neurotoxic (cause brain and neurologic damage), carcinogenic (cause cancer), mutagenic (cause permanent genetic changes to cells), endocrine disruptors (disrupt normal hormonal function) and teratogens (cause birth defects).

The National Cancer Institute estimates childhood acute lymphoblastic leukemia and brain tumors (effecting about 16,000 adults and children) will continue to rise at the rate of one percent per year, and researchers have found a direct link to childhood leukemia and parents exposed to

---

1 "Green This! Volume 1: Greening Your Cleaning" by Deirdre Imus, Simon & Schuster, 2007.

pesticides and chemicals[2]. The World Health Organization says indoor air pollution is responsible for over one million deaths per year. The EPA has rated indoor air pollution one of the top five risks to human health linked to SIDS or sudden infant death syndrome. It has also been linked to reduced birth weight, miscarriage, infertility, reduced lung function, asthma, cancer and neurocognitive function.

Common Household Toxins

The following is a list of common household products and cleaners, some of the chemical toxins they contain and some of the effects of those toxins.

Air Fresheners

Most air fresheners interfere with the ability to smell by coating the nasal passages with an oil film, or by releasing a nerve-deadening agent. Known toxic chemicals found in air fresheners:

1. Formaldehyde: Highly toxic, known carcinogen.
2. Phenol: When phenol touches your skin it can cause it to swell, burn, peel, and break out in hives. Can cause cold sweats, convulsions, circulatory collapse, coma and even death.

Ammonia is a very volatile chemical; it is very damaging to the eyes, respiratory tract and skin.

Bleach is a strong corrosive. It will irritate or burn the skin, eyes and respiratory tract. It may cause pulmonary edema or vomiting and coma if ingested. Warning: never mix bleach with ammonia it may cause fumes which can be deadly.

Most **Carpet and Upholstery Shampoo** formulas are designed to over power the stain itself; they accomplish the task but not without using highly toxic substances. Some include:

1. Perchlorethylene: Known carcinogen; Can cause liver, kidney and nervous system damage.
2. Ammonium Hydroxide: Corrosive, extremely irritable to eyes, skin and respiratory passages.

Dishwasher Detergents contain chlorine in a dry form that is highly concentrated. Chlorine is the number one cause of child poisonings according to poison control centers.

Most **Drain Cleaners** contain lye, hydrochloric acid or trichloroethane.

1. Lye: Caustic burns to skin and eyes, if ingested will damage esophagus and stomach.
2. Hydrochloric Acid: Corrosive, eye and skin irritant, damages kidneys, liver and digestive tract.
3. Trichloroethane: Eye and skin irritant, nervous system depressant; damages liver and kidneys.

Furniture Polish

1. Petroleum Distillates: Highly flammable, can cause skin and lung cancer.
2. Phenol: (See Air fresheners, Phenol.)
3. Nitrobenzene: Easily absorbed through the skin, extremely toxic.

Mold and Mildew Cleaners

1. Sodium Hypochlorite: Corrosive irritates or bums skin and eyes, causes fluid in the lungs, which can lead to coma or death!
2. Formaldehyde: Highly toxic, known carcinogen. Irritant to eyes, nose, throat, and skin. May cause nausea, headaches, nosebleeds, dizziness, memory loss and shortness of breath.

---

2 "Green This! Volume 1: Greening Your Cleaning" by Deirdre Imus, Simon & Schuster, 2007.

Oven Cleaner

Sodium Hydroxide (Lye): Caustic and a strong irritant, which can cause burns to both skin and eyes. Inhibits reflexes, will cause severe tissue damage if swallowed.

Antibacterial Cleaners

Triclosan: Absorption through the skin can be tied to liver damage. When exposed to excessive heat or sunlight, triclosan turns into the deadly poison dioxin.[3]

Laundry Room Products

1. Sodium or Calcium Hypocrite: Highly corrosive; irritates or burns skin, eyes or respiratory tract.
2. Linear Alkylate Sulfonate: Absorbed through the skin. Known liver damaging agent.
3. Sodium Tripolyphosphate: Irritates skin and mucous membranes, causes vomiting. Easily absorbed through the skin from clothes.

Toilet Bowl Cleaners

1. Hydrochloric Acid: Highly corrosive, irritant to both skin and eyes. Damages kidneys and liver.
2. Hypo Chlorite Bleach: Corrosive, irritates or burns eyes, skin and respiratory tract. May cause pulmonary edema, vomiting or coma if ingested. Contact with other chemicals may cause chlorine fumes, which may be fatal.

Most **Pesticides** have ingredients that affect the nervous system of insects. Imagine what these extremely poisonous chemicals do to the body, or a baby's body.

1. Dimpylate: Better known as Diazinon, extremely toxic. Impairs the central nervous system.
2. Chlorinate Hydrocarbons: Suspected carcinogen and mutantagen. Accumulates m food and m fatty tissue. Will attack the nervous system.
3. Organophosphates: Toxic and poisonous. If you can smell it, your lungs are absorbing it.

Lice Shampoo

***Children are especially vulnerable[4].**

Lindane: inhalation, ingestion, or absorption through the skin causes vomiting, diarrhea, convulsions and circulatory collapse. May cause liver damage, stillbirths, birth defects and cancer.

Car Wash and Polish

Petroleum Distillates: Associated with skin and lung cancer, irritant to skin, eyes, nose and lungs. Entry into the lungs may cause fatal pulmonary edema, most marked "Danger -Harmful or Fatal."

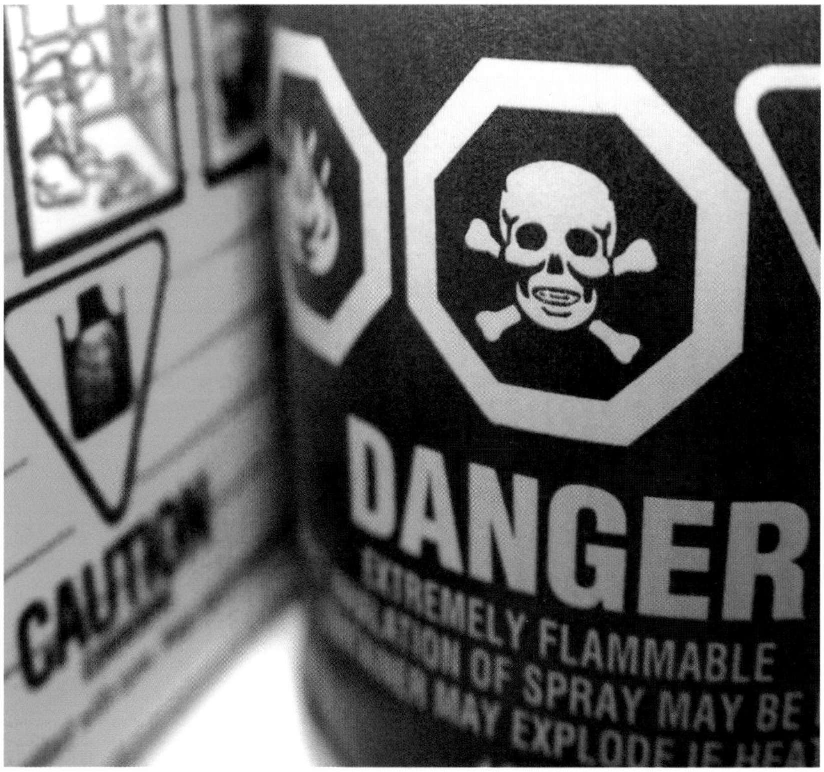

3 "Green This!" by Deirdre Imus. Simon & Schuster. 2007.

4 For a safe, natural way to get rid of lice, contact the editor@growinghealthyhomes.com.

Read the Labels!

If a product has a warning on the label, **it is poison!** Here are the warning labels required by the U.S. EPA, Office of Pesticides and Toxic Substances and a definition of what they mean.

DANGER – Harmful or Fatal if absorbed by or through the skin, ingested or inhaled. One taste to a teaspoon can be FATAL to an adult!

WARNING – Harmful or Fatal if absorbed by or through the skin, ingested or inhaled. One teaspoon to an ounce can be FATAL to an adult!

CAUTION – Harmful or Fatal if absorbed by or through the skin, ingested or inhaled. One ounce to a pint can be FATAL to an adult!

30 Ways To Poison Yourself Before Breakfast

We spend every night breathing vapors from chemical poisons in the mattress or pillow and sleeping between sheets washed in toxins. A typical U.S. family might start the day grooming with a shower/bath, shampoo, condition, brush teeth, shave, as well as using colognes, perfumes, hairsprays and etc. Typically these poisonous ingredients are used in an enclosed area. Then they dress with clothes washed in poison.

What is the cumulative effect on our health after using many, many products that contain small amounts of dangerous poisonous chemicals?

According to the U.S. government and the product manufacturers, the following is only a partial list of chemical poisons found in products that are inhaled, absorbed, or ingested by the body before breakfast is even eaten. This list does not include the additional use of common household cleaners. The numbers next to the products correspond to the numbered list of chemical toxins following the chart.

Product								
Air Freshener	1			4			7	8
Bath Soap			3	4	5	6	7	8
Body Wash			3	4	5	6	7	8
Hair Shampoo	1		3	4				8
Hair Conditioner	1			4				8
Skin Cream	1		3	4	5	6	7	8
Lotion	1		3	4	5	6	7	8
Shaving Cream			3	4				8
Aftershave Lotion	1			4				8
Skin Rash Lotion	1		3	4	5	6	7	8
Ache Medication	1		3	4	5	6	7	8
Moisturizers	1			4	5		7	8
Antiperspirants	1			4	5		7	8
Cologne	1			4			7	8
Underarm Deodorant	1			4		6	7	8

Product								
Hair Spray				4			7	
Toothpaste			3	4	5	6		
Mouthwash				4	5	6		8
Foot Deodorant				4		6		8
Plastic Glass to Rinse Mouth								8
Laundry Detergent	1		3	4	5	6	7	
Fabric Softener			3	4	5		7	
Chlorine Bleach	1	2						
Dry Cleaned Clothes	1						7	
Make-up	1		3	4	5		7	8
Feminine Deodorant				4			7	
Sanitary Napkins				4			7	
Perfumes	1			4			7	8
Facial Cleanser			3	4				8
Nail Polish				4	5		7	8

1. **Alcohol's - Acid & Alkali:** rashes, muscle weakness, headaches, dizziness, nerve damage, vision problems, sleeping problems, stomach cramps, disorientation, depression, coughing, respiratory problems, anemia, organ damage, fatigue, heart damage, cancer, death.
2. **Chlorine's:** headaches, mental function difficulties, pulmonary edemas and heart disease, anemia, diabetes, gastrointestinal and urinary tract cancer, organ and gland cancer, severe eye problems, immune system breakdown, child development problems and more.
3. **Detergents/Emulsifier's:** strip skin of protective oils, skin irritation, scalp eruptions, interference with nutrient absorption, hair loss, allergic reaction, cataract formation, organ damage, reproductive damage, blindness, cancer.
4. **Synthetic Fragrance and Dyes:** allergic reactions, skin rashes, stomach upsets, muscular aches and pains, violent coughing and sneezing, irritability, vertigo, hyperactivity, convulsions, emotional and behavioral problems, Leukemia, Hodgkin's, emotional problems, ADD, multiple tumors, reproductive damage, headaches, dizziness, organ damage, depression, cancer.
5. **Heavy Metals:** Abdominal cramps, nausea, joint and bone pain, muscle weakness, mouth sores, muscle, joint, and bone pain; cancer, motor difficulties, reduced intelligence, brain disorders, short attention span, hyperactivity, short attention span, emotional disorders, immune disorders, genetic damage, aging.
6. **Pesticides and Fungicides:** Flu-like symptoms (fatigue, muscle and joint pain), stomach cramps, nervous system disorders, insomnia, memory loss, swelling of body parts, dizziness, genetic mutations, birth defects, gland tumors, organ damage, cancers, death.
7. **Petrochemicals:** inhibit skin functions, pimples, rashes, splitting nails, sensitivity to sun, headaches, premature aging, allergic reactions, depression, fatigue, intestinal gas, asthma, respiratory failure, immune system disorders.
8. **Preservatives** (synthetic): headaches, shin rashes, eye damage, asthma, respiratory problems, tumors, cancer, digestive problems, mental confusion, organ damage, muscle weakness & cramps, loss of motor control, joint pain, reproductive damage, etc.

(*) Anti-bacterial products contain poisonous pesticides and fungicides as ingredients that create more serious health risks.

Get Rid of the Toxins!

All of these toxins in the home together cause so many illnesses, such as asthma, allergies, upper respiratory conditions and a myriad of other health issues. Resolve to rid the home of all toxic substances and replace them with natural, safe, botanical alternatives. This will save money, provide peace of mind, and in a short while allow a family to begin reaping the benefits of using safe cleaning products.

Just be aware, that many so-called natural cleaners still contain hazardous ingredients. Watch out for all the popular "green" marketing out there. Many natural cleaners, even those sold in health food stores, are simply environmentally safe and do not test on animals, but they still use toxic ingredients. What may be safe and "green" for the home may not be safe for the people living in it. And what is safe for the home and family might not be getting rid of the germs in the home.

The standard should be - if you can't drink it, don't clean with it. If it isn't safe enough in a babies room, don't use it! Plus it has to work, be cost effective and easy to use.

Very few products out there safely clean and rid the house of germs while being completely safe for the family. The authors use one product that does both — Young Living's Thieves Household Cleaner®. It contains therapeutic-grade essential oils that kill germs while being completely safe for children. We not only endorse it, but use it confidently every day.

Get rid of the toxic chemicals and reap the benefit of better health!

Natural Cleaner Recipes

There are numerous Web sites on "Cleaning Green" that list lots of recipes. All we really need is a few simple ingredients for a toxic free, clean home. Housecleaning does not have to make us sick.

Below are a few recipes that are family safe and easy to make and use.

Laundry Soap

1 cup finely grated pure soap or soap flakes
1 cup washing soda
½ cup borax
Combine in a plastic tub container, add ½ cup to the wash cycle. Recipe may be doubled, tripled, etc.

Laundry Rinse

2 cups vinegar
10 drops lemon oil, eucalyptus, lavender[5] (whitens)

Combine in a glass jar, use ½ cup in the rinse cycle. Recipe may be doubled, tripled, etc.

Pre-treatment

Especially good around collars and for underarm stains.

Combine ¼ white vinegar, four drops lemon oil, one teaspoon baking soda and use an old toothbrush to scrub on area, then launder as usual.

Clove, lemon or Thieves will help prevent and kill mold in towels.

5 Only use the Young Living® brand of essential oils to be assured of quality, purity, and potency.

Spot Remover
As soon as the stain happens, combine two tablespoons cream of tarter, two drops eucalyptus oil or lemon oil and some water to make a paste. Spread the paste over the stain and let completely dry before washing.

Fabric Softener
1 gallon white vinegar, 30 drops essential oil your choice for smell and disinfectant - lavender, rosewood, cedarwood, Thieves oil
Use ½ cup of the mixture in the rinse cycle

Disinfecting Formula for Walls
1 cup water
1 cup vinegar
5 drops thyme oil
5 drops lemon oil

Combine in a spray bottle. Lightly spray the surface and wipe clean.

Abrasive Cleaner
One cup each of table salt (the cheap kind will do), borax and baking soda (large boxes are found in the laundry section of most stores).

Stir in 20 drops essential oil - Purification, Lemon, Melrose or Thieves[6]. Place in a sealed glass jar. For convenience, place one cup of this blend in a pizza cheese shaker and it is ready to use.

Carpet Freshener
Combine ½ cup baking soda with 10 drops essential oil, place in a pizza cheese shaker and sprinkle on carpet, let sit a few minutes and then vacuum. Or place five drops of a favorite essential oil on a tissue and place in the vacuum bag.

Chrome, stainless steel, steel sink, copper and tin polish
Combine one tablespoon baking soda with one drop lemon oil, rub on with a damp soft cloth. Then, rinse in warm water and dry.

Vinegar
With five percent acetic acid, white distilled vinegar is great to remove stains, dissolve hard water mineral deposits and grease. It can also remove wax buildup and mildew. Use in a 50/50 dilution with water.

Table Salt
Removes rust by adding a drop of lemon oil to a spoonful of salt to clean copper, or let sit around rust areas with a damp cloth covering for several hours. Wipe clean.

All Purpose Cleaner
Of course, our first choice is Thieves Household Cleaner, but here are some other homemade varieties.

Combine one quart distilled water, 20 drops essential oil (lemon, spruce, clove, cinnamon, orange, rosemary - use one or a combination) and five drops of dishwashing liquid or shampoo. Shake gently to combine. The dish soap helps disperse the oils.

6 These are Young Living® essential oil blends.

Windows and Mirrors

Vinegar and water (25/75% dilution) wiped on with a sponge, then dried with crumpled newspaper or removed with a squeegee.

Air Freshener

Diffusing therapeutic-grade essential oils is the first choice. Another method is combining 10 drops lemon, six drops bergamot, five drops grapefruit, five drops orange in some baking soda. Place in small jars in bathrooms for a clean fresh scent.

Mothballs

Moths and bugs in general hate the smell of many essential oils. Make up a sachet with the one or more of the following oils on a cotton ball or pad wrapped in colorful cloth. Lavender, lemongrass, Western Red Cedar, rosemary, and rose are good choices.

Additional Resources

Books:

"Green This! Volume 1: Greening Your Cleaning," by Deidre Imus, Simon & Schuster, 2007.

Appendix T: Are Toxins in Your Personal Care Products?

Everyday our skin comes into contact with possibly hundreds of potentially harmful chemicals. Many of these could be avoided if we spent a little time learning about the harmful chemicals found in bath and body care products.

The cosmetic and personal care products industry is largely unregulated, resulting in products which contain a multitude of chemicals that have very little to do with personal care. Allergies, skin sensitivities and other serious health conditions can be a result of using toxic chemicals on the skin. Most people think the government would not allow toxins in the products we use. Surprisingly, according to, Doris J. Rapp, M.D, author of "Our Toxic World: A Wake-Up Call" over 80,000 chemicals presently are used in the U.S. and less than 10 percent even have been partially evaluated for safety by the U.S. government. As a board certified environmental medical specialist and pediatric allergist, Dr. Rapp warns that none of these known chemicals "have been properly studied on effects on human immune, nervous, endocrine and reproductive systems."

Baby Care Products

The Environmental Working Group Study of October 2007[1] surveyed 3,300 parents and compared the baby care products they used to lists of chemicals known to cause allergies, hormone disruption, damage to the nervous system and cancer. The study found that, on a daily basis, children are exposed to 27 chemical ingredients that have never been assessed for safety – not by the industry, nor by the government.

Dr. Rebecca Sutton, the environmental scientist who conducted the study, points out that baby products in American markets create allergies, skin irritations and in certain products, break down to form new cancer-causing agents. Dr. Sutton reports that Desitin diaper cream contains sodium borate, which can collect in a child's brain and liver, causing detrimental health effects.

Surprisingly, 89 percent of products labeled "Recommended by doctor" are actually some of the worst offenders, containing what Dr. Sutton considers as dangerous chemicals.

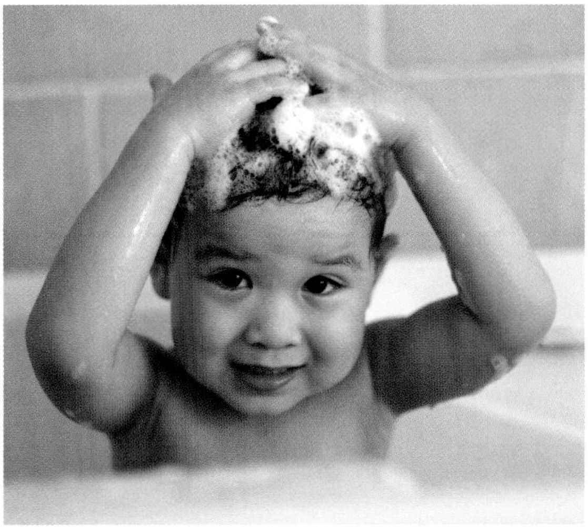

Here are just some of the products available on the market today that may be harmful to our health: diaper cream, body lotions, shampoos, bath soap, household cleaners, carpet shampoo, air fresheners, hand sanitizers, toothpaste, over-the-counter ache, pain, cough and cold remedies, perfumes, nutritional supplements, food and clothing.

Replacing these with quality, life-enhancing, cost-effective products will provide greater peace of mind and wellness. Choosing such products often can be confusing as many manufacturers recognize that customers are more aware of environmental dangers and use packaging that contains misleading information. There are ways of decoding these marketing tactics.

1 Go to The Environmental Working Group's website at www.ewg.org for more studies with shocking findings.

Fragrances

Most every personal care product uses a fragrance to enhance the smell of the product. Some even boast on the label that their product is all natural. Fragrances pose a serious health risk. Over 5,000 chemicals are used in the manufacture of fragrances, and according to a report from the National Institute of Occupational Safely and Health, 900 were identified as toxic with 95 percent of them petro-chemically derived. Yet the labeling can lead a person to believe that the essential oil or other fragrance is natural and safe. Some of the best known perfumes and fragrances are banned in Europe due to phthalates, which cause infertility in men and genital abnormalities.

Truly pure, natural and safe essential oils with therapeutic properties come from organically grown plants that have been harvested at a particular time and have been painstakingly distilled. Due to their delicate growing and distillation process, such essential oils are quite expensive, are very hard to come by and would not be easily found in just any products or added just for their fragrance [2].

Cosmetics

Adolescence is a fragile age for young girls as they become vulnerable by experimenting with make-up and body care products containing dozens, if not hundreds, of chemicals. As the body is undergoing many hormonal changes, a toxic onslaught of chemicals poses a huge threat to physical, mental and emotional changes. At this age the reproductive system is maturing as is the immune, blood and adrenal hormone systems. Major changes to brain structure and function, as well as rapid bone growth, is occurring at this age of a young female.

During adolescence, hormones present in the body at a mere one part per billion and even one part per trillion lead the body's changes into adulthood. Trace chemicals with hormone-like properties can wreak havoc to a young girl's body, especially at this age.

In September of 2008, the Environmental Working Group tested blood and urine samples of 20 teenage girls ages 14 to 19. The tests found 16 chemicals from four chemical families – phthalates, triclosan, parabens and musks -- linked to cancer and hormone disruption. Two types of parabens – methylparaben and polyparaben – were found in every teen.

As teens use more personal care products than the average adult woman, young girls should be advised to use as little products as they can. Parents are encouraged to research common personal care product ingredients and find out what is dangerous and what is safe. For lists of ingredients in common skin care products and their safety, go to the Environmental Working Group's Cosmetic Safety Database at www.cosmeticsdatabase.com.

Household Cleaning Products

Household cleaning products are among the most toxic substances we encounter daily. In one study conducted over a 15-year period, women who cleaned their own homes had a 54 percent higher death rate from cancer than women who did not. The study concluded that the increased death rate was due to daily exposure to hazardous chemicals found in ordinary household products.

Of the 80,000 chemicals being used commercially in this country, the EPA considers more than 75 percent of them to be potentially, if not definitely, hazardous to human health. We are exposed to more toxins in one day, than our grandparents were in a lifetime. Refer to Appendix S: Labels and Household Toxins for a list of potentially hazardous products in the home.

---

2 The authors recommend personal care products containing therapeutic-grade essential oils from Young Living®, which is the only company that both grows and distills their own essential oils.

The 2004 Body Burden Study by the Environmental Working Group tested the umbilical cords of 100 infants for 418 chemicals and found:

- 287 chemicals
- 208 of the chemicals were known to cause birth defects
- 180 of the chemicals were known to cause cancer
- All traced to mothers' diets

Chemicals to avoid in personal care products

Here is a list of some of the main toxic chemicals and the products in which they are commonly found. A product may be labeled all natural and still contain these because they are derived from petroleum products and petroleum is naturally occurring in our environment.

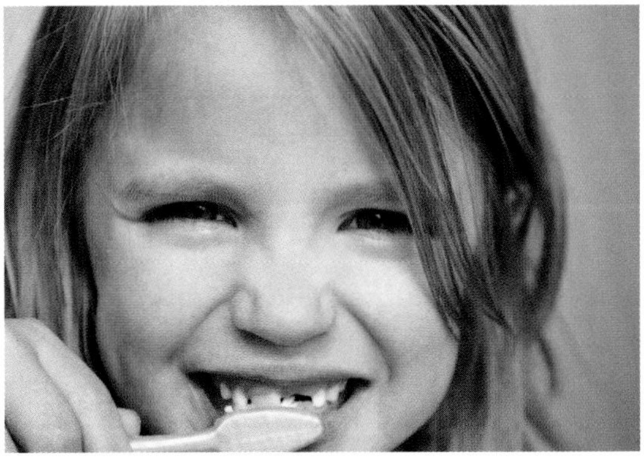

Sodium Lauryl Sulfate and **Sodium Laureth Sulfate** (SLS) irritates skin, corrodes hair follicles and impairs the ability to grow hair, can damage the immune system and can cause permanent eye damage. SLS enters and maintains residual levels in the heart, liver, lungs and brain from skin contact[3]. SLS is found in toothpaste, liquid soap, shampoos, conditioners and lotions.

Propylene Glycol is a suspected carcinogen. It is implicated in contact dermatitis, kidney damage and liver abnormalities; can inhibit skin cell growth in human tests and can damage cell membranes causing rashes, dry skin and surface damage. Acute effects include harm by inhalation, ingestion or skin absorption. Exposure can cause gastro-intestinal disturbances, nausea, headache and vomiting and central nervous system depression[4].

A published clinical review in The American Academy of Dermatologists, Inc. in January of 1991 showed that propylene glycol causes a significant number of reactions and was a primary irritant to the skin even in low levels of concentrations. It is commonly used in anti-freeze and is also found in shampoos, conditioners, soaps, lotions, make-up, contact cleaner solution and is now even added to processed food such as cake mixes.

Even with propylene glycol's known affects of nausea, vomiting and gastro-intestinal disturbances and companies now putting it into foods, it's no wonder so many Americans have gastro-intestinal issues like Irritable Bowel Syndrome (IBS).

"After going to the eye doctor, I was given a new bottle of my regular contact cleaning solution. For several days, I experienced severe itching and irritation in my eyes. I finally compared the new bottle of contact solution to the old one I had kept. To my surprise, there was a new ingredient in my contact solution – propylene glycol. I quickly changed solutions to one that did not contain it, and I experienced immediate relief." – Sera Johnson

Diethanolamine (DEA) is a known carcinogen as stated by the U.S. Department of Health and Human Services' National Toxicology Program. It is found in shampoos, conditioners, bubble baths, lotions, cosmetics, soaps, laundry and dishwashing detergents.

Talc is chemically similar to asbestos. A study by the American Journal of Epidemiology found a possible link to ovarian cancer. Talc is found in baby powder, feminine powder and feminine deodorants.

3 Journal of the American College of Toxicology; Vol. 2, No. 7, 1983.
4 Material Safety Data Sheets (MSDS)

Aluminum has been linked to Alzheimer's and is found in antiperspirants, especially aerosol antiperspirants.

So what products are safe? It is important to be a label reader and trust the sources of such products. Just purchasing items at a health food store does not guarantee that they are free of chemicals. The authors and their families choose Young Living Essential Oil products and recommend them to their friends and loved ones.

Therapeutic-Grade Essential Oils good for the Skin[5]

Lavender (Lavandula angustifolia) - Good for all skin types, gentle antiseptic, great on bee stings, sunburns, muscle cramps.

Geranium (Pelargonium graveolens) - Very soothing to the skin, especially good for the pain of shingles.

Rose (Rosa damascena) - the number one oil to combat wrinkles.

Juniper (Juniperus osteosperma and J. scopulorum) - Good antiseptic, nerve regenerator, especially helpful in cases of eczema and oily acne. Often used in the treatment of cellulite.

Lemongrass (Cymbopogon flexuosus) - Great for normal to oily skin because it is mildly astringent. Also good for sagging skin, especially great for smokers as it helps detoxify the skin.

Orange (Citrus sinensis) - Recommended for all skin types except very dry. May cause skin photo-sensitivity.

Oregano (Origanum compactum) - Be sure to use diluted for warts, fungal infections and insect bites.

Peppermint (Mentha piperita) - A refreshing and cooling astringent. Mix with lavender in a spray bottle with water for a cooling, refreshing facial spray any time of day.

Thyme (Thymus vulgaris) - Strong antiseptic, highly recommended.

Tea tree (Melaleuca alternafolia) - powerful antiseptic and antifungal. Makes a good addition to most cleansers.

For a complete list of personal care products that the authors not only recommend but regularly use for their family, contact the editor@growinghealthyhomes.com.

Our families' health is so important. With the many recent reports in the news about chemical related health issues found in children, it is more important than ever to start getting the toxins out of your home!

If you don't take action today, how will you feel years down the road when you or your child is diagnosed with a health concern directly related to the use of cheap, synthetic, hazardous products you used.

Additional Resources

Books:
"Saving Face," by Dr. Sabina DaVita, Wellness Institute of Living and Learning, 2003.
"Our Toxic World: A Wake-Up Call," Doris Rapp, M.D., Environmental Medical Research Foundation, 2004

5 Only use the Young Living® brand of essential oils to be assured of quality, purity, and potency.

Appendix U: Nail Health Guide

Remember when the doctor used to look into your eyes and at your hands when you went in for a check-up? Why? Because the fingernails are a window into the body's health, changes in the look, shape, or color of fingernails can indicate a nutritional deficiency or disease somewhere in the body long before other symptoms manifest. Though your doctor may not do this anymore, you can use the following guide to evaluate your overall health. Don't ignore your nails, they can serve as an early warning signal for your health. If you are used to polishing your nails, give them a break, let them breath and take a look at what they are telling you.

Healthy nails are pink on the nail bed indicating a rich blood supply. Nails are made of keratin, a type of protein and sulfur. It takes approximately seven months to fully grow a fingernail, at a rate of about .05 to 1.2 millimeters a week. The following are some of the nutritional deficiencies that can show up in the nails and the health issues associated with each.

- White fingernails with pink coloring near the tips can be a sign of cirrhosis of the liver. If the entire nail is white it could mean kidney or liver disorders or anemia.
- White lines across the nail may indicate a protein deficiency or liver disease, while white lines in a horizontal fashion may indicate heart disease, high fever or arsenic poisoning. A half white nail with dark spots on the tip could indicate a kidney disorder.
- If the moon part of the nail area turns red, heart problems are suspect. If the moon area turns blue, then possible heavy metal poisoning or lung problems may exist.
- Cuts and cracks in nails may indicate the need for more water intake.
- Two white lines that do not seem to move as the nail grows indicate hypoalbuminemia which is a protein deficiency in the blood.
- Abnormally thick nails might be due to the blood not circulating properly in the vascular system.
- Yellow nails can mean there are problems with your liver, diabetes, respiratory disorders or problems with the lymphatic system.
- Dark nails that are flat and/or thin, or are spoon shaped, can be a sign of vitamin B12 deficiency or anemia.
- Brittle nails are often a sign of iron deficiency and thyroid problems. You could also have impaired kidneys or problems with circulation.
- Nails that are very bendable could be a sign of rheumatoid arthritis.
- Pitted brown spots or split fingernail tips may mean you have psoriasis or that vitamin C, folic acid or protein are needed.

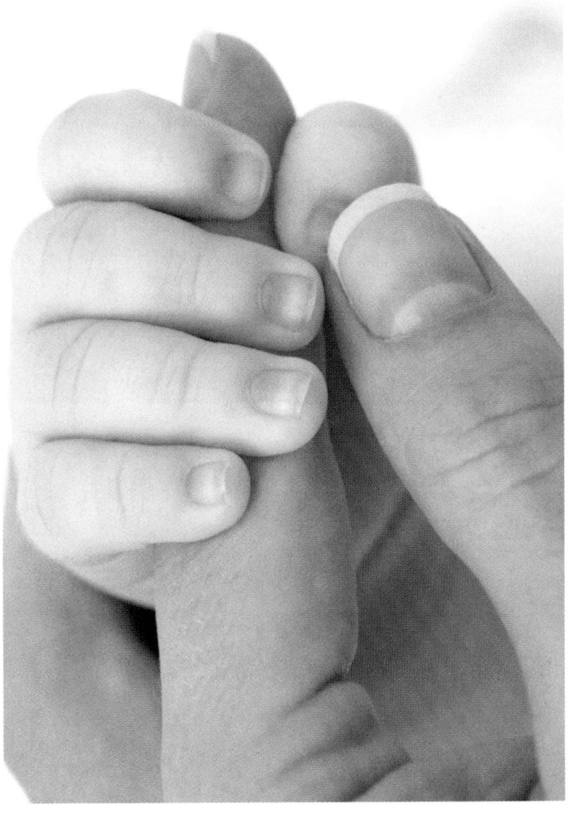

- Very deep blue nail beds can indicate pulmonary obstruction or emphysema.

- Nail's that crack, peel and chip easily mean a general nutritional deficiency and insufficient hydrochloric acid production which facilitates the digestion and absorption of protein. More protein and minerals may be needed in your diet.

- Thyroid problems can be seen in nails that are brittle, soft, shiny, without a moon, separate from the nail bed, have ridges or like a bumpy road.

- Nails with brass coloring may indicate a tendency toward partial or total hair loss.

- Flat nails can indicate Raynaud's disease. This disease affects the circulatory system, which in turn affects the limbs. It leaves hands and feet continually cold.

- Unusually wide nails that are square can mean a hormonal disorder.

- Red skin at the very bottom of your nail bed could indicate a connective tissue disorder.

- Greenish tints to nails can signify a fungal infection of the nail or a bacterial infection in the body. Additional good friendly gut bacteria - probiotics - may be needed.

- Black splinter like bits under the nails can indicate infectious endocarditis, a serious heart infection. Black bands from the cuticle outward to the end of the nail, can be an early sign of melanoma. In either case you should seek professional help immediately.

- Lack of B vitamins causes nails to become fragile, especially indicated with ridges. Lack of vitamins, minerals or protein causes hang nails.

- Dryness and brittleness together often indicate a lack of Vitamin A and calcium. Zinc deficiencies can show up as small white spots on the nails. Iron deficiency may result in "spoon" shaped nails or vertical ridges.

- Lack of sufficient gut bacteria can contribute to nail fungal infections.

Many women with not-so lovely nails often have acrylic nails glued on top of their natural nails. This is an extremely bad practice. The glues and acrylics are toxic and can penetrate into the bloodstream; the fake nails cut off oxygen to the nail making it weak and thin; and many a nail fungus had it's beginning with a manicure or pedicure. The area where the acrylic nail attaches to the natural nail bed is a breeding ground for bacteria.

For the sake of your health, let your natural nails grow out and take steps to make them strong and healthy by getting your whole body in balance and eating nail supporting foods (See Unit 4 Chapter 3). For a while you will have soft nails. Keep them cut short and they will improve in a short while.

Excessive exposure to water and detergents or soaps can cause the nails to swell. When they dry, they shrink, which results in loose, brittle nails. Rubber gloves should be used when washing the dishes or getting your hands in lots of water.

Herbs that provide the body with nutrients specific for the nails include alfalfa, black cohosh, burdock root, horsetail, oatstraw, dandelion, Gotu kola and yellow dock, royal jelly, spirulina and kelp which are all rich in minerals and silica.

Carrier oils such as warm olive, flaxseed or borage oil mixed with high-quality therapeutic-grade essential oils can be applied topically and will nourish the nail. Choose from the following essential oils: lemongrass, frankincense, lemon and myrrh. See recipes at the bottom for more choices.

Here are a couple of simple recipes that nourish the nails[1].

Nail Butter

2 Tbs. beeswax
2 Tbs. cocoa butter
3 Tbs. jojoba oil
1 Tbs. grape seed oil
20 drops essential oils - rose, carrot, rosemary, geranium and sandalwood - 4 drops each.

Combine beeswax, cocoa butter and jojoba oil in a saucepan and warm on low heat in a double-boiler until cocoa butter and beeswax have melted. Remove from heat and add the essential oils. Stir well, let cool slightly and pour into jars. Use a Q-tip swab or orange stick to get a small amount of the cream from the jar. Apply to nails and massage with your fingers.

Nail Ointment

1 jar Young Living Rose Ointment
10 drops olive oil or Young Living V6 oil
4 drops geranium oil
4 drops Palo Santo
4 drops Citrus Fresh
4 drops myrrh

Scoop out Rose ointment into a stainless steel double boiler. Warm the ointment until it melts. Remove from heat and pour into glass measuring cup with a pouring spout. Add V6 oil and essential oils, swirl gently with a toothpick. Pour back into Rose ointment jar, re-label or pour into smaller jars, label and give as gifts. Using a cotton swab, apply a small amount to nail bed and massage in, twice daily.

Quick Nail Growth Oil

10 drops frankincense
10 drops lemon oil
10 drops myrrh
Combine in a small vial or bottle. Apply with a paint brush to bare nails twice per day.

Therapeutic-Grade Essential Oils that soften cuticles

Eucalyptus and peppermint

Therapeutic-Grade Essential Oils for fungal infections

Melaleuca alternafolia, oregano, Purification, Thieves, thyme and Ravensara

1 Authors' recommend using only Young Living® therapeutic-grade essential oils as they are properly grown, harvested, distilled, contain no added ingredients and may be ingested, used topically and inhaled.

Appendix V: Reproductive Health

The endocrine system is comprised of the reproductive glands and the corresponding hormones they produce. They are vital to the body's health by regulating metabolism, tissue function, growth, puberty and development.

Both females and males naturally produce both estrogen and testosterone and must have both hormones in balance for their bodies to function properly.

In order to cover into this topic with sensitivity, we first will discuss the female reproductive system and then the male reproductive system.

Female Reproductive System Health Issues

The **female reproductive glands** are the **ovaries**, but when pregnant the **uterus** and **placenta** also are considered glands because they secrete hormones. In addition to producing several hormones, including **estrogen**, the ovaries produce eggs. The following issues are associated with a female endocrine system:

Endometriosis occurs when the lining of the uterus begins to grow on the outer wall of the uterus, ovaries, vagina, fallopian tubes and even on the abdominal wall. This extra growth is not shed during normal menstruation and the cause is largely unknown, though many theories exist. Because of this, cysts and fibroids will often form and can cause heavy periods, back pain and in some instances can be a contributing factor in infertility. Traditional treatments of choice include surgery or prescription birth control pills, but many women have gained relief and completely eliminated endometriosis naturally by balancing their hormones, supplementing with large doses of completely safe fibrin and scar tissue digesting enzymes and the use of certain topical essential oils.

Fibroids of the uterus are benign, meaning non-cancerous tumors, which grow from the muscle layers of the uterus. They can be very small or grow to the size of a large grapefruit. Uterine fibroids are more common in overweight women. Generally, symptoms relate to the location of the lesion and its size and include abnormal gynecological bleeding, heavy or painful periods, abdominal discomfort or bloating, back ache, urinary frequency or retention, and in some cases, infertility. The three most common treatments involve surgery, embolization of the uterus or high frequency ultrasound. The natural approach is to follow the PCOS diet below and use the same high potency enzyme formula as used with endometriosis.

Cysts can occur any where on the body and are believed by naturopathic healthcare professionals to be largely accumulated pockets of mucous. Ovarian cysts form for numerous reasons. The most common type is a follicular cyst, which results from the growth of a follicle, but a corpus luteum cyst, which is related to the menstrual cycle. If it is determined that there is no heath problem associated with the cyst, it is left alone. Otherwise surgery is the typical treatment offered. Many women find relief with diet changes, but if more help is needed, many herbal remedies have been shown helpful. These would include blood cleansing herbs, such as red clover and enzymes, and the favorite female herbal tonic and astringent herb red raspberry leaf.

Premenstrual Syndrome (PMS) is the most common hormone related condition of women. With symptoms of mood swings, sadness, anger, headaches, fatigue, memory loss, depression, breast tenderness and several others beginning two weeks before menstruation, PMS has been associated not only with hormone imbalance, but diet and the stress of Western culture. Many women are helped by taking a multivitamin every day that includes folic acid, calcium and vitamin D. Lifestyle factors that can have a positive impact include regular exercise, at least eight hours of sleep, eating healthy foods, refraining from smoking, finding healthy ways to deal with stress and avoiding salt, sugary foods, caffeine, and alcohol, especially when symptoms persist.

Polycystic ovarian syndrome (PCOS) also is known as Stein-Leventhal syndrome and chronic an-ovulatory hyper-androgenism. It is a disorder that affects approximately six percent of women who have not reached menopause. While the reported cases are rare, there are probably many as yet undiagnosed cases. In addition to causing infertility, PCOS also is usually accompanied by physical characteristics that can damage self-esteem. There is little agreement in the medical community as to whether insulin-resistance causes PCOS, although many doctors blame obesity as the primary cause.

The natural alternative is to address the problem at its root. Losing weight, if a woman is more than 15 pounds overweight, is the first step. In addition, it is crucial to use a progesterone cream to support the female organs and balance hormones, as well as an estrogen-boosting supplement containing the herb clary sage, flaxseed or soy. Finally, regular aerobic exercise is necessary at least three times per week.

Infertility is on the rise in America. Factors include diet, stress and waiting later in life to start a family. Causes of female infertility may be exacerbated by formaldehyde, excessive consumption of caffeine, monosodium glutamate (MSG) and trans-fatty acids, and excessive consumption of alcohol or tobacco smoke. Overexposure to fluoride and mercury also may increase the risk of female infertility. In addition, pharmaceuticals such as chorionic gonadotrophic hormone and Clomiphene may reduce the chances of becoming pregnant. Health conditions that may have an adverse affect include Celiac disease, hypothyroidism, endometriosis, Luteal Phase Defect, ovarian cysts, PCOS or uterine fibroids.

Although there are not a lot of answers, happily about one-third of all couples who seek either natural or traditional surgery or drug fertility treatments go on to have at least one child. Natural fertility options are varied in scope, but start with a great diet, cleansing routines, stress management, lots of prayer and finding a health professional to work with will be sure all of the bases are covered to overcome possible causes of infertility. Substances that may alleviate female infertility include DHEA (Dehydroepiandrosterone) 80 mg per day, melatonin and progesterone cream applied topically. Vitamins and minerals that may help include inositol, potassium chloride, vitamins B6, B12, C, D and E, and para aminobenzoic acid.

Foods and herbs that may cause female infertility

Fungi, Chinese black tree fungus, green peas (in large quantities, carrots (over a pound of carrots a day)

Foods and herbs that may alleviate female infertility

Thyroid extract, chaste berry (Vitex), Dong Quai, ginsengs, maca, Mexican wild yam

Menopause is the permanent cessation of the female menstrual cycle and can occur at anytime generally between the ages of 35 and 60. At the beginning of menopause, often referred to as perimenopause, the cycles may be erratic for many years before completely stopping. Symptoms may include night sweats, hot flashes, decreased libido, vaginal and urinary complications, depression, and mood swings. In some women the hormone progesterone declines making them at more risk for breast and uterine cancers. Once hormone levels are known, the proper herbs and natural therapies can be employed. Progesterone creams are used to balance and/or increase progesterone levels; and herbs such as red clover, Dong Quoi, clary sage and soy isolates can improve estrogen levels without any harmful side effects of synthetic and even bio-identical hormone replacement.

Female reproductive cancers - ovarian, breast and cervical

Female cancers that are hormone-related or estrogen-receptor positive are some of the most aggressive and difficult to treat. In the U.S., traditionally approved methods for treating any cancer are chemotherapy, radiation and surgery. As with any health condition, prevention is always better than even the smallest amount of treatment.

For more information on cancer and nutritional support, see Appendix W. For a more complete list of nutrients and foods that best support the endocrine glands and system, see Unit 6 Chapter 2.

Soy contains phytoestrogens that mimic estrogen in the body which infants, children, teens, men and most women do not need and should not consume. The only exception is with women with certain hormone issues who may need an estrogen supplement and should seek the advice of a health care professional.

Male Reproductive System Health Issues

The primary **male reproductive glands** are the **testes**, which produce estradiol, inhibin and adrogens, the primary one being testosterone. The prostate is another gland necessary for reproduction. Pumpkin seeds with their high zinc content have always been a good food for male prostate health.

Other than cancer, most men over the age of 50 will experience some inflammation of the prostate gland called **Benign Prostate Hyperplasia** (BPH). Natural progesterone creams to balance reduced levels of the male hormone testosterone have been used as a natural therapy successfully, as have the herbs saw palmetto and phygeum africanum.

Infertility is the inability in a male to induce conception. Possible culprits are excessive consumption of amino acids and MSG, electromagnetic radiation, environmental toxins like dioxin and some pesticides, excessive levels of the hormone prolactin, excessive consumption of caffeine, prolonged use of pharmaceutical drugs and excessive amounts of minerals, such as cadmium, fluoride, lead or mercury, as well as m-xylohydroquinone, abundant when green peas are consumed in large quantities. In addition, excessive consumption of alcohol, marijuana and tobacco smoking may increase the risk of male infertility.

Natural fertility options are similar to those for women and are varied in scope, but start with a great diet, cleansing routines, stress management, lots of prayer and finding a health professional to work with will be sure all of the bases are covered to overcome possible causes of infertility. Amino acids and carotenoids that may alleviate male infertility include arginine (8,000 mg per day), carnitine (400 to 3,000 mg per day), taurine, astaxanthin and lycopene (at least 4 mg per day). Gonadotrophic hormones are synthesized and released by the pituitary gland and act on the testes to promote the production of sperm. Melatonin may be useful for the treatment due to its ability to increase sperm motility. Minerals and vitamins that may be helpful include: chromium orotate (10 to 20 mg per day), selenium (100 mcg per day), zinc (50 to 100 mg per day), folic acid, inositol, vitamins A, B12 (1,000 to 6,000 mcg per day), C (5 grams per day) and E. Other factors that may contribute to male infertility include metabolism, excessive endurance exercise, free radicals, Celiac disease and male hypogonadism.

Foods, herbs and oils that may cause male infertility
Cottonseed oil, papaya seeds in excess, raw garlic in excess, green peas in large quantities
Foods, herbs and oils that may alleviate male infertility
Ashwagandha, caterpillar fungus, Korean ginseng, passion flower, rosemary, siberian ginseng, tribulus, terrestris, velvet beans, fish oils, flaxseed oil, alpha-linolenic acid, shark liver oil

Male reproductive cancers - testes and prostate

Testicular cancer forms in the tissues of the testis, one of the two glands inside the scrotum that make sperm. It usually occurs in young or middle aged men. According to the National Institutes of Health, only 8,000 cases were estimated to be diagnosed in 2008, resulting in less than 400 deaths.

Prostate cancer is the abnormal growth of cells in the prostate gland. It is more common in men over 65. The cause is again largely unknown, but risk factors include age, genetics and eating a high-fat diet.

Scientists are tracing the higher incidence of hormone-dependent cancers of the prostate and testes to exposure to endocrine disrupters in the environment. Petrochemical contamination from DDT, PCB, pesticides, the phylate DBP, and synthetic steroids in meat, are all implecated in interfering with hormone receptor sites, rendering them unable to function properly, eventually leading to cancer.

For more information on cancer and nutritional support, see Appendix W. For more information on nutritional support for the endocrine glands and system, see Unit 6 Chapter 2.

Appendix W: Cancer

Cancer – a six letter word that strikes fear in the heart of many, even though heart disease is the number one killer of Americans.

So what is cancer? Why do some people get cancer and others do not? Are there ways to reduce the risk or prevent cancer? Are there natural healing modalities that work to bring about a healing if you should get cancer?

The American Cancer Society regards a person as a cancer survivor if he or she is living five years after they are declared cured. The truth is though, that many people die after the five year period of heart complications from chemotherapy treatment or their cancer returns elsewhere.

Just about everyone has known or knows someone with cancer, possibly even someone who lost their life to cancer. It now affects one out of every two Americans, and is growing rapidly among children.

What is cancer?

Cancer is essentially a healthy cell that stops functioning and reproducing properly. It is theorized that the cell DNA mutates and then reproduces incorrectly, again and again. These newly mutated cells then begin to reproduce uncontrollably no longer in harmony with the rest of the body. Some experts also believe that tumors become surrounded by fungi and yeast that inhibits the possibility of surgery and the effectiveness of chemotherapy treatments.

Cancer is now considered to be *the* disease of our time. Look at all the foundations and fund raising events that center on cancer and finding a cure. American's have been waging a war on cancer for some 30 years. While finding a cure is certainly a good idea, preventing cancer is even more important for the future. The adages "an ounce of prevention is worth more than a pound of cure" and "a good offense is better than a defense" are true strategies when dealing with cancer.

There are currently 150 types of cancer in five major groups.

- Carcinomas that form in epithelial cells on the skin surface or on the cells of various organs.
- Sarcomas form in soft bone and connective tissue surrounding organs. These also are solid tumors and are the most rare and deadly.
- Leukemia forms in the blood and bone marrow. Many in the natural health profession link leukemia with depression.
- Lymphomas are cancers in the lymph glands.
- Myelomas are rare tumors of the cells that produce blood cells in tissue and bone marrow.

Staging is the term used as an index to determine how much cancer exists in the body, its size, location and containment of any metastasis. Stage one is better than stage four for example and stage five is generally a fully metastasized, meaning spread everywhere, cancer. The medical establishment offers little hope to late stage cancer patients.

Research has shown links to toxic chemicals, food and nutrition, viruses, fungus, parasites, poor detoxification channels, decreased thyroid function, free radicals, excess alcohol, excess caffeine, toxic emotions, chronic stress, excess iron intake, excess fat intake and more. There is no one way to get cancer, which means that there is no one answer, medically or naturally, to prevent or cure cancer. It is a combination of preventive measures or, in the case of disease, holistic treatments.

Early detection of a cancer can mean the difference in survival or not. The medical field does an exceptional job in this area. Changes in skin health, unexplained pain, lumps under the skin, blood in stool or urine, headaches – any sudden unexplained changes in a person's health – should be investigated. We should take advantage of the wide range of medical and non-conventional tests, such as:

PSA – prostate
Pap smear – cervical and uterine
Mammogram and DITI – breast
AMAS – antibody test for early detection (www.amascancertest.com)
Dark field or live cell microscopy

No cancer treatment should be undertaken without consulting a licensed medical practitioner. The natural therapies, products and applications listed here can be used to complement the effectiveness of conventional cancer therapies. These applications should continue until the cancer is in remission. Traditional oncologists, medical doctors who specialize in cancer treatment, will most likely not understand a natural approach to treating cancer. If you choose to incorporate these ideas into your cancer protocol, you will need to be educated yourself and be armed with the books and data to support your decision to use natural therapies.

Reducing Risk and Prevention:

1. **Thoughts.** Toxic thoughts – anger, frustration, grief, sadness, etc. – continuously produce hormones the body doesn't really need. Over time these hormones can cause physical changes in the body. Doing an Internet search on the phrase "emotions and cancer" will yield a plethora of information supporting the link between thoughts and physical health. Henry Wright, author of "A More Excellent Way," has done extensive research into the spiritual connection and emotions in regards to cancer.

2. **Food.** Most naturally minded health professionals recommend a mostly vegetarian diet, rich in fresh vegetables, including juices, fruit, whole grains, sprouts, nuts and seeds. A brief list of nutrients shown to lower a persons cancer risk include: beta-carotene, vitamin B6, C and E, selenium, calcium, folic acid, iodine, magnesium, zinc, and Omega-3's. Fiber is important to keep the colon clean. The immune system should be supported with vitamin C, zinc and beta glucans. A landmark German study found that vegetarians had twice as high NK cell activity as meat eaters. NK cells are among the immune systems prime cancer fighting cells.

3. **Cleaning supplies.** An EPA study stated that the indoor air pollution in many homes due to common household cleaners containing carcinogenic, volitile organic compounds (VOC's) was 10 times greater than outdoor pollution even in areas located near petrochemical plants.[1] Safe and effective cleansers can be made at home without harmful chemicals. Use borax and baking soda and essential oils for scrubbing cleaners. Furniture polishes can be concocted with beeswax or olive oil and essential oils. The very concentrated Thieves Household Cleaner® cleans walls, floors, tubs, showers, windows, counter tops, siding, porch furniture, carpet and much, much more. These costs pennies to use and are safe enough to drink.

4. **Personal care products.** Most shampoo, rinses, lotions, and cosmetics contain petrochemicals. In 1998 the U.S. Department of Health and Human Services announced that diethanolamine, when applied to the skin, resulted in clear evidence of carcinogenic activity. However, it still is used in the cosmetic and personal care industry and in home cleaners; it is found in over 600 products in the name – DEA and

1 U.S. Environmental Protection Agency, Office of Acid Deposition, Environmental Monitoring and Quality Assurance. Project Summary: The Total Exposure Assessment Methodology (TEAM) Study. EPA-600-S6-87-002, 1987.

Cocamide DEA. Another reason to read a label. Propylene glycol, the main ingredient in anti-freeze, is not only used in cosmetics, cleansers but now food products. It is the most widely used base for liquid "natural" flavorings. Propylene glycol has been linked to kidney damage, contact dermatitis, inhibit skin cell growth, rashes and more. The article Labels and Household Toxins in Appendix S is a guide to help identify the toxic products in every home.

5. **Increase free-radical protection.** Max Gerson M.D., founder of the famous Gerson Institute, found that cancer cells grow in an environment low in oxygen and fermentation. A believer that only a detoxified body has the power and resistance to heal itself of cancer, Dr. Gerson stated that proper sodium/potassium ratios where key to cancer prevention and reversal. He said "Cancer is not a single cellular problem, it is an accumulation of deteriorating metabolism, liver impairment and numerous damaging factors.[2]" Dr. Bruce Ames of the University of California at Berkley estimates that our cells are attacked by free-radial 10,000 per day, and it is this lifetime of free-radical assault that causes DNA damage, aging and possibly cancer. An Italian study looked at more than 2,500 women ages 20 to 74. One group with cancer, one without. Those with cancer had a significantly lower intake of antioxidants.

6. **Detoxification.** The colon, kidneys, liver – all the body organs can accumulate waste and toxins – and the blood can and should be detoxified. This can be done on a small scale daily by incorporating some form of cleaning food, nutrient or protocol. All successful, natural cancer-healing protocols use massive, extensive cleansing routines on patients.

7. **Supplements.** While not a remedy, proper supplementation may be a critical component to well being and cancer prevention. Important ones for the diet include: probiotics for healthy gut flora, and amino acids, the building blocks of protein. Excess animal protein with improper digestion and elimination can be a contributing factor in cancer, amino acids from plants (fruits and vegetables) have shown anticancer activity. One amino acid l-glutathione is critical in liver cleansing and found in abundance in NingXia Red and both lemon and orange essential oils. Enzymes for both digestion and blood cleaning aid the body in riding itself of undigested foods and toxins. Supplementing selenium amplifies NK cell production and stimulates DNA repair enzymes. One great source is Brazil nuts. Omega-3 fatty acids from both fish oils and plants tend to inhibit certain tumor producing substances. Woman with high concentrations of Omega-3 in breast tissue were five times less likely to develop deadly metastasis. See Appendix DD regarding choosing supplements.

8. **Herbs.** These have long been used to aid people with cancer. Rene Cassia, a nurse, made Essiac tea famous for its ability to arrest many cancers. The tea is also known as Ojibway tea, named for a native tribe in North America or present-day Canada. The herbs used are burdock, turkey rhubarb, sheep sorrel and slippery elm. Essential oils, the most potent form of an herb, have a great deal of research as to their benefit in cancer prevention and healing. Essential oils from lemon and orange contain limonene which stimulates two primary phases of liver detoxification.

Ground breaking research published in 2004 at Brigham Young University for the first time identified essential oils which effectively kill cancer cells while being non-toxic to normal cells (non neoplastic cells). Some of the most effective oils studied included sandalwood essential oil which inhibited growth by up to 90 percent of several different types of cancer cells (cervical, breast, skin and prostate), while having little or no harmful effect on normal cells. Sandalwood showed excellent action even at very small concentrations (100 ppm). Tsuga, thyme, grapefruit, and thyme linalool also showed low normal cell toxicity and strong anticancer action.

---

2 "A Cancer Therapy: Results of Fifty Cases and the Cure of Advanced Cancer" Max Gerson, M.D., Gerson Inst; 6th edition.

Oils rich in limonene, such as lemon, orange, tangerine, and Idaho balsam fir have been shown in clinical studies to have potent anticarcinogenic effects. According to a study at the Indiana University-Purdue University at Indianapolis, "monoterpenes would appear to act through multiple mechanisms in the chemoprevention and chemotherapy of cancer.[3]" Studies using one to 15 grams a day of limonene in very advanced cancer patients resulted in almost 20 percent of the patients going into remission. To enhance the action of essential oils, strong cleansing and nutritional building programs are required.

On March 17, 2009, researchers with the University of Oklahoma Health Sciences Center and Oklahoma City VA Medical Center reported that they had found that the frankincense essential oil from the Somalian frankincense herb Boswellia carteri killed off bladder cancer cells. Published in the BioMed Central Complementary and Alternative Medicine, the study tested the frankincense oil on human bladder cancer cells and normal human bladder cells and found that the frankincense was able to descriminate between normal and cancerous bladder cells. "Frankincense oil may represent an inexpensive alternative therapy for patients currently suffering from bladder cancer," researcher H.K. Lin said in a statement.[4] The frankincense oil used in the study was from Young Living Essential Oils.

Books related to cancer:

- Cancer Verses Essential Oils – Essential Science Publishing
- Rub A Dub Dub, is Cancer in your Tub booklet– Young Living Essential Oils
- Cancer Diagnosis: What to do Next – by W. Lee Cowden, Burton Goldberg, W. John Diamond, published by Future Medicine Pub.
- Definitive Guide to Cancer: An Integrative Approach to Prevention, Treatment, and Healing by Lise Alschuler, ND and Karolyn A. Gazella, published by Celestial Arts (expanded version of the above book with many alternative medical physician's guidelines to prevention and healing protocols)
- NingXia Red, the Ultimate Superfood – Essential Science publishing
- Cancer: Curing the Incurable -- William Kelly, D.D.S., M.S.

So to reduce risk, we must be proactive and start making changes today. We must take care of our bodies as if they will last for a 100 more years.

---

3 "Prevention and therapy of cancer by dietary monoterpenes" Crowell P. Journal of Nutrition. 1999 Mar;129(3):775S-778S
4 http://www.biomedcentral.com/content/pdf/1472-6882-9-6.pdf

Appendix X: Sleep

Sleep is the time our bodies cleanse and rejuvenate. While we sleep the body is at work feeding and replenishing our glands and organs. It is widely known that people with interrupted sleep patterns, known as sleep apnea, rob the heart of needed oxygen and many have heart issues later in life. Sleep also recharges us mentally and physically.

How much sleep do we need? Is there a certain time we should be sleeping?

According to the National Sleep Foundation, there are over 70 sleep disorders suffered by nearly 40 million Americans. Moodiness, irritability, flat emotional responses, impaired coordination and memory loss are all signs a person could be suffering from lack of sleep. Stress is the number one cause of disrupted sleep and is usually resolved as the stressful event passes.

Truck drivers and night shift workers make up a large percentage of adults suffering from a lack of sleep. Every year in America falling asleep while driving is responsible for at least 100,000 automobile accidents resulting in 71,000 injuries and 1,550 deaths. Young people particularly are susceptible to the effects of chronic sleep loss and are involved in more than 50 percent of the fall-asleep crashes on American highways each year.

Did you know?

The cause of the infamous 1989 grounding of the oil tanker Exxon Valdez in Prince William Sound offshore Alaska was attributed to the crew's sleep deprivation by the National Transportation Safety Board. As a result, an estimated 11 million gallons of crude oil spilled into the sensitive ecosystem, affecting 28 fish and wildlife species.

Sleep loss also interferes with the learning of young people in our nation's schools. A majority of grade school and high school children reported that they are tired during the daytime and 15 percent of them admitting to falling asleep in class. Additionally, preschool children with poor sleep patterns were twice as likely to use drugs, tobacco and /or alcohol.[1]

There are a few people who manage to get by on very little sleep, six hours or less; however, the majority of people need more than six hours of sleep. Infants will sleep up to 18 hours during a 24-hour time period; toddlers about 12; teens should have eight to 10 and adults seven to nine.

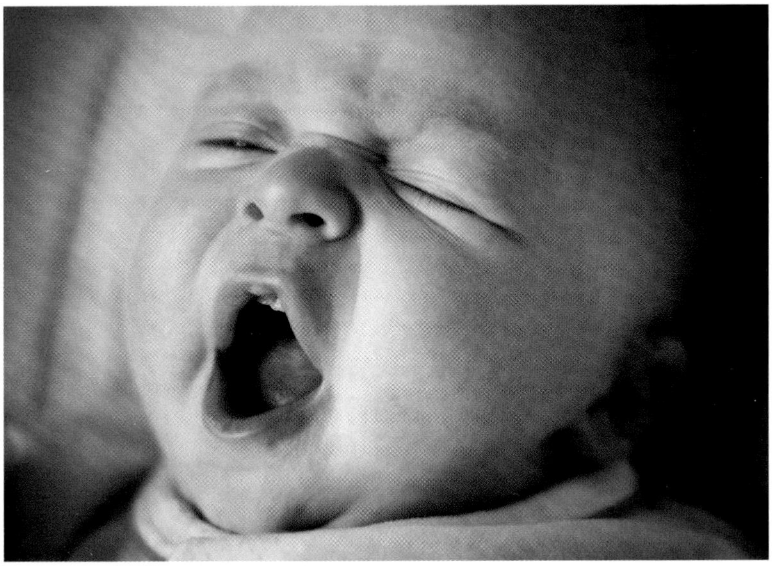

The adrenal glands are one of the first body organs to be affected by sleep. Many will turn to coffee or other caffeinated beverage first thing in the morning to wake-up tired adrenals. According to Chinese Traditional Medicine, the adrenal glands refortify themselves between the hours of 10 p.m. and 2 a.m., so it is important that some of your sleep is within this time period.

1 University of Michigan Health System, 2004 issue of Alcoholism: Clinical and Experimental Research

According to leading sleep researchers, there are techniques to combat common sleep problems:

- Keep a regular sleep/wake schedule.
- Refrain from drinking or eating caffeine four to six hours before bed and minimize daytime use.
- Do not smoke, especially near bedtime or if awake in the night.
- Avoid alcohol and heavy meals before sleep.
- Get regular exercise.
- Minimize noise, light and excessive hot and cold temperatures in the sleeping environment.
- Develop a regular bedtime and go to bed at the same time each night.
- Try to wake up without an alarm clock.
- Attempt to go to bed earlier every night for a certain period of time to readjust your sleep cycle.

Fun Fact

Look into my eyes. One easy way to see if the adrenal glands may need some support is to look in your eyes. Face a mirror close up. Look at one eye, paying attention to the pupil. Does it slowly expand and contract as the eye focuses, or does it appear to have its own heart beat? Is it about one-third the size of the iris, or larger? If it seems to have it's own heart beat or is larger than half the circumference of the iris, your adrenals may need supplementation with vitamin C and pantethenic acid as well as better sleep.

Sleep vs. Test Cramming

According to the Secondary School Admission Testing, cramming is not as useful or effective as learning at the traditional, and presumably more thorough, pace established at school.

What will help us learn are: good nights of sleep, a nutritious diet, exercise and good study skills and habits.

Fun Fact

Cramming for a test all night long in lieu of a good night's sleep is worthless. Cramming information places it into our brains short-term memory storage. In order to learn, we have to transfer information into long-term memory. Once there, it can be retrieved far easier over a longer period of time.

For more information on a learning program of study skills suitable for all ages go to: www.newamericanschool.com and select Products.

- Adjust studying strategies over a broad range of learning needs.
- Understand the meaning and significance of what is learned rather than simply rote learning information.
- Think more and work less.
- Assimilate a significant amount of their textual material in a minimum of time.
- Quickly target the most important information needing to be learned.
- Apply multiple note-taking techniques.
- Prepare to take notes in class and while reading text.
- Manage study time to become more effective and efficient.

Debra's note: This is the program that my homeschool daughter used to complete high school two years ahead of schedule, and I personally have used in my professional life with great success.

Appendix Y: Microwaves

Microwave ovens were first introduced in 1967 and have become ingrained in our culture, supplying heated food with little or no preparation for our fast-paced, on-the-go American lifestyle. However, this convenience was not without controversy. Many experts were concerned that the microwave would further decrease interest in healthy food and move families further away from the dinner table. Now scientific evidence is mounting against this once-loved appliance, proving what its opponents feared.

Before nuking, consider the following facts:[1]

Microwaving:

- Causes foods lose 60 to 90 percent of the vital-energy field and microwaving accelerates the structural disintegration of foods.
- Creates cancer-causing agents within milk and cereals.
- Alters elemental food-substances, causing digestive disorders.
- Alters food chemistry, which can lead to malfunctions in the lymphatic system and degeneration of the body's ability to protect itself against cancerous growths.
- Altered the breakdown of elemental substances when raw, cooked, or frozen vegetables were exposed for even a very short time and free radicals were formed.
- The microwave field next to a microwave oven caused a slew of health problems as well.

Microwaved foods:

- Caused stomach and intestinal cancerous growths, a general degeneration of peripheral cellular tissues, and a gradual breakdown of the digestive and excretive systems in a statistically high percentage of people.
- Lead to a higher percentage of cancerous cells in the bloodstream.
- Lowered the body's ability to utilize B-complex vitamins, vitamin C and E, essential minerals and lipotropics.

Safe alternatives to microwaves are:

- Stove-top heating for liquids or frozen items. A small amount of water will provide enough steam to heat frozen foods.
- Toaster ovens, an inexpensive appliance that heats food electrically with high-resistant heating element.
- Convection ovens, also known as fan ovens or turbo ovens, cook food like a traditional oven, but use a fan to circulate heated air for quicker cooking. They come in traditionally sized ovens or in single, counter top size.
- A saucepan lid over a dinner plate of food will keep it warm until the late-comer gets home. Another option is to put the plate on top of a simmering pan of water to keep it warm without drying it out.
- A warming drawer, available in some conventional oven models, keep leftovers warm without heating the entire oven.

1 Lubec, G. et al. (1989): Aminoacid Isomerisation and Microwave Exposure. The Lancet, 2 (8676): 1392-93; and The World Foundation for Natural Science : "Are Microwave Ovens a Source of Danger?," Microwave Oven Critique" http://www.natural-science.org/en/frames.html , and "The Hidden Hazards of Microwave Cooking," http://www.nexusmagazine.com/microwave.html, from Nexus Magazine; and "Healing with Whole Foods" by Paul Pitchford, pg. 20.

Further research

The World Foundation for Natural Science : "Are Microwave Ovens a Source of Danger?," Microwave Oven Critique" http://www.naturalscience.org/en/frames.html, and "The Hidden Hazards of Microwave Cooking," http://www.nexusmagazine.com/microwave.html, from Nexus Magazine

The World Foundation for Natural Science : "Are Microwave Ovens a Source of Danger?," Microwave Oven Critique" http://www.naturalscience.org/en/frames.html

Science News, 4/25/1992 issue and "The Hidden Hazards of Microwave Cooking," http://www.nexusmagazine.com/microwave.html, from Nexus Magazine

Health, Wealth & Happiness, "MICROWAVED FOOD: It's Like Eating Nuclear Waste!."

http://www.relfe.com/microwave.html

Lubec, G. et al. (1989): Aminoacid Isomerisation and Microwave Exposure. ? The Lancet, 2 (8676): 1392-93; and The World Foundation for Natural Science : "Are Microwave Ovens a Source of Danger?," Microwave Oven Critique" http://www.naturalscience.org/en/frames.html , and "The Hidden Hazards of Microwave Cooking," http://www.nexusmagazine.com/microwave.html, from Nexus Magazine; and "Healing with Whole Foods" by Paul Pitchford, pg. 20.

Appendix Z: Cadmium - A Silent Culprit

Cadmium is a trace mineral element found in soil. It is also present in the smoke from cigarette, cigar and pipe smoking. Cadmium can be seen as the blue color in a smoke-filled room or smog over large industrialized cities.

Found in refined flour products, coffee, tea and some seafood, cadmium is one of the most toxic substances known to mankind.

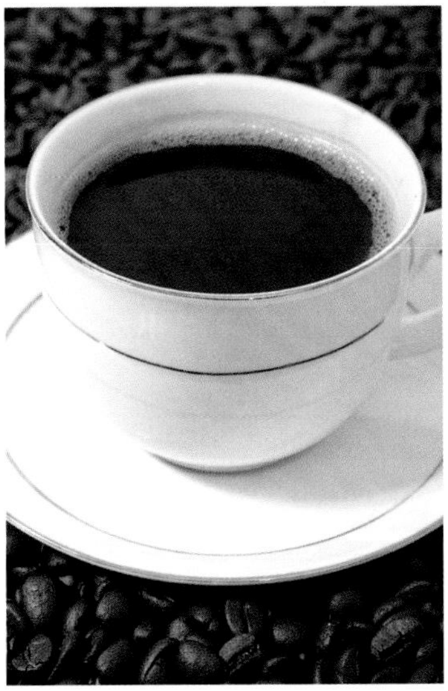

It has been discovered that cadmium is involved in all eight processes that develop cancer. These eight processes are responsible for the over 800 named types of cancer. Cadmium facilitates the progression of every one of these. It accumulates in most malignant cells – in prostate cancer there is a direct correlation between the grade of malignancy and cadmium content. It has a half life in the human body of 15 to 20 years and is considered to be one of the most insidious and dangerous heavy metals found in the human body.

Crustaceans, such as crabs and lobsters, and mollusks, such as clams and oysters, have higher cadmium levels; though many are also high in zinc, which helps balance the cadmium somewhat. Cadmium also is a component of alloys, used in electrical materials, and is present in ceramics, some older dental materials and storage batteries. Because it has a unique capacity to form close bonds with chloride compounds, cadmium is used in many fertilizers, pesticides and herbicides.

Cadmium acts like a stress agent and has been implicated in learning disorders. Alone, cadmium is highly toxic, combined with other agents – it could be deadly! When exposed to other chemical toxins, the cadmium helps transfer these toxic chemicals from the tissue through the lipid membrane of the cells to increase the ratio of bad to good minerals.

However, cadmium exposure is countered by keeping the beneficial essential and trace minerals – zinc, copper and magnesium – optimal in the body, leaving no room for the cadmium, and it is excreted.

During the growth of grains such as wheat and rice, cadmium from the soil is concentrated in the core, or endosperm of the kernel, while zinc is found mostly in the germ and bran coverings. Using the whole wheat berry allows us to receive 100 percent of the nutrients God placed in the grain, including the proper ratio of cadmium to zinc, which causes no harm. However, when processed into white flour, 30 percent of the nutrients are removed, particularly the outer layer and germ, and the only mineral left in the starchy endosperm is cadmium. Processing gets rid of the zinc and copper, which was in a 200:1 ratio to cadmium. Eating whole grains, gives the body minerals in proper proportion and leaves no cadmium overexposure in the endosperm.

Cadmium occurs naturally in the wheat berry is to control insects. When an insect begins to nibble on a wheat berry and reaches the endosperm ingesting the cadmium, they die. This is one reason cadmium is found in many commercial fertilizers and insect control products.

The zinc-cadmium ratio is very important, as cadmium toxicity and storage are greatly increased with zinc deficiency, and good levels of zinc protect against tissue damage by cadmium. Cadmium levels in humans tend to increase with age, most likely because of chronic subtle exposure, usually peaking at around age 50 and then leveling off. Interestingly, no cadmium is present in newborns, as cadmium does not cross the placenta-fetal barrier, nor the blood-brain barrier like lead and mercury do. So cadmium is not toxic to unborn babies, nor does it cause the mental or brain symptoms of lead and mercury toxicity.

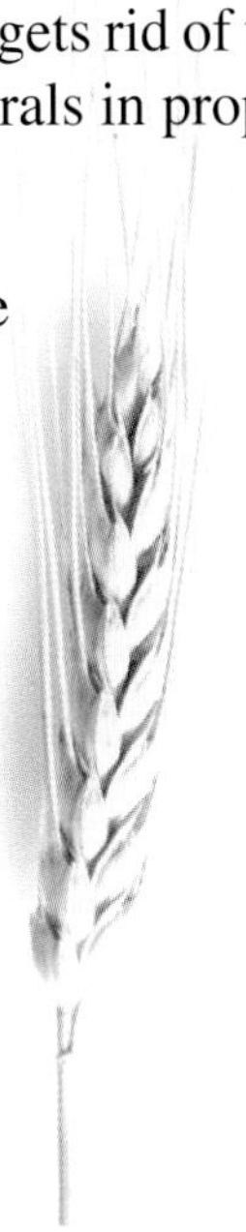

Cadmium is excreted mainly by the kidneys. This mineral is stored primarily in the liver and kidneys. As zinc has an affinity for the testes, cadmium also is stored there in higher concentrations than in other tissues. With aging, cadmium accumulates in the kidneys and may predispose a person to hypertension. In one study of a group of men with hypertension and lowered zinc levels, their hypertension went away when adequate zinc levels were restored.

This hypertension is likely related to the reduced zinc-cadmium ratio. The cadmium effect may contribute not only to hypertension, but to heart disease as well. In rat studies, higher levels of cadmium are associated with an increase in heart size, higher blood pressure, progressive atherosclerosis and reduced kidney function. In humans, cadmium toxicity is worse with zinc deficiency and reduced with higher zinc intake.

One pack of cigarettes contains about 20 microgram (mcg) of cadmium, or about 1 mcg per cigarette. About 30 percent of that goes into the lungs and is absorbed, and the remaining 70 percent goes into the atmosphere to be inhaled by others or to contaminate the environment. With long-term smoking, the risk of cadmium toxicity is increased. Though most of it is eliminated, a little bit is stored every day, making life-long smokers and second-hand smoke breathers more at risk for cadmium-related disease.

Water pipes can be a source of cadmium concentration. Cadmium often is used to protect metals from corrosion. Galvanized (zinc) pipes usually contain some cadmium, as does the solder used to hold them together. Soft or acid water is corrosive and causes the metals in the pipes to break down, releasing cadmium and other minerals from them. Hard water containing calcium and magnesium salts actually coats the pipes and protects against the leaching of other minerals.

Though cadmium has no known useful biological function, it competes with zinc for binding sites and can therefore interfere with some of zinc's essential functions. In this way, it may inhibit enzyme reactions and utilization of nutrients.

Cadmium may be a catalyst to oxidation reactions, which can generate free-radical tissue damage.

Cadmium also affects the bones. It has been known to cause bone and joint aches and pains. This syndrome, first described in Japan, where it was termed the itai-itai, or ouch-ouch, disease, was caused by cadmium pollution there. It also was associated with weak bones that lead to deformities, especially of the spine, or to more easily broken bones. This disease was fatal in many cases.

We may be seeing an increase in emphysema due to cadmium exposure. Anemia also seems to be a problem connected with cadmium overload. Most of these potential cadmium toxicity problems, including its immuno-suppressant actions and its role in cancer, hypertension, and heart and kidney disease, need to be substantiated by more research. Knowing this, it is safe to say we all need to reduce our exposure to this mineral.

So how do we get rid of excess cadmium in the body?

1. Intravenous and oral EDTA chelation has been shown to be effective in increasing cadmium elimination, though this probably is indicated only at more toxic levels. This can be very costly and take about six months of weekly office visits costing as much as $10,000. Tests checking mineral loss and kidney function often are part of the protocol as chelation does not discriminate between good and bad mineral removal.

2. Bio-electric field enhancement (BEFE) hydrotherapy uses ionizing foot baths to produce a significant output of cadmium. Taking about 45 minutes per session and involving multiple sessions, this can be very time consuming and costly as well.

3. Heavy metal oral chelators are the preferred choice for both cost and effectiveness.

4. High intake of zinc, as well as of calcium and selenium will protect against further cadmium absorption. In addition, adequate body levels of zinc may displace some tissue cadmium. Iron, copper, selenium, and vitamin C have been shown to increase cadmium elimination as measured by urine levels.

5. As cadmium can generate free radicals, taking both water and fat soluble antioxidants should be a standard part of our nutritional routines. Because cadmium is excreted generally through the kidneys, it is imperative that proper kidney function be maintained.

What steps should we take to prevent further cadmium toxicity?

1. Exposure to cadmium through air contamination usually is minimal compared to that from food and water – the most important steps to changing lifestyle and diet. Avoid cadmium exposure and intake primarily by eliminating smoking and exposure to cigarette smoke. Also avoid refined foods (white flour products), shellfish in moderation and coffee. Traditional teas should be replaced with good water or herbal tea, and soft water should be filtered. While organic coffee no doubt contains less than commercial grown and fertilized coffee, the risk factors for future problems are greater.

2. Eating high zinc foods, such as whole grains, legumes, and nuts, help abate cadmium. Be aware that when learning about foods high in zinc that those that are equally high in cadmium should be eaten in moderation. For example, oysters are high in zinc but also high in cadmium. Other foods high in zinc but not cadmium are pumpkin seeds, wheat germ, sesame seeds, sage, hot peppers, celery seed, mustard seeds and basil.

3. Proper supplementation is key. Taking additional zinc, 15 to 30 mg. daily in a supplement will offer further protection against cadmium problems and may be necessary for some individuals with already compromised health. Antioxidant rich foods will help to fight the free radical damage cadmium toxicity can cause.

Appendix AA: Spices for Good Health

Most people add great flavor to the food they prepare with a variety of culinary spices. While some spices are mostly for flavor, many common spice herbs also are medicinal. The following spices have been proven historically to be of nutritional value and should become a valuable part of daily nutrition. The information below is for using the powdered, fresh, flake or essential oil forms.

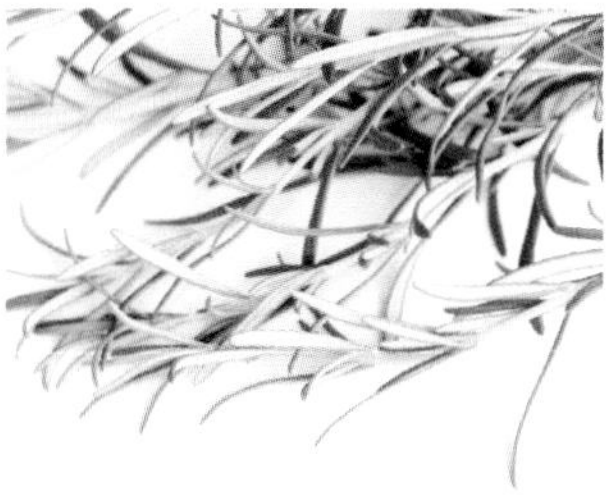

Rosemary is thought to promote memory and fidelity. It was often used in wreaths and garlands at weddings. It is known as a blood thinner and strengthens heart muscles and weak stomachs. Many people describe its flavor as warm and spicy with a fragrance of pine and nutmeg combined. It is commonly added to meat dishes of lamb, veal and pork and gives a robust flavor to vegetables. It is thought to improve the immune system, promote youthfulness and is helpful in cases of Candida (yeast). Rosemary tea is a good hair rinse to promote growth, relieve dandruff and restore hair color. Rosemary stimulates circulation and eases pain by increasing blood flow when applied. Rosemary essential oil commonly is used to enhance memory function and cleanse the liver. Until recently French hospitals used rosemary to disinfect the air. Rosemary oil also may help with infectious diseases, hepatitis, hair loss and shows promise in Alzheimer's.

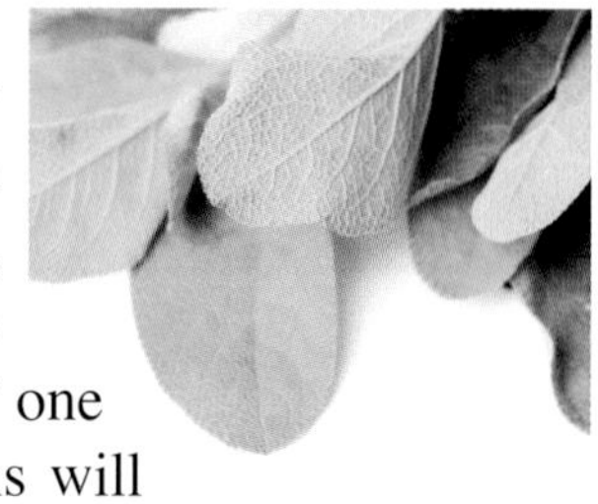

Basil was said to have been found growing at Christ's tomb and even today many churches use basil in the preparation of holy water. Its aromatic influence is said to help a person have an open mind. Basil is regarded as brain food and is said to aid in depression, nervous exhaustion and mental fatigue. Basil may help fight viruses and may be used to fight colds, flu, indigestion, kidney problems, cramps and constipation. A tea made of one ounce of basil simmered in a pint of water for 20 minutes with six black peppercorns will relieve most fevers. Basil is an insect repellent, and when the oil or juice is applied to the skin it is reported to relieve the sting of insect bites, as well as itching and ringworm. Another topical use for basil essential oil is as a pain reliever for lower back ailments and migraines.

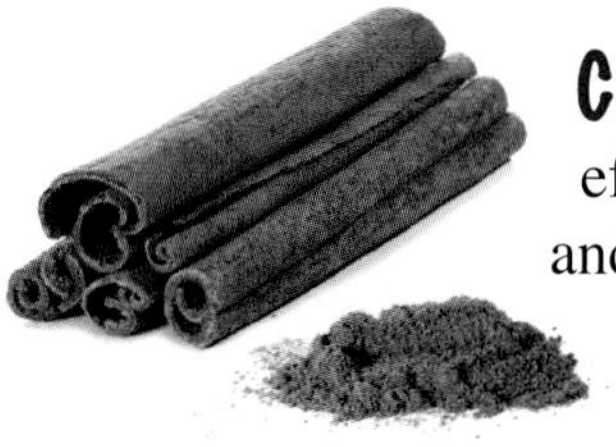

Cinnamon is an ancient spice used throughout history to warm the body. It has a calming effect and is said to have a frequency that attracts wealth. Cinnamon is used for fighting viral and infectious diseases. Viruses, bacteria and fungus cannot live in the presence of cinnamon oil.[1] Cinnamon is a germicide, blood conditioner and helps circulation. For bleeding bowels drink one half cup cinnamon tea four times daily. To remove fallout, radiation and lead poisoning, sprinkle a generous amount of cinnamon on toasted whole wheat bread and eat. For colds, combine cinnamon, sage, bay leaves and cloves in apple juice. Bring to a boil, turn off heat, stir and cover. Let it cool slightly and then drink. Cinnamon oil can be quite hot when applied undiluted to the skin or placed in the mouth full strength. Taken in capsules with meals or other oils it is not hot to the digestive tract. Cinnamon bark oil is widely used to lower blood sugar. Its cousin – **cassia oil**, mentioned numerous times in the Bible, can be taken orally providing a great breath freshener. Cassia may help fight fungal infections and also may reduce inflammation and swelling while acting like a COX 2 inhibitor. Once you start putting a drop of cassia on your tongue, you'll likely continue – it is fresh and invigorating.

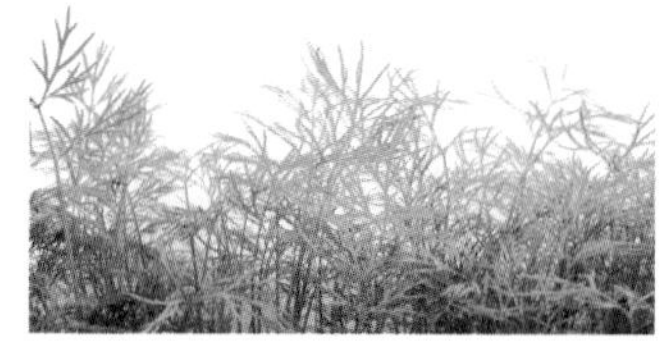

Dill tea can be made from one teaspoon of dill seeds and eight ounces of water that are brought to a boil and steeped 20 minutes then strained. This helps to relieve gas, cramps and colic. The seeds can be chewed to freshen the breath. Additionally, dill

1 "The Ultimate Antiseptics: 12 Essential Oils that Wipe Out Disease-causing Bacteria, Molds and Viruses." Demarco, Carolyn, M.D. Essential Science Publishing. 2006

seeds are thought to be beneficial for children with learning disabilities. Simmer dill seeds in olive oil and rub on your forehead to promote better sleep. To overcome hardened bowel movements, simmer one teaspoon of dill seed in one cup boiling water. Strain the seeds and spread them on whole wheat bread and eat. Drink the remaining tea for improvement in digestion. Dill oil commonly is used in the Middle East for blood sugar disorders.

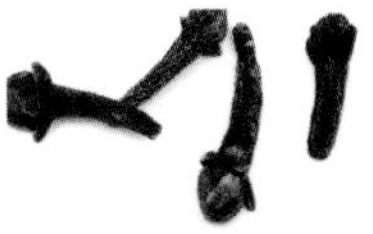

Cloves are also known as Peruvian Balm. A few cloves in a cup of water helps if you suffer from mucus in the chest, nausea, vomiting and eczema with ulceration. Cloves will help settle loud chest rattles. Cloves may expel worms. It freshens breath when chewed. Cloves are beneficial to the liver when it is swollen and hard, damaged or contains tumors. For a paper cut on the hand, wet the finger and apply powdered cloves. The pain will quickly disappear as cloves act like an anesthetic on the skin. Clove essential oil has medical research showing its benefit to prevent blood clotting, equally effective as prescription drugs. Clove is the highest antioxidant spice/herb yet discovered with an Oxygen Radical Absorbance Capacity (ORAC) rating of 1,078,700.

Thyme is an herb with many therapeutic properties. It is antiseptic in nature and has been used in tea to treat roundworm, tapeworm, threadworm and hookworm. It stimulates the production of white blood cells. Thyme is a digestive tonic, improves sluggish digestion, colic, gas and indigestion. Thyme tea is a reliable folk remedy for relieving phlegm and shortness of breath. It has been used as a skin antiseptic for lice, scabies, insect and snake bites. It may help heal wounds and is thought to stop hair loss. Thyme promotes blood circulation and relieves muscular pain. Thyme oil is also used for back pain and may help fight viruses.

Anise was originally brought to America by the colonists as a medicinal herb. It made a great tea for indigestion and colic in babies. Chronic asthma cases are aided by anise tea. In olden times, anise was used to heal kidney stones. They would put one tablespoon of anise in a quart of grape juice and simmer for 30 minutes. They would drink seven ounces of this, three times per day. Twelve drops of anise oil is said to improve liver function.

Bay leaves have been used for centuries. The Roman's used bay leaves for prophecy and for healing. Bay leaves spread around the pantry will keep the bugs "at bay." Bay leaf is a digestive aid. The oil of bay leaves massaged into joints and muscles brings relief for pain. Bay leaves have been combined with cinnamon, sage and cloves in a tea as a natural cold remedy.

Cayenne was introduced to the Western world in 1548 from India. Books have been written as to the medicinal properties of cayenne making it possibly the most written about and researched herb. Cayenne is a stimulant herb benefiting the heart and preventing a heart attack. Cayenne binds bile and cholesterol in the intestinal tract for elimination. When used as a poultice, cayenne will draw out toxins under the skin. Cayenne ointment, salve or even hot cayenne fomentations can be applied to sore muscles and will provide quick relief. Use cayenne daily in a tea, capsule, tincture, powder or raw fruit and see amazing good health return.

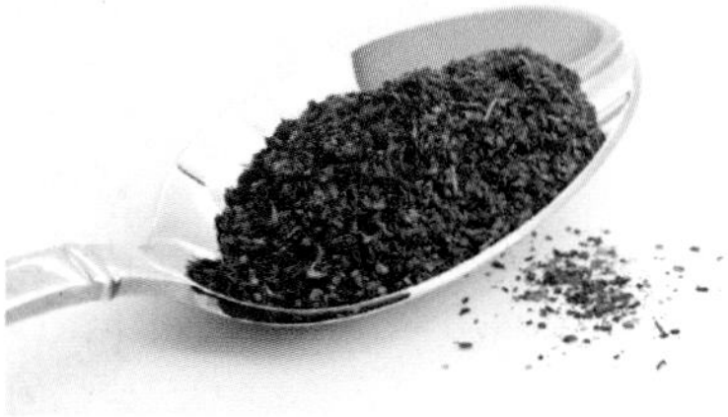

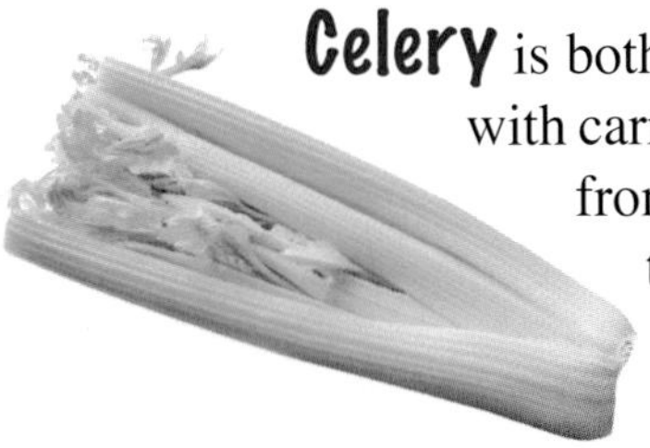

Celery is both an important food and medicinal spice. Celery contains organic sodium. Juiced with carrots it not only makes a delicious drink, but the sodium balances the loss of minerals from exercise. Organic sodium in celery will suspend inorganic calcium deposits in the body's water until they can be flushed from the system. Celery increases uric acid excretion and has been used as a kidney cleanser and for the removal of urinary tract stones.

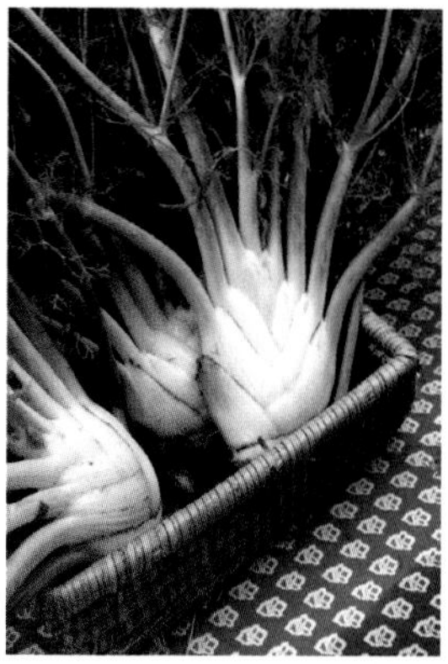

Fennel seed is naturally sweet and delicious. It has been used to prevent obesity by chewing on the seeds when a person is hungry. Used as a mouthwash, fennel is thought to help with loose teeth and gum disease. Fennel and catnip tincture applied to a sore tooth often brings relief. Fennel is added routinely to colic tonics for babies. When a nursing mother drinks fennel tea, it may also ease colic in her infant. It has hormonal properties that aid in relieving premenstrual and menopausal symptoms. Fennel has been strewn in beds and pet areas to repel fleas. Steamed fennel stalks served with vinegar and pepper is a favorite Italian dish called cartucci. Often, it is used with laxatives to prevent gripping and gas. Fennel is available as an essential oil and is used in combination with other herbs in the treatment of blood sugar disorders.

Lemon balm was used medicinally by the Greeks over 2,000 years ago. It has been used in preparations for maintaining youth and is thought to strengthen the brain and ease depression. Lemon balm is antibacterial and anti-viral in nature because of the tannins it contains. When taken at the onset of a cold, it appears to stop a cold in its tracks. Steam inhalation of lemon balm leaves will relieve bronchial catarrh (congestion) and sore throats. Applied externally it often brings relief to insect bites. Lemon Balm oil is referred to as Melissa – one of the most potent herbs against viruses. One drop on a cold sore, fever blister or herpes outbreak may help them go away fast.

Nutmeg used sparingly stops fainting spells and will help weak heartbeats. When the digestive enzymes of the pancreas cannot reach the duodenum, people often complain of a swollen pancreas. Nutmeg is most helpful in these cases. Take six to seven ounces of hot water and add one teaspoon of cloves and one quarter teaspoon of nutmeg. Drink for immediate relief. Nutmeg is said to make teenage girls more self-reliant, just by adding a heaping teaspoon of nutmeg to the bath water. Nutmeg tea inspires sleep and is thought to overcome nervous fatigue. *Don't be afraid of nutmeg, but use this spice sparingly as* ***large*** *doses can be toxic and cause miscarriage*. Nutmeg essential oil is often used in thyroid formulations.

Poppy seed and its flowers can be steamed and the vapor inhaled to bring sinus relief. Poppy seeds eaten in breads, cakes, dressings or with a bit of honey will carry excess inorganic nickel away from the body. Excess nickel, which we unknowingly ingest if we consume foods containing hydrogenated oils,[2] can impair the spinal cord and cause paralysis in extreme cases. If you find the seeds irritating, take a tablespoon of poppy seed and soak overnight in water or juice. In the morning strain and drink the liquid. Do again at evening using only water.

The next time you read a recipe that calls for one of these spices, you will know that the flavor of your dish will be enhanced, and so might your health. Many spice herbs are available in the form of a therapeutic-grade essential oil. In the oil form, they are more economical than their powdered or flaked counterparts and free of all irradiation and chemical processing in their purest form. See Appendix DD for more information.

2 "Nickel-- Finely divided nickel dissolves 17 times its own volume of hydrogen, and is extensively used as a catalyzer in hydrogenation of oils" Van Nostrand's Scientific Encyclopedia, 4th Edition, 1968, p. 1186.

Appendix BB: Nutrition 101: Choose Life! Top Foods

Top Foods and Food Ingredients to Avoid - Be A Label Reader!

1. Alcohol

2. Nitrates - sodium nitrite, sodium nitrate - found in processed meats, sandwich meats, hot dogs and sausages.

3. Artificial Sweeteners - Splenda (sucralose), aspartame, saccharine, etc. - found in diet sodas, juice, desserts, ice cream, bread, yogurt, pasta sauce, ketchup, most grocery items labeled "Sugar Free".

4. High Fructose Corn Syrup and Corn Syrup - found in sodas, juices, sports drinks, bread, salad dressing, cake mix, most packaged and processed food items.

5. Refined white sugar - sucrose, sucrose syrup (I saw this one on the label of the new Gatorade "G"), and the other words for sugar (I can't think of them off hand) - found in most packaged and processed food items.

6. Trans Fats - partially hydrogenated oils (any kind), hydrogenated oils, shortening - found in margarines, fried foods, bread, pastries, packaged desserts, salad dressings, most packaged and processed food items.

7. Propylene Glycol - found in breads, boxed cake mixes, dressings, artificial food colorings and processed food items.

8. Artificial colorings and preservatives - found in most processed and packaged foods.

9. White Flour – enriched bleached flour, enriched flour – found in bread and baked goods and packaged pre-baked goods, soups, crackers, cookies and most processed foods.

10. Margarines - contain partially hydrogenated and hydrogenated oils.

11. Soda/soft drinks – all kinds

12. Fried foods

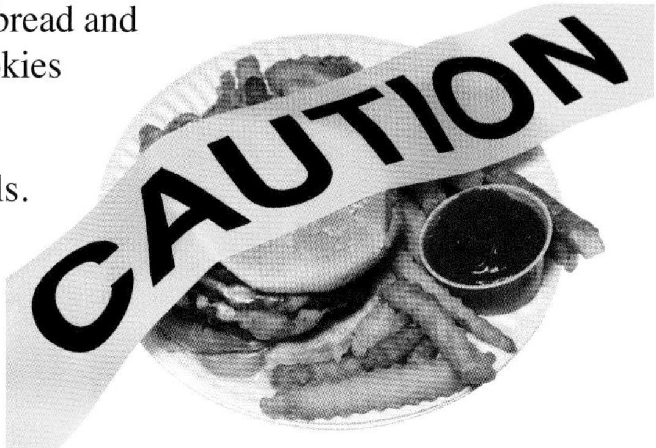

Top 40 Foods to Enjoy!

God gave us His foods to enjoy. The following list of top 40 foods was compiled by the authors of **Nutrition 101: Choose Life!** based on foods readily available in the United States, ease of preparation (raw or cooked), high nutritional value, and, yes, great taste. Enjoy every one of these weekly and enjoy better health and vitality. Each contains more detail to understand why they are our top picks.

1. **Almonds** – These really are fruits, though we classify them and use them as nuts. Almonds have research supporting their benefit in preventing colon cancer, lowering serum cholesterol, and preventing DNA damage. High in vitamin B3, fiber, Omega-6 fats, protein, zinc and potassium.

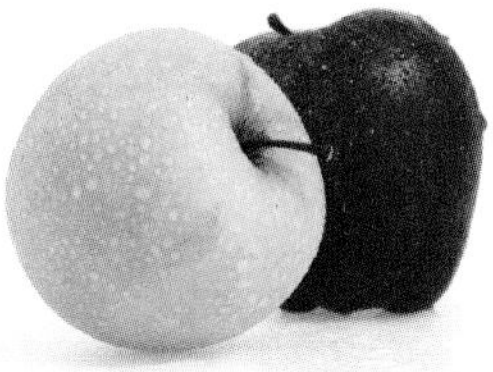

2. **Apples** – Due to their high quercetin content, pectin and other nutrients, apples have been proven supportive in preventing asthma, lung, and colon cancer, as well as in inhibiting various viruses, including polio. Apples are in the top twelve most contaminated fruits and vegetables containing pesticides[1], so please select only organic apples.

1 "The Shopper's Guide to Pesticides in Produce" by the Environmental Working Group, October 4, 2006.

3. **Artichoke, Globe** – With edible leaves and hearts, artichoke is used as food and in many herbal preparations, especially those benefiting the liver. Artichoke may help to prevent atherosclerosis and alleviate various ailments of the kidneys. When infusion applied topically to the hair globe artichoke is claimed to lighten the color of hair.

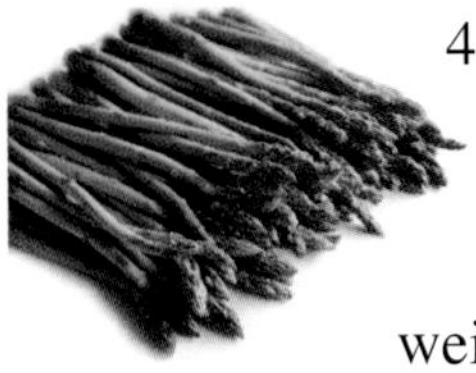

4. **Asparagus** – An excellent source of folate, highly alkaline and a good source of vitamin C, thiamine and vitamin B6, asparagus also is high in glutathione. It has been observed to reduce bone loss, possess cancer cell killing ability and strengthen the cardiovascular system. Asparagus also helps inhibit starch digestion which can be beneficial for diabetics and for weight balance.

5. **Avocado** – It may inhibit the development of some types of cancer, especially prostate, due to its mannoheptulose content inhibiting the glucokinase enzyme and by inhibiting the uptake of glucose into cancer cells. High in vitamin K, folate, lutein, zeaxanthin, beta-carotene and potassium, raw avocado sliced on salads or made into guacamole is delicious and nutritious.

6. **Blueberries** – Loaded with anti-oxidants, blueberries also contain ellagic acid that may inhibit tumor growth. Blueberries are high in vitamin C, lutein, zeaxanthin, flavonoids, beta-carotene, manganese and fiber.

7. **Broccoli** – High in vitamins C and A, folate, calcium, chromium and anti-cancer compounds indoles and isothiocynates, broccoli also contains some of the highest amount of health-promoting sulfur compounds supporting liver health. Broccoli also may inhibit the growth of ulcers with its anti-bacterial compound sulforaphene.

8. **Brussels sprouts** – Rich in vitamins A and K, potassium, phosphorus and calcium, Brussels sprouts, like broccoli, contain high sulfur compounds, increase the liver's detoxification ability and are very low in calories.

9. **Cabbage** – A relative of Brussels sprouts, cabbage is the ultimate digestive and immune system food containing vitamins and fiber. With several varieties, red, Chinese, green and savoy, cabbage may be eaten raw, cooked or fermented. Cabbage also may protect against many cancers, ulcers and viruses.

10. **Cantaloupe** – An excellent source of vitamin A and C, and powerful antioxidants, the distinctive orange color of this sweet melon provides a wealth of beta-carotene.

11. **Carrots** – An excellent source of carotenes, particularly beta-carotene, one cup of carrots provides roughly 686.3 percent of the RDA for vitamin A. Carrots are also a good source of fiber, manganese, niacin, potassium, vitamins B6 and C. Studies show that as little as one carrot a day could cut the rate of lung cancer in half.[2]

12. **Cauliflower** – Full of fiber and vitamins C and K, as well as B vitamins biotin and folate, cauliflower also contains a phytochemical called sulforaphane, which helps the liver produce enzymes that block cancer-causing chemicals from damaging the body. Cauliflower may prevent several types of cancers, such as bladder, breast, colon, lung and stomach.[3]

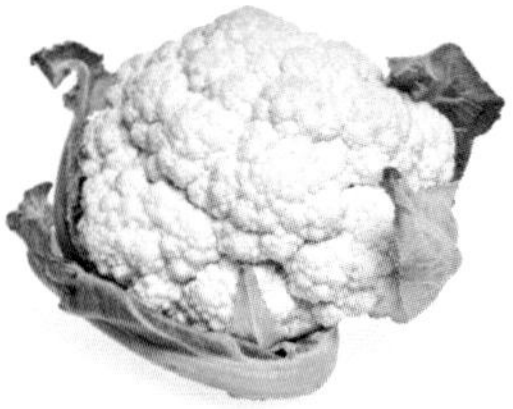

13. **Chia seed** - Chia Seeds contain the highest known proportion of alpha-linolenic acid of any seed. Chia seed oil contains 60 to 63 percent alpha-linolenic acid.

14. **Cucumbers** – High in nutrients, low in calories and very filling, cucumbers are for weight control. A very

---

2 Michaud DS, Fesknich D, Rimm EB, et al. intake of specific carotenoids and risk of lung cancer in 2 prospective US cohorts. *Am J Clin Nutr.* 2000;72(4):990-997. Ylonen K, Alfthan G, Groop, L et al. Dietary intakes and plasma concentrations of carotenoids and tocopherol in relation to glucose metabolism in subjects at high risk of Type 2 diabetes: The Bontnai Dietary Study. Am J Clin Nutr. 2003 June;77(6):1434-1441.

3 Verhoeven, D., et al. A review of mechanisms underlying anticarcinogenicity by brassica vegetables. Chemico-Biological Interactions. 103(2):79-129, 1997.

good source of vitamin C and A, molybdenum, potassium and manganese, these true fruits – because they contain seeds that reproduce – are great for the skin and kidneys.

15. **Flaxseed** – A rich source of Omega-3 fatty acids, flaxseed[4] is an excellent source of soluble and insoluble fiber, beneficial for regulating cholesterol, blood glucose and digestion. A pilot study conducted in India evaluated the effect of flaxseed oil on behavior in children with Attention Deficit Hyperactivity Disorder. There were significant improvements in their symptoms, reflected by reduction in total hyperactivity scores.

16. **Garlic** – Rich sources of vitamin and mineral such as manganese, B6, and vitamin C, garlic also contains unique sulfur compounds that contribute to its health benefits. The evidence is particularly strong for a link between garlic and prevention of prostate and stomach cancers[5].

17. **Grapefruit** – An excellent source of vitamin C, the pink and red varieties are the best because they are 50 times higher in carotenoids, which act as powerful antioxidants. A half a of grapefruit contains more that 150 phytonutrients, mostly flavonoids, believed to help the body fight against aging, allergies, infection, cancer, ulcers and heart disease.

18. **Grapes** – An excellent source of manganese, grapes also are high in vitamin C, B1 and potassium. With a small amount of fiber and a high amount of flavonoids, red grapes contain the carotenoid lycopene, which may help in fighting breast and prostate cancers. A rat study found that the consumption of anthocyanin-rich grape extract blocks breast cell DNA damage.[6]

19. **Green beans** – Green beans are high in vitamins A, C and K and high in minerals manganese, potassium, iron. A good source of dietary fiber, they contain carotenoid phytonutrients, such as beta-carotene, lutein and zeaxanthin, which provide anti-inflammatory properties. High in nutrients and low in calories this makes green beans a great food for weight loss.

20. **Green peas** – True legumes, green peas are a rich source of B vitamins, including B1, B2, B3, B6 and folate, which are essential for the proper metabolism of fats, proteins and carbohydrates. They are also rich in health protective carotenoid phytonutrients, which provide antioxidant protection against the oxidative damage to cellular structures that can be used by free radicals.

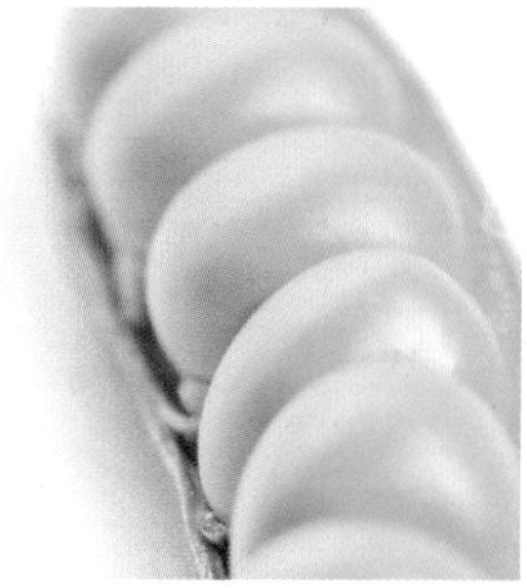

21. **Hazelnuts** - Also known as filberts, hazelnuts are a high source of protein and the amino acid arginine, which supports blood vessel health, and folate. Hazelnut oil applied topically is said to eliminate cellulite.

22. **Kale** – Unfortunately, the primary use of kale in the U.S. is for garnishing. What a shame because kale is one of the healthiest foods a person can add to his or her diet. With only 36 calories per cup (cooked), kale is an excellent source of vitamins A, C and K, potassium and manganese.

23. **Kiwi** – The most nutrient-dense of the 27 most commonly eaten fruits, kiwi has more vitamin C than any other. Kiwis are high in fiber, potassium, and vitamin E and also contains lutein, which is a phytochemical that may reduce the risk of cancer, heart disease and cataracts.

24. **Legumes** – Legumes are common beans such as kidney, black, navy and lentils. More and more people are substituting legumes for meat because of their high supply of low fat protein and they are less expensive than meat. Nutrient-rich, legumes contain vitamins, minerals, phytonutrients, amino acids and dietary fiber.

25. **Lemons** – A member of citrus family lemons are alkaline in nature and when metabolized by the body. An excellent source of vitamin C, they also contain vitamin A, folate, calcium, potassium. limonene and flavonoids, the most common antioxidant found in fruits and vegetables.

4 Because flax contains phyto-estrogen, it may not be recommended to use with certain types of hormone related cancers.
5 "A historical perspective on garlic and cancer" Molner, JA. *J. Nutrition*. 2001. 131:1027s-1031s.
6 Singletary, K. W., et al. J Med Food. 10(2):244-251, 2007

26. **Olives** – More than 80 percent fat, of which approximately 79 percent is made up of oleic acid, a health-promoting monounsaturated fat that supports heart health, olives are a good source of vitamin E, iron, copper and dietary fiber.

27. **Onions** – Containing quercetin, a powerful flavonoid antioxidant which has anti-inflammatory benefits and has been suggested to promote heart health, onions are an excellent source of fiber, vitamin C, chromium and folate. Phytochemicals found in onions, particularly allyl sulfides, appear to reduce the risk of some cancers. An in-vitro study found that onion extract can destroy tumor cells in the test tube and can arrest tumor growth when tumor cells are implanted in rats[7].

28. **Pears** – One medium size pear contains as much vitamin C and potassium as one half cup to orange juice. An average pear contains about four grams of fiber, much of which is made up of soluble pectins and lignans. It is also packed with powerful phytochemical antioxidants.

29. **Prunes** – These are a good source of fiber, potassium, copper and vitamin A. In a study conducted by Tufts University, prunes outranked all other fruits and vegetables tested for their antioxidant values. Phenolic and carotenoid phytonutrients found in prunes, such as chlorogenic acid and neocholrogenic acid, beta-carotene, alpha-carotene and beta-cryptoxanthin, provide powerful antioxidant protection against the oxidative damage caused by free radicals.

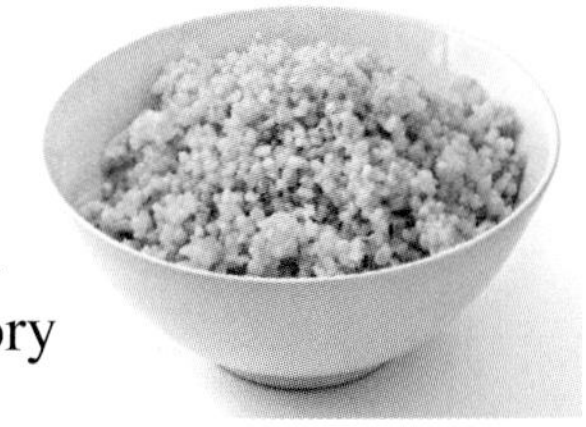

30. **Quinoa** - This small seed of the goosefoot plant is a relative of spinach and Swiss chard. Quinoa comes in colors of pale yellow, red and black. This gluten-free grain is soft and creamy and found in cereals, pasta, flour and breads. Quinoa contains at least 16 different terpine saponins, which may have anti-cancer and anti-inflammatory properties as well as inhibit cholesterol absorption.

31. **Raspberries** – An excellent source of manganese, vitamin C, folate and dietary fiber, raspberries are unusually rich in health-promoting nutrients that provide powerful antioxidant protection from free radicals that can damage cellular structures, including DNA. Ellagic acid and flavonoids such as quercetin, kaemperol and anthocyanins give red raspberries their deep red color.

32. **Rice** - Whole grain brown rice contains all three layers of kernel – the bran, germ and endosperm, which provide superior nutrition values over white rice. Brown rice is rich in lignans, phytoestrogens and phenolic compounds that are high in antioxidant activity and is five times the fiber of white rice. It also may help reduce cholesterol and the risk of breast and colon cancers.[8]

33. **Romaine lettuce** – One of the most nutritious of all lettuces, romaine is an excellent source of vitamins K, A, C, folate, manganese, and chromium. Rich in lutein and zeaxanthin, which are carotenoids found naturally in the eye that fight age-related macular degeneration.

34. **Sesame seeds** – Unhulled seeds that are darker in color and have their bran intact are a great source of calcium. They are more nutritious than the hulled (white) sesame seeds so commonly seen. They are rich in unique lignan phytonutrients, sesamin and sesamolin, which also are found to have anti-inflammatory properties.

35. **Spinach** – An excellent plant-based source of iron that, in comparison to meat sources, is low in calories and virtually fat-free. It also is an excellent source of fiber, vitamins A, C, B2, B6, K and folate, manganese, magnesium, calcium, potassium and tryptophan and rich in glycolipids, powerful phytochemicals known to have cancer cell growth suppression and antiproliferation qualities[9].

---

7 "Can allium vegetables prevent cancer?" Ernst, E. Phytomedicine. 4(1):79-83, 1997.

8 Hudson, E. A., et al.

9 "Inhibitory effects of glycolipids fraction from spinach on mammalian DNA polymerase activity and human cancer cell proliferation" Kuriyama, I., et al. J Nutr Biochem. 2005.

36. **Strawberries** – A serving of eight strawberries contains more vitamin C than an orange. Rich in folate, potassium and fiber, strawberries are second only to plums as the richest fruit in phenolics and antioxidants, being especially high in cancer- and heart disease-fighting flavonoids, anthocyanins, ellagic acid, quercetin, catechin and kaempferol. Harvard researchers found strawberries to have protective qualities for a variety of cancers[10].

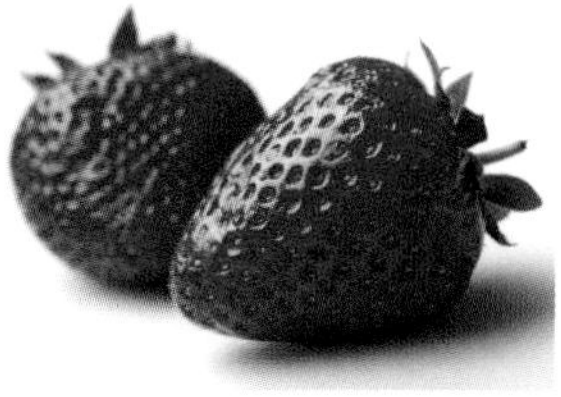

37. **Summer squash** – This vegetable can be grown any time during the warm, frost free season. Also known as Italian marrow, it is an excellent source of vitamin C and manganese, which helps facilitate protein and carbohydrate metabolism and activate enzymes that are responsible for the utilization of important nutrients such as biotin, thiamin and choline.

38. **Sweet potatoes** – Not a part of the nightshade vegetables, this potato makes a good food choice. Rich in vitamin A and beta-carotene, and a good source of vitamins C, B6, manganese, copper, potassium, and fiber. The red variety is an excellent source of the phytochemical lycopene, which my help fight heart disease and breast and prostate cancer.

39. **Tomatoes** – Rich in vitamins C, A and K and potassium, tomatoes are a good source of plant chemicals such as phytosterols, beta-carotene, and lycopene, a protent antioxidant that becomes more abundant when tomatoes are cooked. Tomatoes also contain polyphenols which have been shown effective in halting growth against liver and prostate cancer in cell line studies[11].

40. **Watermelon** – Containing a rich source of heart-healthy nutrients, such as vitamin C and the carotenoid phytonutrient, watermelon gets its reddish-pink distinctive coloration from lycopene. Lycopene, along with beta-carotene and vitamin A, provides powerful antioxidants protection. One cup of watermelon contains only 49 calories.

References

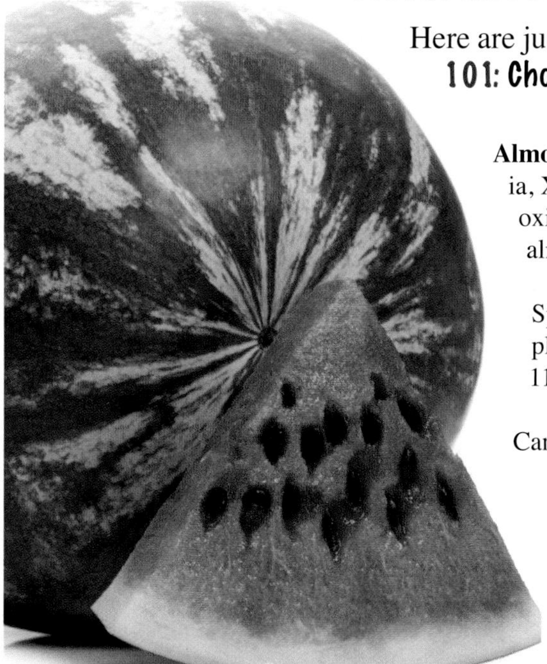

Here are just a few of the references that support the main reasons why **Nutrition 101: Choose Life!** picked these foods as the Top 40 Foods list.

Almonds - www.almondsarein.com

ia, X., et al. A pilot study on the effects of almond consumption on DNA damage and oxidative stress in smokers. Nutrition & Cancer. 54(2):179-183, 2006. (3 – 6 ounces almonds daily)

Spiller, G. A., et al. Effect of a diet high in monounsaturated fat from almonds on plasma cholesterol and lipoproteins. Journal of the American College of Nutrition. 11(2):126-130, 1992. (4 ounces raw almonds)

Cancer Letters. 165:27-33, 2001. (4 ounces)

Apples - www.allaboutapples.com

Chan, A., et al. Apple juice concentrate maintains acetylcholine levels following dietary compromise. Journal of Alzheimer's Disease. 287-291, 2006.

Shaheen, S. O., et al. Dietary antioxidants and asthma in adults: population-based case-control study. American Journal of Respiratory and Critical Care Medicine. 164(10 Part 1):1823-1828, 2001.

10 "Berry extracts exert different antiproliferative effects against cervical and colon cancer cells grown in vitro" McDougall, G. J., et al. J Agric Food Chem 2008

11 "The relationship between dietary carotenoids and prostate cancer risk in Southeast Chinese men" Binns, C. W., et al. Asia Pac J Clin Nutr. 13(Supplement):S117, 2004.

Atichokes, Globe - www.artichokes.org
Zapolska-Downar, D., et al. Protective properties of artichoke (Cynara scolymus) against oxidative stress induced in cultured endothelial cells and monocytes. Life Sciences. 71(24):2897-2908, 2002
Kuoroda, T., et al. Bile acids in hepatic bile in liver disease. Acta Hepato Gastroenterol. 21:120-126, 1974. Globe artichoke preparations were shown to increase the flow of bile from the liver to the gallbladder (choleresis).

Gebhardt, R. Hepatoprotection through artichoke extracts. Pharmazeutische Zeitung. 140:34-37, 1995.

Gebhardt, R. Antioxidative and protective properties of extracts from leaves of the artichoke (Cynara scolymus L.) against hydroperoxide-induced oxidative stress in cultured rat hepatocytes. Toxicol Appl Pharmacol. 144(2):279-286, 1997.

Kraft, K. Artichoke leaf extract: recent findings reflecting effects on lipid metabolism, liver and gastrointestinal tracts. Phytomedicine. 4:369-378, 1997.

Maros, T., et al. The effect of Cynara scolymus extracts on the regeneration of the rat liver. Arzneim Forsch. 16:127-129, 1966.

Asparagus - www.asparagus.org
Clark R, et al. Hyperhomocystenemia: an independent risk factor for. New England J Med 324 (1991(: 1149-55

Mathews JN, Flatt PR, Abel-Wahab YH. Asparagus adscendens (Shweta musali) stimulates insulin secretion, insulin action and inhibits startch digestion. Br J Nutr. 2006 March:95(3):576-581

Avocado - www.avocado.org
Board, M., et al. High Km glucose-phosphorylating (glucokinase) activities in a range of tumor cell lines and inhibition of rates of tumor growth by the specific enzyme inhibitor mannoheptulose. Cancer Res. 55(15):3278-3285, 1995.

Klotter, J. Sugar & cancer - connection between high blood sugar and tumor growth. Townsend Letter for Doctors and Patients. June, 2002.

Quillin, P. Cancer's sweet tooth. Nutrition Science News. April 2000.

Segala, M. (editor). Disease Prevention and Treatment 3rd Edition. Life Extension Media. Florida, USA. 2000:137.

Blueberry - www.blueberry.org
Galli, R. L., et al. Blueberry supplemented diet reverses age-related decline in hippocampal HSP70 neuroprotection. Neurobiol Aging. 2005. Neuroscience Laboratory, USDA-ARS Human Nutrition Research Center on Aging at Tufts University., Boston, MA, USA.

Wilson, M. A., et al. Blueberry polyphenols increase lifespan and thermotolerance in Caenorhabditis elegans. Aging Cell. 5(1):59-68, 2006. Laboratory of Neurosciences, National Institute on Aging, Intramural Research Program, Baltimore, MD, USA.

Bickfored, P. Nutritional support for adult stem cells: guidelines for the clinical practice. Proceedings Report from the American Nutraceutical Association's Fall 2007 CME Conference held in Memphis, Tennessee. Journal of the American Nutraceutical Association. 11(1):12-18, 2008.

Department of Neurosurgery, College of Medicine, University of South Florida, Tampa, Florida, USA.

Broccoli - www.answers.com/topic/broccoli
Beecher, C. W. Cancer preventive properties of varieties of Brassica oleracea: a review. American Journal of Clinical Nutrition. 59(5 Supplement):1166S-1170S, 1994.

Kall, M. A., et al. Effects of dietary broccoli on human in vivo drug metabolizing enzymes: evaluation of caffeine, estrone and chlorzoxazone metabolism. Carcinogenesis. 17(4):793-799, 1996.

Zhang, Y., et al. A major inducer of anticarcinogenic protective enzymes from broccoli: isolation and elucidations of structure. Proceedings of the National Academy of Sciences, USA. 89(6):2399-2403, 1992.

Brussels sprouts - http://www.whfoods.com/genpage.php?tname=foodspice&dbid=10
Beecher, C. W. Cancer preventive properties of varieties of Brassica oleracea: a review. American Journal of Clinical Nutrition. 59(5 Supplement):1166S-1170S, 1994.

Zhu, C. Y., et al. Effect of chemopreventive compounds from Brassica vegetables on NAD(P)H:quinone reductase and induction of DNA strand breaks in murine hepa1c1c7 cells. Food Chem Toxicol. 41(4):455-462, 2003.

Cabbage - www.answers.com/topic/sauerkraut
Monograph: Glutamine. Alternative Medicine Review. 6(4), 2001.

Albert, P. M. Physiological effects of cabbage with reference to its potential as a dietary cancer-inhibitor and its use in ancient medicine. Journal of Ethnopharmacology. 9(2-3):261-272, 1983.

Beecher, C. W. Cancer preventive properties of varieties of Brassica oleracea: a review. American Journal of Clinical Nutrition. 59(5 Supplement):1166S-1170S, 1994.

Verhoeven, D., et al. A review of mechanisms underlying anticarcinogenicity by brassica vegetables. Chemico-Biological Interactions. 103(2):79-129, 1997.

Cantaloupe - http://plantanswers.tamu.edu/vegetables/cantalou.html
Altman, R., et al. Identification of platelet inhibitor present in the melon (Cucurbitacea Cucumis melo). Thrombosis and Haemostatis. 53(3):312-313, 1985.

Carper, Jean. The Food Pharmacy. Simon & Schuster, London. 1990:225.

Carrots - www.carrotmuseum.co.uk/nutrition2.html
Slattery, M., et al. Carotenoids and colon cancer. American Journal of Clinical Nutrition. 71(2):575-582, 2000.

Amin, M., et al. Carrot phytoalexin alters the membrane permeability of Candida albicans and multilamellar liposomes. Journal of General Microbiology. 134(Pt 1):241-246, 1988.

Cauliflower - www.dolenutrition.com/Facts_ae.aspx
Verhoeven, D., et al. A review of mechanisms underlying anticarcinogenicity by brassica vegetables. Chemico-Biological Interactions. 103(2):79-129, 1997.

Lukaczer, D. Nutritional Q&A: cruciferae vs. cancer. Nutrition Science News. November 1998.
Mindell, Earl R. Earl Mindell's Food as Medicine. Simon & Schuster, New York, USA. 1994:110.

Chia seeds - www.living-foods.com/articles/chia.html
Ayerza, R., et al. Ground chia seed and chia oil effects on plasma lipids and fatty acids in the rat. Nutrition Research. 25:995-1003, 2005.

Office of Arid Lands Studies. The University of Arizona. Tucson , Arizona USA.

Cucumbers - www.cucumbergrowingtips.com
Murray, Michael T. The Healing Power of Foods. Prima Publishing, Rocklin, California, USA. 1993:111-112.

Flax - www.flaxcouncil.ca; www.flaxrd.com
Prasad, K. Dietary flax seed in prevention of hypercholesterolemic atherosclerosis. Atherosclerosis. 132(1):69-76, 1997.

Department of Physiology, College of Medicine, University of Saskatchewan, Saskatoon, Canada.

Clark, W. F., et al. Flaxseed: a potential treatment for lupus nephritis. Kidney Int. 48(2):475-480, 1995.

Department of Medicine, University of Western Ontario, London, Canada. Flaxseed is rich in alpha-linolenic acid (alpha-LA) which has anti-atherogenic properties, and lignans which are platelet activating factor (PAF)-receptor antagonists. 30 g flaxseed/day was well tolerated and conferred benefit in terms of renal function as well as inflammatory and atherogenic mechanisms important in the pathogenesis of lupus nephritis.

Garlic - http://anrcatalog.ucdavis.edu/pdf/7231.pdf

Oi, Y., et al. Garlic supplementation increases testicular testosterone and decreases plasma corticosterone in rats fed a high protein diet. Journal of Nutrition. 131(8):2150-2156, 2001.

Hanafy, M. S., et al. Effect of garlic on lead contents in chicken tissues. DTW Dtsch Tierarztl Wochenschr. 101(4):157-158, 1994.

Grapefruit - www.floridajuice.com/grapefruit_juice.php
Gorinstein, S., et al. Red grapefruit positively influences serum triglyceride level in patients suffering from coronary atherosclerosis: studies in vitro and in humans. J Agric Food Chem. 54(5):1887-1892, 2006.

Baig, M. M., et al. Studies on the role of citrus in health and disease. ACS Symposium Series. 143:25-41, 1980.

Grapes - www.tablegrape.com
Konowalchuk, J., et al. Virus inactivation by grapes and wines. Applied Environmental Microbiology. 32(6):757-763, 1976.

Park, Y. K., et al. Daily grape juice consumption reduces oxidative DNA damage and plasma free radical levels in healthy Koreans. Mutat Res. 529(1-2):77-86, 2003. Department of Food and Nutrition, Hannam University, Daejeon, South Korea.

Green beans - www.producepete.com/shows/beans.html
Murray , Michael N.D. The Encyclopedia Of Healing Foods.
New York: Atria Books, 2005.

Centers For Disease Control And Prevention-5 A Day. http://www.cdc.gov/nccdphp/dnpa/5aday/.

Green peas - www.whfoods.com/genpage.php?tname=foodspice&dbid=55
National Agricultural Library-USDA. http://www.nal.usda.gov.

Wikipedia The Free Encyclopedia. http://www.wikipedia.org.

Hazel nuts - www.hazelnutcouncil.org
Bayer A et al. Doxorubin induced cataract formation and the inhibitory effects of hazel nut, a natural antioxidant. Med Sci Monit. 2005 Aug;11 (8):br300-304

Kale - http://www.whfoods.com/genpage.php?tname=foodspice&dbid=38
Seddon, J., et al. Dietary carotenoids, vitamins A, C, and E, and advanced age-related macular degeneration. Journal of the American Medical Association. 272:18:1413-1420, 1994.

Verhoeven, D., et al. A review of mechanisms underlying anticarcinogenicity by brassica vegetables. Chemico-Biological Interactions. 103(2):79-129, 1997.

Kiwi - www.kiwifruit.org
Duttaroy, A. K., et al. Effects of kiwi fruit consumption on platelet aggregation and plasma lipids in healthy human volunteers. Platelets. 15(5):287-292, 2004.

Legumes - http://waynesword.palomar.edu/ecoph33.htm
Shutler S. M. et al. The cholesterol lowering effects of legumes: effects of the major nutrients. Human Nutrition: Food Sciences & Nutrition. 41F:71-86.

Venn, B. J., et al. Cereal grains, legumes and diabetes. Eur J Clin Nutr. 2004.

Lemon - www.hort.purdue.edu/newcrop/morton/lemon.html
Murray, Michael T. The Healing Power of Foods: Nutrition Secrets for Vibrant Health and Long Life. Prima Publishing, Rocklin, California, USA. 1993:144.

Vigushin, D. M., et al. Phase I and pharmacokinetic study of d-limonene in patients with advanced cancer. Cancer Research Campaign Phase I/II Clinical Trials Committee. Cancer Chemotherapy & Pharmacol. ;42:111-17, 1998.

Wattenberg, L W. Inhibition of neoplasia by minor dietary constituents. Cancer Research. 43(supplement):2448s-2553s, 1983.

Olives - www.calolive.org
Aldini, G., et al. Antioxidant activity of polyphenols from solid olive residues of c.v. Coratina. Fitoterapia. 2006.

Machowetz, A., et al. Effect of olive oils on biomarkers of oxidative DNA stress in Northern and Southern Europeans. FASEB J. 2006.

Onions - www.onions-usa.org
Hu, J., et al. Diet and brain cancer in adults: a case-control study in northeast China. Int J Cancer. 81(1):20-23, 1999.

Department of Epidemiology, Harbin Medical College, Heilongjiang, China. Campos, K. E., et al. Hypoglycaemic and antioxidant effects of onion, Allium cepa: dietary onion addition, antioxidant activity and hypoglycaemic effects on diabetic rats. Int J Food Sci Nutr. 54(3):241-246, 2003.

Department of Chemistry and Biochemistry, Institute of Biological Sciences University of Sao Paulo State, UNESP Sao Paulo.

Pears - www.usapears.com
Conceicao de Olivercerica M. Sihieri R, and Moura AS. Weight loss associated with a daily intake of three pears daily among over weight women. Nutrition. 2003; 19:253-256

Mink PJ. Flavinoid intake and cardiovascular disease mortality; a prospective study in postmenopausal women. Am J Clin Nutr. 2007 Mar; 85(3): 895-090.

Prunes - www.whfoods.com/genpage.php?tname=foodspice&dbid=103
Tinker, L. F., et al. Consumption of prunes as a source of dietary fiber in men with mild hypercholesterolemia. Am J Clin Nutr. 53(5):1259-1265, 1991. Department of Nutrition, University of California, Davis, USA. 12 prunes daily.

Stacewicz-Sapuntzakis, M., et al. Chemical composition and potential health effects of prunes: a functional food? Crit Rev Food Sci Nutr. 41(4):251-286, 2001. Department of Human Nutrition and Dietetics, University of Illinois at Chicago, USA.

Quinoa - www.quinoa.net
Berti C, Riso P, Brusamolino A, Porrini M. Effect on appetite control of minor cereal and pseudoceral products. Br J Nutr. 2005 Nov:94(5):850-858

Estrada A, Li B, Laarveld B. Adjuvany action o Chenopodium quinoa saponins on the induction of antibody responses to intragastric and intranasal administered antigens in mice. Comp Immunol Microbiol Infect Dis. 1998 Jul;21(3):225-36.

Raspberries - www.raspberries.us
Liu, M., et al. Antioxidant and antiproliferative activities of raspberries. J Agric Food Chem. 50(10):2926-2930, 2002. Department of Food Science and Institute of Comparative and Environmental Toxicology, Stocking Hall, Cornell University, Ithaca, New York, USA. Raspberries are rich in phenolic phytochemicals.

Hope Smith, S., et al. Antimutagenic activity of berry extracts. J Med Food. 7(4):450-455, 2004. Department of Microbiology, Clemson University, Clemson, South Carolina, USA.

Rice - www.usarice.com
Hudson, E. A., et al. Characterization of potentially chemopreventive phenols in extracts of brown rice that inhibit the growth of human breast and colon cancer cells. Cancer Epidemiol Biomarkers Prev. 9(11):1163-1170, 2000. Medical Research Council Toxicology Unit, University of Leicester, United Kingdom.

Newborg, B. Disappearance of psoriatic lesions on the rice diet. North Carolina Medical Journal. 47(5):253-255, 1986.

Romaine lettuce - www.produceoasis.com/Items_folder/Vegetables/Romaine.html
Feskanich, D., et al. Vitamin K intake and hip fractures in women. American Journal of Clinical Nutrition. 69(1):74-79, 1999.

Nicolle, C., et al. Health effect of vegetable-based diet: lettuce consumption improves cholesterol metabolism and antioxidant status in the rat. Clin Nutr. 23(4):605-614, 2004.

Sesame seeds - www.recipezaar.com/library/getentry.zsp?id=344
Wu, W. H., et al. Sesame ingestion affects sex hormones, antioxidant status, and blood lipids in postmenopausal women. Journal of

Nutrition. 136(5):1270-1275, 2006. Department of Obstetrics and Gynecology, Taipei City Hospital-Yang Ming Branch, Taipei, Taiwan. Hypertens Res. 24(6):735-742, 2001.

Spinach - http://urbanext.illinois.edu/veggies/spinach1.html
Chasan-Taber, L., et al. A prospective study of carotenoid and vitamin A intakes and risk of cataract extraction in US women. American Journal of Clinical Nutrition. 70(4):509-516, 1999.

Marshall, J. R., et al. Diet and smoking in the epidemiology of cancer of the cervix. Journal of the National Cancer Institute. 70(5):847-851, 1983.

Strawberries - www.calstrawberry.com
Hannum, S. M. Potential impact of strawberries on human health: a review of the science. Crit Rev Food Sci Nutr. 44(1):1-17, 2004. Nutritional Sciences, University of Illinois, USA.

Chatterjee, A., et al. Inhibition of Helicobacter pylori in vitro by various berry extracts, with enhanced susceptibility to clarithromycin. Mol Cell Biochem. 265(1-2):19-26, 2004. Department of Pediatrics, Creighton University Health Sciences Center, Omaha, NE, USA.

Summer Squash

www.whfoods.com/genpage.php?tname=foodspice&dbid=62

Sweet potato - www.sweetpotato.org
Ludvik, B., et al. Efficacy of Ipomoea batatas (Caiapo) on diabetes control in Type 2 diabetic subjects treated with diet. Diabetes Care. 27(2):436-440, 2004. Department of Medicine, Division of Endocrinology and Metabolism, University of Vienna, Vienna, Austria.

Tomatoes
O'Kennedy, N., et al. Effects of tomato extract on platelet function: a double-blinded crossover study in healthy humans. American Journal of Clinical Nutrition. 84(3):561-569, 2006.

Romieu, I., et al. Fruit and vegetable intakes and asthma in the E3N study. Thorax. 61(3):209-215, 2006.

Watermelon
Murray, Michael T. The Healing Power of Foods: Nutrition Secrets for Vibrant Health and Long Life. Prima Publishing, Rocklin, California, USA. 1993:149. The author claims that watermelon possesses excellent diuretic properties.

Binns, C. W., et al. The relationship between dietary carotenoids and prostate cancer risk in Southeast Chinese men. Asia Pac J Clin Nutr. 13(Supplement):S117, 2004. School of Public Health, Curtin University of Technology, Perth,WA, Australia.

Appendix CC: How to Choose an Enzyme Supplement

Choosing the right enzyme requires knowledge of their individual purposes. Below is a list of enzymes and their uses in enzyme therapy.

Alpha-Galactosidase
- Breaks down carbohydrates
- Helpful with raw vegetables and beans

Amylase (Carbohydrase)
- Breaks down carbohydrates, starch and glycogen
- Regulates histamine when taken on an empty stomach
- Reduces food cravings
- Increases blood sugar

Bromelain
- Breaks down protein
- Beneficial as an anti-inflamatory

Catalase
- Acts as an antioxidant by breaking down hydrogen peroxide into water and oxygen
- Found in nearly every cell of the body

Cellulase
- Breaks down cellulose and chitin, a cellulose-like fiber found in the cell wall of Candida
- Helps free nutrients in both vegetables and fruits with its action on the cell wall

Diastase and Maltase (Malt Diastase)
- Breaks down carbohydrates, malt and grain sugars and both complex and simple sugars

Glucoamylase
- Breaks down carbohydrates, polysaccharides or long chains of carbohydrates

Glucoreductase
- Breaks down blood glucose

Hemicellulase
- Breaks down carbohydrates; especially sucrose and maltose

Invertase (Sucrase)
- Breaks down carbohydrates; sucrose and maltose

Lactase
- Breaks down lactose
- Used to treat lactose intolerance

Lipase
- Breaks down lipids and improves fat utilization
- Helps reduce cholesterol and supports weight loss, hormone production, and gallbladder function

Mucolase
- Breaks down mucus; helpful for congestion and sinus infections

Papain
- Breaks down protein
- Beneficial as an anti-inflammatory

Pectinase
- Breaks down carbohydrates and pectin found in many fruits and vegetables

Phytase
- Breaks down carbohydrates and phytic acid found in the leaves of plants

Protease
- Breaks down protein
- Bonds with alpha 2-macroglobulin to support immune function when taken on an empty stomach
- Necessary for proper immune function because everything a white blood cell must digest is either protein (bacteria or parasites) or protected by protein (viruses or cancer cells). A deficiency in protease would cause a break down in immune function.
- Reduces inflammation and increases circulation

Seaprose
- Breaks down mucus, helps with congestion and sinus infection

Serrationpeptidase
- Anti-inflammatory

Xylanase
- Breaks down soluble fiber

Appendix DD: Choosing Nutritional Supplements

by Debra Raybern, N.D., M.H., C.N.C., I.C.A.

Synthetic, whole food; liquid, capsules, tables; individual or blends – there are thousands of supplements available in grocery, supermarket health food stores, Internet companies and in the offices of health professionals. With so many choices, how do you choose? How do you know which ones will be effective and which ones are a waste of your money?

After years of personal and client usage of many, many different brands of nutritional, vitamin and mineral supplements, green drinks, protein powders, essential oils, and even personal care and home cleaning products, the feedback from customers has narrowed the choices I recommend to my clients. If you have a favorite and are happy with the results you achieve with your brand, feel free to continue using it. This study mentions several brand names I believe are most effective and give the best buy for the money. If your brand is not listed, is does not necessarily mean it is of poor quality or bad; it simply means it has not made my favorites list for one reason or another.

Here are some suggestions for choosing health and wellness products and supplements:

Cleansing supplements: Choose products that specifically support and detoxify the organs involved in elimination and are enhanced with herbs that are rich in vitamins, minerals, enzymes, amino acids, and fiber. Productive cleanses give users increased energy and promote continued nutritional balance. I recommend Young Living 5 Day Nutritive Cleanse™ - NingXia Red®, Digest + Cleanse™, Balance Complete™. Young Living Cleansing Trio™ - Comfortone™, ICP™ and Essentialzyme™

Enzyme supplementation: Knowing the type of enzyme you need is the first step when choosing the right enzyme supplement. To start, choose a supplement that meets the following criteria:

- Find a company that tests the product after encapsulated or tabulated.
- Choose a company that understands the functions of enzymes especially when looking at the ingredients on the label called proprietary blends.
- Select the enzyme for the healing therapy needed for body function.
- Look for an enzyme that adds a delivery system of the enzymes into the cells. The very best delivery system of enzymes into the body and cells is therapeutic-grade essential oils.
- Look for the potency of the blends of protease, lipase, cellulose or amylase enzymes, which will allow the breakdown of more protein, fat and carbohydrate.

Essential oils: Use only Young Living therapeutic-grade essential oils, which are pure, unadulterated and most can be ingested, applied topically and inhaled. There are many reasons to choose the Young Living brand, if you are interested please contact editor@growinghealthyhomes.com for the articles "The World Leader in Essential Oils" and "Choosing the Right Essential Oil Company," by David Stewart, Ph.D, D.N.M.

Eyesight nutritional supplements: Never place anything in the eye for natural or medication without consulting your health care provider.

"In 2002 Eurofins Scientific, an independent lab, tested dried NingXia wolfberry for its carotenoid content. The results were stunning.

1. They found both lutein and zeaxanthin in the wolfberries, but the ratio and amount was almost unbelievable. There were 278 micrograms of zeaxanthin and two micrograms of lutein per gram of dried wolfberries. This concentration of zeaxanthin was unheard of in natural foods. As the chart shows, it is 17 times the zeaxanthin content of red peppers and 92 times that of raw spinach.[1]

A further positive discovery was that the zeaxanthin found in the NingXia wolfberries was in ester form. This esterified zeaxanthin (zeaxanthin dipalmate) is far more bioavailable to the human body than ordinary zeaxanthin.[2]*"*
- excerpt from "NingXia Wolfberry: Preserving and Protecting Your Vision" by Dr. John Barry Glenn, Jr. M.D.

The NingXia wolfberry is the primary ingredient in Young Living NingXia Red nutrient infusion drink.

In addition, therapeutic-grade essential oils have provided relief from many eye ailments such as glaucoma, sty, pink eye and even failing vision.

Fish oil supplement: Look for purity, freshness, absorption and compliance. **Purity:** Use the right fish (smaller, oily fish like mackerel, sardines and anchovies with rich sources of omega oils), caught in pristine waters free of chemical dioxins, mercury, lead and polychlorinated biphenyls, commonly known as PCBs. **Freshness:** Manufactuers that quickly and minimally handle the omega oils to minimize oxidative damage and enhanced with only 100 percent therapeutic-grade pure essential oils to further protect the fish oil in the capsule, in the body and to protect stability up to 10 times of other brands. The oils clove, lemongrass, myrrh and German Blue Chamomile are added to the Omega Blue from Young Living. **Compliance:** There are only two reasons why people do not benefit from taking Omega-3's – they do not take enough or they won't take due to the fishy after taste. Choose one that is enteric coated to be released in the intestines, not the stomach and with the addition of the essential oils absorption is tripled so smaller doses are give effective results. **Absorption:** When fish oils are delivered through the intestines, absorption is up to three times greater that if released in the stomach. Look for a fish oil with the proper ratio of the two key Omega-3's – EPA and DHA at 14 to 18 percent. Higher ratios can indicate the fish oil has undergone further processing which increases its fishy flavor. My choice is Omega Blue from Young Living.

Intestinal health supplements: For children six and under — Kid-e-Reg, a Dr. Christopher original formula. For adults — Comfortone™ (Young Living); Quick Colon #1, formerly Intestinal Corrective #1 (Dr. Christopher); and Int. Formula 1 (Dr. Schulze). For infants, children and adults — Di-Gize™ therapeutic-grade essential oil blend (Young Living) applied topically or taken as an oral supplement and charcoal caplets or tablets.

Magnesium: Many magnesium supplements can cause loose stools so they are not well tolerated. The form magnesium glycinate, found through health professionals, will eliminate this problem. Using a form properly combined with calcium and in a bioavailable form the body uses more easily, means less does the same job as high doses.

Natural sweetners: Organic Blue Agave, from Young Living®, is much sweeter than sugar, but with a glycemic index (GI) of only 11. The GI of sugar ranges from 68 to 85, while the GI for honey ranges from 55 to 83. It is used like honey as a substitute in recipes for sugar (typically 1/2 to 3/4 cup agave in place of 1 cup sugar). Refer to Appendix P for a complete list of sugar replacements.

Probiotic supplementation: Most probiotics work as long as you take them, but what about when you stop? Have they assisted your body to establish a permanent colony in the gut so that if you miss a week of taking them you'er still covered? For years clients and I tested brand after brand. Some of course worked better

1 Ibid., Young, Lawrence and schreuder, p. 255.

2 Breithaupt DE, ìComparison of plasma responses in human subjects after the ingestion of 3R,3Rí-zeaxanthin diplamitate from wolfberry (Lycium barbarum) and non-esterified 3R-3Rí- zeaxanthin using shiral high-performanceliquid chromatography.î Br J Nutr. 2004 My;91(5):707-13.

than others, but none provided any adhesion strains to establish a permanent colony of beneficial bacteria – until I found Life 5™ capsules from Young Living. Life 5 which contains five strains of bacteria, three of which are considered super strains – Howaru™ Bifido (Bifidobacterium lactis), Howaru™ Rhamnosus (Ld. rhamnosus) and L. acidiophulis (LA-14), plus strains that establish that colony.

The world's greatest super food is the NingXia wolfberry. As the highest ranked antioxidant food ever tested (per Brunswick Laboratories), the NingXia wolfberry is high in lutein and zeaxanthin for eye health as well as vitamin A, C, calcium, protein, fiber and many other vitamins, minerals and amino acids.

Vitamin C supplements abound, from fizzy drink mixes, fortified juices, chewable tablets and more, vitamin C tops the list of supplements marketed and sold. Look for whole food sourced vitamin C. It may be labeled as ascorbic acid, but as long as it is derived from whole food sources it is a good choice. It is quite difficult to take too much vitamin C as it will give the body loose stools in excess. When taking vitamin C, spread it out over the course of the day.

Zinc is best taken in a combination multi-whole food vitamin. True Source is a three capsule, whole food multi with sufficient zinc.

Karen Hopkins Diabetic Success Story

Karen Hopkins, B.S., developed diabetes and early onset dementia at a young age due to S.A.D (Standard American Diet). Traditional nutrition courses did not prepare her for the onslaught of processed, fast food easily available to a college student and then a busy mother of three. Forced to face the reality of a short lifespan due to excessively high blood sugar (225 mg/dl+ with medications), she reversed the prognosis in six short months with a very intense and specific nutrition and supplement protocol and exercise. This is what Karen did to overcome diabetes:

Karen's Extreme Diet for Severe Diabetes[3]

- Raw food diet consuming only vegetables for 30 days[4] along with therapeutic-grade essential oils.[5]
- After the raw foods diet, 75 percent raw foods with no meat until the critical stage of getting her blood sugar level below 200ml/dm was over. Then she added a little fish, poultry, eggs and goat yogurt and cheese in limited quantities. .
- Master Cleanse by Stanley Burroughs for 10 days.

Supplements and Young Living® Products used

- Six to eight ounces of Ningxia Red juice infusion drink daily
- Essential oils of cinnamon bark, coriander, fennel, dill, Thieves - three drops of each to fill a vegetable capsule and up to 5 or 6 capsules a day. Also rubbed over pancreas and inhaled.
- Alkalime - Used as directed three times a day
- Essentialzyme – Two to four tablets with each meal.
- Immupro – Two to four tablets at night.

Detoxification

- Master Cleanse by Stanley Burroughs
- Cleansing Trio from Young Living

---

3 Consult the professional health practitioner of your choice before beginning any diet.
4 www.rawfor30days.com
5 See Appendix DD for more specifics and authors' recommendations.

Exercise – It has been suggested by Ron Rosedale, M.D. that exercise is a must to reverse diabetes.[6]

- 30 minutes to one hour daily walking or other aerobic exercise.

At the beginning of her program Karen's fasting glucose was 225 mg/dl and her A1C was 11.9 with diabetic medications. After six weeks on the program, she no longer needed her medication. At the end of eight months, her AIC was 6.3, which is pre-diabetic. Now a full year and half later **without** medication her blood glucose levels remain on average under 100 mg/dl and her A1C is 6.1, which is normal. She continues to drink NingXia Red, take Essentailzyme, use the essential oils and maintain a healthy diet. She now travels cross country to share with people how the Lord healed her through natural means.

Emotions and Essential Oils

Chapter 4 titled "Emotions" in Unit 6 provides additional information about the impact of negative emotions on the body. Therapeutic-grade essential oils are routinely used by either putting a a few drops in the hand and breathing deeply, wearing the oil as a perfume and applying it to the feet. Select a Bible verse or make a statement or affirmation about the fear to help tell the body that it is no longer bound by that emotion.
Here are some beneficial oils in dealing with the following emotions:

Recommended Young Living oils for fear are the blends **Valor®, Present Time™, Hope™, White Angelica™, Trauma Life™, Transformation™, Gratitude™ and Highest Potential™**.

Anger can be combated by using the blends **Release™, Valor, Sacred Mountain™, Joy™, Harmony™, Forgiveness™, Present Time, Trauma Life™, Surrender™, Christmas Spirit™** and **White Angelica™.** Single oils include **frankincense, lavender, sandalwood** and **cedarwood**.

Oils for grief are the blends **Trauma Life, Release, Inspiration™, Gathering™, Harmony™, Present Time, Magnify Your Purpose™** and **Gratitude.** Single oils are **frankincense, clary sage** and **lavender.**

6 "The Rosedale Diet" Ron Rosedale, M.D. and Carol Colman, Harper Collins, New York, NY, 2004.

Appendix EE: Healthy Home Resources

The following are tools to further enhance a family's study of whole health, including natural and supernatural healing.

"Gentle Babies: Essential Oils and Natural Remedies for Pregnancy, Childbirth and Infant Care," Debra Raybern N.D., M.H., C.N.C., I.C.A., 2008 – Be confident in safely and effectively using essential oils, herbs, supplements and natural therapies during this special time in your life. **www.GrowingHealthyHomes.com**

"101 Foods That Could Save Your Life," David Grotto, Bantam Books, 2008 – Each of the hundred foods includes a brief history, cultivation and origin and therapeutic benefits. Available online or at your local bookstore.

"Essential Oils Desk Reference," 4th Edition – *The* how-to manual when it comes to learning about essential oils and essential oil enhanced products. This book is YL product specific. **www.essentialscience.net** or 1-800-336-6308

"The World's Healthiest Foods," George Mateljan, 2007, 800 pages of the world's healthiest foods with recipes to help you eat healthy. **www.whfoods.com**

"Green This!" Deirdre Imus – Well-known proponent of using chemical-free products in the home including home-healthy cleaning recipes. Available online or at your local bookstore.

"Discovery of The Ultimate Superfood," Gary Young N.D., Ronald Lawrence M.D., Ph.D., Marc Schreuder – Everything you ever needed to know about the NingXia wolfberry and why it truly is the world's most powerful superfood infusion. **www.essentialscience.net**

"Healing Oils of the Bible," David Stewart, Ph.D. – A Biblically based study on the history of essential oils, how they were used in ancient times and instruction on true Biblical anointing. **www.essentialscience.net**

"Chemistry of Essential Oils Made Simple: God's Love Manifest in Molecules," David Stewart, Ph.D. – Many complex issues are summarized for non-technical readers, as Dr. Stewart guides the reader through how essential oils work, why they work and why we must use them today. **www.essentialscience.net**

"A More Excellent Way," Pastor Henry Wright – A Christian perspective on emotional healing. Although he does not offer natural remedies, his insight into emotional issues and physical health is excellent. **www.beinhealth.com**

"Nature's Mold RX: the Non-Toxic Solution to Toxic Mold," Edward R. Close, Ph.D., and Jacquelyn Close, R.A. – After having to battle mold in his own house, Dr. Close, a world-recognized expert in environmental science, found what works best and is safer than any chemical. Complete with research and a mold eradication plan. **www.essentialsciencc.net**

"Hyperhealth Pro CD-ROM - The World's Most Comprehensive Encyclopedia of Nutrition and Natural Health." Based on published scientific research, Hyperhealth is the most credible and trusted content used by health conscious consumers, researchers, physicians and health care professionals worldwide. Equal to a 40,564 page book with 59,287 references. Contains 5,300 topics. **www.hyperhealth.com**

Young Living Essential Oils - The world leader in therapeutic-grade essential oils with global farms and distilleries. When only the best will do for your family's health and home. Contact **editor@growinghealthyhomes.com.**

Index

B

C

D

E

H

M

N

O

P

Q

R

S

X

Y

Z